Principles of
Addiction
Medicine

THE ESSENTIALS

Principles of
Addiction
Medicine

THE ESSENTIALS

Christopher A. Cavacuiti, MD, FCFP, MHSc, ASAM

Assistant Professor
University of Toronto
Staff Physician, Department of Family and
   Community Medicine
St. Michael's Hospital
Toronto, Ontario

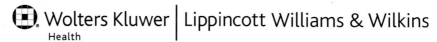
Wolters Kluwer | Lippincott Williams & Wilkins
Health

Philadelphia · Baltimore · New York · London
Buenos Aires · Hong Kong · Sydney · Tokyo

Acquisitions Editor: Charles Mitchell
Product Manager: Tom Gibbons
Vendor Manager: Alicia Jackson
Senior Manufacturing Manager: Benjamin Rivera
Marketing Manager: Brian Freiland
Design Coordinator: Stephen Druding
Production Service: SPi Global

Library of Congress Cataloging-in-Publication Data
  Principles of addiction medicine : the essentials / [edited by] Chris Cavacuiti.
     p. ; cm.
  ISBN 978-1-60547-776-3
  1. Substance abuse—Handbooks, manuals, etc. I. Cavacuiti, Chris. II. American Society of Addiction Medicine.
  [DNLM: 1. Substance-Related Disorders—therapy—Handbooks. 2. Behavior, Addictive—Handbooks. 3. Substance-Related Disorders—diagnosis—Handbooks. WM 34]

  RC564.15.P75   2010
  362.29—dc22

                                                                                         2010031296

Care has been taken to confirm the accuracy of the information presented and to describe generally accepted practices. However, the authors, editors, and publisher are not responsible for errors or omissions or for any consequences from application of the information in this book and make no warranty, expressed or implied, with respect to the currency, completeness, or accuracy of the contents of the publication. Application of the information in a particular situation remains the professional responsibility of the practitioner.

The authors, editors, and publisher have exerted every effort to ensure that drug selection and dosage set forth in this text are in accordance with current recommendations and practice at the time of publication. However, in view of ongoing research, changes in government regulations, and the constant flow of information relating to drug therapy and drug reactions, the reader is urged to check the package insert for each drug for any change in indications and dosage and for added warnings and precautions. This is particularly important when the recommended agent is a new or infrequently employed drug.

Some drugs and medical devices presented in the publication have Food and Drug Administration (FDA) clearance for limited use in restricted research settings. It is the responsibility of the health care provider to ascertain the FDA status of each drug or device planned for use in their clinical practice.

To purchase additional copies of this book, call our customer service department at (800) 638-3030 or fax orders to (301) 223-2320. International customers should call (301) 223-2300.

Visit Lippincott Williams & Wilkins on the Internet: at LWW.com. Lippincott Williams & Wilkins customer service representatives are available from 8:30 am to 6 pm, EST.

10 9 8 7 6 5 4 3 2 1

To the three generations of women who have been with me every step of the way— my mother Margaret, my wife Aleksandra, and my daughters Sasha and Emma.

FOREWORD

From the time ASAM was founded, ASAM's members and leaders have addressed a recurrent question with no simple answer: "What is addiction medicine?"

Consider that in the 1950s, when Dr. Ruth Fox and her colleagues founded ASAM, there were few physicians and lay persons who shared their vision. There was no infrastructure for demonstrating that addiction truly *is* a disease. There was no group of physicians within organized medicine to treat the disease of addiction and to advocate for the patients who suffered from it. In those days, nearly everyone—physicians and laypersons alike—viewed alcoholism and other drug addictions as moral weaknesses. The Federal and State governments had little, if any, interest. And there certainly was no concept of a special field called "addiction medicine."

Yet that small handful of pioneers—led by Drs. Ruth Fox, Stanley Gitlow, LeClair Bissell, Percy Ryberg, Marty Mann, Brinkley Smithers and others—held a conviction that impelled them to action. As a result, 56 years later, ASAM is a vibrant national organization of more than 3,000 members—physicians who are dedicated to the belief that the treatment of addiction should be granted parity with the treatment of any other chronic medical disorder, that all physicians should receive education in addiction medicine, and that physicians who wish to do so should be trained and board-certified in addiction medicine.

In 1954, there was no textbook of addiction medicine. In 2010, ASAM published the Fourth Edition of its *Principles of Addiction Medicine*, which in 1,570 pages reflects the vast body of scientific knowledge that now enriches our field.

As a result of these accomplishments and the formation of the new American Board of Addiction Medicine (ABAM), addiction and addiction treatment have become topics of great interest to government agencies, law enforcement, and mainstream medicine.

Yet the question persists. In fact, the larger and more complex our current body of knowledge about addiction, the more difficult it is to distill the essential knowledge that constitutes the core of addiction medicine. Addiction research and treatment modalities have multiplied so rapidly over the past few years that it is difficult to ascertain what information is clinically essential and necessary to provide competent and appropriate care to patients who suffer from addictive disorders.

To answer the question, ASAM now offers *Principles of Addiction Medicine: The Essentials*. The developers of *Essentials* have served as "translators" by selecting and condensing information from the more comprehensive *Principles* so as to make it accessible to primary care physicians and other nonaddiction specialists.

Thus, *Principles of Addiction Medicine: The Essentials* provides a new answer to the old question—what is Addiction Medicine?—in a way that should resonate with all caregivers who wish to identify, manage, and appropriately refer patients suffering from addictive disorders. With *Essentials*, ASAM and its members forge yet another link in the partnership that binds us together with our primary care colleagues, so that together we can provide the best possible care to the patients we mutually serve.

Louis E. Baxter, Sr., MD, FASAM

PREFACE

Our mission in creating *Principles of Addiction Medicine: The Essentials* was to provide a valuable companion guide to ASAM's *Principles of Addiction Medicine*.

Principles of Addiction Medicine is quite rightly considered one of the most comprehensive and authoritative sources of information in its field. However, it was clear to ASAM that busy clinicians also needed a trusted source for more distilled information. The aim of this handbook is to meet that need.

During our work on this textbook, our three key goals were

1. To convey up-to-date and clinically relevant information in a clear and concise form.
2. To keep as much of the existing structure as possible from *Principles of Addiction Medicine* (so that readers could quickly switch back and forth from the distilled information in one book to the comprehensive information in the other).
3. To make the information pertinent and accessible to a wide variety of addiction medicine practitioners (including physicians, trainees, counsellors, nurses, and the many other health professionals who work in this challenging and rewarding field).

We hope that you will find that this textbook meets these goals and that it will find a home on the desks and shelves of health professionals whose patients experience substance use problems.

When it comes to the field of addiction medicine, it is never easy to decide what information to keep and what to leave out. Our group faced many tough choices in our effort to maintain a tight focus on the essentials of this fascinating subject. One such choice that deserves special mention is our decision to omit any suggested readings and/or formal citations at the end of each chapter. It was our feeling that readers who were looking for this more comprehensive information could find it in *Principles of Addiction Medicine*. Our group would like to make it very clear that our decision to omit this information was made in order to keep the book small and portable, not out of a failure to recognize the important contributions that other authors have made to this field. We have nothing but the utmost respect to the many outstanding writers and researchers who have contributed to our knowledge and understanding of addiction.

Readers should be aware that while the original chapters from *Principles of Addiction Medicine*, 4th edition, were written by world-renowned experts in their particular fields, the authors who created these chapter summaries are all front-line addiction medicine physicians, just like many of the people we anticipate will read this book. It was a leap of faith for ASAM to decide that those well-placed to know what is essential information for front-line doctors are the front-line doctors themselves. All of us who worked on these chapters are very grateful for the trust ASAM placed in us.

We are also grateful for the invaluable assistance and expertise offered by so many of the original *Principles of Addiction Medicine* authors. The support these authors gave to our project was tremendous. It should also be noted that while we made every effort to reflect the views of the original authors, these chapter summaries do not necessarily reflect the views of the *Principles of Addiction Medicine*, 4th edition authors.

As the lead editor on this book, I would like to take this opportunity to thank the many people who made this textbook possible. First and foremost, I would like to thank all of the individuals with substance use disorders who have been my patients and who have placed their trust in me over the years. The changes I have seen you make in your lives are a constant source of hope and inspiration and fill me with faith that each and every one of us is capable of transformation. Second, I would like to thank the American Society of Addiction Medicine for the generous support and encouragement they have given. Third, I am grateful for the wonderful editorial expertise provided by the staff at Lippincott Williams & Wilkins, particularly Tom Gibbons. Fourth, I am thankful to my fellow staff in the Department of Family and Community Medicine at St. Michael's Hospital; I am truly lucky to have such a wonderful group of colleagues to work with.

Christopher A. Cavacuiti

CONTRIBUTORS

Sharon Cirone, MD, CCFP(EM), ASAM
Board Member, Canadian Society of Addiction
    Medicine (C.S.A.M.)
Staff Physician, SHOUT Clinic for Homeless and
    Street-Involved Youth
Addictions Consultant, Child and Adolescent
    Mental Health Team
St. Joseph's Health Centre
Toronto, Ontario

Ashok Krishnamurthy, MD, CM, CCFP, ABAM
Adjunct Lecturer
University of Toronto
Staff Physician, Department of Family and
    Community Medicine
St. Michael's Hospital
Toronta, Ontario

Agnes Kwasnicka, MSc, MD, CCFP
Lecturer
University of Toronto
Staff Physician, Family Health Team
Sherbourne Health Centre
Toronto, Ontario

Christopher Sankey, BA, MD, CCFP(EM)
Adjunct Lecturer
University of Toronto
Vice Chair of Ontario Medical Association, Section
    of Addiction Medicine
Staff Physician, Satellite Comprehensive Addictions
    Treatment Centre
Medical Director, First Step Clinics
Supervisor, Assessor and Methadone Maintenance
    Preceptor, CPSO member of Minister of Health's
    Task Force on Methadone Maintenance
Toronto, Ontario

Aleksandra Vasic, BA
Resource Coordinator
Self Help Resource Center
Toronto, Ontario

Thea Weisdorf, MD, FCFP, ASAM, ABAM
Assistant Professor
University of Toronto
Staff physician, Department of Family and
    Community Medicine
St. Michael's Hospital
Toronto, Ontario

John Young, MD
Toronto, Ontario

EDITORS AND CONTRIBUTORS TO *PRINCIPLES OF ADDICTION MEDICINE*, 4TH EDITION

SENIOR EDITOR

Richard K. Ries, MD, FAPA, FASAM
Professor of Psychiatry
Director, Division of Addictions
Department of Psychiatry and Behavioral Sciences
University of Washington
Medical Director, Harborview Addictions and
  Rehabilitation Psychiatry Programs
Harborview Medical Center
Seattle, Washington

ASSOCIATE EDITORS

David A. Fiellin, MD
Associate Professor of Medicine and Investigative
  Medicine
Department of Internal Medicine
Yale University School of Medicine
New Haven, Connecticut

**Shannon C. Miller, MD, FASAM, FAPA,
CMRO**
Medical Director, Integrated Dual Diagnosis and
  Sobriety Plus Clinics
Program Director, VA Advanced Fellowship in
  Addiction Research/Medicine
Cincinnati VA Medical Center
Associate Director of Education, Training, and
  Dissemination
Center of Excellence for Treatment, Research, and
  Education in Addictive Disorders (CeTREAD)
Addiction Sciences Division
Associate Professor of Clinical Psychiatry, Affiliated
Department of Psychiatry and Behavioral
  Neuroscience
University of Cincinnati School of Medicine
Cincinnati, Ohio

**Richard Saitz, MD, MPH, FACP,
FASAM**
Professor of Medicine and Epidemiology
Director, Clinical Addiction Research and
  Education (CARE) Unit
Section of General Internal Medicine, Department
  of Medicine
Boston Medical Center/Boston University Schools
  of Medicine and Public Health
Boston, Massachusetts

SECTION EDITORS

Peter Banys, MD
Clinical Professor of Psychiatry
University of California, San Francisco
VA Medical Center
San Francisco, California

Edward C. Covington, MD
Director, Neurological Center for Pain
Cleveland Clinic Foundation
Cleveland, Ohio

John A. Dani, PhD
Professor of Neuroscience
Baylor College of Medicine
Houston, Texas

Robert L. DuPont, MD, FASAM
Clinical Professor of Psychiatry
Georgetown University
President, Institute for Behavior and Health
Rockville, Maryland

David A. Fiellin, MD
Professor of Medicine
Department of Internal Medicine
Yale University School of Medicine
New Haven, Connecticut

Peter D. Friedmann, MD, MPH
Professor, Departments of Medicine & Community Health
Alpert Medical School of Brown University
Director, Center on Systems, Outcomes & Quality in Chronic Disease & Rehabilitation
Providence Veterans Affairs Medical Center
Rhode Island Hospital
Providence, Rhode Island

Marc Galanter, MD, FASAM
Professor and Director, Division of Alcoholism and Drug Abuse
NYU School of Medicine
New York, New York

R. Jeffrey Goldsmith, MD
Professor of Clinical Psychiatry
College of Medicine, University of Cincinnati
Staff Psychiatrist
Mental Health Care Line
Cincinnati VA Medical Center
Cincinnati, Ohio

Adam J. Gordon, MD, MPH, FACP, FASAM
Assistant Professor of Medicine and Advisory Dean
University of Pittsburgh School of Medicine
Associate Clinical Director, Mental Illness Research & Education Center
Center for Health Equity Research and Promotion
VA Pittsburgh Healthcare System
Pittsburgh, Pennsylvania

David A. Gorelick, MD, PhD
Intramural Research Program
National Institute on Drug Abuse, National Institutes of Health
Adjunct Professor, Department of Psychiatry
University of Maryland School of Medicine
Baltimore, Maryland

J. Harry Isaacson, MD, FACP
Associate Professor of Medicine
Director of Clinical Education
Cleveland Clinic Lerner College of Medicine
Cleveland Clinic
Cleveland, Ohio

John R. Knight, MD
Associate Professor of Pediatrics
Harvard Medical School
Director, Center for Adolescent Substance Abuse Research
Children's Hospital Boston
Boston, Massachusetts

Thomas R. Kosten, MD
Professor of Psychiatry and Neuroscience
Baylor College of Medicine
Director and Vice Chair, Psychiatry, Addictions, and Neuroscience
Michael E. DeBakey Veterans Administration Medical Center
Houston, Texas

Margaret M. Kotz, DO
Professor of Psychiatry and Anesthesiology
Case Western Reserve University School of Medicine
Director, Addiction Recovery Services
Case Medical Center
University Hospitals of Cleveland
Cleveland, Ohio

Theodore V. Parran, Jr., MD, FACP
Associate Clinical Professor, Department of Internal Medicine
Case Western Reserve University School of Medicine
Associate Medical Director, Rosary Hall Addiction Services
St. Vincent Charity Hospital
Cleveland, Ohio

Richard K. Ries, MD, FAPA, FASAM
Professor of Psychiatry
Director, Division of Addictions, Department of Psychiatry and Behavioral Sciences
University of Washington
Medical Director, Harborview Addictions and Rehabilitation Psychiatry Programs
Harborview Medical Center
Seattle, Washington

Richard N. Rosenthal, MD
Antenucci Professor of Clinical Psychiatry and Senior Associate Dean
Columbia University College of Physicians and Surgeons
Chairman, Department of Psychiatry and Behavioral Health
St. Luke's–Roosevelt Hospital Center
New York, New York

Seddon R. Savage, MD, MS, FASAM
Director, Dartmouth Center on Addiction Recovery and Education (DCARE)
Pain Consultant, Manchester VA Medical Center
Associate Professor of Anesthesiology, Dartmouth Medical School, Adjunct Faculty
Hanover, New Hampshire

Andrew J. Saxon, MD
Professor of Psychiatry & Behavioral Sciences
University of Washington
Director, Addiction Patient Care Line, Mental
 Health Service
VA Puget Sound Health Care System
Seattle, Washington

Deborah R. Simkin, MD
Section Head, Division of Child and Adolescent
 Psychiatry
Residency Training Director, Adjunct Associate
 Professor
University of South Alabama Medical School
Mobile, Alabama

Ramon Solhkhah, MD
Director, The Child and Family Institute
Chief, Division of Child and Adolescent Psychiatry
St. Luke's–Roosevelt Hospital Center
Assistant Professor of Clinical Psychiatry
Columbia University College of Physicians and
 Surgeons
New York, New York

Bonnie B. Wilford, MS
Executive Director, Coalition on Physician
 Education in Substance Use Disorders (COPE)
Senior Principal and Director, Center for Health
 Services and Outcomes Research
JBS International, Inc.
Easton, Maryland

Joan E. Zweben, PhD
Clinical Professor of Psychiatry
University of California, San Francisco
Executive Director
East Bay Community Recovery Project
Oakland, California

CONTRIBUTORS

Daniel P. Alford, MD, MPH, FACP, FASAM
Associate Professor of Medicine
Boston University School of Medicine
Medical Director, MASBIRT and OBOT Programs
Boston, Massachusetts

Marie E. Armentano, MD
Psychiatrist
Belchertown, Massachusetts

Ashraf Attalla, MD
Clinical Assistant Professor of Psychiatry
Emory University School of Medicine
Director
Institute of Behavorial Medicine
Smyrna, Georgia

Sanford Auerbach, MD
Associate Professor of Neurology, Psychiatry and
 Behavioral Neurosciences
Boston University School of Medicine
Director, Sleep Disorders Center
Boston Medical Science
Boston, Massachusetts

Sudie E. Back, PhD
Associate Professor, Department of Psychiatry
Clinical Neuroscience Division, Medical University
 of South Carolina
Charleston, South Carolina

Robert L. Balster, PhD
Butler Professor of Pharmacology and Toxicology
Director, Institute for Drug and Alcohol Studies
Virginia Commonwealth University
Richmond, Virginia

Kristen L. Barry, PhD
Research Associate Professor
Department of Psychiatry
University of Michigan
Department of Veterans Affairs
Serious Mental Illness Treatment Research and
 Evaluation Center (SMITREC)
Ann Arbor VAMC
Ann Arbor, Michigan

Andrea G. Barthwell, MD, FASAM
Chief Executive Officer
Two Dreams Outer Banks Comprehensive
 Wellness Center
Corolla, North Carolina

Robert Gordon Batey, MD, FRACP, FRCP (UK), FAChAM
Conjoint Professor of Medicine
University of Sydney
Senior Staff Specialist, Addiction Medicine
Royal Prince Alfred Hospital
Camperdown, New South Wales, Australia

Neal L. Benowitz, MD
Professor of Medicine, Psychiatry, and
  Biopharmaceutical Sciences
University of California, San Francisco
Chief, Division of Clinical Pharmacology
San Francisco General Hospital
San Francisco, California

Nicolas Bertholet, MD, MSc
Clinical Epidemiology Center
Institute of Social and Preventive Medicine
Centre Hospitalier Universitaire Vaudois
Alcohol Treatment Center
Department of Community Medicine and Public
  Health
Lausanne University, Switzerland

Aurelia N. Bizamcer, MD, PhD
Assistant Professor of Psychiatry
Medical Director, Outpatient Psychiatry
Temple University School of Medicine
Philadelphia, Pennsylvania

Anton C. Bizzell, MD
Vice President, Health and Clinical Services
DB Consulting Group, Inc.
Silver Spring, Maryland
Clinical Instructor, Community Health and Family
  Practice
Howard University Hospital
Washington, District of Columbia

Richard D. Blondell, MD
Professor of Family Medicine
University at Buffalo
Attending Physician
Erie County Medical Center
Buffalo, New York

Frederic C. Blow, PhD
Department of Psychiatry
University of Michigan
Department of Veterans Affairs
Serious Mental Illness Treatment Research and
  Evaluation Center (SMITREC)
Ann Arbor VAMC
Ann Arbor, Michigan

Lisa Borg, MD
Senior Research Associate, The Laboratory of the
  Biology of Addictive Diseases
The Rockefeller University
Associate Attending Physician
The Rockefeller University Hospital
New York, New York

Gilbert J. Botvin, PhD
Professor of Public Health and Psychiatry
Weill Cornell Medical Center
Attending Psychologist
Department of Psychiatry
The New York Presbyterian Hospital
New York, New York

Andria Botzet, MA
Research Program Coordinator
Department of Psychiatry
University of Minnesota
Minneapolis, Minnesota

Carol J. Boyd, PhD, MSN, RN, FAAN
Professor of Nursing
Director, Institute for Research on Women and Gender
University of Michigan
Ann Arbor, Michigan

Katharine A. Bradley, MD, MPH
Associate Professor of Medicine
University of Washington
General Internist
VA Primary and Medical Care Services, Division of
  General Internal Medicine
VA Puget Sound & University of Washington
Seattle, Washington

Kathleen T. Brady, MD, PhD
Professor of Psychiatry
Medical University of South Carolina
Charleston, South Carolina

Lawrence S. Brown, Jr., MD, MPH, FASAM
Clinical Associate Professor of Public Health
Weill Medical College, Cornell University
Executive Senior Vice President
Medical Services, Research & Information
  Technology
Addiction Research & Treatment Corporation
New York, New York

Richard A. Brown, PhD
Professor of Psychiatry and Human Behavior
Warren Alpert Medical School at Brown
  University
Director of Addictions Research
Butler Hospital
Providence, Rhode Island

John C.M. Brust, MD
Professor, Department of Neurology
Columbia University
Director of Neurology
Harlem Hospital Center
New York, New York

John S. Cacciola, PhD
Adjunct Associate Professor, Department of
 Psychiatry
University of Pennsylvania School of Medicine
Senior Scientist
The Treatment Research Institute (TRI)
Philadelphia, Pennsylvania

James W. Campbell, MD, MS
Professor of Family Medicine
Case Western Reserve University
Chairman, Family Medicine/Geriatrics
Metro Health
Cleveland, Ohio

Victor A. Capoccia, PhD
Senior Scientist
Center for Health Enhancement System Studies
Network for the Improvement of Addiction
 Treatment
University of Wisconsin
Madison, Wisconsin

Kathleen M. Carroll, PhD
Professor, Department of Psychiatry
Yale University School of Medicine
New Haven, Connecticut

Domenic A. Ciraulo, MD
Professor and Chairman, Department of Psychiatry
Boston University School of Medicine
Psychiatrist-in-Chief
Boston Medical Center
Boston, Massachusetts

H. Westley Clark, MD, JD, MPH, CAS, FASAM
Director, Center for Substance Abuse Treatment
Substance Abuse and Mental Health Services
 Administration
Department of Health and Human Services
Rockville, Maryland

Jeffrey S. Cluver, MD
Associate Professor of Psychiatry
Medical University of South Carolina
Assistant Chief, Mental Health Service
Ralph H. Johnson VAMC
Charleston, South Carolina

Peggy Compton, RN, PhD, FAAN
Professor, School of Nursing
University of California, Los Angeles
Los Angeles, California

Katherine Anne Comtois, PhD, MPH
Associate Professor, Department of Psychiatry and
 Behavioral Sciences
University of Washington
Clinical Director, Dialectical Behavior Therapy
 Program
Harborview Mental Health Services
Harborview Medical Center
Seattle, Washington

Edward C. Covington, MD
Director, Neurological Center for Pain
Cleveland Clinic Foundation
Cleveland, Ohio

Rosa M. Crum, MD, MHS
Professor
Department of Epidemiology, Psychiatry and
 Mental Health
Welch Center for Prevention, Epidemiology &
 Clinical Research
Johns Hopkins Medical Institutions
Baltimore, Maryland

Dennis C. Daley, PhD
Professor of Psychiatry
University of Pittsburgh
Chief, Addiction Medicine Services
Western Psychiatric Institute and Clinic
Pittsburgh, Pennsylvania

John A. Dani, PhD
Professor of Neuroscience
Baylor College of Medicine
Houston, Texas

Itai Danovitch, MD
Director, Addiction Psychiatry Clinical Services
Associate Director, Addiction Psychiatry Fellowship
Department of Psychiatry and Behavioral
 Neurosciences
Cedars-Sinai Medical Center
Los Angeles, California

Jose Carlos T. DaSilva, MD, MPH
Assistant Clinical Professor, Department of
 Medicine
Boston University School of Medicine
Staff Physician, Commonwealth Nephrology
 Association
Boston, Massachusetts

Linda C. Degutis, Dr.PH, MSN
Associate Professor, Emergency Medicine and Public
  Health
Department of Surgery
Yale University
New Haven, Connecticut

**William E. Dickinson, DO, FASAM,
FAAFP, ABAM**
Medical Director, Providence Behavioral Health
  Services
Providence Regional Medical Center-Everett
Everett, Washington

Linda A. Dimeff, PhD
Chief Scientific Officer
Behavioral Tech Research, Inc.
Seattle, Washington

Carson V. Dobrin, BS
Graduate Student
Neuroscience Program
Wake Forest University School of Medicine
Winston-Salem, North Carolina

Edward F. Domino, MD
Professor of Pharmacology
University of Michigan
Ann Arbor, Michigan

Gail D'Onofrio, MD, MS
Professor and Chief, Section of Emergency Medicine
Yale University
Chief, Department of Adult Emergency Services
Yale-New Haven Hospital
New Haven, Connecticut

Antoine Douaihy, MD
Associate Professor of Psychiatry
University of Pittsburgh School of Medicine
Medical Director, Addiction Medicine Services
Director of Addiction Psychiatry Fellowship
Western Psychiatric Institute and Clinic
Pittsburgh, Pennsylvania

Robert L. DuPont, MD, FASAM
Clinical Professor of Psychiatry
Georgetown University
President, Institute for Behavior and Health
Rockville, Maryland

Paul H. Earley, MD, FASAM
Medical Director
Talbott Recovery Campus
Atlanta, Georgia

Jon O. Ebbert, MD
Associate Professor of Medicine
Mayo Clinic
Rochester, Minnesota

Steven J. Eickelberg, MD, FASAM
President, Performax, P.C.
Sport Psychiatry
Addiction Psychiatry
Paradise Valley, Arizona

Tamara Fahnhorst, MPH
Research Program Coordinator
Department of Psychiatry
University of Minnesota
Minneapolis, Minnesota

**Kathleen J. Farkas, PhD, LISW-S,
ACSW**
Associate Professor
Mandel School of Applied Social Sciences
Case Western Reserve University
Cleveland, Ohio

Sergi Ferré, MD, PhD
Principal Investigator
Behavioral Neuroscience Branch
National Institute on Drug Abuse
Baltimore, Maryland

David A. Fiellin, MD
Professor of Medicine
Department of Internal Medicine
Yale University School of Medicine
New Haven, Connecticut

John W. Finney, PhD
HSR&D Center for Health Care Evaluation
VA Palo Alto Health Care System
Palo Alto, California
Stanford University School of Medicine
Menlo Park, California

Marc Fishman, MD
Assistant Professor of Psychiatry
Johns Hopkins University
Medical Director
Mountain Manor Treatment Center
Baltimore, Maryland

Michael F. Fleming, MD, MPH
Professor of Family Medicine
Northwestern University Feinberg School of
  Medicine
Chicago, Illinois

Keith Flower, MD
Scientist
Addiction Pharmacology Research Lab
California Pacific Medical Center Research Institute
St. Luke's Hospital
San Francisco, California

P. Joseph Frawley, MD
Co-Medical Director, Intensive Outpatient Program
Recovery Road Medical Center
Assistant Medical Director
Cottage Residential Treatment Center
Santa Barbara Cottage Hospital
Santa Barbara, California

Howard S. Friedman, MD
Clinical Professor of Cardiology
New York University School of Medicine
New York, New York

Peter D. Friedmann, MD, MPH
Professor, Departments of Medicine & Community
  Health
Alpert Medical School of Brown University
Director, Center on Systems, Outcomes & Quality in
Chronic Disease & Rehabilitation
Providence Veterans Affairs Medical Center Rhode
  Island Hospital
Providence, Rhode Island

Marc Galanter, MD, FASAM
Professor and Director
Division of Alcoholism & Drug Abuse
NYU School of Medicine
New York, New York

Rollin M. Gallagher, MD, MPH
Deputy National Program Director for Pain
  Management
Veterans Health System
Director for Pain Policy Research and Primary Care
Penn Pain Medicine
Clinical Professor of Psychiatry and Anesthesiology
University of Pennsylvania
Philadelphia, Pennsylvania

Joseph E. Galligan, MA
Focal Therapist, Men's Treatment Team
Hazelden Springbrook
Newberg, Oregon

Gantt P. Galloway, PharmD
Scientist, Addiction Pharmacology Research Laboratory
California Pacific Medical Center Research Institute
San Francisco, California

Aaron M. Gilson, PhD, MS, MSSW
Senior Scientist, Pain & Policy Studies Group
Carbone Cancer Center
University of Wisconsin School of Medicine and
  Public Health
Madison, Wisconsin

Richard A. Glennon, PhD
Professor and Chair, Department of Medicinal
  Chemistry
Virginia Commonwealth University
Richmond, Virginia

Mark S. Gold, MD
Distinguished Professor and Chairman
Department of Psychiatry
University of Florida
McKnight Brain Institute
Gainesville, Florida

Linn Goldberg, MD, FACSM
Professor and Head, Division of Health Promotion
  and Sports Medicine
Oregon Health & Science University
Portland, Oregon

Bruce A. Goldberger, PhD, DABFT
Professor and Director of Toxicology
Departments of Pathology, Immunology &
  Laboratory Medicine, and Psychiatry
University of Florida College of Medicine
Gainesville, Florida

R. Jeffrey Goldsmith, MD
Professor of Clinical Psychiatry
College of Medicine, University of Cincinnati
Staff Psychiatrist
Mental Health Care Line
Cincinnati VA Medical Center
Cincinnati, Ohio

David A. Gorelick, MD, PhD
Intramural Research Program
National Institute on Drug Abuse
National Institutes of Health
Adjunct Professor
Department of Psychiatry
University of Maryland School of Medicine
Baltimore, Maryland

Jon E. Grant, MD, JD, MPH
Professor, Department of Psychiatry
University of Minnesota Medical School
Minneapolis, Minnesota

Kenneth W. Griffin, PhD, MPH
Associate Professor of Public Health
Weill Cornell Medical College
New York, New York

Roland R. Griffiths, PhD
Professor, Department of Psychiatry and Behavioral
  Sciences
Department of Neuroscience
Johns Hopkins University School of Medicine
Baltimore, Maryland

Paul J. Gruenewald, PhD
Senior Research Scientist
Prevention Research Center
Pacific Institute for Research and Evaluation
Berkeley, California

Nady el-Guebaly, MD
Professor and Head, Addiction Division
University of Calgary
Consultant, Addictions Program
Alberta Health Services
Calgary, Alberta

David H. Gustafson, PhD
Professor
center for Health Enhancement Studies
University of Wisconsin
Madison, Wisconsin

Paul S. Haber, MD, FRACP, FAChAM
Head, Discipline of Addiction Medicine
University of Sydney
Director, Drug Health Services
Royal Prince Alfred Hospital
Camperdown, New South Wales, Australia

Karen J. Hartwell, MD
Assistant Professor of Psychiatry
Medical University of South Carolina
Charleston, South Carolina

J. David Hawkins, PhD
Professor, School of Social Work
University of Washington
Seattle, Washington

J. Taylor Hays, MD
Associate Professor, Department of Internal Medicine
College of Medicine, Mayo Clinic
Associate Director, Nicotine Dependence Center
Mayo Clinic
Rochester, Minnesota

Derya Bora Hazar, MD
Assistant Clinical Professor of Medicine
Tufts University School of Medicine
Section Chief of Nephrology
Carney Hospital
Boston, Massachusetts

Stephen T. Higgins, PhD
Professor, Departments of Psychiatry and Psychology
University of Vermont
Burlington, Vermont

Harold D. Holder, PhD
Senior Scientist, Prevention Research Center
Pacific Institute for Research and Evaluation
Berkeley, California

Hon. Peggy Fulton Hora, JD
Judge of the Superior Court of California (Retired)

Ryan Horvath, BA
Graduate Student in Pharmacology/Toxicology
Dartmouth Medical School
Hanover, New Hampshire

Matthew O. Howard, PhD
Frank A. Daniels Distinguished Professor, School of
  Social Work
University of North Carolina
Chapel Hill, North Carolina

Richard D. Hurt, MD, FASAM
Professor of Medicine
Director
Nicotine Dependence Center
Mayo Clinic
Rochester, Minnesota

Mark Hrymoc, MD
Clinical Instructor, Department of Psychiatry
Cedars-Sinai Medical Center
Los Angeles, California

Jerome H. Jaffe, MD
Clinical Professor, Department of Psychiatry
Division of Alcohol and Drug Abuse
University of Maryland
Baltimore, Maryland

Steven L. Jaffe, MD
Professor Emeritus of Child and Adolescent Psychiatry
Emory University
Clinical Professor of Psychiatry
Morehouse School of Medicine
Atlanta, Georgia

Alain Joffe, MD, MPH
Associate Professor of Pediatrics
Johns Hopkins University School of Medicine
Johns Hopkins Hospital
Baltimore, Maryland

Laura M. Juliano, PhD
Associate Professor,
Department of Psychology
American University
Washington, DC

Christopher W. Kahler, PhD
Professor (Research) of Community Health
Center for Alcohol and Addiction Studies
Brown University
Providence, Rhode Island

Lori D. Karan, MD, FACP, FASAM
Associate Clinical Professor of Medicine
University of California, San Francisco
San Francisco, California

Jason R. Kilmer, PhD
Research Assistant Professor, Psychiatry and
    Behavioral Sciences
Assistant Director of Health and Wellness for
    Alcohol and Other Drug Education
Division of Student Life
University of Washington
Seattle, Washington

Clifford M. Knapp, PhD
Associate Professor, Department of Psychiatry
Boston University School of Medicine
Boston, Massachusetts

John R. Knight, MD
Associate Professor of Pediatrics
Harvard Medical School
Director, Center for Adolescent Substance Abuse
    Research
Children's Hospital Boston
Boston, Massachusetts

Patricia K. Kokotailo, MD, MPH
Professor of Pediatrics
University of Wisconsin School of Medicine and
    Public Health
University of Wisconsin Hospitals and Clinics
Madison, Wisconsin

Thomas R. Kosten, MD
Professor of Psychiatry and Neuroscience
Baylor College of Medicine
Director and Vice Chair, Psychiatry, Addictions,
    and Neuroscience
Michael E. DeBakey Veterans Administration
    Medical Center
Houston, Texas

Margaret M. Kotz, DO
Professor of Psychiatry and Anesthesiology
Case Western Reserve University School of Medicine
Director, Addiction Recovery Services
Case Medical Center
University Hospitals of Cleveland
Cleveland, Ohio

Henry R. Kranzler, MD
Treatment Research Center
University of Pennsylvania
Philadelphia, Pennsylvania

Igor Kravets, MD
Instructor of Clinical Investigation
Laboratory of Addictive Diseases
The Rockefeller University
Associate Attending Physician
The Rockefeller University Hospital
New York, New York

Mary Jeanne Kreek, MD
Professor and Head, Laboratory of the Biology of
    Addictive Diseases
The Rockefeller University; Senior Physician
Rockefeller University Hospital
New York, New York

**Donald J. Kurth, MD, MBA, MPA,
FASAM**
Associate Professor, Departments of Psychiatry and
    Preventive Medicine
Loma Linda University
Chief of Addiction Medicine, Psychiatry Department
Loma Linda University Behavioral Medicine Center
Redlands, California

Maritza Lagos-Saez, MD, DABAM
Assistant Professor and Director of Medical Student
    Education
Department of Psychiatry
Michigan State University College of Human Medicine
Kalamazoo Center for Medical Studies
Attending Physician, Borgess Medical Center
Kalamazoo, Michigan

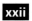

Bruce D. Lamb, JD, MA
Partner, Ruden McClusky
Tampa, Florida

Mary E. Larimer, PhD
Professor of Psychiatry and Behavioral Sciences
Clinical Psychologist
University of Washington
Seattle, Washington

David Y-W. Lee, PhD
Associate Professor of Psychiatry
Harvard Medical School
Director, Bio-Organic and Natural Products Lab
McLean Hospital
Boston, Massachusetts

Elizabeth Mirabile Levens, MD
Waterbury Pulmonary Associates
Waterbury, Connecticut

Adam M. Leventhal, PhD
Assistant Professor of Preventive Medicine and
  Psychology
University of Southern California
Division of Health Behavior Research
USC Keck School of Medicine
Los Angeles, California

Frances R. Levin, MD
Kennedy-Leavy Professor of Clinical Psychiatry
Columbia University
Research Psychiatrist
New York State Psychiatric Institute, Division on
  Substance Abuse
New York, New York

Sharon Levy, MD, MPH
Assistant Professor of Pediatrics
Harvard Medical School
Medical Director, Adolescent Substance
  Abuse Program
Children's Hospital Boston
Boston, Massachusetts

Ting-Kai Li, MD
Director
National Institute on Alcohol Abuse and
  Alcoholism
National Institutes of Health
Bethesda, Maryland

**Michael R. Liepman, MD, FASAM,
DLFAPA, DABAM**
Professor and Director of Research
Department of Psychiatry
Michigan State University, College of Human Medicine
Kalamazoo Center for Medical Studies
Medical Director
Jim Gilmore Jr. Community Healing Center
Kalamazoo, Michigan

Marsha M. Linehan, PhD
Professor, Department of Psychology
Director, Behavioral Research & Therapy Clinics
  (BRTC)
University of Washington
Seattle, Washington

Scott E. Lukas, PhD
Professor of Psychiatry and Pharmacology
Harvard Medical School
Boston, Massachusetts
Director, Neuroimaging Center
Director, Behavioral Psychopharmacology Research
  Laboratory
McLean Hospital
Belmont, Massachusetts

Alan Ona Malabanan, MD, FACE
Assistant Professor of Medicine
Harvard Medical School
Attending Physician
Endocrinology, Diabetes and Metabolism
Beth Israel Deaconess Medical Center
Boston, Massachusetts

Issam A. Mardini, MD, PhD
Assistant Professor, Departments of Anesthesiology
  and Critical Care
University of Pennsylvania
Attending, Penn Pain Medicine Center and
  Department of Anesthesiology
University of Pennsylvania Health System
Philadelphia, Pennsylvania

John J. Mariani, MD
Assistant Professor of Clinical Psychiatry
Columbia University
Psychiatrist II
New York State Psychiatric Institute, Division on
  Substance Abuse
New York, New York

G. Alan Marlatt, PhD
Professor of Psychology
University of Washington
Seattle, Washington

Judith Martin, MD
Medical Director
BAART Turk Street Clinic
San Francisco, California

W. Alex Mason, PhD
Research Associate Professor
Social Development Research Group
School of Social Work
University of Washington
Seattle, Washington

Martha A. Maurer, MSW, MPH, PhD
Assistant Researcher
Pain & Policy Studies Group
University of Wisconsin School of Medicine and
    Public Health
Madison, Wisconsin

Michael F. Mayo-Smith, MD, MPH
Network Director
VA New England Health Care System
Bedford, Massachusetts

Elinore F. McCance-Katz, MD, PhD
Professor of Psychiatry
University of California, San Francisco
San Francisco, California

Dennis McCarty, PhD
Professor
Department of Public Health & Preventive Medicine
Oregon Health & Science University
Portland, Oregon

Richard A. McCormick, PhD
Senior Scholar
Center for Health Care Research and Policy
Case Western Reserve University
Cleveland, Ohio

Barbara S. McCrady, PhD
Distinguished Professor of Psychology
Director, Center on Alcoholism, Substance Abuse
    and Addictions (CASAA)
University of New Mexico
Albuquerque, New Mexico

James R. McKay, PhD
Professor of Psychiatry
University of Pennsylvania
Director, Center of Excellence in Substance Abuse
    Treatment and Education
VA Medical Center
Philadelphia, Pennsylvania

A. Thomas McLellan, PhD
Director, Penn Center for Substance Abuse
    Solutions
Professor of Psychiatry
University of Pennsylvania School of Medicine
Philadelphia, Pennsylvania

Mary G. McMasters, MD
Assistant Professor of Addiction Medicine and
    General Internal Medicine
University of Virginia
Co-Medical Director
Pantops Clinic (MMT)
Charlottesville, Virginia

David Mee-Lee, MD
Consultant
DML Training and Consulting
Davis, California

John Mendelson, MD
Senior Scientist, Addiction Pharmacology Research
    Laboratory
California Pacific Medical Center Research
    Institute
San Francisco, California

Delinda E. Mercer, PhD
Clinical Coordinator
Behavioral Health Unit
Regional West Medical Center
Scottsbluff, Nebraska

Lisa J. Merlo, PhD, MPE
Assistant Professor
Department of Psychiatry
University of Florida
Director of Research
Professionals Resource Network, Inc.
Gainesville, Florida

Shannon C. Miller, MD, FASAM, FAPA, CMRO
Medical Director, Integrated Dual Diagnosis and
  Sobriety Plus Clinics
Program Director, VA Advanced Fellowship in
  Addiction Research/Medicine
Cincinnati VA Medical Center
Associate Director of Education, Training, and
  Dissemination
Center of Excellence for Treatment, Research, and
  Education in Addictive Disorders (CeTREAD)
Addiction Sciences Division
Associate Professor of Clinical Psychiatry, Affiliated
Department of Psychiatry and Behavioral Neuroscience
University of Cincinnati School of Medicine
Cincinnati, Ohio

Rudolf H. Moos, PhD
Professor Emeritus, Department of Psychiatry and
  Behavioral Sciences
Stanford University School of Medicine
Health Research Science Specialist, Research Service
Department of Veterans Affairs Health
  Care System
Palo Alto, California

Hugh Myrick, MD
Associate Professor of Psychiatry
Medical University of South Carolina
Director, Mental Health Service Line
Ralph H. Johnson VAMC
Charleston, South Carolina

Eric J. Nestler, MD, PhD
Nash Family Professor and Chair
Department of Neuroscience
Mount Sinai School of Medicine
New York, New York

Edward V. Nunes, MD
Professor of Clinical Psychiatry
Columbia University College of Physicians and
  Surgeons
New York State Psychiatric Institute
Associate Attending Psychiatrist
New York Presbyterian Hospital
New York, New York

Patrick G. O'Connor, MD, MPH
Professor of Medicine
Chief, Section of General Internal Medicine
Yale University School of Medicine
Yale-New Haven Hospital
New Haven, Connecticut

Brian L. Odlaug, BA
Research Associate, Department of Psychiatry
Graduate Student, School of Public Health
University of Minnesota
Minneapolis, Minnesota

James A.D. Otis, MD
Associate Professor
Department of Neurology
Boston University School of Medicine
Director, Pain Management Group
Boston Medical Center
Boston, Massachusetts

Theodore V. Parran, Jr., MD, FACP
Associate Clinical Professor, Department of Internal
  Medicine
Case Western Reserve University School of
  Medicine
Associate Medical Director, Rosary Hall Addiction
  Services
St. Vincent Charity Hospital
Cleveland, Ohio

Rebecca A. Payne, MD
Resident, Department of Psychiatry and Behavioral
  Sciences
Clinical Neuroscience Division
Medical University of South Carolina
Charleston, South Carolina

J. Thomas Payte, MD
Medical Director
Drug Dependence Associates
San Antonio, Texas

Michael Perloff, MD
Resident, Department of Neurology
Boston University, Boston Medical Center
Boston, Massachusetts

Karran A. Phillips, MD, MSc
Staff Clinician
Intramural Research Program
National Institute on Drug Abuse
National Institutes of Health
Adjunct Assistant Professor
Division of General Internal Medicine
Johns Hopkins School of Medicine
Baltimore, Maryland

Marc N. Potenza, MD, PhD
Associate Professor
Department of Psychiatry and Child Study
Yale School of Medicine
New Haven, Connecticut

Vladimir Poznyak, MD, PhD
Coordinator, Management of Substance Abuse
Department of Mental Health and Substance Abuse
World Health Organization (WHO)
Geneva, Switzerland

James O. Prochaska, PhD
Professor and Director, Cancer Prevention Research
  Center
University of Rhode Island
Kingston, Rhode Island

Terri L. Randall, MD
Instructor, Department of Psychiatry and Human
  Behavior
Division of Child and Adolescent Psychiatry
Assistant Director, Child and Adolescent Psychiatry
  Fellowship Program
Thomas Jefferson University
Philadelphia, Pennsylvania

Lillian G. Remer, MA
Associate Research Scientist
Prevention Research Center
Pacific Institute for Research & Evaluation
Berkeley, California

Richard K. Ries, MD, FAPA, FASAM
Professor of Psychiatry
Director, Division of Addictions, Department of
  Psychiatry and Behavioral Sciences
University of Washington
Medical Director, Harborview Addictions and
  Rehabilitation Psychiatry Programs
Harborview Medical Center
Seattle, Washington

David C.S. Roberts, PhD
Professor
Department of Physiology and Pharmacology
Wake Forest University School of Medicine
Winston-Salem, North Carolina

Randall E. Rogers, PhD
Addictions Treatment Program Director
Harry S. Truman Memorial Veterans Hospital
Columbia, Missouri

Richard N. Rosenthal, MD
Antenucci Professor of Clinical Psychiatry and
  Senior Associate Dean
Columbia University College of Physicians and
  Surgeons
Chairman, Department of Psychiatry and
  Behavioral Health
St. Luke's–Roosevelt Hospital Center
New York, New York

Bruce J. Rounsaville, MD
Professor of Psychiatry
Yale University School of Medicine
Director, New England Mental Illness Research
  and Education Center
VA Connecticut Healthcare
New Haven, Connecticut

Stanley Sacks, PhD
Director, Center for the Integration of Research &
  Practice
National Development & Research Institutes, Inc.
New York, New York

**Richard Saitz, MD, MPH, FACP,
FASAM**
Professor of Medicine and Epidemiology
Director, Clinical Addiction Research and
  Education (CARE) Unit
Section of General Internal Medicine, Department
  of Medicine
Boston Medical Center/Boston University Schools
  of Medicine and Public Health
Boston, Massachusetts

Michael E. Saladin, PhD
Associate Professor
Department of Health Sciences and Research and
  Department of Psychiatry and Behavioral Sciences
Clinical Neuroscience Division
Medical University of South Carolina
Charleston, South Carolina

Jeffrey H. Samet, MD, MA, MPH
Professor of Medicine and Community Health
  Sciences
Boston University Schools of Medicine and Public
  Health
Chief, General Internal Medicine
Boston Medical Center
Boston, Massachusetts

Jussi J. Saukkonen, MD
Associate Professor of Medicine
Department of Pulmonary and Critical Care
  Medicine
Boston University School of Medicine
Boston, Massachusetts

Seddon R. Savage, MD, MS, FASAM
Director, Dartmouth Center on Addiction Recovery
  and Education (DCARE)
Pain Consultant, Manchester VA Medical Center
Associate Professor of Anesthesiology, Dartmouth
  Medical School, Adjunct Faculty
Hanover, New Hampshire

Andrew J. Saxon, MD
Professor of Psychiatry and Behavioral Sciences
University of Washington
Director, Addiction Patient Care Line
Mental Health Service
VA Puget Sound Health Care System
Seattle, Washington

Hon. William G. Schma, (Ret)
Kalamazoo Circuit Court
Kalamazoo, Michigan

Jerome E. Schulz, MD, FASAM
Medical Director
Hazelden Center for Youth and Family
Plymouth, Minnesota

Neil Sharma, MD
Chief Resident Department of Internal Medicine
University of South Florida
Attending/Chief Resident
James A. Haley VA Hospital
Tampa, Florida

Steven J. Shoptaw, PhD
Professor, Department of Family Medicine
University of California, Los Angeles
Los Angeles, California

Gerald D. Shulman, MA, MAC, FACATA
President
Shulman & Associates, Training and Consulting in Behavioral Health
Jacksonville, Florida

Diana I. Simeonova, Dipl-Psych, MA
Associate Director
Institute for Behavioral Medicine
Smyrna, Georgia

Deborah R. Simkin, MD
Program Director, Psychiatry
Section Head, Division of Child and Adolescent Psychiatry
Residency Training Director
Adjunct Associate Professor
University of South Alabama Medical School
Mobile, Alabama

David A. Smelson, PsyD
Professor/Vice Chair of Clinical Research
Department of Psychiatry
University of Massachusetts Medical School
Worcester, Massachusetts

Ramon Solhkhah, MD
Director, The Child & Family Institute
Chief, Division of Child and Adolescent Psychiatry
St. Luke's–Roosevelt Hospital Center
Assistant Professor of Clinical Psychiatry
Columbia University College of Physicians and Surgeons
New York, New York

Crystal R. Spotts, MEd
Senior Research Principal
Department of Psychiatry
University of Pittsburgh Medical Center
Western Psychiatric Institute and Clinic
Pittsburgh, Pennsylvania

Marc L. Steinberg, PhD
Assistant Professor of Psychiatry
Robert Wood Johnson Medical School
New Brunswick, New Jersey

Randy Stinchfield, PhD
Associate Director
Center for Adolescent Substance Abuse Research
Department of Psychiatry
University of Minnesota
Minneapolis, Minnesota

Susan M. Stine, MD, PhD
Associate Professor, Department of Psychiatry and Behavioral Neurosciences
Wayne State University School of Medicine
Director, Addiction Psychiatry Residency Program
Wayne State University School of Medicine and Detroit Medical Center
Detroit, Michigan

Amanda M. Stone, BS
Medical Student
University of Florida
Gainesville, Florida

Carol A. Sulis, MD
Associate Professor of Medicine, Division of Infectious Diseases
Boston University School of Medicine
Hospital Epidemiologist
Attending Physician
Boston Medical Center
Boston, Massachusetts

Maria A. Sullivan, MD, PhD
Associate Professor of Clinical Psychiatry
Columbia University
Research Psychiatrist, Division on Substance
  Abuse
Columbia College of Physicians and Surgeons
New York State Psychiatric Institute
New York, New York

Zebulon Taintor, MD
Professor of Psychiatry
New York University School of Medicine
Consulting Attending Psychiatrist
Bellevue Hospital
New York, New York

Jeanette M. Tetrault, MD
Assistant Professor of Medicine
Department of Internal Medicine
Yale University School of Medicine
New Haven, Connecticut

Jennifer W. Tidey, PhD
Associate Professor (Research) of Psychiatry and
  Human Behavior
Center for Alcohol and Addiction Studies
Brown University
Providence, Rhode Island

Juana Maria Tomás-Rosselló, MD, MPH
Treatnet Coordinator, Southeast Asia
Regional Centre for East Asia and the Pacific
United Nations Office on Drugs and Crime
Vienna, Austria

J. Scott Tonigan, PhD
Research Professor, Department of Psychology
Center on Alcoholism, Substance Abuse, and
  Addictions (CASAA)
University of New Mexico
Albuquerque, New Mexico

Andrew J. Treno, PhD
Research Scientist
Prevention Research Center
Pacific Institute for Research and Evaluation
Berkeley, California

Himanshu P. Upadhyaya, MD, MBBS, MS
Associate Professor, Department of Psychiatry and
  Behavioral Sciences
Medical University of South Carolina
Charleston, South Carolina

Adrienne D. Vaiana, BS
Research Coordinator II
Department of Psychiatry
University of Massachusetts Medical School
Worcester, Massachusetts

Nora D. Volkow, MD
Director
National Institute on Drug Abuse
Chief
Laboratory of Neuroimaging
National Institute on Alcohol Abuse and Alcoholism
Bethesda, Maryland

Angela E. Waldrop, PhD
Assistant Professor
Department of Psychiatry
University of California, San Francisco
Staff Psychologist, PTSD Clinical Team
San Francisco VA Medical Center
San Francisco, California

Hong Wang, MD, PhD
Instructor of Psychiatry
Harvard Medical School
Bio-Organic and Natural Products Lab
McLean Hospital
Belmont, Massachusetts

Elizabeth A. Warner, MD
Associate Professor of Internal Medicine
University of South Florida College of Medicine
Medical Director, Ambulatory Services
Tampa General Hospital
Tampa, Florida

Michael F. Weaver, MD, FASAM
Associate Professor of Internal Medicine and
  Psychiatry
Virginia Commonwealth University
Medical Director, Substance Abuse Consult
  Service
Medical College of Virginia Hospital
Richmond, Virginia

Melissa Weddle, MD, MPH
Associate Professor of Pediatrics
Doernbecher Children's Hospital
Oregon Health and Science University
Portland, Oregon

Roger D. Weiss, MD
Professor of Psychiatry
Harvard Medical School
Boston, Massachusetts
Chief, Division of Alcohol and Drug Abuse
McLean Hospital
Belmont, Massachusetts

Sandra P. Welch, PhD
Professor
Department of Pharmacology and Toxicology
Virginia Commonwealth University
Richmond, Virginia

Joseph J. Westermeyer, MD, MPH, PhD
Professor of Psychiatry
University of Minnesota
Medical Director, Addictive Disorders Service
Minneapolis VA Medical Center
Minneapolis, Minnesota

David B. Wexler, JD
Professor of Law
University of Puerto Rico
San Juan, Puerto Rico

William L. White, MA
Senior Research Consultant
Lighthouse Institute
Chestnut Health Systems
Bloomington, Illinois

Ursula Whiteside, MSD
NIAAA Postdoctoral Fellow
Department of Psychology
University of Washington
Seattle, Washington

Paula L. Wilbourne, PhD
Addiction Treatment Service
VA Palo Alto Health Care System
Palo Alto, California

Bonnie B. Wilford, MS
Executive Director, Coalition on Physician
  Education in Substance Use Disorders (COPE)
Senior Principal and Director, Center for Health
  Services and Outcomes Research
JBS International, Inc.
Easton, Maryland

Jeffery N. Wilkins, MD
Professor, Department of Psychiatry and
  Biobehavioral Sciences
David Geffen School of Medicine at UCLA
Vice Chair and Lincy/Moynihan-Heyward Chair in
  Addiction Medicine
Cedars-Sinai Medical Center
Los Angeles, California

Mark L. Willenbring, MD
Director, Division of Treatment and Recovery
  Research
National Institutes on Alcohol Abuse and
  Alcoholism
Bethesda, Maryland

Emily C. Williams, MPH
Doctoral Student, Health Services
University of Washington
Seattle, Washington

Vern Williams, MD
Medical Director
Hazelden Springbrook
Newberg, Oregon

Kevin C. Wilson, MD
Assistant Professor of Medicine
Boston University School of Medicine
Attending Physician, Pulmonary, Critical Care, and
  Allergy
Boston Medical Center
Boston, Massachusetts

Bruce J. Winick, JD
Professor of Law, School of Law
Professor of Psychiatry and Behavioral Sciences
University of Miami
Coral Gables, Florida

Ken C. Winters, PhD
Professor of Psychiatry
University of Minnesota Medical School
Minneapolis, Minnesota

Alex Wodak, AM, MB BS, FRACP, FAChAM
Director, Alcohol and Drug Service
St. Vincent's Hospital
Sydney, New South Wales, Australia

John J. Woodward, PhD
Professor, Department of Neurosciences,
    Department of Psychiatry and Behavioral Sciences
Center for Drug and Alcohol Programs
Medical University of South Carolina
Charleston, South Carolina

Tara M. Wright, MD
Assistant Professor of Psychiatry
Medical University of South Carolina
Staff Psychiatrist, Medical Health Service Line
Ralph H. Johnson VAMC
Charleston, South Carolina

Martha J. Wunsch, MD, FAAP, FASAM
Medical Director
The TASL Clinic
Blacksburg, Virginia

Stephen A. Wyatt, DO
Medical Director, Dual Day Treatment Program
Department of Psychiatry
Middlesex Hospital
Middletown, Connecticut

Sarah W. Yip, BA, MSc
PhD Student, Department of Psychiatry
University of Oxford
Warneford Hospital
Oxford, United Kingdom

Christine Yuodelis-Flores, MD
Clinical Associate Professor of Psychiatry and
    Behavioral Sciences
University of Washington
Attending Psychiatrist
Harborview Medical Center
Seattle, Washington

Anne Zajicek, MD, PharmD
Pediatric Medical Officer, Associate Branch Chief
Obstetric and Pediatric Pharmacology Branch
Center for Research for Mothers and Children
Eunice Kennedy Shriver National Institute of Child
    Health and Human Development
National Institutes of Health
Bethesda, Maryland

Aleksandra Zgierska, MD, PhD
Assistant Professor
Department of Family Medicine
University of Wisconsin Hospital and Clinics
    Center for Addictive Disorders
University of Wisconsin School of Medicine and
    Public Health
Madison, Wisconsin

Douglas M. Ziedonis, MD, MPH
Professor and Chairman, Department of Psychiatry
UMass Memorial Health Care and University of
    Massachusetts Medical School
Worcester, Massachusetts

Joan E. Zweben, PhD
Clinical Professor of Psychiatry
University of California, San Francisco
Executive Director
East Bay Community Recovery Project
Oakland, California

CONTENTS

Section 7.

Pharmacologic Interventions

Section 8.

Behavioral Interventions

Section 12.

Pain and Addiction

Section 13.

Children and Adolescents

Section 14.

Ethical, Legal, and Liability Issues in Addiction Practice

CHAPTER

1

Summary Author: Christopher Sankey
Nora D. Volkow • Ting-Kai Li

Drug Addiction: The Neurobiology of Behavior Gone Awry

Repeated drug use leads to long-lasting changes in the brain that undermine voluntary control. Psychoactive drugs (both legal and illegal) are used and misused for various reasons including the following:

- Pleasurable effects
- Altering mental state
- Improving performance
- Self-medicating a mental disorder

The aberrant behavioral manifestations that occur during addiction have been viewed by many as "choices" of the addicted individual. However, recent studies have revealed an underlying disruption to brain regions that are important for the normal processes of motivation, reward, and inhibitory control in addicted individuals. **From a neurobiological perspective, drug addiction is a disease of the brain and the associated abnormal behavior is the result of dysfunction of brain tissue.**

ADDICTION: A DEVELOPMENTAL DISORDER

Normal adolescent-specific behaviors (such as risk taking, novelty seeking, and response to peer pressure) increase the propensity to experiment with legal and illegal drugs. This behavior may be due in part to the incomplete development of brain regions (e.g., myelination of frontal lobe regions) that result in "executive functions" such as decision making and motivation. In addition, **drug exposure during adolescence might result in different neuroadaptations from those that occur during adulthood** (e.g., exposing adolescent rodents to nicotine leads to significant changes in nicotine receptors; this does not occur in adult rodents). Individuals who start using psychoactive drugs in adolescence are at higher risk of addiction than those who start using drugs later in life.

NEUROBIOLOGY OF DRUGS OF ABUSE

Dopamine has been consistently associated with the reinforcing effects of most drugs of abuse. **Drugs of abuse increase extracellular dopamine concentrations in limbic regions, including the nucleus accumbens (NAc).** Drugs of abuse provide longer and larger (5–10-fold) increases in dopamine than natural reinforcers such as food and sex. Some drugs (such as cocaine, amphetamine, methamphetamine, and ecstasy) increase dopamine directly (by inhibiting dopamine reuptake or promoting dopamine release). Other drugs (such as nicotine, alcohol, opiates, and marijuana) work indirectly via other neuron receptors that modulate dopamine levels.

Dopamine is involved in many aspects of reward and pleasure, including the prediction of reward and salience. Salience refers to stimuli or environmental changes that are arousing or that elicit an attentional-behavioral switch. Salience affects the motivation to seek the anticipated reward and facilitates conditioned learning. This suggests that drug-induced increases in dopamine will inherently motivate further procurement of more drug (regardless of whether or not the effects of the drug are consciously perceived to be pleasurable). Salience also leads to a situation in which sensory stimuli (sights, sounds, etc.) that are associated with the drug or with drug taking can increase dopamine by themselves and elicit the desire for the drug. This explains also why the addicted person is at risk of relapsing when exposed to an environment where he or she has previously taken the drug.

NEUROBIOLOGY OF DRUG ADDICTION

From a neurobiologic perspective, addiction probably results from neurobiologic changes that are associated with recurrent supraphysiologic perturbations in the dopamine system. **Chronic drug exposure alters the morphology of neurons in dopamine-regulated circuits.** At a *cellular* level, drugs have been reported to alter the expression of certain transcription factors (nuclear proteins that bind to regulatory regions of genes, thereby regulating their transcription into mRNA), as well as a wide variety of proteins involved in neurotransmission in brain regions that are regulated by dopamine. At the *neurotransmitter* level, addiction-related adaptations have been documented not only for dopamine but also for glutamate, GABA, opiates, serotonin, and various neuropeptides. In people with addictions, abnormal neurotransmitter levels are found in the mesocortical region of the brain. This brain region contains the orbiofrontal cortex, which is involved in compulsive behavior, as well as the cingulate gyrus, which regulates disinhibition. These adaptations are believed to play a significant role in aberrant addictive behaviors such as compulsive drug administration and poor inhibitory control, and relapse.

VULNERABILITY TO ADDICTION

Genetic Factors
It is estimated that 40% to 60% of the vulnerability to addiction is attributable to genetic factors. In humans, several chromosomal regions have been linked to drug abuse, but only a few specific genes have been identified with polymorphisms (alleles) that either predispose to or protect from drug addiction. While much of this research is still in its infancy, some of the best-known examples of addiction-related polymorphisms are as follows:

- The genetic alterations of alcohol dehydrogenase are protective against alcoholism.
- The genetic alterations of cytochrome P450 2A6 are protective against nicotine addiction.
- The genetic alterations of cytochrome P450 2D6 are protective against codeine abuse.
- The CHRNA5/A3/B4 gene cluster that is associated with nicotine dependence
- The genetic alterations of GABA type A that predispose to alcoholism
- The genetic alterations of D2-receptor that are linked to higher vulnerability to drug addiction in general

Environmental Factors
Environmental factors that have been consistently associated with the propensity to self-administer drugs include low socioeconomic class, poor parental support, and drug availability. Imaging techniques now allow us to investigate how environmental factors affect the brain and how these, in turn, affect the behavioral responses to drugs of abuse. For example, in nonhuman primates, social status affects D2-receptor expression in the brain. Animals that achieve a dominant status in the group show increased numbers of D2 receptors. High D2 receptor levels have been shown to lead to marked decreases in drug consumption in primates.

Comorbidity with Mental Illness
The risk for substance abuse and addiction in individuals with mental illness is significantly higher than for the general population. The high comorbidity probably reflects, in part, overlapping environmental, genetic, and neurobiologic factors that influence drug abuse and mental illness. It has been proposed that comorbidity might be due to the use of the abused drugs to self-medicate the mental illness. In addition, chronic exposure to psychoactive drugs could lead to neurobiologic changes, which might explain the increased risk of mental illness. This highlights the relevance of the early evaluation and treatment of mental diseases as an effective strategy to prevent drug addiction that starts as self-medication.

STRATEGIES TO COMBAT ADDICTION

The knowledge of the neurobiology of drugs and the adaptive changes that occur with addiction is guiding new strategies for prevention and treatment.

Preventing Addiction

As we gain knowledge of the genes (and the proteins that they encode) that make a person more or less vulnerable to taking drugs and to addiction, we will become better at tailoring interventions for those at higher risk. For example, our understanding of the greater neurobiologic vulnerability of adolescents underscores why prevention of early exposure to drugs during adolescence is such an important strategy to combat drug addiction.

Treating Addiction

The adaptations in the brain that result from chronic drug exposure are long lasting; therefore, **addiction must be viewed as a chronic disease.** Long-term treatment will be required for most cases, just as for other chronic diseases (such as hypertension, diabetes, and asthma). This "chronic disease" perspective should modify the expectations of treatment:

- Discontinuation of treatment, as for other chronic diseases, is likely to result in relapse.
- Relapse should not be interpreted as a failure of treatment (as is the view in most cases of addiction), but instead as a temporary setback because of lack of compliance or tolerance to an effective treatment
- Rates of relapse and recovery in the treatment of drug addiction are very similar to those of other chronic medical diseases
- As with other "multisystem" chronic disease, addiction treatment requires the involvement of multiple brain circuits (reward, motivation, learning, inhibitory control, and executive function), and their associated disruption of behavior indicates the need for a multimodal approach in the treatment of the addicted individual.

Pharmacologic Intervention

Pharmacologic interventions can be grouped into two classes:

- Those that interfere with the reinforcing effects of drugs of abuse. Potential mechanisms for this include
  - Interfering with drug binging
  - Reducing or eliminating drug-induced dopamine increase
  - Reducing or eliminating postsynaptic dopamine responses
  - Decreasing the drug's delivery to the brain
  - Medications that trigger aversive responses.
- Those that compensate for the adaptations that either predated or developed after long-term use, that is, medications that
  - Decrease the prioritized motivational value of the drug
  - Enhance the saliency value of natural reinforcers
  - Interfere with conditioned responses, stress-induced relapse, or physical withdrawal

Table 1.1 summarizes proven medications and medications for which there are preliminary clinical data.

TABLE 1.1	Medications for Treating Drug and Alcohol Addition[a]	
Clinical target	**Medication**	**Biological target**
Alcoholism		
FDA approved	Disulfiram (Antabuse; Wyeth-Ayerst)	Aldehyde dehydrogenase (triggers aversive response)
	Naltrexone	μ opioid receptor (antagonist; interferes with reinforcement)
	Acamprosate	Glutamate related
	[a]Topiramate (Topamax; Ortho-McNeil)	GABA/glutamate
Under investigation	[a]Valproate	GABA/glutamate
	Ondansetron	5-HT$_3$ receptor
	Nalmefene	μ opioid receptor (antagonist)

(Continued)

TABLE 1.1   **Medications for Treating Drug and Alcohol Addition[a] (Continued)**

Clinical target	Medication	Biological target
	Baclofen (Lioresal; Novartis)	GABA$_B$ receptor (agonist)
	Pyrrolopyrimidine compound (Antalarmin; George Chrousos et al.)	CRF1 receptor (inhibits stress-triggered responses)
	Rimonabant (Acomplia; Sanofi-Synthelabo)	CB1 receptor (antagonist)
Smoking cessation		
FDA approved	Nicotine replacement	Nicotinic receptor (substitution with different pharmacokinetics)
	Varenicline	Nicotinic receptor ($\alpha4\beta2$ partial agonist)
	Bupropion	DA transporter blocker (amplifies DA signals)
Under investigation	Deprenyl	MAO-B inhibitor (inhibits metabolism of DA)
	Rimonabant (Acomplia; Sanofi-Synthelabo)	CB1 receptor (antagonist)
	Methoxsalen	CYP2A6 (inhibits nicotine metabolism)
	Nicotine conjugate vaccine (NicVax; Nabi Biopharmaceuticals)	Blocks entry into brain
	Naltrexone	μ opioid receptor (antagonist)
Heroin/opiate addiction		
FDA approved (84)	Naltrexone	μ opioid receptor (antagonist)
	Methadone	μ opioid receptor (substitution with different pharmacokinetics)
	Buprenorphine	μ opioid receptor (substitution)
Cocaine addiction		
Under investigation	[a]Topiramate (Topamax; Ortho-McNeil)	GABA agonist
	[a]γ-vinyl GABA (GVG) (Sabril; HoechstMarionRoussel)	GABA transaminase (inhibits GABA metabolism)
	[a]Gabapentin (Neurontin; Parke-Davis)	GABA/glutamate (synthesis)
	[a]Tiagabine (Gabitril; Abbott)	GABA transporter (inhibitor)
	Baclofen (Lioresal; Novartis)	GABA$_B$ receptor (agonist)
	Modafinil	Glutamate (?)
	Disulfiram (Antabuse; Wyeth-Ayerst)	Unknown for cocaine
	Cocaine vaccine (TA-CD; Xenova)	Blocks entry into brain
	N-acetylcysteine	Glutamate (?)

Medications used for physical withdrawal are not included.
[a]Antiepileptic drugs that have been shown to decrease drug induced DA increases as well as conditioned response.
FDA, Food and Drug Administration; GABA, γ-aminobutyric acid; GABA$_B$, GABA type B; 5HT$_3$, 5-hydroxytryptamine (serotonin) receptor subtype 3; MAO-B, monoamine oxidase B.

Cognitive–Behavioral Intervention

In a similar fashion, behavioral interventions can be classified by their intended remedial function, such as to strengthen inhibitory control circuits, provide alternative reinforcers, and strengthen executive function. Dual approaches that pair cognitive-behavioral strategies with medications to compensate for or counteract the neurobiologic changes induced by chronic drug exposure might, in the future, provide more robust and longer lasting treatments for addiction than either given in isolation.

CHALLENGES FOR SOCIETY

In most cases, **drug abuse and addiction alienate the individual from both family and community, increasing isolation, and interfering with treatment and recovery.** Because both the family and the community provide integral aspects of effective treatment and recovery, this identifies an important challenge: to reduce the stigma of addiction that interferes with intervention and proper rehabilitation. Recognition of addiction as a chronic disease resulting from neurological abnormalities is essential for large-scale prevention and treatment programs that require the participation of the medical community. Existing barriers to more medical involvement include

- The lack of treatment resources (detoxes, treatment centers, etc.)
- The lack of reimbursement by many private medical insurance policies for the evaluation or treatment of drug abuse and addiction
- The limited involvement of the pharmaceutical industry in the development of new medications.

CHAPTER 2

Summary Author: Christopher Sankey
Rosa M. Crum*

The Epidemiology of Substance Use Disorders

SOME EPIDEMIOLOGIC PRINCIPLES

Epidemiology is the study of how diseases are distributed in populations and quantifies the determinants of disease and health. Some general definitions follow.

- Incidence = No. of new cases/at-risk population over a given period
- Prevalence = No. of cases at the time of sample/total population
- Prevalence takes into account both the incidence and the duration of a disease, because it depends not only on the proportion of newly developed cases over time but also on the length of time the disease exists in the population—it is affected by the degree of recovery and death from the disease. Incidence generally is taken to represent the risk of disease, whereas prevalence is an indicator of the public health burden the disease imposes on the community.
- Relative risk (RR) = Incidence of disease X in population with trait A/incidence of disease X in population without trait A

RR is a measure of the strength of association between a particular characteristic and the development of disease. An RR of one implies no effect of the studied variable, while values above or below one indicate that the characteristic is associated with increased risk or is associated with reduced risk, respectively.

Types of Studies
1. Observational
2. Experimental

Observational studies may include cross-sectional, case-control, or cohort studies. In cross-sectional studies or surveys, individuals are assessed (e.g., by interview or physical examination) at a particular point in time. Analytic studies usually are classified as case-control (retrospective) or cohort (longitudinal, prospective). Analytic studies generally test a hypothesis of a suspected association between a particular exposure (risk factor) and a disease or other outcome. In all observational studies, the investigator observes the study participants and gathers information for analysis. In contrast, experimental studies, such as randomized clinical trials, are designed by the investigator, study groups are selected, and often an intervention (such as a new type of treatment) is given to one group of participants. The study participants are followed and the outcomes of each group are measured and compared.

PREVALENCE OF ALCOHOL USE DISORDERS

Prevalence of addiction has been typically measured using definitions for "substance abuse and /or dependence" as defined in DSM-IV and ICD.

---

*All the citations for the data and scientific statements presented below are included in Chapter 2 of the *Principles of Addiction Medicine* textbook.

Abbreviations used in this guide:

AAb = Alcohol abuse
ADp = Alcohol dependence
AUD = Alcohol use disorder
Drug Ab = Drug abuse
Drug Dp = Drug dependence
LT Prev = Lifetime prevalence
1Y Prev = 1 year prevalence

The earliest prevalence study (1980s) was the National Institute of Mental Health's Epidemiologic Catchment Area (ECA) Study—surveying more than 20,000 adult participants in five metropolitan areas of the United States. Overall prevalence of alcohol use disorders in the baseline ECA survey was 13.5% (lifetime prevalence), 4.8% (6-month prevalence), and 2.8% (1-month prevalence).

More recently, the National Comorbidity Survey (NCS), completed between 1990 and 1992 based on DSM-III-R criteria, found higher numbers: lifetime prevalence for alcohol abuse was 12.5% in males and 6.4% in females, and lifetime prevalence of dependency was 20.1% and 8.2%, respectively. The NCS also has revealed that approximately one third of adolescent drinkers will transition to alcohol abuse or dependence. Data from the 2001-02 National Epidemiologic Survey on Alcohol and Related Conditions (NESARC), a nationally representative sample survey sponsored by the National Institute on Alcohol Abuse and Alcoholism, provide lifetime and 12-month estimates of alcohol use disorders based on DSM-IV criteria using the Alcohol Use Disorder and Associated Disabilities Interview Schedule (AUDADIS). Twelve-month prevalence of alcohol abuse from the NESARC was found to be 6.9% among men and 2.6% among women. For alcohol dependence, the estimates were 5.4% for men and 2.3% for women. Overall lifetime prevalence of DSM-IV alcohol abuse and dependence using data from the NESARC was 17.8% and 12.5%, respectively. Most studies have found that the prevalence of alcohol use disorders is highest among young adults and generally decreases among older age groups.

Many factors can influence study results; variations in diagnostic definitions, study samples (such as a statistically different age distribution), or preselection/exclusion with "gated protocols" can influence prevalence estimates.

INCIDENCE OF ALCOHOL USE DISORDERS

Data from the Swedish Lundby study provide one of the few estimates of incidence of alcohol abuse and dependence over a prolonged follow-up period. The Lundby community was interviewed for the first time in 1947, reinterviewed in 1957 (with 1% lost to follow-up), and then examined again in 1972. Of the 2,550 participants in the original survey, 98% of those still alive in 1972 were reinterviewed.

Results

- Overall male age-adjusted annual incidence of AAb or ADp was 0.3%.
- Sharp decline in incidence after 30 years old
- Highest annual incidence of AUD was in men 10 to 19 years old (0.67%).
- Only 3 of 925 women in 1972 survey had AUD.

Various studies in the United States have yielded different numbers yet similar trends—incidence of AUD higher for males than females and highest in young adulthood.

- From the ECA surveys, the overall annual incidence of AAb per 100 person-years is 3.7 for men and 0.6 for women.

Fillmore examined longitudinal data from population-based samples. Drinking problems were identified using scales which included measures of binge drinking; drinking to cope; loss of control of alcohol use; belligerence; and drinking-related problems involving one's spouse, friends, job, finances, and the law. Fillmore's findings also indicated different patterns of drinking by gender. For example, women tended to develop problems associated with drinking later in life than men, and women were found to have higher rates of remission across all age groups than did men.

The recent prospective data from the NESARC have provided annual incidence rates for DSM-IV alcohol abuse (1.0 per 100 person-years) and alcohol dependence (1.7 per 100 person-years) and also indicate that the greatest risk for alcohol use disorders occurs during young adulthood.

PREVALENCE OF DRUG USE DISORDERS

Although several major surveys estimate the prevalence of drug use in the United States, there are fewer population-based studies that have examined the prevalence and incidence of drug use disorders or drug addiction. Results from NCS surveys are as follows:

- LT Prev of Drug Ab without Drug Dp = 5.4% (m) and 3.5% (f)
- LT Prev of Drug Dp = 9.2% (m) and 5.9% (f)
- Approximately 50% of drug using adolescents developed Drug Ab or Drug Dp.

The 2001–2002 NESARC survey results:

- LT Prev of Drug Ab (7.7%) and Drug Dp (2.6%)
- 1Y Prev of Drug Ab (1.4%) and Drug Dp (0.6%)
- Prev rates higher for males

Since 2000, the National Survey on Drug Use and Health (NSDUH) has gathered information on substance use disorders within the prior year based on DSM-IV criteria. From the 2006 survey, prevalence of illicit drug use disorders in the year before the survey was reported to be 2.8% overall, with the largest prevalence among young adults aged 18 to 25 years (8.1%). Differences in data collection methodology as well as diagnostic instrumentation may account for some of the variations found in prevalence estimates reported for these large national surveys.

NICOTINE

Lifetime prevalence of nicotine dependence, estimated from the NCS, has been reported to be 24%. From the 2006 NSDUH, we know that 25% of the population is current tobacco cigarette smokers. Data from the 2001–2002 NESARC indicate that 12.8% of the population meets DSM-IV criteria for nicotine dependence in the year before the survey. A greater proportion of males (14.1%) than females (11.1%) have current nicotine dependence. The vast majority of the individuals with dependence use tobacco cigarettes (93.7%).

INCIDENCE OF DRUG USE DISORDERS

There is a relative paucity of information regarding the incidence of drug use disorders as a group, with less information available for specific drugs. Early findings from the 1-year prospective ECA data showed

- Annual incidence of Drug Ab and Dp = 1.09/100 person-years (men = 1.66) (women = 0.66)
- Highest incidence in 18 to 25 year olds, dropping sharply after young adulthood, and being close to zero after 65

Recent analyses of the 3-year NESARC prospective data:

- Drug Ab in general US population = 0.28/100 person-years
- Drug Dp in general US population = 0.32/100 person-years

CORRELATES AND SUSPECTED RISK FACTORS

Many risk factors or traits associated with drug and alcohol have been identified.

Gender and Alcohol Use Disorders

Alcohol dependence is twice as common in men as women, and women drinkers are less likely to transition to alcohol dependence or to have persistent dependence after it develops.

Differences in prevalence and incidence between men and women have been attributed to a number of factors. Cultural norms, societal standards, and body size and differences in the metabolism of alcohol all may contribute to the finding that women appear to use less alcohol and to have lower rates of alcohol addiction. Recently, there appears to have been a rise in AUD in women, and this is thought to be due to many factors.

Many characteristics (e.g., marital status, full-time employment, ethnicity, age, occupation, educational level), as well as the occurrence of life events, and the presence of other psychopathology (such as depression) may play a role in gender variability with respect to alcohol consumption and the development of alcohol disorders.

Wilsnack and Wilsnack found that there was an increase in alcohol involvement in certain subgroups of American women. These included younger women, those in nontraditional jobs, and unmarried women cohabiting with a partner. Other researchers have identified physical or sexual violence and history of childhood sexual abuse as being associated with alcohol involvement in women.

Gender and Drug Use Disorder

As discussed for alcohol, males (boys and men) generally are more likely to use illicit drugs and may have a higher prevalence and incidence of drug use and disorders than females. However, gender differences will differ by the specific substance and the age of use. For example, in the 2006 Monitoring the Future survey, prevalence of cigarette and alcohol use was higher for female adolescents in some grades.

The social or cultural restrictions that are possible explanations for the reduced prevalence of alcohol use among women also may apply to some types of illicit drug use. However, some, but not all, data show that among drug users, the proportion of males and females who develop dependence is similar. In more recent analyses, using data from the NCS Replication, sex differences in the risk of progression from first use to dependence have been found for cannabis with relatively smaller differences found for other substances such as cocaine.

In the 2006 NSDUH, the overall proportion of substance use disorder in the past year (abuse or dependence) among participants 12 years of age or older was approximately twice as large for males (12.3%) as females (6.3%). However, in the subgroup aged 12 to 17, the proportion with substance abuse or dependence was very similar (8.0% and 8.1% for boys and girls, respectively).

Age and Alcohol Use Disorder

Age prevalence of alcohol use disorders is generally lower among older adults. This may be due to both reduced incidence and duration of alcohol use disorders in older adults. If the duration of the disorder is reduced, it may be a result of an increase in remission with age or a reduction in survival. Explanations for a decreased prevalence with age also may include (i) a reduced tolerance to alcohol with age, (ii) poorer recall among older adults, or (iii) a cohort effect. Further, alcohol problems and disorders may be under-recognized in older adults. Other age-related findings include the following:

1. Increased problems related to alcohol use at lower doses in the elderly
2. Decreased incidence of AUD with age
3. Highest hazard rate for AUD is 19 years of age and decreases steadily after this.
4. The earlier the first use of alcohol, the higher the associated risk of AAb, ADp, motor vehicle accidents (MVAs), violence, and drinking to address stressors.
5. Early smoking is associated with increased AAb and ADp.
6. Highest incidence for illicit drug use is in late adolescents and early adults.
7. Earlier use of drugs is associated with increased risk of subsequent DAb and DDp.
8. There seems to be a rise in AUD and drug use disorders since WWII.
9. Increase in use of cannabis, cocaine, and other street drugs in childhood and early adolescence among more recent cohorts.

Social factors may contribute to age-related findings. For example, the current cohort of older adults had no access to crack cocaine in their youth. When evaluating changes in the frequency of a disorder (in this case, drug and alcohol addiction), distinctions need to be made between changes that uniformly occur for all age groups during a particular historic period (period effect), changes that occur with age as the individual matures (age effect), and a cohort effect that reflects differences in disease rate for individuals born in different years.

Factors Relating to Race and Ethnicity and Alcohol Use Disorders

The relationship between race, ethnicity, and substance use is generally unclear. This is due to limited studies and many confounding variables. Some findings are listed below:

1. Among African Americans, the onset of heavy drinking appears to begin later, rates of consumption and prevalence of disorders tend to be lower, and abstention rates are higher than in whites.
2. Although the odds of alcohol dependence are lower for blacks compared with whites, after it develops, it is more likely to be chronic.
3. In addition, frequent heavy drinking (drinking five or more drinks at one sitting at least weekly) has declined faster among whites.

4. Compared with whites, African Americans tend to suffer more medical consequences from drinking, including higher mortality and psychiatric comorbidity.
5. Acculturation to US society tends to result in increased use of alcohol among Hispanic women.
6. Prevalence of alcohol abuse and dependence is lower for Hispanics relative to whites, yet alcohol dependence may be more persistent after it develops.
7. Mortality from liver cirrhosis is higher for Hispanic populations.
8. Asian Americans generally have the lowest levels of alcohol consumption and lowest prevalence of alcohol use disorders. This may be due to genetically linked variations in aldehyde dehydrogenase resulting in uncomfortable flushing with alcohol consumption.
9. Native Americans historically have had the highest prevalence of alcohol use disorders in the United States, with high drinking-related death rates. However, it is not accurate to generalize to all Native American populations, as drinking practices are varied across tribal groups, and cultural factors as well as socioeconomic factors play a role.

When socioeconomic factors are taken into account, race is often not a risk factor for alcohol and other substance use.

Factors Relating to Race and Ethnicity and Drug Use Disorders

Patterns of drug use and drug disorders also vary by racial/ethnic group; however, less information is available for drug addiction than for alcoholism. A sample of some finding appears below.

1. Data from the NCS show that whites are more likely than African Americans or Hispanics to use drugs but are less likely to have persistent dependence once the disorder develops.
2. The occurrence of past year illicit drug abuse and dependence was highest among Native Americans (classified as American Indian or Alaskan Native in the NSDUH) and lowest for the Asian American subgroup.
3. Black, Asian, and Hispanic subgroups were less likely and Native Americans more likely than whites to report use and to have lifetime abuse or dependence to sedatives, tranquilizers, opioids, and amphetamines.

As with alcohol, race and ethnicity may not be an independent predictor—one study found that, although national survey data indicated a higher prevalence of crack cocaine smoking among some ethnic minorities, when area of neighborhood residence was taken into account, differences in the prevalence of drug use between racial groups were attenuated.

Addiction and Genetics

Addiction in a family member is a known predictor of risk. Twin studies and adoption studies have shown that this may not simply be due to exposure (nurture). Linkage studies have provided evidence for specific genes that may be involved in alcohol dependence. However, many individuals whose parents drink do not become alcoholic themselves, and many who develop alcohol disorders do not have a family history of alcoholism. Some similar genetic liabilities have been found regarding nicotine, caffeine, cannabis, cocaine, hallucinogens, stimulants, and opioids.

Other Characteristics

Numerous other traits have been found to be associated with addiction. For example, alcoholism is more common in unemployed persons. Even this association may be more complex as early drinking in youth may be causally related to poorer employment in adulthood. Also, working long hours may itself be associated with increased drinking in adolescents. Similarly, some studies show a higher prevalence of AUD in "blue collar" jobs, while others show an increase in "high status" occupations.

With few exceptions, it is often difficult to know which developed first; that is, whether lack of employment led to heavy drinking or drug use, or whether alcohol or drug problems resulted in job loss, inability to obtain work, or selection into a particular type of occupation. Marital status also has been found to be related to the occurrence of alcohol disorders and drinking behavior, but understanding the temporal relationships may be difficult. Alcohol and drug addiction may predate the time that individuals make decisions about marriage, and problems associated with drinking and drug use may be the reason some individuals remain single or become separated or divorced.

As with employment, studies into marital status and alcohol have yielded a variety of results:

1. Individuals who never married or are separated, divorced, or widowed are less likely than married or cohabiting couples to have prevalent or incident alcohol use disorders.
2. Persons in stable marriages or cohabiting had the lowest 12-month prevalence of alcohol use disorders (6.1%), as opposed to adults who had never married (15.9%).

3. The incidence of alcohol disorder symptoms is higher among single or divorced participants than in those who are married.
4. The risk of problem drinking is higher for women with spouses or partners who drink heavily.

Lifetime prevalence rates of illicit drug disorders also have been found to vary by marital status. Early data from the ECA surveys showed:

1. For both men and women and generally across all ages, individuals who lived with a partner but had never married had the highest lifetime prevalence of drug disorders.
2. Cohabiting unmarried men had a 30.2% lifetime prevalence of an illicit drug disorder, compared with a 3.6% prevalence for married men.
3. Cohabiting women had a lifetime prevalence of 19.9%, compared with 1.8% among women with a stable marital history.
4. From the NESARC data: Individuals who never married (classified separately from those that are cohabiting) are the group with the highest prevalence of drug use disorders.
5. The severity of alcohol and drug use affects marital functioning and is associated with risk of partner violence.

Educational level often is included as part of broader socioeconomic or social class characteristics, and studies of the relationship between educational level and the development of alcohol abuse and dependence may yield conflicting results.

COMORBIDITY OF ALCOHOL AND DRUG USE DISORDERS

Many clinical studies and assessments from household survey samples document the comorbid occurrence of substance use disorders with psychopathology. Data from the NCS show that the majority of people with an alcohol use disorder had at least one psychiatric disorder. Analyses of the NESARC found positive associations for mood, anxiety, and personality disorders with most substance use disorders. Close to half of all individuals with a current drug use disorder also have at least one personality disorder; antisocial personality disorder is strongly associated with drug dependence. Furthermore, the prevalence of alcohol and other substance use disorder comorbidity is typically high. Treatment outcomes tend to be worse for individuals with co-occurring psychiatric and substance use disorders.

With respect to studies of the stages of drug use, patterns of progression have been described that begin with the use of tobacco or alcohol with progression to marijuana and the use of other illicit drugs. For example, among most cocaine and crack users, marijuana use is an antecedent. There are also gender differences with regard to the significant role of the early use of alcohol for young men and cigarettes for young women. Further, there may be differences by gender with respect to the pathways that lead to substance use disorders, as well as in the type and severity of comorbid psychopathologies.

Summary Author: Christopher Sankey
Carson V. Dobrin • David C.S. Roberts

The Anatomy of Addiction

NEUROANATOMY OF DRUG REINFORCEMENT AND ADDICTION

To understand the neuroanatomy and psychopharmacology of addiction, we must understand the normal processes and structures involved in motivation, reward, decision making, and impulse control. From here, we can examine the compulsivity, excessive consumption, and the resultant harm, which are central to addiction.

PRIMER ON NEUROANATOMY

The structures most often mentioned in the context of drug abuse are closely associated with the limbic system, lateral hypothalamus, basal ganglia, and frontal cortical regions.

The limbic system has been characterized as highly interconnected, phylogenetically older regions of the forebrain that appear to form the only major route for information transfer between the neocortex and the hypothalamus. The main structures denoted by "the limbic system" are the limbic lobe (subcallosal area, cingulate, and parahippocampal gyri), amygdala, hippocampus, parts of the basal ganglia, anterior thalamic nucleus, parts of the hypothalamus, the habenula, and olfactory cortex (Fig. 3.1). The structures associated with the limbic system (such as the hypothalamus, hippocampus, and amygdala) are essential not only for learning and memory but also for the emotional context and the affective response to learned associations.

As will be detailed, many drugs of abuse have their sites of action within the limbic system and the neurochemistry within these structures is altered during the addiction process. This may help explain why decisions surrounding drug seeking and drug taking seem to be driven more by emotion and instinct rather than by logic.

The basal ganglia are traditionally thought of as a motor system; however, the idea that this system deals only with motor function while the limbic system deals with reinforcement and emotion is oversimplified. As more is learned about how the basal ganglia and limbic system communicate, it is becoming increasingly clear that the two systems are jointly involved in coordinating motivated behavior. The largest mass associated with the basal ganglia is the striatum (caudate-putamen). The dorsal portion has long been considered part of the basal ganglia, while the ventral striatum (also called the accumbens) is considered to be part of the limbic system. Mogenson famously described the accumbens as "the place where motivation is translated into action."

The prefrontal cortex (PFC) is thought to be the "hub" of executive function in the brain. The PFC in humans is subdivided into three main regions: (a) the orbitofrontal (OFC) and the ventromedial areas (vm-PFC), which are thought to be involved in processing reward; (b) the dorsolateral prefrontal cortex (dl-PFC), more broadly involved in decision making; and (c) the anterior and ventral cingulate cortex, which help to control whether or not a particular behavior will be performed, and to what intensity.

PSYCHOSTIMULANTS

Cocaine binds to dopamine, noradrenaline, and serotonin (DA, NA, and 5-HT) transporters and blocks the reuptake of these neurotransmitters. Amphetamine acts additionally as a releasing agent. Both of these actions result in an increased concentration of monoamine neurotransmitters in the synapse.

Figure 3.2 demonstrates how the origins and projections of the main neuronal mass are associated with NA, 5-HT, and DA. All start in the brainstem and project upward. The catecholaminergic NA fibers start in the

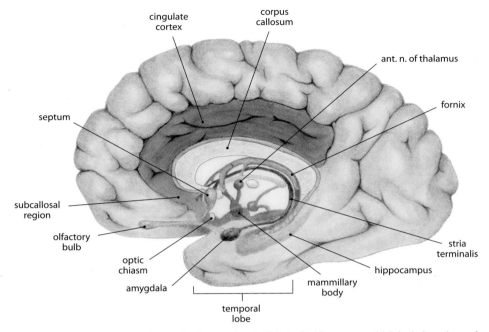

cingulate cortex

corpus callosum

ant. n. of thalamus

fornix

septum

subcallosal region

olfactory bulb

optic chiasm

amygdala

stria terminalis

hippocampus

mammillary body

temporal lobe

FIGURE 3.1 Regions of the human brain associated with the limbic system, which includes a loop of cortex extending from the subcallosal region through cingulate cortex to the parahippocampal gyrus. Also shown are the hippocampal formation, septum, amygdala, and mammillary bodies.

locus coeruleus and spread diffusely. The DA system is more contained—originating in the ventral tegmental area (VTA) and the substantia nigra.

The extensive reach and overlap of the DA, NA, and 5-TH systems throughout the brain makes research complex. While for many years it was thought that drug use and addiction was confined to humans, and thus attributed to the neocortex, subsequent research on animals demonstrated that self-administration of drugs will occur in other mammalian species such as rat, dog, cat, rabbit, and nonhuman primates. This supports neuroanatomical findings that addiction arises in subcortical, evolutionary residual regions of the brain—that is, limbic and brainstem areas.

This anatomical understanding may help us to understand the complex nature of reinforcement—while patients may describe the alterations in consciousness associated with a specific substance as the "reason" for ongoing use, the mechanics behind use, abuse, and addiction are more complex and involve subcortical, unconscious factors.

Dopamine plays a central role in reward and drug addiction. Studies by Roy Wise demonstrated that treatment with DA antagonists produced an increase in cocaine or amphetamine intake in animals previously trained to self-administer these drugs. The use of the dopaminergic neurotoxin 6-OH-DA has been a useful tool in highlighting the role of DA. Removing the DA input to the NAcc (nucleus accumbens—now called the ventral striatum)—or destroying the DA cell bodies in the VTA (ventral tegmental area) resulted in diminution or abolition of cocaine self-administration in animals. Denervation of NA systems to the entire forebrain had no effect. The data demonstrate that the DA projects from the VTA to limbic areas are critical for the reinforcing effects of cocaine and amphetamines.

Both ablation and stimulation studies confirm that the striatum is responsible for motor behavior: the ventral area for locomotion and the dorsal for stereotypy. The appearance of Parkinsonian side effects of neuroleptics confirms the involvement of DA in motor pathways involved in stereotypic repetitive motor behaviors. Any behavior can become reinforced, and the more frequently an action occurs, in the setting of drug use, the more likely it will become stereotyped. As such behaviors increase, others are excluded—thus limiting the behavioral range of the animal. In the case of a person with addiction, the frequent behaviors associated with drug seeking and drug taking become repetitive and ritualistic.

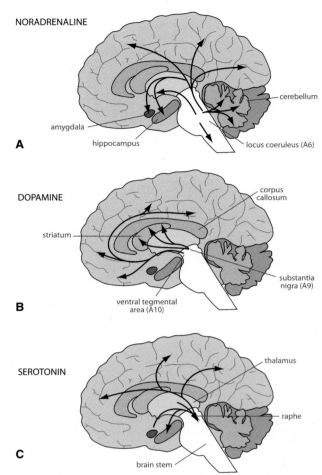

FIGURE 3.2 Schematic diagram illustrating the distribution of the main central neuronal pathways containing noradrenaline (**A**), dopamine (**B**), and serotonin (**C**). The location of cell bodies of origin is indicated by *circles* with the projections indicated by *arrows*.

The great body of research showing VTA-DA neurons' role in drug use and with primary reinforcing stimuli such as food, drinking, and sex has led to the term "Mesolimbic Reward Pathway." Interestingly, there is no direct connection between this region and visual, auditory, or somatosensory systems. It appears instead that the VTA is a part of, and receives inputs from, a widespread collection of neurons that belong to the "isodendritic core." This system is a network of neurons stretching from brainstem to telencephalon. It would appear that this network serves an integrative function and responses to changes in the environment that are biologically significant. At present, it remains unclear whether the VTA-DA neurons respond differentially than others in the network and whether they are specifically activated by reward or more generally by any other important stimulus.

Opioids

Opioid receptors are expressed throughout the brain, especially in limbic and limbic-related structures. There are three different types of G protein–coupled opioid receptors; μ, κ, and δ, which are acted on by both endogenous and exogenously applied opioids. Selective μ agonist drugs, such as morphine, heroin, and most clinically used opioid analgesics, produce analgesia, euphoria, respiratory depression, emesis, and antidiuretic effects. Selective κ agonist drugs, such as the experimental compounds ethylketazocine and bremazocine, produce analgesia, dysphoria, and diuretic effects, but no respiratory depression. There is less known about the direct role of δ receptors. Agonists at μ receptor are more likely to have abuse liability than κ agonists.

Almost all that is known about the neurobiology of opioid reinforcement is derived from animal models. Three approaches have been used to investigate the involvement of various brain regions in opioid reward:

(a) intracerebral self-administration of opioid agonists, (b) blockade of IV heroin self-administration by intracerebral injections of opioid antagonists, and (c) disruption of IV heroin self-administration by lesions. Generally, the focus has been on areas associated with the mesolimbic DA system (ventral striatum and VTA). Self-administration of drugs directly into various brain regions would seem to be the most straightforward test of their involvement in reinforcement processes; however, the procedures have a number of technical problems that limit their appeal. The main areas supporting opioid self-administration are the ventral striatum, NAcc and VTA—with the latter being the most responsive. Interestingly, while injection of μ and δ opioid agonists into the VTA is strongly reinforcing, injection of antagonist into the VTA has little effect. This is especially surprising given that intracranial injections of antagonists into other areas of the brain can produce strong and predictable reactions.

When systemic naloxone is given, a compensatory increase in opioid self-administration is noticed. Similarly, increase in IV heroin self-administration is noticed when low-dose opioid antagonists are injected into the NAcc, periaqueductal gray, stria terminalis, and lateral hypothalamus, but not the PFC.

Lesion studies offer further support of the key role played by the NAcc in opioid reinforcement—kainic acid injected into the NAcc correlated with impaired heroin self-administration, yet did not have this effect when injected into other areas. Further studies suggest that the NAcc core is far more responsive than the shell, viz. opioid self-administration. Similar site-specific effects have been found when β-FNA (an irreversible opioid antagonist) is injected into the caudal, but not rostral NAcc.

The role of the mesolimbic DA system in opioid reinforcement is unclear. DA antagonists reduced self-administration of cocaine but not heroin, and opioid antagonists reduce heroin but not cocaine use. However, it has been shown that opioids indirectly affect DA cell firing through inhibition of GABA interneurons in the VTA. This disinhibition can result in enhanced DA release in the NAcc. Heroin self-administration increases DA in the accumbens, and this has been argued to be the mechanisms of action for heroin reinforcement. It appears that DA innervation to the VTA is very important to opioid reinforcement, while altering such innervation to the NAcc has little effect. In contrast, reducing DA innervation to the NAcc results in dramatic reduction in cocaine reinforcement.

Cannabinoids

Two cannabinoid receptors (CB1 and CB2) have been identified. Both are G protein–coupled receptors and function to inhibit adenylate cyclase. They are acted on by endogenous cannabinoids and exogenous activators such as marijuana (Fig. 3.3).

There remains limited understanding about the reinforcing neuroanatomy of cannabinoids—this being due to difficulties in study designs with inhaled marijuana. The use of IV Δ9-tetrahydrocannabinol for self-administration studies on animals and the use of synthetic cannabinoid agonists have shown some reinforcing effects. It appears that both opioid and DA mechanisms may interact with cannabinoid reinforcement.

Neuroanatomy of Drug Addiction

The research questions that can be addressed by using animal models are necessarily different than those that can be asked with human subjects. The former allow for invasive interventions, surgical manipulations not possible with humans, while the latter provides insight into the uniquely human aspects of addiction. Addiction is a disease that lives in the real world and thus encompasses many different facets, such as poly drug use, comorbidity with other disorders, predisposition, drug use history, and environmental context. Thus, the literature on human drug abuse offers quite different insights.

The neuroanatomy of addiction in human subjects has been studied using positron emission tomography (PET) and functional magnetic resonance imaging (fMRI). PET uses a radioisotope that is introduced into the body and binds to specific receptors, transporters, and enzymes. Specific ligands can be visualized, thereby offering insights into drug distribution and changes in receptor mechanism in vivo. fMRI offers much greater temporal resolution. Changes in the fMRI signal can be assessed on the order of seconds rather than minutes, making it possible to detect metabolic changes associated with transient cognitive demands or craving states.

Volkow et al. used PET to demonstrate decreased relative cerebral blood flow in the PFC of chronic cocaine users, and metabolic changes varying with time from last use (increased in the 1st week of withdrawal). PET has also been used to show high cocaine binding in the corpus striatum in non–drug-using human subjects, and to show that striatal dopamine D2 receptor binding is reduced in cocaine, heroin, and methamphetamine abusers and also in alcohol dependence. This area of work is in good concordance with nonhuman primate PET studies showing decreased D2 receptor availability in animals that are more susceptible to the reinforcing aspects of cocaine.

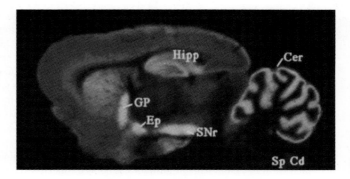

FIGURE 3.3   Cannabinoid receptor expression in the rat brain.

fMRI studies have demonstrated increased activity in the NAcc and decrease in amygdala in cocaine users during cravings, and increase in activity in the ventral tegmentum (VTA and substantia nigra), pons, basal forebrain, caudate, and cingulate that correlated with self-reported feelings of "rush" following cocaine use. Drug users also show increases in brain activity in limbic areas and the PFC following the presentation of drug-associated cues (such as pictures of drugs and drug paraphernalia) when compared with nondrug users, and decreased responsiveness when presented with nondrug reinforcers (e.g., sexually evocative cues).

Remarkably, drug-associated cues can produce limbic activation in cocaine users even when these stimuli are not consciously perceived. Childress et al. presented stimuli for only 33 ms. Although this short presentation was too brief for the image to be correctly identified, the drug-related stimuli nonetheless produced a strong increase in activity in the ventral pallidum and amygdala. The intensity of this response strongly predicted the magnitude of the subject's affective response when later shown visible versions of the same cues. These data suggest that drug cues can stimulate drug craving even before there is conscious awareness. Childress et al. speculate that "by the time the motivational state is experienced and labeled as conscious desire, the ancient limbic reward circuitry already has a running start." Medical imaging technology has thus provided concrete evidence of limbic involvement in drug craving that fits well with the wealth of evidence for animal studies.

Summary Author: Christopher Sankey
Eric J. Nestler

From Neurobiology to Treatment: Progress Against Addiction

The compulsive, obsessive, ongoing participation in a physically, psychologically, and socially harmful activity that defines addiction is one of our most serious national health issues. Current medical interventions remain inadequate, however through increased understanding and ongoing research into the neurobiology of addiction significant improvements in treatments are emerging.

Considerable progress has been made in understanding how chronic exposure to drugs leads to chemical and structural changes in the brain. The initial protein targets for almost all drugs of abuse are known (Table 4.1). Also, several circuits in the brain, containing these drug targets, are known to be instrumental in the process of addiction. The VTA and its dopaminergic input into the NAcc (also called ventral striatum) are known to be essential to reward and addiction, as are, to a lesser extent, the amygdala, prefrontal and other limbic cortical regions, hippocampus, and hypothalamus. These components of the "reward pathway," which have evolutionary importance in reinforcing natural rewards (food, sex, social interaction, etc.), are subverted by chronic exposure to specific chemicals.

Prolonged drug exposure leads to reduction in the reinforcing effects of natural rewards, reduced motivation, and depression. Given the reduced effects of natural rewards, and the simplicity and repetition of drug ingestion, the latter behavior dominates. In addition, addiction results in deeply ingrained memories capable of creating intense urges in patients exposed to triggers even after years of nonuse. Such triggers can be emotional stress, or any sensory cue associated with drug acquisition or use.

While managing physical dependence can be an important aspect of treating many addictions, they are distinct entities. Dependence is defined by tolerance and withdrawal, while addiction by a loss of control and ongoing participation in intrusive and harmful behaviors. Physical dependence per se is neither necessary nor sufficient to cause addiction: some drugs of abuse do not cause appreciable physical dependence, and some medications used in general medicine cause physical dependence but are not addictive (e.g., β-adrenergic antagonists such as propranolol). Moreover, physical dependence and withdrawal syndromes are largely mediated to a great extent by different central nervous system regions than those important for addiction.

Increased understanding of the cellular effects of drugs of abuse and medications has resulted in improved management of withdrawal. Clonidine (an α_2-adrenergic agonist) produces cellular effects similar to opioid receptor activation and is used to reduce withdrawal symptoms. The ability of benzodiazepines to activate γ-aminobutyric acid (GABA) receptor function similar to alcohol has led to their routine use to prevent the life-threatening sequelae of alcohol withdrawal. Unfortunately, treatment of the core symptoms of addiction has proved much more difficult than treatment of physical withdrawal syndromes.

BLOCKADE OF DRUG TARGETS

Naltrexone is an opiate receptor blocker that can be used in some highly motivated patients to maintain opioid abstinence. It can also be useful in assisting with nicotine and alcohol abstinence as both of these compounds impose their reinforcing effects via activation of endogenous opioidergic neurons. Although some efficacy has been observed clinically, the effects of naltrexone are relatively small in magnitude. Naltrexone will, however, precipitate extreme

TABLE 4.1	Acute Actions of Some Drugs of Abuse	
Drug	**Action**	**Receptor signaling mechanism**
Opiates	Agonist at μ, δ, and κ opioid receptors[a]	Gi
Cocaine	Indirect agonist at dopamine receptors by inhibiting dopamine transporters[b]	Gi and Gs[c]
Amphetamine	Indirect agonist at dopamine receptors by stimulating dopamine release[b]	Gi and Gs[c]
Ethanol	Facilitates $GABA_A$ receptor function and inhibits NMDA glutamate receptor function[d]	Ligand-gated channels
Nicotine	Agonist at nicotinic acetylcholine receptors	Ligand-gated channels
Cannabinoids	Agonist at CB_1 and CB_2 cannabinoid receptors[e]	Gi
Phencyclidine	Antagonist at NMDA glutamate receptor channels	Ligand-gated
Hallucinogens	Partial agonist at $5HT_{2A}$ serotonin receptors	Gq
Inhalants	Unknown	

Data from Nestler EJ. Molecular basis of neural plasticity underlying addiction. *Nat Rev Neurosci.* 2001;2:119–128.
[a]Activity at μ (and possibly) δ receptors mediates the reinforcing actions of opiates; κ receptors mediate aversive actions.
[b]Cocaine and amphetamine exert analogous actions on serotonergic and noradrenergic systems, which may also contribute to the reinforcing effects of these drugs.
[c]Gi couples D_2-like dopamine receptors, and Gs couples D_1-like dopamine receptors, both of which are important for dopamine's reinforcing effects.
[d]Ethanol affects several other ligand-gated channels, and at higher concentrations voltage-gated channels, as well. In addition, ethanol is reported to influence many other neurotransmitter systems, including serotonergic, opioidergic, and dopaminergic systems. It is not known whether these effects are direct or achieved indirectly via actions on various ligand-gated channels.
[e]Activity at CB_1 receptors mediates the reinforcing actions of cannabinoids; CB_2 receptors are expressed predominantly in the periphery. Endogenous ligands for the CB_1 receptor include the arachidonic acid metabolites, anandamide, and 2-arachidonylglycerol.

withdrawal if given to an actively opioid-dependent person. Also, its blockade of the body's endogenous opioid peptides (enkephalin, dynorphin, endorphin) can cause negative emotional effects (such as depressed mood).

Cocaine works by inhibiting presynaptic dopamine transporters. Efforts at developing a compound to block this effect without altering their normal function have not produced viable medications as yet. An alternative to such a "cocaine antagonist" is the "cocaine vaccine," which would block cocaine's entry into the brain through immunologic approaches. This has shown some success in animals—resulting in increased cocaine clearance and attenuation of behavioral effects. Even if effective, immunological approaches would have limitations; patients may just switch to an alternate stimulant not blocked by the cocaine-specific vaccine.

Cannabinoids, the active ingredients in marijuana, act through the stimulation of CB1 receptors. Opioids and alcohol also activate endogenous cannabinoids in the brain (Table 4.1). It has been speculated that Rimonabant—a CB1 antagonist, approved in Europe for the treatment of obesity—might be effective in treating drug addiction. The presence of depressive side effects and insufficient evidence call for more research.

Mimicry of Drug Action

While blockade may prevent a compound from stimulating the receptor (Naltrexone blocking the opioid receptors), the resultant extreme withdrawal limits the utility of this as an acute treatment maneuver. Mimicry of effect—such as the use of methadone in patients with chronic refractory opioid addiction—is one way to decrease street drug use, encourage patients into treatment, and work to address the larger bio/psycho/social issues. Methadone and Buprenorphine are effective, not just because they stimulate the same receptors as street opioids, but they have a long duration of action—thus avoiding the rapid on/off effect of other opioids.

Although the effectiveness of drug mimicry has been documented clinically, it is poorly understood at the neurobiologic level. Decades of experience have documented the safety and efficacy of methadone. A variation in this theme is buprenorphine—a high-affinity partial agonist that binds to opioid receptors to produce a mild agonist effect. Its low intrinsic activity results in a ceiling effect—where higher doses do not result in significantly stronger results, while its high receptor affinity means that it prevents other opioids from accessing the receptors. This can discourage street opioid use. While far from perfect, opioid substitution, combined with addiction counseling, is the treatment of choice for chronic refractory opioid addiction.

Nicotine replacement delivery systems are another example of mimicry to achieve a therapeutic outcome. While the sustained release of low levels of nicotine dampens cravings, most patients are unable to achieve cessation. Research is underway on varenicline, which selectively stimulates cerebral nicotinic receptors in an attempt to increase success rates.

Stimulation of dopaminergic transmission in the nucleus accumbens and elsewhere seems to be the most important mechanism of stimulant action and contributes to the actions of other drugs of abuse as well. Activation of opioid, cholinergic, or cannabinoid receptors increases dopaminergic transmission in these brain regions. Based on this knowledge, there has been intense effort to use dopamine receptor antagonists and agonists in the treatment of addiction. The goal is to develop agents that regulate the general process of addiction, which might be equally effective for all drugs of abuse. The use of dopamine antagonists is based on the notion that inhibition of drug effects would limit drug use, whereas the use of dopamine agonists is based on the notion that mimicry of drug effects would be more efficacious. The former approach has not been promising. Although dopamine receptor antagonists can block acute drug effects, there is no evidence that they limit drug craving or self-administration in the long term. They may even make animals and humans more sensitive to drugs of abuse via adaptive increases in dopamine receptor signaling efficacy. In contrast, there is some promise for the use of D1 receptor agonists and D2 receptor partial agonists, which dampen cocaine craving and relapse in animal models. Studies in humans are a high priority but are limited by the lack of availability of suitable compounds for human use.

Glutamate is essential for learning and memory functions, as well as for functions of the NAcc and VTA. Research into a possible therapeutic role for glutamatergic agents is being studied. For example, a drug that enhances glutamatergic transmission, and therefore, new memory formation, given in concert with behavioral extinction trials, might be a novel approach to treating addiction-related memories that are thought to underlie aspects of craving and relapse.

A great deal has been learned over the past decade about the changes that drugs of abuse cause in the brain's reward pathways to produce addiction. While progress is being made, we are still at a very early stage in developing therapeutic compounds to effectively treat addiction.

CHAPTER 5

Summary Author: Christopher A. Cavacuiti
Sarah W. Yip • Marc N. Potenza

Understanding "Behavioral Addictions": Insights from Research

The term *addiction* is derived from the Latin word *addicere*, meaning "bound to" or "enslaved by." In its original formulation, the word was not linked to substance use behaviors. Several hundred years ago, the term began to be applied to alcohol and then other substances and by the late 20th century was used almost exclusively to describe excessive substance use. Interestingly, the past decade has seen a growing movement to revert back to the earlier definition of "addiction" that would include nondrug behaviors such as gambling, sex, and eating.

Addiction is often described as having four components (the "four Cs"): (a) continued engagement in a behavior despite adverse Consequences, (b) loss of self-Control over engagement in the behavior, (c) Compulsive engagement in the behavior, and (d) an appetitive urge or Craving state before the engagement in the behavior. Behavioral addictions include all of these core features.

IMPULSE CONTROL DISORDERS: "BEHAVIORAL ADDICTIONS"?

Many disorders that might be considered behavioral addictions are currently categorized in the *DSM* as "Impulse Control Disorders (ICDs) not Elsewhere Classified." The ongoing debate among research workgroups is whether the "behavioral addictions" might be best categorized as ICDs, or with substance use disorders (SUDs) as addictions, or as obsessive-compulsive disorders (OCDs).

PATHOLOGIC GAMBLING

The ICDs within the "not elsewhere categorized" section include intermittent explosive disorder (IED), kleptomania, pathologic gambling (PG), pyromania, trichotillomania, and ICD not otherwise specified. A particular emphasis will be placed on PG because it is arguably the best studied of the ICDs to date. However, for a more detailed description of the clinical features of PG and its treatment, we direct you to Chapter 38, "Pathologic Gambling: Clinical Characteristics and Treatment."

PG and SUDs share clinical characteristics and diagnostic criteria. Individuals with PG often experience withdrawal, craving, tolerance, and failed attempts to reduce or abate gambling behaviors—all common features of SUDs.

A Nonsubstance Addiction?

SUDs and PG share a number of phenomenologic features:

- Both typically begin in adolescence.
- Incidence and prevalence decrease with age.
- The time between initiation and problematic engagement in the addictive behavior is shorter in females than in males.

These commonalities suggest that there may be shared genetic and environmental vulnerabilities for both disorders. This is further supported by the high (39%) rate of comorbid SUDs in clinical samples of individuals with PG.

Neurocognition

Neurocognitive research provides evidence of dysregulation of the ventromedial prefrontal cortex (vmPFC) and orbitofrontal cortex (OFC) in individuals with PG. These areas are also known to be dysregulated in SUDs. Individuals with PG display impaired performance on tasks involving risk/reward decision making (such as the Iowa Gambling Task); other populations with impaired performance on such testing include individuals with SUDs, schizophrenia, or vmPFC lesions.

Delay Discounting

Individuals with PG often make disadvantageous decisions, selecting small immediate rewards over larger delayed rewards. This has been termed *delay discounting*, because rewards are more steeply discounted as the reward is delayed. Like their PG counterparts, individuals with substance abuse discount rewards more rapidly than do healthy controls.

Delay discounting involves aspects of reward evaluation, and multiple brain regions contribute to reward processing in humans. Among the most widely implicated brain regions in reward processing is the nucleus accumbens (NAcc), situated in the ventral striatum. The NAcc is also strongly implicated in neurocognitive research of SUDs.

The Neurobiology of PG

Neurocircuitry Research suggests that there is a dysregulation of the mesocorticolimbic dopamine (DA) system in PG. The mesocorticolimbic DA system, often referred to as the *reward pathway*, has long been implicated in reward processing in SUDs.

Neurochemistry

Serotonin (5-HT) Serotonin neurons project from the raphe nucleus of the brain stem to multiple brain regions including the hippocampus, amygdala, and prefrontal cortex (PFC). It has been hypothesized that dysregulated 5-HT functioning may mediate behavioral inhibition and impulsivity in PG. Other pharmacologic studies support the hypothesis that there is a dysregulation of the 5-HT system in PG. Serotonin reuptake inhibitors (SRIs) have been found to improve social functioning and reduce gambling behaviors and thoughts about gambling.

Dopamine Psychopharmacologic data suggest that the DA system may influence impulsive behavior, which is characteristic of both SUDs and behavioral addictions, although the precise manner is not completely understood. DA agonists (such as those used in the treatment of Parkinson disease) have been associated with PG and other ICDs in Parkinson disease.

Norepinephrine and Arousal in PG Dysregulation of norepinephrine (NE)—a neurotransmitter implicated in arousal, attention, and sensation-seeking behavior—has been reported in individuals with PG. Individuals with PG have elevated urinary concentrations of NE, as well as elevated Cerebrospinal Fluid (CSF) levels of a metabolite of NE.

Opioids Research implicates the opioid system in PG. Naltrexone and nalmefene (which are opioid receptor antagonists) have been found to reduce gambling-related thoughts and behaviors in individuals with PG.

Population Genetics Family and twin-based studies of addiction indicate that genetic factors are important in both SUDs and behavioral addictions. Twin study data suggest that one third to two thirds of the variance for meeting criteria for PG is attributable to inherited factors. This is very similar to the degree of heritability seen with SUDs. Other research supports the notion that there are shared genetic and environmental contributions for both PG and SUDs.

Conclusion

Although the precise neurobiology of PG is incompletely understood, data from neurocognitive, neurochemical, neuroimaging, and genetic research suggest similarities with other disorders involving impaired impulse control, such as SUDs. There are important treatment implications inherent in these similarities. For example, the biologic similarities between SUDs and PG could help to guide treatment development.

BINGE EATING

Introduction

Changes in eating patterns are frequently observed in substance use and abuse, for example

- Weight loss associated with amphetamine and heroin use
- Weight gain with smoking cessation
- Increased food intake with marijuana

A growing body of data suggests that SUDs and eating behaviors may be modulated by the same motivational neurocircuitry.

Eating disorders include anorexia nervosa, bulimia nervosa, and binge-eating disorder (BED). BED is distinct from bulimia nervosa as it does not include compensatory behaviors such as purging. Given that BED has an important element of episodic behavioral dyscontrol similar to many SUDs, this section will focus primarily on the neurobiology of this disorder. BED is characterized by unsuccessful attempts to stop binge eating, and negative physical and social consequences related to binge eating. These are also two important criteria for SUDs.

The Biology of Eating Behaviors

Existing data suggest a number of shared neurobiological mechanisms in eating and substance use behaviors.

Leptin and DA-Regulated Reward Processing
Leptin, an adipose-derived hormone, is a chemical modulator involved in the maintenance of energy homeostasis and feeding behaviors. In addition to its metabolic function, leptin may help to modulate mesolimbic reward circuits that may relate to both palatability and substance use. Research suggests that leptin acts directly on brain regions associated with reward, including the substantia nigra pars compacta and ventral tegmental area (VTA) of the midbrain. Functional MRI studies demonstrate that the consumption of palatable food leads to increases in the activation of the same mesolimbic reward pathways that are implicated in substance use and dependence.

Orexins
Partially modulated by adipose-derived hormones such as leptin and ghrelin, the hypothalamic neuropeptides orexin A and orexin B—also referred to as hypocretin 1 and hypocretin 2—are important modulators of eating behavior and help to maintain energy homeostasis. Data suggest that orexins increase DA levels within the mesolimbic pathways and that it is associated with increases in brain stimulation of reward, suggesting a negative regulation of reward circuits. This is further supported by studies showing that the administration of orexins reinstates both opioid- and cocaine-seeking behaviors.

Ghrelin
Ghrelin is a gastrointestinal hormone that helps to maintain energy homeostasis. Unlike leptin and orexin, which are anorexigenic, ghrelin is orexigenic and increases food intake and body weight. Preclinical research has identified a ghrelin receptor in the reward areas of the brain and ghrelin has been linked to increased synapse formation and DA turnover in the NAcc. Further investigation is needed to determine the extent to which ghrelin is involved in other reward-seeking behaviors.

The NAcc: Opioid and Endocannabinoid Encoding of Palatability
Research suggests that increased endogenous and exogenous opioid levels within the NAcc region of the brain enhance food palatability. In contrast, administration of an opioid antagonist reduces food preference. This effect appears to be independent of the caloric or nutritional value of the food administered, suggesting that opioids may play a role in general food habit formation or basic motor control of feeding behaviors, rather than in basic appetite control.

Human and animal studies also implicate the endocannabinoid system of the NAcc in eating behaviors. Cannabinoids have long been associated with rewarding psychotropic effects and are additionally associated with increases in food intake.

Prefrontal Cortex
Research from neuroimaging, neurocognitive, and lesion studies implicates the PFC in the modulation of eating behaviors. The PFC is generally considered the "decision-making" section of the brain, and PFC lesions are characterized by a variety of behavioral changes including eating, substance use, and sexual behaviors.

Positron emission tomography (PET) study data suggest that successful dieters have different patterns of PFC activation compared with unsuccessful dieters. Further investigation is required to fully understand interactions between PFC regions in relation to eating behaviors.

As with PG and SUD, individuals with eating disorders often display impairments in reward-related decision making such as *delay discounting* and a disregard for future negative consequences in favor of immediate short-term gains.

Serotonin (5-HT) Increases in both exogenous and endogenous serotonin (5-HT) are associated with a reduction of food intake and weight gain and an increase in energy expenditure. D-fenfluramine/phentermine (also known as Fen-Phen) may exert its anorexigenic effects via 5HT2C receptor activation. 5-HT is also thought to be implicated in food preference. Drugs that increase 5-HT availability (such as SSRIs) selectively inhibit carbohydrate intake, but have no significant effect on fat or protein intake. Some of these drugs have also been shown to improve various aspects of disordered eating. Sibutramine, a drug that blocks serotonin reuptake, is approved by the U.S. Food and Drug Administration for the treatment of obesity.

Conclusion

Binge eating and comorbid obesity are increasingly common phenomena with wide-ranging public health implications. There is mounting evidence to suggest that binge eating is a brain-based disorder that may share many of the same neurobiological features of SUD.

COMPULSIVE SEXUAL BEHAVIOR

Clinically relevant "addictive" sexual behaviors may be divided into paraphilic and nonparaphilic behaviors. In paraphilic sexual behaviors, there is a disturbance in the object selection (e.g., an animal, unwilling person, inanimate object). In nonparaphilic compulsive sexual behavior, there is disordered impulse control characterized by excessive, obsessive, or compulsive engagement in socially normative sexual behaviors.

Paraphilic disorders are a distinct category of disorders, already included in the current *DSM-IV-TR*, and are outside the scope of this chapter. The focus here is on nonparaphilic compulsive sexual behavior, hereafter referred to as "CSBs." Nonparaphilic impulsive or compulsive sexual disorders are not specifically listed in the *DSMIV-TR*.

Epidemiology

There has been no systematic epidemiological study of compulsive sexual behavior, although estimates of 5% to 6% in the adult population have been reported. Individuals with CSB have high levels of psychiatric comorbidity, including mood and anxiety disorders, SUDs, ICDs, and Attention-Deficit Hyperactivity Disorder (ADHD).

Defining the Disorder

Coleman has identified seven distinct CSB categories, all with their own unique constellation of symptoms: (a) compulsive cruising and multiple partners, (b) compulsive multiple love relationships, (c) compulsive sexuality in a relationship, (d) compulsive use of erotica, (e) compulsive autoeroticism, (f) compulsive use of the Internet, and (g) compulsive fixation on an unattainable partner.

Kinsey et al. created the frequency measure of "total sexual outlet," defined as the number of orgasms per week. Kafka later redefined total sexual outlet as: # of orgasms/# of weeks. According to Kafka's criteria, a total sexual outlet score >7 is associated with both paraphilic and nonparaphilic (i.e., CSB) disorders.

Other instruments, such as the Minnesota Impulsive Disorders Inventory and Voon's diagnostic model, more closely resemble the diagnostic criteria for other ICDs.

Neurobiology of CSB

DA, serotonin, NE, and the opioid system all contribute to human sexual behavior. However, no systematic studies of neurotransmitter systems involvement in CSB have been published to date. Lithium, tricyclic antidepressants, selective serotonin reuptake inhibitors (SSRIs), nefazodone, naltrexone, and atypical antipsychotics have all been used to treat CSB. However, their efficacy in treating CSB has not been systematically examined.

PROBLEMATIC INTERNET USE

Diagnostic Criteria

There are no uniformly agreed on diagnostic criteria for problematic Internet use. Based on the *DSM-IV* definitions of SUDs, Young proposed the following criteria for "Internet addiction": withdrawal, tolerance, preoccupation with the Internet, longer than intended spent on the Internet, risk to significant other relationships or employment, lying about Internet use, and repeated, unsuccessful attempts to stop Internet use.

Co-Occurring Disorders

Greater amounts of Internet use have been associated with vocational impairment, financial impairment, legal problems, decreased social involvement, loneliness, and depression.

COMPULSIVE BUYING DISORDER

Classically referred to as "oniomania," compulsive shopping behavior has been clinically recognized for almost a century. Research on CBD is very limited. There are case reports suggesting that naltrexone may have efficacy in CBD populations.

KLEPTOMANIA

Epidemiology

Individuals with kleptomania suffer from a diminished ability to inhibit impulses to steal unnecessary or unwanted items, resulting in negative personal and professional consequences and experiences of regret and distress. Kleptomania has been reported to have a prevalence approaching 1%. Kleptomania generally begins in adolescence or early adulthood and appears more commonly in women than men.

Neurobiology

Neurocognitive and neuroimaging research suggest frontal lobe involvement in kleptomania. Performance deficits in neuropsychologic tasks associated with prefrontal regions have been found to correlate with kleptomania symptom severity. A number of case reports have described individuals developing kleptomania after frontal lobe damage.

Neurochemistry

There have been several small trials and case reports reporting successful pharmacologic treatment of kleptomania. Agents used in these studies include SSRIs, opioid antagonists, and antiepileptics.

TRICHOTILLOMANIA

Hair twirling, lip and nail biting, skin picking, and other mildly uncomfortable or painful behaviors are common among the general population and are generally benign. Trichotillomania involves the pulling out of hair, most frequently from the scalp, although axillary, pubic, and perirectal regions may also be targeted. Trichophagia (eating hair) may co-occur with trichotillomania.

Phenomenologic aspects of trichotillomania seem similar to those of SUDs. Hair pulling is generally preceded by a sense of tension or experience of craving, and individuals report feeling unable to inhibit behaviors and experiencing of pleasure/relief during hair pulling.

OCD and Trichotillomania

Elevated levels of OCD have been reported in subjects with trichotillomania and their first-degree relatives. Interestingly, individuals with both OCD and trichotillomania generally report their hair pulling as a negative "ego-dytonic" experience, while those with trichotillomania and no OCD more often report hair pulling as an enjoyable "ego-sytonic" experience. Naltrexone and SRIs may have efficacy in the treatment of trichotillomania.

PATHOLOGIC SKIN PICKING (PSP)

Introduction

Skin picking is currently listed in the *DSM-IV* under stereotypic movement disorder with self-injurious behavior. Stereotypic movement disorder is defined as repetitive, seemingly goal-directed but nonfunctional motor behavior, resulting in self-inflicted injury or disruption to daily activities. Stereotypic movement disorder is most prevalent in individuals with mental retardation, and approximately 25% of adults institutionalized for mental retardation meet criteria. We will use the term pathologic skin picking (PSP) to describe a pathologic attention to, and duration of, skin-picking behavior that is impulsive, ritualistic and repetitive. A recent study of ICD prevalence among adolescent psychiatric inpatients found that 12% met the criteria for skin picking.

Epidemiology

As with trichotillomania, PSP most commonly occurs in females. There have been no widespread epidemiological studies of PSP, but data suggest that 3.8% of college students meet the criteria for PSP and that 2% of dermatology patients meet the criteria for skin picking.

Psychopharmacology

Some, but not all, individuals with PSP may be successfully treated with SSRIs, anticonvulsants, antipsychotics, or opioid antagonists.

INTERMITTENT EXPLOSIVE DISORDER

Introduction

IED is characterized by a failure to inhibit aggressive impulses that are out of proportion to any precipitating stressor resulting in destruction of property or serious physical assault. A diagnosis of IED is only given if the aggressive behavior cannot be explained by another mental disorder, such as a personality disorder or manic episode, or by substance use. Based on data from the National Comorbidity Survey Replication, it has been estimated that as many as 7.3% of adult Americans meet lifetime criteria for IED, and 3.9% meet criteria for previous 12-month IED.

Neurobiology

Current research suggests that many of the same areas of the brain implicated in substance use are also implicated in IED. The areas include the OFC, vmPFC, DLPFC, anterior cingulate cortex, and amygdale. At the neurochemical level, corticotrophin releasing factor, NE, and 5-HT all seem to play a role in IED.

CHAPTER

6

Summary Author: Christopher A. Cavacuiti
Lori D. Karan • Elinore McCance-Katz • Anne Zajicek

Pharmacokinetic and Pharmacodynamic Principles

Pharmacokinetics describes the movement of a drug within the body and especially how a drug's concentration in blood, body fluids, and tissues varies over time. *Pharmacodynamics* describes the biochemical and physiologic effects of drugs and their mechanisms of action. To put it another way, pharmacokinetics can be explained as "what the body does to the drug," pharmacodynamics can be thought of as "what the drug does to the body."

PHARMACOKINETICS

Absorption

Psychoactive drugs can be inhaled, smoked, sniffed, taken orally, transdermally, sublingually, or rectally or they can be injected (intravenously, subcutaneously, or intramuscularly).

The more rapidly a psychoactive drug is delivered to its site of action in the central nervous system, the greater is its reinforcing effect. Smoked and inhaled drugs bypass the venous system and thus have the most rapid rate of delivery.

With illicit drugs, dose often is difficult to determine because of the presence of adulterants in the preparations as well as imprecise measurement of the amount consumed (as compared to the quantity of active ingredients in prescription medications, which is known precisely).

Bioavailability is defined as the fraction of unchanged drug that reaches the systemic circulation after administration by any route. The *bioavailability factor* (F) takes into account the portion of the administered dose that is able to enter the circulation unchanged. For intravenously administered drugs, F = 1.0 (100%).

First-pass metabolism is the metabolism that occurs before a drug reaches the systemic circulation. First-pass metabolism is particularly important for drugs administered by oral and deep rectal routes. After absorption across the gut wall, the portal blood delivers the drug to the liver before it enters into the systemic circulation. Metabolism by the gut and liver can significantly reduce a drug's bioavailable fraction. First-pass metabolism is relatively unimportant for drugs administered through the intravenous, sublingual, intramuscular, subcutaneous, and transdermal routes.

Upon absorption, when drug concentrations are graphed against time, a peak drug concentration (C_{max}) is reached at a particular time (T_{max}). The trough concentration (C_{min}) is reached at a particular time (T_{min}). The **A**rea **U**nder the concentration-time **C**urve (AUC) is a measure of drug exposure that can be calculated (as the sum of trapezoids) and quantified.

Distribution

Once absorbed, a drug is distributed to the various organs of the body. Distribution is influenced by how well each organ is perfused with blood, the organ's size, binding of the drug within the blood and in the tissues, and the permeability of tissue membranes. Different drugs distribute to different body compartments and tissues and have different *volumes of distribution* (V_d). This volume has no direct physical equivalent because it describes the amount of serum, plasma, or blood that would be required to account for all drug in the body if the entire dose of that drug were spread uniformly throughout. V_d can be thought of as the amount of drug in the body (D=dose) divided by the concentration of drug (C) in the plasma. Drugs that are tightly bound to plasma proteins, or have a high molecular weight may only distribute to the intravascular space and may have V_d of approximately 5 L. Drugs can have large V_d values up to 50,000 L if they are highly bound to tissue sites or are lipophilic.

The activity of a drug depends not on its total quantity but on the concentration of free drug at its site of action. This free concentration is clinically relevant for drugs such as phenytoin, warfarin, and thyroxine, which are >90% bound to plasma proteins.

The rate of blood flow delivered to specific organs and tissues is important. Well-perfused tissues can receive large quantities of drug, provided that the drug can cross the membranes or other barriers present between the plasma and tissue.

The endothelial cells lining brain capillaries have tight junctions (the *blood–brain barrier*) that do not permit larger molecules to pass through. To enter the brain, drugs must cross the two membranes of the endothelial cell. Specific active transport systems enable compounds such as glucose, amino acids, and nucleotides to gain access to the brain. Many drugs cross these membranes by passive diffusion. Because the endothelial cell membrane is composed of lipids, drugs can only diffuse across the blood–brain barrier if they are lipid soluble and most psychoactive drugs enter the brain in this manner.

Metabolism

Metabolism is the process by which lipophilic drugs and foods are mostly transformed to more polar products that are more readily eliminated. Compared with the parent drug, drug metabolites usually have a diminished volume of distribution and diminished ability to penetrate cellular membranes. Not all metabolites are inactive or nontoxic; some biotransformation products have enhanced activity or toxic properties, including mutagenicity, teratogenicity, and carcinogenicity.

Drugs can be metabolized by Phase I and/or Phase II reactions. Phase I reactions (such as cytochrome P450 metabolism) are nonsynthetic reactions in which the drug is chemically altered and oxidized. Phase II reactions (such as glucuronidation) are synthetic reactions in which the drug is conjugated with another moiety, such as glucuronide.

Phase I oxidations can take place by cytochrome P450–dependent and –independent mechanisms. More than 50 individual cytochrome P450 subtypes (CYPs) have been identified in humans. Not only do CYPs that metabolize medications have a tremendous capacity to oxidize a large number of structurally diverse compounds but they can also metabolize a single compound at different positions on that molecule. CYP3A4 alone is responsible for metabolizing >50% of clinically prescribed drugs.

Genetic variability in drug-metabolizing enzymes can influence drug response. For example, the metabolism of codeine (which produces little analgesia) to the potent analgesic, morphine, is determined by CYP2D6 genotype. Those with genotypes associated with an enzyme with reduced metabolic function can result in patients not obtaining effective analgesia with codeine administration. The new discipline of pharmacogenetics aims to elucidate cytochrome and other drug-metabolizing enzyme polymorphisms, the degrees of expression of these polymorphisms, and the functional significance of such expression.

Many drugs, foods, and environmental chemicals can induce and/or inhibit the activity of the cytochromes, speeding up or slowing down their own metabolism and that of other CYP-metabolized compounds.

To take just one example, methadone is a substrate of CYP3A4. *Inhibitors* of CYP3A4 (including erythromycin, diltiazem, ketoconazole, and saquinavir) slow the metabolism of methadone and increase methadone levels. *Inducers* of CYP3A4 (such as carbamazepine, phenobarbital, efavirenz, and St. John's wort) speed the metabolism of methadone and decrease methadone levels.

Drug interactions also can cause altered *biotransformation*. For example, when cocaine is used in conjunction with ethanol, there is an ethyl transesterification of cocaine to cocaethylene, which is a biologically active compound that causes a prolonged and enhanced euphoric effect.

Drug metabolism may influence risk of addiction, with relative protection for persons who experience adverse drug reactions at lower drug doses. The Lys487 and Arg47 alleles of the aldehyde dehydrogenase 2 (ALDH2) enzyme can lead to the accumulation of acetaldehyde when alcohol is consumed. This accumulation of acetaldehyde causes flushing, nausea, and headache, and individuals carrying one or both of these alleles have a reduction in the risk of alcoholism. Persons of South Asian descent are likely to carry both alleles, whereas those with Jewish ancestry often carry the Arg47 allele.

Although drug metabolism occurs largely in the liver, most other tissues and organs, including the brain, lungs, gastrointestinal tract, skin, and kidneys, carry out varying degrees of drug metabolism.

Elimination and Excretion

Elimination refers to disappearance of the parent and/or active molecule from the bloodstream or body, which can occur by metabolism and/or excretion. *Excretion* is the process of removing a compound from the body. Drugs can be excreted through the urine or feces, exhaled through the lungs, or secreted through sweat or salivary glands.

The *half-life* ($t_{1/2}$) of a drug is a measure of time required for a drug to arrive at or decay from steady state. This measure is such that 1 half-life represents a 50% change, and 2, 3, 4, and 5 half-lives represent 75%, 87.5%, 93.7%, and 96.8% changes, respectively. Half-life is dependent on clearance and volume of distribution. Clearance is a rate that represents a theoretical volume that is completely cleared of drug in a given period of time. As clearance decreases because of aging or a disease process, half-life would be expected to increase. However with aging and disease, there may also be alterations in body water and lipid content influencing the volume of distribution.

Most drugs display *first-order elimination* kinetics. The *fraction or percentage* of the total amount of drug present in the body that is removed at any one time remains constant and is independent of dose. When first-order kinetics are graphed, there is an exponential decay in the rate of elimination of the drug so that the concentration of drug in the body diminishes logarithmically over time.

In contrast, drugs with *zero-order elimination* kinetics eliminate a constant amount of drug (rather than a constant fraction of drug). In most cases, the maximal rate of metabolism and/or elimination is due to the saturation of a key enzyme. Because the half-life depends on the variable clearance, it too is not constant. Therefore, half-life is not particularly useful for drugs eliminated by zero-order kinetics. Ethanol is an example of a drug with *zero-order elimination* kinetics. It is eliminated at a constant rate no matter how much ethanol is in the system.

THERAPEUTICS BASED ON PHARMACOKINETIC CALCULATIONS

Pharmacokinetics explores the relationship between the drug dose and the time-varying concentration of drug at its site(s) of action. A rational dosage regimen is based on the assumption that there is a target concentration that will produce a desired therapeutic effect. This target drug concentration falls within a therapeutic range whose lower bounds are a minimal therapeutic concentration and whose upper bounds are a minimum toxic concentration.

PHARMACODYNAMICS

The study of pharmacodynamics is the study of the biochemical and physiologic effects of drugs on the body. This study includes an understanding of the mechanisms of drug action, dose response phenomena, and the body's regulatory response to this activity. Most drugs act on specific endogenous targets, not to create new effects but rather to modulate the rate and extent of the body's endogenous functions.

Receptor Physiology

Receptors contain at least two functional domains: a ligand-binding site and an effector or message propagation (i.e., signaling) area. Receptors can be grouped according to four common types. These are (a) ligand-gated ion channels, (b) G protein–coupled receptor signaling, (c) receptors with intrinsic enzymatic activity, and (d) receptors regulating nuclear transcription.

Ligand-Gated Ion Channels

These receptors selectively gate the flow of ions through channels into the cell. Each unit of these multisubunit proteins spans the plasma membrane several times. The association of the subunits allows the formation of a wall or a pore. Binding to single or multiple subunits then enables these subunits to rapidly and cooperatively control channel opening and closing to alter cell membrane voltage potential. *Excitatory neurotransmitters* result in a net inward current of cations (such as Na^+, Ca^{2+}, and K^+) that depolarize the cell and increase the generation of action potentials. Inhibitory neurotransmitters result in the inward flux of anions such as Cl^-, which hyperpolarize the cell and decrease the generation of action potentials.

G Proteins and Second Messengers

G protein receptors have an extracellular amino (N) terminal and an intracellular carboxyl (C) terminal and commonly transverse the plasma membrane seven times (and hence are often referred to as "serpentine" receptors). When agonists bind to a G protein receptor, a change of confirmation occurs that is transmitted to the serpentine loops of the G protein receptor that in turn activates the appropriate G protein. Several serpentine receptors exist as dimers or larger complexes. G proteins modify the activity of regulatory proteins and/or ion channels, which in turn alter the activity of intracellular second messengers that enable signal transduction and amplification. Among the well-established second messenger systems are cyclic adenosine monophosphate (cAMP), cyclic guanosine monophosphate, and phosphoinositides.

G protein receptors undergo pharmacodynamic tolerance. They acutely attenuate their response by reversible and rapid desensitization.

It is now believed that G protein–coupled receptors can exist in multiple conformational states including ones that are active, inactive, partially active, and selectively active. The relative affinity of the drug for various conformations of the receptor will determine the extent to which the equilibrium is shifted toward the active state. *Full agonists* have a higher affinity for the active conformation and drive the equilibrium toward the active state. *Partial agonists* bind to the receptor with only moderately more affinity for the active than for the inactive receptor. Buprenorphine is an example of a highly potent μ opioid G protein receptor partial agonist. *Antagonists* have no effect upon response when used alone. They bind with equal affinity to the active and inactive conformations and prevent an agonist from inducing a response. Competitive antagonists may be reversed by adding excess agonist, but noncompetitive antagonists cannot be counteracted in this manner.

Receptors with Intrinsic Enzyme Activity

These receptors typically consist of an extracellular domain that binds to growth factors or hormones and an intracellular enzyme domain that catalyzes the activity of cytoplasmic proteins.

Receptors Regulating Nuclear Transcription

Receptors that regulate nuclear transcription are lipid-soluble DNA-binding proteins that bypass the plasma membrane to reach their intracellular targets.

A Mechanistic Classification of Selected Drugs of Abuse

Abused drugs generally activate the mesolimbic system by (a) interacting with ion channel receptors, (b) binding to G_{io}-coupled receptors, or (c) interfering with monoamine transporters. Substances acting through the first two mechanisms tend to inhibit γ-aminobutyric acid (GABA) inhibitory interneurons, resulting in a net release of dopamine. Drugs that interfere with monoamine transporters block the reuptake or stimulate nonvesicular release of dopamine.

Potency, Efficacy, and Dose Response

Potency is a function of the amount of drug required for its specific effect to occur. *Efficacy* measures the maximum strength of the effect itself. Because drug doses are readily adjusted, it is the maximal efficacy that is more often clinically relevant.

Animal experiments can be used to discern a given drug's *median effective dose* (ED_{50}), *median toxic dose* (TD_{50}), and *median lethal dose* (LD_{50}). The *therapeutic index* is defined as the ratio of the TD_{50} to the ED_{50}. Because it is unethical to design experiments using a full range of drug doses to determine these indices in humans, the range of therapeutic drug concentrations and the margin of safety are estimated more broadly through extrapolation from animal studies, human drug trials, and clinical experience.

TOLERANCE, SENSITIZATION, AND PHYSICAL DEPENDENCE

Tolerance and sensitization reflect changes in the way the body responds to a drug *when it is used repeatedly*. Tolerance is the reduction in response to a drug after its repeated administration. Sensitization indicates an increase in drug response after its repeated administration.

Tolerance and sensitization develop more readily to some drug effects than to other effects of the same drug. For example, tolerance to the euphoria produced by cocaine occurs much more rapidly than does tolerance to its cardiovascular effects. The discrepancy between tolerance to the "rush" experienced by drug users and tolerance to a drug's cardiovascular and respiratory effects can be an important cause of mortality in the user who overdoses.

There are several mechanisms by which tolerance can occur. *Pharmacokinetic tolerance* most often occurs as a consequence of increased metabolism of a drug after its repeated administration, resulting in less drug available at the receptor for drug activity. *Pharmacodynamic tolerance* refers to the adaptive changes in receptor density, efficiency of receptor coupling, and/or signal transduction pathways that occur after repeated drug exposure.

Learned tolerance refers to a reduction in the effects of a drug because of compensatory mechanisms that are learned. A common example of learned tolerance is the ability for roofers and workers at heights to walk in a straight line despite motor impairment from alcohol intoxication. *Conditioned tolerance*, which is a subset of learned tolerance, occurs when specific environmental cues such as sights, smells, or circumstances are paired with drug administration so that, when the drug is taken in the presence of the specific environmental cue, a state of expectation occurs. *Cross-tolerance* occurs when tolerance to the repeated use of a specific drug in a given category is generalized to other drugs in that same structural and mechanistic category.

Physical dependence is a state that develops as a result of the adaptation produced by resetting homeostatic mechanisms after repeated drug use. Withdrawal signs and symptoms can occur in a physically dependent person when drug administration is abruptly stopped.

Patients who take prescribed medications for appropriate medical indications can show tolerance, physical dependence, and withdrawal if the drug is stopped abruptly, even though they do not exhibit the compulsive drug use and negative consequences characteristic of drug addiction.

The conclusions in this paper represent the views of the authors and do not necessarily represent the views of NICHD or NIH.

Summary Author: Christopher A. Cavacuiti
John J. Woodward

The Pharmacology of Alcohol

DEFINITION

Alcohol is a chemical name for a group of related compounds that contain a hydroxyl group (-OH) bound to a carbon atom. The form of alcohol that is voluntarily consumed by humans is ethyl alcohol or ethanol and consists of two carbons and a single hydroxyl group (written as C_2H_5OH or C_2H_6O). Unless otherwise noted, the term *alcohol* will be used throughout this chapter to mean ethanol.

FORMULATIONS AND METHODS OF USE

In the United States, a standard alcoholic drink is defined as one that contains 0.6 fluid ounces of alcohol. Thus, this amount of alcohol is typically contained in 12 oz of beer, 5 oz of wine, or 1.5 oz of distilled spirits (40% ethanol by volume), although this can vary depending on the specific type of beverage. Although most alcohol is consumed orally, there are isolated cases of individuals injecting ethanol intravenously. In addition, ethanol vapor can be inhaled, using an *AWOL* (alcohol without liquid) device. A number of US states have now banned the sale or use of these devices.

CLINICAL USES

In addition to its use as a topical antiseptic, alcohol has several clinical indications including treatment of accidental or voluntary ingestion of methanol or ethylene glycol. Ethanol has a higher affinity for alcohol dehydrogenase (ADH) than methanol or ethylene glycol. Ingestion of alcohol can therefore reduce the formation of toxic methanol ethylene glycol metabolites. For both indications, hemodialysis is the recommended first line of treatment.

BRIEF HISTORICAL FEATURES

Alcohol is one of the oldest psychoactive substances used by humans. Consumption of alcohol containing beverages predate recorded human history, while written records of its use are found in Chinese and Middle Eastern texts as far back as 9,000 years ago.

EPIDEMIOLOGY

The lifetime exposure to alcohol is high, with nearly 88% of the US population reporting using alcohol at least once in their lifetime. In 2006, current alcohol use (defined as use in the past 30 days) ranged from 3.9% among 12- to 13-year-olds to nearly 70% of 21- to 25-year-olds. Prevalence decreased among older groups although it was nearly 50% among 60- to 64-year-olds. Annual alcohol-related costs in terms of lost productivity and health care are estimated at $185 billion.

Clinical studies of alcohol abuse and alcoholism have led to the idea that there may be several types of alcohol use disorders, based on the appearance and severity of certain alcohol-related problems. Two particularly well-known examples of these classifications are the type I and type II forms proposed by Cloninger et al. and the Type A and B forms proposed by Babor. Cloninger's type II and Babor's type B share several similarities including the following:

1. Familial alcoholism
2. Earlier onset of alcohol-related problems
3. More incidents of alcohol-related problems or violence, and
4. Higher preference for risk taking/novelty seeking.

PHARMACOKINETICS

Alcohol is a small, water-soluble molecule that is rapidly and efficiently absorbed into the bloodstream from the stomach, small intestine, and colon. The rate of absorption depends on the gastric emptying time and can be delayed by the presence of food in the small intestine.

Women have less gastric metabolism of alcohol than men. When body weights are equivalent, women show a 20% to 25% higher blood alcohol level than men after ingestion of the same amount of alcohol.

In the liver, alcohol is broken down by ADH and CYP2E1. ADH converts alcohol to acetaldehyde, which subsequently can be converted to acetate by the actions of acetaldehyde dehydrogenase. The rate of alcohol metabolism by ADH is relatively constant, as the enzyme is saturated at relatively low blood alcohol levels and thus exhibits zero-order kinetics (constant amount oxidized per unit of time). Levels of CYP2E1 may be increased in chronic drinkers.

PHARMACODYNAMICS

Central Nervous System

Acutely, alcohol acts as a central nervous system (CNS) depressant. During the initial phase when blood alcohol levels are rising, a period of disinhibition often occurs, and signs of behavioral arousal are common. At higher blood levels, alcohol acts as a sedative and hypnotic, although the quality of sleep often is reduced after alcohol intake.

Other Organ Systems

Acute alcohol ingestion usually produces a feeling of warmth as cutaneous blood flow is increased. This is accompanied by a reduction in core body temperature. Gastric secretions usually are increased. Alcohol generally decreases sexual performance in both men and women. Alcohol consumption is also associated with an increased risk of tumors in the GI system as well as in other tissues including lung and breast. Chronic alcohol ingestion is associated with increased fat accumulation in the liver as well as mitochondrial toxicity from acetaldehyde accumulation. The resulting liver damage can progress to severe liver disease and cirrhosis. Small amounts of alcohol are believed to a protective effect on cardiovascular tissue.

DRUG–DRUG INTERACTIONS

Alcohol potentiates the CNS depressant properties of a number of centrally acting drugs such as such as opioids, barbiturates, benzodiazepines, general anesthetics, and anticonvulsants. Alcohol also enhances the sedative effects of antihistamines that are commonly used in the treatment of nasal congestion. Combining these medications with alcohol can result in significant CNS depression and reduced ability to safely carry out normal functions such as automobile driving.

NEUROBIOLOGY (MECHANISMS OF ADDICTION)

All drugs of abuse, including alcohol, affect reward pathways by enhancing the release of dopamine from midbrain dopaminergic projections. The DA neurons involved in this action originate in the midbrain ventral tegmental area (VTA) and project to multiple areas of the forebrain. The initial reinforcing actions of alcohol appear to involve excitation of VTA dopamine neurons. Acutely, alcohol enhances the firing rate of midbrain DA neurons. Rats that self-administer alcohol show significant dose-dependent increases in extracellular dopamine levels in the nucleus accumbens.

Molecular Sites of Alcohol Action

Psychostimulants such as cocaine and amphetamine or opiates such as heroin and morphine all produce their primary effect by binding to specific protein receptors expressed on brain neurons. Alcohol, in contrast, is rather indiscriminate and interacts with a wide variety of targets, including both lipids and proteins. While it was previously thought that alcohol's actions were due to alcohol's effects on the lipid cell membranes on CNS neurons, a consensus has emerged that specific ligand-gated and voltage-gated ion channels represent a likely site for many of the acute effects of alcohol on neuronal function, though how alcohol actually produces its effect on these proteins is not yet clear.

γ-Aminobutyric acid (GABA) and Glycine Receptors

There are distinct families of subunits that make up GABA and glycine receptors. Different subunit combinations can give rise to a variety of GABA and glycine receptors that show variable sensitivity to pharmacologic agents, including alcohol. Alcohol generally enhances GABA and glycine receptor function.

Glutamate-Activated Ion Channels

Glutamate is the major excitatory neurotransmitter in the brain and activates two major subtypes of ion channels called AMPA/Kainate and NMDA receptors. NMDA receptors are antagonized by alcohol, whereas AMPA/Kainate receptors are generally insensitive to alcohol and the concentrations that are associated with intoxication and sedation. The antagonism of NMDA receptors by alcohol may also be involved in its rewarding properties because NMDA antagonists (including alcohol) have been shown to increase levels of dopamine in the nucleus accumbens. It has also been demonstrated that chronic exposure to alcohol (which is an NMDA antagonist) increases the density and clustering of NMDA receptors, leading to heightened NMDA sensitivity. The increased sensitivity of NMDA receptors during withdrawal is thought to play a major role in alcohol withdrawal and seizures.

OTHER ION CHANNEL SUBTYPES

5-HT$_3$ Receptors

5-HT$_3$ receptors are ligand-gated ion channels activated by serotonin. Alcohol appears to potentiate currents carried by 5-HT$_3$. Human studies using the 5-HT$_3$ antagonist ondansetron (Zofran) have generally found the drug reduces drinking.

Acetylcholine Nicotinic Receptors

Alcohol has been shown to both potentiate and inhibit acetylcholine nicotinic receptors. This effect appears to result from expression of different subtypes of acetylcholine nicotinic receptors by brain neurons that show a differential response to ethanol. It is not yet clear if or how these different effects of ethanol on neuronal nicotinic receptors are manifested at the behavioral level.

Calcium-activated and G protein–gated Potassium Channels

Calcium-activated potassium channels and G protein–gated potassium channels are also affected either directly or indirectly by alcohol. These channels serve as a brake on excitatory glutamatergic transmission by hyperpolarizing the membrane and thus are critical regulators of neuronal activity. The activity of at least some potassium channel subtypes is enhanced by alcohol. This enhancement may contribute to the inhibition of vasopressin and the resulting diuresis that accompanies alcohol ingestion.

Pharmacologic Studies Implicating Neurotransmitters

Alcohol not only affects receptors and ion channels (as discussed above), but also alters neurotransmitter levels. A brief review of this literature is presented here.

Adenosine

Adenosine is a major inhibitory neurotransmitter in the brain and may serve as an endogenous antiepileptic because of its ability to inhibit neuronal function. Alcohol has been shown to inhibit the function of a nucleoside transporter, leading to increased extracellular adenosine levels.

Dopamine

Alcohol increases the firing of dopamine-containing neurons, located in the VTA, leading to enhanced dopamine release in the nucleus accumbens and the prefrontal cortex. The mechanism underlying this effect of alcohol is not precisely known.

Opioids

Mice that are genetically modified to lack the mu-opioid do not self-administer alcohol or respond to the rewarding effects of opiates, nicotine, or cannanbinoids. Naloxone and naltrexone, two opioid receptor antagonists, reduce alcohol intake in both animals and humans. These agents are thought to work by blocking alcohol-induced increases in β-endorphin, thus reducing the acute rewarding effects of alcohol. However, the clinical efficacy of opiate antagonists in treating alcohol dependence is rather modest, suggesting that other factors may be important

Serotonin (5-HT)

5-HT and 5-HT–metabolite levels are reduced in the cerebrospinal fluid of many alcoholics, suggesting that reduced 5-HT levels or a reduction in 5-HT–mediated neurotransmission may play a role in uncontrolled drinking. However, pharmacologic agents that enhance 5-HT neurotransmission (such as serotonin selective-uptake inhibitors) appear to have limited efficacy in the treatment of alcohol dependence.

Endocannabinoids

The endogenous cannabinoid (EC) system has also been shown to be an important modulator of ethanol drinking in mice. CB1 antagonists reduce ethanol preference in wild-type mice and murine strains that lack CB1 receptors show reduced alcohol preference

ADDICTION LIABILITY

Lifetime prevalence of alcohol dependence is approximately 13% and the risk of developing alcohol dependence shows a strong inverse correlation with the age at which heavy drinking begins. Chronic use of alcohol produces several neuroadaptive changes that may be important in the development of alcohol addiction.

Sensitization

Sensitization is defined as an increase in the pharmacologic and physiologic response to a drug after repeated exposures. Another form of sensitization is characterized by an increase in the severity and intensity of withdrawal signs after multiple episodes of alcohol intoxication and withdrawal. This form of sensitization has been suggested to be similar to the "kindling" phenomena observed after repeated seizures and may involve some of the same mechanisms.

Tolerance and Dependence

Tolerance is manifested as a reduced sensitivity to alcohol. In human alcoholics, tolerance to the sedative and even lethal effects of alcohol can be profound. For example, while the lethal dose of 50% (LD50) in nontolerant humans is approximately 400 to 500 mg%, blood levels exceeding these values are often reported in individuals arrested for driving under the influence of alcohol. Dependence is defined by the occurrence of symptoms that appear after the cessation of alcohol drinking. These withdrawal symptoms include both physical (tremors, convulsions) and psychologic (negative emotions, craving) components. Although reward mechanisms are undoubtedly important in the development of heavy alcohol use, processes and brain areas that underlie the development of dependence may be critical for maintaining continued drinking through negative reinforcement (anxiety, stress) generated during withdrawal.

Toxicity States

Alcohol is metabolized under zero-order kinetics such that it is independent of dose and time and blood alcohol levels fall at a rate of about 20 mg/dL/hour. Alcohol produces a well-studied progression of behavioral symptoms that are highly correlated with blood alcohol levels. In nontolerant individuals

- Low levels (10–50 mg%)—decreased anxiety, a feeling of well-being, increased sociability
- Increased levels (80–100 mg%)—impaired judgment and motor function
- Higher levels (150–200 mg%)—marked ataxia, reduced reaction time, blackouts
- Anesthetic level (300–400 mg%)—severe motor impairment, decreased level of consciousness, vomiting
- Lethal level (400–500 mg%)

Medical Complications

Alcohol affects nearly all tissue and organ systems studied, and heavy drinkers show skeletal fragility and damage to tissues such as brain, liver, and heart and increased susceptibility to some cancers.

Brain tissue effects of alcohol include increases in cortical cerebrospinal fluid, damage to frontal lobes and cerebellar gray matter, volume deficits of the anterior hippocampus (in Korsakoff syndrome), damage to the corpus callosum (in both prenatal and adult exposure to alcohol), reduced brain glucose metabolism, and decreased blood perfusion of frontal lobes; animal studies suggest that even brief episodes of heavy drinking, or binges, also cause neuron loss

Heavy alcohol use during pregnancy can lead to a variety of birth defects and alterations in normal growth and development of the newborn.

Despite these negative effects, beneficial effects of moderate alcohol intake have been demonstrated; these include a reduced risk of coronary heart disease in individuals classified as light to moderate drinkers (two or fewer drinks per day for men and one or fewer per day for women). The amount of alcohol (if any) that is safe in pregnancy remains unknown.

Summary Author: Christopher A. Cavacuiti
Domenic A. Ciraulo • Clifford M. Knapp

The Pharmacology of Nonalcohol Sedative Hypnotics

Sedative-hypnotic drugs represent a diverse group of chemical agents that suppress central nervous system (CNS) activity. They are used therapeutically as anxiolytics, hypnotics, anticonvulsants, muscle relaxants, and anesthesia induction agents. Substances discussed in this chapter include benzodiazepines, nonbenzodiazepine hypnotics, barbiturates, and miscellaneous related compounds.

FORMULATIONS AND CHEMICAL STRUCTURE

The basic structure of the benzodiazepines is the 1,4-benzodiazepine nucleus. Various substitutions alter the efficacy, potency, and other properties of individual benzodiazepines. More recently, four nonbenzodiazepine hypnotics have been introduced: (a) zopiclone, a cyclopyrolone; (b) eszopiclone, a stereoselective isomer of zopiclone; (c) zaleplon, a pyrazolopyrimidine; and (d) zolpidem, an imidazopyridine. Although these agents exert their hypnotic effects at the γ-aminobutyric acid (GABA$_A$) receptor, their actions are not identical to classic benzodiazepines.

Benzodiazepines have largely replaced the use of barbiturates because benzodiazepines have greater safety and less potential for abuse; however, barbiturates continue to be used in some circumstances. Barbiturates continue to be used in general anesthesia and for the treatment of seizures. In the practice of addiction medicine, phenobarbital (a barbiturate) is used to treat difficult cases of sedative-hypnotic withdrawal.

BRIEF HISTORICAL FEATURES

Barbituric acid was first prepared in 1864 by von Baeyer. Although not a central depressant itself, several of its derivatives have been used in medicine since the early 1900s. Barbital was introduced in 1903 and phenobarbital in 1912. With respect to benzodiazepines, in the mid-1930s, Sternbach synthesized several heptoxdiazines, although it wasn't until 1955 when one of these quinazolines was treated with methylamine that an active compound was developed. Nonbenzodiazepine hypnotics have been the most recent addition and may offer some advantages of lower abuse liability.

EPIDEMIOLOGY

In clinical populations, most patients take benzodiazepines for periods of <1 month. Between 7.4% and 17.6% of the US population use a benzodiazepine for medical purposes at least once during a 1-year period, with about 1% using the medication for a year or longer. Studies both in the United States and Europe indicate that long-term users are more likely to be older, women, and report high levels of chronic health problems and emotional difficulties. Benzodiazepine abuse is particularly high among alcoholics and methadone-treated patients.

Eight percent of the US population 12 years old or older have used tranquilizers for nonmedical purposes at some time in their life. Benzodiazepines were mentioned in 27% of suicide attempts.

PHARMACOKINETICS

Many benzodiazepines are metabolized by cytochrome P450 (CYP450), with CYP450 3A4 being the most common subtype involved in benzodiazepine metabolism. CYP3A4 also plays a role in the biotransformation of the nonbenzodiazepine sedative-hypnotic agents, eszopicione, zaleplon, and zolpidem. The final phase of metabolism for most benzodiazepines consists of conjugation of either the parent drug or their metabolites with glucuronide.

As is true with other classes of addictive drugs, benzodiazepines with a more rapid onset of action are generally associated with more euphoria and generally have a higher addiction liability. However, other yet to be discovered factors also appear to be involved in determining the addiction liability of benzodiazepines.

PHARMACODYNAMICS

Benzodiazepines exert their clinical effects through agonist activity at the $GABA_A$ receptor. The $GABA_A$ receptor is a pentameric protein structure surrounding a central chloride channel. Benzodiazepines act as indirect agonists. They do not activate the GABA receptor themselves. Instead, they function by enhancing the binding of GABA to the receptor and thereby lead to an increased frequency of the opening of the central chloride channel. As GABA is the major inhibitory neurotransmitter system in the brain, positive modulation of the receptor by benzodiazepines is responsible for sedative, anticonvulsant, hypnotic, and amnestic effects of the drug.

Barbiturates share some pharmacodynamic properties with the benzodiazepines. At low concentrations, barbiturates act as positive modulators of the $GABA_A$ receptor via an allosteric mechanism (i.e., barbiturates bind to a site on the GABA protein other than the active site, resulting in a change in confirmation at the active site). However, at higher concentrations, barbiturates act as direct $GABA_A$ receptor agonists by prolonging the duration of the opening of the chloride channel.

Several nonbenzodiazepines compounds, which are commonly referred to as "the Z drugs," have been identified that act as positive modulators of the effects of GABA agonists on the $GABA_A$ receptor. These agents include zolpidem, zaleplon, and zopiclone. (Zopiclone is marketed in the United States only as the more active S-enantiomer, eszopicione.) As would be expected, these drugs share many of the pharmacologic actions with the classic benzodiazepine agents including sedative-hypnotic, anxiolytic, myorelaxant, and anticonvulsant effects, although their selectivity for these actions differs. The Z drugs may differ from the classic benzodiazepines in that their amnestic effects may be less pronounced and tolerance is less likely to develop to their pharmacologic actions. Dissimilarities in the activity between individual Z drugs or between Z drugs and the classic benzodiazepines may arise, in part because of differences in the affinity of these drugs for the different subtypes of $GABA_A$ receptors.

DRUG–DRUG INTERACTIONS

The most serious drug–drug interactions occur when sedative hypnotics are combined with alcohol or other drugs that depress CNS activity. Benzodiazepines do not induce their own metabolism; however, those that are metabolized through CYP3A4 are subject to altered plasma levels by agents that inhibit/induce this metabolic pathway. Common CYP3A4 inhibitors included atazanavir, indinavir, nelfinavir, ritonavir, saquinavir, macrolide antibiotics (erythromycin, clarithromycin, telithromycin, troleandomycin), azole antifungals (fluconazole, itraconazole, ketoconazole, voriconazole), nefazodone, fluoxetine, cimetidine, grapefruit, and grapefruit juice.

Common CYP3A4 inducers include rifabutin, rifampicin, rifapentine, carbamazepine, phenobarbital, phenytoin, and St. John's wort.

Barbiturates present a serious risk of CNS depression, coma, and death when taken in high doses or with ethanol or other sedative hypnotics. They induce their own metabolism (pharmacokinetic tolerance) and induce CYP2B6, CYP2C9, and CYP3A4, resulting in enhanced metabolism of drugs that are substrates of these cytochromes, reducing therapeutic effects. Patients taking phenobarbital may experience decreased effects of anticoagulants, oral contraceptives, corticosteroids, some antibiotics, and other drugs.

MECHANISM OF ADDICTION

Although the paths to sedative-hypnotic addiction are complex and vary among individuals, it is helpful to consider three characteristics of the drug class that are related to misuse: (a) hedonic effects, (b) tolerance, and (c) the withdrawal syndrome. The use of benzodiazepines purely for the hedonic value, that is, to achieve a pleasurable or euphoric mood change, is rare unless they are used in combination with other drugs such as opioids (including methadone), which results in a "boost." Benzodiazepines with a rapid onset of action, such as alprazolam or diazepam, probably present the greatest risk for this type of abuse.

Tolerance of clinical effects may lead some patients to escalate the dosage. The risk appears greatest when the drugs are used as hypnotics because tolerance of sedation occurs rapidly, whereas tolerance to the other effects of sedative hypnotics occurs more slowly and to a lesser extent.

The withdrawal syndrome that appears upon decreasing dosage or abrupt discontinuation of treatment may produce uncomfortable mental and physical states that make it difficult for patients to terminate drug use. Rebound insomnia is a particular problem for patients who discontinue benzodiazepines.

Although the mechanism of therapeutic action is well known for benzodiazepines and barbiturates, the neurophysiologic basis of their reinforcing effects are not well understood.

ADDICTION LIABILITY

Benzodiazepines are the most widely used and abused drugs of the sedative-hypnotic class. In animal models and human laboratory studies, they occupy an intermediate position of abuse liability that is lower than barbiturates, but higher than anxiolytics that do not act at the $GABA_A$ receptor complex (e.g., buspirone, antidepressants, ramelteon). Many authorities believe that the Z-drugs have lower potential for abuse than classic benzodiazepines; however, there are case reports of tolerance, withdrawal, and abuse of these agents. More controversial is the issue of relative abuse liability among the benzodiazepines themselves.

Sedative-hypnotic abuse is more common among individuals with opioid dependence and alcohol dependence than in those with anxiety.

TOXICITY STATES AND THEIR MEDICAL MANAGEMENT

With respect to sedative hypnotics, benzodiazepines provide a greater margin of safety than barbiturates and older agents. Despite the improved safety profile, prescription of benzodiazepines is associated with acute and chronic risks. Acute toxicity of benzodiazepines includes sedation, psychomotor impairment, and memory problems. Benzodiazepines produce anterograde amnesia, difficulty acquiring new learning. It is unclear if tolerance develops to the toxic effects. Although many studies have found no cognitive impairment associated with long-term benzodiazepine treatment, others have reported persistent problems in psychomotor function, learning, concentration, and visuospatial skills. Greater impairment is seen in men, the elderly, and individuals taking the highest doses.

Classic benzodiazepines, nonbenzodiazepine hypnotics, SSRI antidepressants, and antipsychotics have all been linked to falls and fractures in the elderly, making the treatment of insomnia in aged patients a challenge. The Z-drugs have been associated with somnambulism and complex nocturnal behaviors, such as eating, shopping, and driving.

There is a higher incidence of motor vehicle accidents in benzodiazepine users. It is not known whether this reflects acute psychomotor impairment, falling asleep at the wheel, or persistent visuospatial impairment.

The risks of benzodiazepines during pregnancy and lactation have been the subject of controversy. There may be an association between cleft palate and maternal benzodiazepine use. In addition, newborns who have been exposed to benzodiazepines in utero during the last trimester or during delivery may present with *floppy baby syndrome*, which is characterized by low Apgar scores, poor sucking, hypotonia, poor reflexes, and apnea. Neonatal withdrawal syndromes have also been reported. Benzodiazepines administered to nursing mothers enter the breast milk but appear in such low concentrations that they do not usually cause adverse effects in infants. Two important exceptions are when the benzodiazepine is given in high doses antepartum and continued postpartum and if infants have impaired hepatic function.

The use of barbiturate anticonvulsants, including phenobarbital, by pregnant women with epilepsy has been associated with congenital malformations, although the findings are not consistent.

MEDICAL COMPLICATIONS

All sedative hypnotics produce effects on a continuum from sedation to deep coma. Barbiturates have a greater risk for respiratory depression than do benzodiazepines. Sedative hypnotics are often combined with ethanol or other CNS depressants in overdoses.

Complications of severe sedative-hypnotic withdrawal can include grand mal seizures, status epilepticus, and psychosis. In general, longer treatment periods, higher doses, sudden drug discontinuation, and psychopathology increase the severity of the abstinence syndrome. All patients who have been taking these drugs for several weeks or longer should have the medication tapered, rather than abruptly stopped.

Some clinicians believe that there is prolonged withdrawal syndrome that persists for several months, but it has not been clearly distinguished from return of original anxiety symptoms.

Summary Author: Christopher A. Cavacuiti
Lisa Borg • Igor Kravets • Mary Jeanne Kreek

The Pharmacology of Long-Acting as Contrasted with Short-Acting Opioids

DEFINITION OF DRUGS IN THE CLASS

Opioids include any substance (agonist, partial agonist, antagonist) that binds to or otherwise affects the (μ, κ, and δ) opioid receptors on the surface of the cell. Opioids include the following:

- The "natural opioids" (also known as "opiates"), which are directly derived from the resin of the opium poppy (*Papaver somniferum*)
- The semisynthetic opioids, which are partially derived from opiates
- The synthetic opioids, which are fully synthesized in labs and not derived at all from opium resin
- Endogenous opioid peptides (β-endorphin, enkephalins, and dynorphin)
- Antagonists such as naloxone (Narcan), naltrexone (Trexan or ReVia), and nalmefene (Revix)

Although all three opioid receptor subtypes (μ, κ, and δ) are involved in mediating both the analgesic and the rewarding effects of opioids, in this chapter, we concentrate on the opioid activity at the μ-receptor as *most* of the clinically relevant activity of opioids occurs at this receptor.

SUBSTANCES INCLUDED IN THE OPIOID CLASS

Heroin

Diacetylmorphine was first synthesized in the 1870s by the Bayer company and marketed by Bayer under the name "heroin." Heroin is considered to be an opiate (natural opioid) as it is derived from the natural opioid morphine. Heroin is a prodrug, which is not itself active; it is rapidly deacetylated to 6-mono-acetylmorphine and morphine, both of which are active at the mu opioid receptor. In the United States, heroin is classified in schedule I (i.e., not available for any therapeutic use), although it is available in some other countries as a pain medication and/ or for treatment of heroin addiction. It is most commonly used intravenously. However, it is not uncommon for heroin to be used intranasally or smoked in the freebase form.

Morphine

Morphine is a natural product of the seeds of the poppy plant. Morphine is prescribed primarily as a high-potency analgesic. It is primarily administered orally or intravenously, though a variety of other routes of administration are possible.

Oxycodone Oxycodone has been used clinically since the early 1900s. It is combined with aspirin or acetaminophen for moderate pain and is available orally without coanalgesic for severe pain. It is a popular drug of abuse, especially in the controlled release formulation, which can be crushed for a potentially toxic, rapid "high."

Codeine While codeine can be extracted from directly from opium, most codeine is synthesized from methyl substitution on the phenolic hydroxyl group of morphine. It is more lipophilic than morphine and thus crosses the blood–brain barrier faster. It also has less first-pass metabolism in the liver, therefore, greater oral bioavailability than morphine, although it is less potent than morphine. Codeine is a prodrug that is metabolized to the active compounds. Approximately 5% to 10% of the population lacks the CYP2D6 enzyme to metabolize codeine to morphine, which is one of its active metabolites. Codeine is less effective for analgesia in these patients.

Meperidine Meperidine is a potent analgesic that is no longer used for long-term analgesia owing to concerns regarding CNS toxicity (seizures, delirium, other neurotoxic effects) of its metabolite. It also has serotonergic activity when combined with monoamine oxidase inhibitors, which can produce serious serotonin toxicity (including clonus, hyper-reflexia, hyperthermia, and even death).

Pentazocine Both parenteral and oral formulations of pentazocine were approved for marketing in the late 1960s. It is one of the initial "agonist-antagonist" medications, a weak antagonist or partial agonist (it has a "ceiling effect"; there is a plateau in maximal effect as contrasted with a full agonist wherein each increment in dose gives a greater effect).

Hydromorphone Hydromorphone is a more potent opioid analgesic than morphine. It is used for the treatment of moderate to severe pain.

Hydrocodone Hydrocodone is a prescription drug frequently prescribed for relatively minor pain (such as dental pain) or cough. It is often used in combination with acetaminophen; thus, there can be hepatotoxicity associated with its abuse

Methadone Methadone is a synthetic long-acting full μ-opioid agonist. It was developed in Germany by Bayer during the World War II and was first used to provide pain relief. While is continues to be used as an analgesic, it is now used primarily as a maintenance treatment for opioid dependence. Pure methadone is a white crystalline powder. When it is used to treat opioid dependence, the powder is dissolved in a fruit-flavored drink, which is usually taken orally once a day.

Levo-alpha-acetylmethadol Levo-alpha-acetylmethadol (LAAM) is a synthetic, longer-acting (48-hour) congener of methadone that also is orally effective. There are concerns that LAAM can cause prolonged QTc intervals and cardiac arrest. This led to a black-box warning being added to the product label. LAAM remains approved for humans in the United States. However, at this time, no company is manufacturing LAAM.

Buprenorphine Buprenorphine (alone and in combination with naloxone) was approved in 2002 by the FDA as an office-based sublingual treatment for opioid dependence. At the same time, buprenorphine was reclassified by the Drug Enforcement Administration (DEA) from a Schedule V to a Schedule III drug. Buprenorphine is a partial agonist with a ceiling effect (i.e., there is a plateau in maximal effect versus that observed with the use of a pure agonist).

EPIDEMIOLOGY OF OPIOID ABUSE AND ADDICTION

The United States represents <5% of the world's population but consumes approximately 80% of the world's opioid supply. According to the 2006 National Survey on Drug Use and Health (NSDUH), between 1999 and 2006, the number of persons aged 12 and older illicitly using prescription pain relievers in the month prior to being surveyed increased from 2.6 million in 1999 to 5.2 million in 2006.

It is estimated that individuals with opioid dependence have a mortality rate 10 to 30 times higher than those who do not use heroin. The main causes of death are HIV/AIDS and overdose. Individuals on opioid replacement therapy (methadone or buprenorphine) have a 70% reduction in mortality compared with those who are not in treatment.

Summary Author: Christopher A. Cavacuiti
David A. Gorelick*

The Pharmacology of Cocaine, Amphetamines, and Other Stimulants

DEFINITION

Stimulants are a class of drugs that stimulate activity in the central and sympathetic peripheral nervous systems, chiefly by enhancing neurotransmitter activity at catecholaminergic synapses.

SUBSTANCES IN THE CLASS

Stimulants include both naturally occurring plant alkaloids, such as cocaine and ephedra, and more than a dozen synthetic compounds, such as the amphetamines and methylphenidate. Most stimulants are variants of the basic phenethylamine chemical structure. This structure is also found in the endogenous catecholamine neurotransmitters norepinephrine and dopamine.

HISTORY

Naturally occurring plant alkaloids have been used for their central nervous system (CNS) stimulant properties for thousands of years. Chinese medicine has used the herbal preparation ma-huang (ephedra) for at least 5,000 years. Chewing of coca leaves has been prevalent in the Andean regions of South America for at least 2,000 years.

In 1860, a German graduate student, Albert Niemann, isolated cocaine as the active ingredient of coca leaf. A nonalcoholic beverage (containing 4.5 mg of cocaine per 6 oz) was introduced in 1886 and quickly became one of the world's most popular soft drinks: Coca-Cola.

With widespread use of cocaine came increasing reports of adverse effects. The first report of cocaine-associated cardiac arrest and stroke was published in 1886. By 1903, cocaine had been removed from Coca-Cola. In 1914, the Harrison Narcotic Act banned cocaine from over-the-counter (OTC) medications, beverages, and foods in the United States, restricting its use to prescription drugs.

Synthetic stimulants first appeared with the synthesis of amphetamine in 1887 (by Edeleau) and of methamphetamine in 1919. During World War II, amphetamine was widely used by the Allied and Axis countries to enhance the performance of troops and factory workers.

EPIDEMIOLOGY

There are substantial geographic and sociodemographic differences in the epidemiology of stimulant use. In 2005, there were an estimated 14.3 million cocaine users worldwide, representing 0.3% of the 15- to 64-year-old population. Almost half (44%) were in North America (6.4 million; 2.2% prevalence), and about one quarter (27%) were in Western and Central Europe (3.9 million, 1.2% prevalence). Central and South America (including the Caribbean) had 2.2 million users (0.8% prevalence). There is very little cocaine use in Eastern Europe, Africa, or Asia.

---

*Dr. Gorelick is supported by the Intramural Research Program, NIH, National Institute on Drug Abuse.

According to the National Survey on Drug Use and Health (NSDUH) data, cocaine is the second most widely used illegal drug in the United States, after marijuana. The 2006 NSDUH estimated that 35.3 million Americans (14.3% of the US population 12 years old or older) had used cocaine at some time during their lifetimes and 2.4 million (1.0%) had used cocaine within the preceding month. 20.1 million (8.2%) were nonmedical users of stimulants other than cocaine at some time during their lifetimes and 1.2 million (0.5%) were current users.

Cigarette smokers or heavy alcohol drinkers are each at least 10 times more likely to use cocaine than are nonsmokers or moderate (nonbinge) drinkers. Current cocaine users are twice as likely to have symptoms of depressive or anxiety disorders than are nonusers.

Stimulant use often is associated with adverse consequences. In the 2005 Drug Abuse Warning Network survey, cocaine was the drug associated most often with visits to hospital emergency departments, with 448,481 visits (30.9% of all drug-related visits), which is almost twice as often as the next most common drug, marijuana (16.7%).

High rates of stimulant abuse have been documented in persons involved with the criminal justice system. A 2002 national study of US inmates found that 20.7% reported using cocaine in the month before their offense and 10.6% had used cocaine at the time of their offense.

FORMULATIONS AND METHODS OF USE AND ABUSE

Plant-Derived Stimulants

Several naturally occurring, plant-derived stimulants are widely available for traditional oral use in many areas of the world. These include cocaine (in South America), ephedra (in North America and East Asia), khat (in East Africa and Arabia), and caffeine (most world regions). Traditional oral use generally adheres to certain cultural sanctions, involves lower potency and/or unpurified stimulants and a slow onset route of administration, and is therefore less often associated with abuse or dependence.

Cocaine Cocaine is a natural plant alkaloid. The leaves of the coca bush, *Erythroxylon coca*, contain 0.2% to 1% cocaine. The name was derived by combining the prefix "coca" with the standard alkaloid suffix -ine, forming *cocaine*. Coca bushes grow at higher altitudes in the Andean region of South America. Preparation of illicit cocaine begins with crushing the coca leaves and heating them in an organic solvent (often kerosene) to extract and partially purify the cocaine. After several more extraction and filtering steps, the coca paste (now 80%–90% pure) is heated in an organic solvent (often ether or acetone) with concentrated acid to convert it to salt form.

Forms of cocaine Cocaine exists in several chemical forms, having different routes of administration. However, regardless of the form of cocaine, the molecule itself exerts the same actions once it reaches the brain or other target organ.

Salts: The salt form of cocaine is a powder, usually cocaine hydrochloride. Cocaine salt is highly water soluble making it easy to dissolve for injection purposes and facilitating absorption across mucus membranes. Therefore, this form of cocaine is most commonly self-administered by snorting or injecting it.

Base: (aka freebase) The salt form of cocaine can be readily converted back to the water insoluble base form by heating it in an organic solvent at basic pH. The base has a relatively low melting point (98°C). Therefore, this form of cocaine is commonly self-administered by smoking it. Cocaine base is relatively insoluble in water, making it difficult to dissolve for injection purposes.

Crack cocaine: "Crack" is a street name for freebase cocaine reportedly derives from the crackling sound made when the impurities are heated during the smoking process.

Cocaine is legally available in the United States only as a 4% or 10% injectable solution (or powder for reconstitution) or viscous liquid for use as a local or topical anesthetic.

An estimated 530 to 710 metric tons of illegal cocaine entered the United States in 2006. The average wholesale (dealer) and retail (user) prices for cocaine in 2005 were $23 and $119 per gram.

Ephedra Ephedrine and pseudoephedrine are naturally occurring alkaloids that are found in several *Ephedraceae* species. Ephedra alkaloids are widely used in East Asia, Europe, and North America, and they have the same range of psychological and physiologic effects as do other CNS stimulants such as cocaine and amphetamines. However, Epedra products are often marketed at being safer than synthetic stimulants because they are "natural" or "herbal." Synthetic forms of ephedrine and pseudoephedrine are also commercially available. Ephedra use has been associated with severe cardiovascular and CNS effects, including death, leading to its banning from the US market in 2006.

Khat *Khat* is the common term for preparations of the *Catha edulis* plant, which is native to East Africa and the southern Arabian peninsula. Fresh khat leaves contain at least two stimulant alkaloids with phenethylamine chemical structures: cathinone (present at 1%–3%) and cathine (norpseudoephedrine). Pure cathinone is a Schedule I controlled substance; cathine is in Schedule IV. Khat use has been a widely accepted social custom for centuries; the leaves are chewed and kept in the cheek for several hours. Moderate use reduces fatigue and appetite. Compulsive use may result in manic behavior or psychotic symptoms such as paranoia or hallucinations. The extent of abuse or dependence is unclear.

Chemically similar to cathinone is the cathinone congener methcathinone (also known as ephedrone in Europe, or "MCat" [pronounced "em-cat"] on the street). It is clandestinely synthesized from ephedrine or pseudoephedrine. It is a Controlled Substances Act (CSA) schedule I drug in the United States and is widely abused in Russia and the Baltic area.

Synthetic Stimulants

More than a dozen synthetic stimulant medications are legally available in the United States, either by prescription (Table 10.1) or over the counter (Table 10.2).

Several of these stimulants are available in extended- or sustained release formulations. Sustained release versions of these stimulants have two theoretical advantages over conventional immediate release formulations:

1. Improved patient compliance and effectiveness because of longer duration of action
2. Reduced abuse liability because of slower onset of action and weaker peak subjective effects

Synthetic stimulants typically are abused by the oral or intravenous route. Amphetamines, especially highly pure crystallized methamphetamine ("ice"), may be used intranasally or smoked. Amphetamines, especially

TABLE 10.1	Stimulants Available by Prescription in the United States				
Drug	**Trade name**	**Street name**	**CSA schedule**	**Typical indications**	**Oral dose (mg/d)**
Amphetamine (as *d*-isomer or racemic mixture)	Adderall, Dexedrine, Dextrostat, generic	Amp, bennies, dex, black beauties	II	ADHD, Narcolepsy, weight control, depression[a]	2.5–60
Lisdexamfetamine (L-lysine-d-amphetamine)	Vyvanse	—	II	ADHD	30–70
Benzphetamine	Didrex	—	III	Weight control	25–150
Cocaine	—	Coke, crack, flake, snow	II	Local or topical anesthetic	—
Diethylpropion	Tenuate	—	IV	Weight control	75–100
Mazindol	Sanorex, Mazanor	—	IV	Weight control	1–3
Methamphetamine	Adipex, Desoxyn, Methedrine	Ice, meth, speed, crank, crystal	II	ADHD, Weight control	5–40 10–15
Methylphenidate (as *d*-isomer or racemic mixture)	Ritalin, Focalin, Concerta	Rits, Vitamin R	II	ADHD, narcolepsy	10–60 10–60
Phendimetrazine	Bontril, Plegine	—	III	Weight control	35–105
Phenmetrazine	Preludin	—	II	Weight control	25–75
Phentermine	Adipex-P, Fastin, Ionamin	—	IV	Weight control	15–90

ADHD, attention deficit/hyperactivity disorder; CSA, U.S. Controlled Substances Act.
[a]Not labeled for this indication by the U.S. Food and Drug Administration.

TABLE 10.2	Stimulants Available as OTC Preparations in the United States		
Drug	**Trade name**	**Indications**	**Typical oral dose (mg/d)**
Caffeine	(Various)	Weight control, alertness	50–250
Ephedrine	Marax, Quadrinal	Decongestant, bronchodilation	50–100
Phenylephrine	Comhist, Dristan, Neo-Synephrine	Decongestant	40–60
Pseudoephedrine	Sudafed, Sine-Aid	Decongestant	90–240
Propylhexedrine	Benzedrex, Dristan, Obesin	Decongestant, weight control	50–150

methamphetamine, usually are synthesized in clandestine laboratories. This can be done with standard chemical reactions applied to legally available precursors. For example, methamphetamine (desoxyephedrine) can be made by reducing ephedrine or pseudoephedrine. For this reason, retail purchases in the United States of products containing ephedrine or pseudoephedrine are limited to 3.6 g per day and 9 g per month and require photographic identification.

Most of these stimulants exist in two (or more) stereoisomer forms. The d- or S-(+) isomer generally has three to five times the CNS activity and about one third the half-life of the l- or R-(–) isomer. For example, d-methamphetamine is a potent CNS stimulant, whereas l-methamphetamine (l-desoxyephedrine) has been used as a decongestant (as in the Vicks nasal inhaler). Methylphenidate exists in four stereoisomeric forms, of which the d-threo enantiomer is the active one.

Clinical Uses

The clinical uses of prescription stimulants are listed in Table 10.1. There are very few long-term, controlled trial data on whether or not the medical use of stimulants at therapeutic doses in appropriately diagnosed patients leads to stimulant abuse or increases the risk of serious adverse events. Prospective, longitudinal studies in children receiving stimulant treatment for attention deficit/hyperactivity disorder (ADHD) found no increased risk of developing substance abuse.

Nonmedical Use, Abuse, and Dependence

Oral stimulants (both prescription and OTC) have been widely used in work, school, military, and sports settings, often without medical supervision, for their alerting, antifatigue, sleep-suppressing, and performance-enhancing properties.

While stimulants may differ in their potency and addiction liability, all stimulants have a potential for misuse, abuse, and dependence. Cocaine, amphetamine, and methamphetamine have high abuse potential, as reflected in their placement in Schedule II. Studies suggest that up to one in six persons who use cocaine and one in nine who use prescription stimulants for other than medical purposes will become dependent.

Twin studies suggest that there is a genetic influence both on initiation and use of stimulants and on stimulant abuse and dependence. Efforts to identify a specific gene or genes responsible for stimulant dependence have not been successful thus far.

Those stimulants that can be administered intravenously or smoked (as opposed to oral and intranasal routes) tend to be more reinforcing (and therefore have a higher risk of addiction) owing to their faster rate of drug delivery and faster onset of psychological effects.

Many stimulant users concurrently use CNS depressants such as benzodiazepines, alcohol, and opioids. Common examples include the concurrent intravenous use of cocaine plus heroin (termed *speedballing),* the combined use of oral amphetamine plus an oral opiate (such as codeine), and the combination of alcohol and cocaine. Studies suggest that the acute psychological effects of stimulants are somewhat enhanced with concurrent administration of a CNS depressant. Furthermore, the use of CNS depressant may ameliorate some of the unpleasant physiologic and psychologic effects of CNS stimulants (such as anxiety, paranoia, restlessness, hypervigilance, and tremor).

PHARMACOKINETICS

Absorption and Distribution

Route of administration has a major effect on the pharmacokinetic characteristics of stimulants. Smoked stimulants (such as cocaine base or methamphetamine) are rapidly absorbed through the lungs and probably reach the brain in 6 to 8 seconds, with a peak effect occurring within minutes of administration. Intravenous administration also produces peak brain uptake in 4 to 7 minutes.

Intranasal and oral stimulants have a slower absorption and onset of effect (30–45 minutes), a longer peak effect, and a more gradual decline from peak.

Metabolism

In humans, 95% of cocaine is metabolized by hydrolysis of ester bonds to benzoylecgonine (the primary urinary metabolite) and ecgonine methylester. This hydrolysis is catalyzed by the action of carboxylesterases in the liver and butyrylcholinesterase in the liver, plasma, brain, lung, and other tissues. The remaining 5% of cocaine is metabolized by CYP3A4.

Amphetamines are metabolized in the liver via three different pathways: deamination to inactive metabolites, oxidation to norephedrine and other active metabolites, and parahydroxylation to active metabolites. Amphetamine itself is the initial metabolite of methamphetamine.

Elimination

Stimulants and their metabolites are largely eliminated in the urine. It is benzoylecgonine (the primary urinary metabolite of cocaine), rather than the parent drug cocaine, that actually is measured in routine urine drug tests for cocaine.

Alkalinization of the GI tract or urine can increase GI absorption of amphetamines and reduce excretion to negligible levels. This fact is exploited by drug users who take large doses of sodium bicarbonate to prolong the action of amphetamines and reduce the amount present in the urine for detection by drug tests.

DRUG–DRUG INTERACTIONS

The primary drug interaction of stimulants that is of clinical concern is with other stimulants or with other medications that also enhance catecholamine activity. Such interactions risk overstimulation of the sympathetic nervous system, with possible cardiac arrhythmia, hypertension, seizure, cardiovascular collapse, and death. The major potential for interaction is presented by monoamine oxidase inhibitors (MAOIs), which are used as antidepressants. Potent prescription stimulants, such as amphetamine and methamphetamine, should not be used within 2 weeks of MAOI use. Stimulants should be used cautiously in conjunction with tricyclic antidepressants, many of which block presynaptic reuptake of catecholamines.

When cocaine is used in combination with alcohol, a new compound, cocaethylene, is formed by transesterification. Cocaethylene appears to produce a more intense and longer lasting feeling of euphoria than cocaine alone.

PHARMACODYNAMIC ACTIONS

Central Nervous System

Intoxication All stimulants produce a similar range of psychological, behavioral, and physiologic effects, with the intensity and duration depending on potency, dose, route of administration, and duration of use. The initial effects include increased energy, alertness, and sociability; elation or euphoria; and decreased fatigue, need for sleep, and appetite. Up to 40% of chronic stimulant users may have sleep disturbance and weight loss (due to appetite suppression). Up to 25% may experience severe paranoia and/or hallucinations.

Tactile hallucinations are especially typical of stimulant psychosis and include the sensation of something (e.g., insects) crawling under the skin (also referred to as delusional parasitosis or formication).

Physiologic effects include tachycardia, pupil dilation, diaphoresis, and nausea. Behavioral effects include restlessness, agitation, tremor, dyskinesia, and repetitive or stereotyped behaviors (also known as punding, tweeking, or being "hung up"). Common stimulant-induced motor stereotypes include picking at the skin or foraging for drug.

Individual differences in tolerance and sensitization to stimulants may account for the poor correlation between stimulant plasma concentrations and toxic effects. Fatal cases of amphetamine or cocaine intoxication may present with 100-fold differences in plasma stimulant concentration.

Chronic Effects   Chronic cocaine or amphetamine abuse is associated with cognitive impairment that may persist for at least several months of abstinence. Most affected are visuomotor performance, attention, inhibitory control, and verbal memory.

Chronic amphetamine or methamphetamine use can cause a psychotic syndrome that may persist for years after the last drug use, even in persons with no personal or family history of psychiatric disorder. Psychotic flashbacks have been reported in methamphetamine abusers up to 2 years after their last drug use.

Withdrawal   Stimulant withdrawal symptoms generally are the opposite of those associated with stimulant intoxication. Symptoms include depressed mood, anhedonia (inability to experience pleasure), fatigue, difficulty concentrating, increased total sleep and rapid eye movement sleep duration (but with poor sleep quality), and increased appetite. While the physiological features of stimulant withdrawal are generally mild and non–life-threatening, the feelings of despair and depression that accompany stimulant withdrawal can be profound and dangerous.

Behavioral Pharmacology   Animals allowed free access to stimulants often self-administer in a "binge-abstinence" pattern similar to the pattern often seen in humans. This pattern is marked by periods of high levels of drug intake (producing stereotyped behavior, hyperactivity, decreased eating, and little sleep), alternating with periods of abstinence, during which behavior returns to normal. Animals given unlimited access to stimulants may self-administer to the point of death during a binge period.

Other CNS Effects   Stimulant administration is associated with increased electroencephalographic activity, and is associated with seizures, even in persons without a preexisting seizure disorder. Cocaine and amphetamine use is associated with cerebral vasoconstriction, cerebrovascular atherosclerosis, cerebrovascular disease, and stroke.

Stimulant use is associated with a variety of movement disorders (including stereotyped behaviors, acute dystonic reactions, choreoathetosis, akathisia, buccolingual dyskinesias, and tardive dyskinesias), presumably as the result of increased dopamine activity in the basal ganglia and other brain areas that control movement.

Cardiovascular System

Stimulants act acutely on the cardiovascular system both directly (by increasing adrenergic activity at sympathetic nerve terminals) and via the CNS to increase heart rate, blood pressure, and systemic vascular resistance. Frequent cocaine users are up to seven times more likely to have a nonfatal heart attack than are nonusers. Cocaine use is also associated with cardiac arrhythmias (such as ventricular tachycardia or fibrillation) and sudden cardiac death. There is also an association with cardiomyopathy and myocarditis. Autopsy series of current cocaine users have found myocarditis in up to 20%.

Pulmonary   Smoked cocaine produces both acute and chronic pulmonary toxicity. Acute respiratory symptoms may develop in up to half of users within minutes to several hours after smoking. Chronic cocaine smoking has been associated in case reports with pulmonary and peripheral eosinophilia, interstitial pneumonitis, and bronchiolitis obliterans.

Renal   Acute renal failure can occur as a result of stimulant-induced renal ischemia or infarction, malignant hypertension, or rhabdomyolysis.

Head and Neck   Intranasal cocaine use ("snorting") is associated with chronic rhinitis, perforated nasal septum and nasal collapse, oropharyngeal ulcers, and osteolytic sinusitis.

Sexual Function   Stimulants are commonly thought of as an aphrodisiac, but chronic use usually impairs sexual function. Men may experience erectile dysfunction or delayed or inhibited ejaculation. Priapism is rare. Women may develop irregular menses.

Reproductive, Fetal, and Neonatal Health Prescription stimulants, including cocaine and amphetamines, are classified by the FDA in pregnancy category C, meaning that risk cannot be ruled out because human studies are lacking. Prenatal (in utero) exposure to cocaine, amphetamines, or methylphenidate has been associated with vaginal bleeding, abruptio placenta, placenta previa, premature rupture of membranes, decreased head circumference, low birth weight, tremulousness, irritability, poor feeding, and autonomic instability. The long-term effects of prenatal exposure to stimulants are unclear.

NEUROBIOLOGY

Mechanisms of Action

Neurotransmitters All stimulants act to enhance monoamine (dopamine, norepinephrine, and serotonin) activity in the central and peripheral nervous systems. Potent stimulants, such as cocaine, amphetamines, mazindol, and methylphenidate, do this indirectly by blocking and inhibiting membrane reuptake pumps (transporters) for monoamines. These effects result in more monoamines being available to cross the synaptic cleft and bind to postsynaptic monoamine receptors. Less potent stimulants (e.g., OTC decongestants) act directly by binding to and activating norepinephrine receptors.

Dopamine Several lines of evidence from animal and human studies suggest that it is the increased synaptic dopamine activity in the mesocorticolimbic reward circuit that primarily mediates the behavioral effects of stimulants. Experimental attempts to block the acute psychological effects of cocaine or amphetamine with antidopaminergic medications have not been successful. These failures may have been due to the inability of subjects to tolerate sufficient doses of medication to influence cocaine's effects.

Norepinephrine and Serotonin The strong correlation between the level of synaptic release of these neurotransmitters and the subjective euphoric effects in humans suggests that both norepinephrine and serotonin play a role in the psychological effects of stimulants. However, available evidence suggests that it is dopamine (rather than norepinephrine or serotonin) that is primarily responsible for the reinforcing effects of stimulants.

Endogenous Opiates Stimulants do not directly interact with opiate receptors but do influence endogenous opiate (endorphin, enkephalin) systems in the brain. A variety of neurotransmitters, including dopamine, have been demonstrated to enhance endogenous opiate release.

Glutamate The acute administration of cocaine or amphetamine increases glutamate release in the reward centers of the brain. A growing body of evidence suggests that drug-related environmental stimuli and cues can enhance glutamate transmission. This suggests that glutamate may play an important role in environmentally induced cravings and relapse.

Neuroadaptation Repeated exposure to stimulants results in two distinct neuroadaptations: sensitization (increased drug response) and tolerance (decreased drug response). The precise pharmacologic, neurobiologic, and behavioral factors that determine sensitization and tolerance are not well understood.

Sensitization The phenomenon whereby prior intermittent (rather than continuous) exposure to a drug results in an enhanced response to a later exposure. Sensitization is the opposite of tolerance and thus sometimes is termed *reverse tolerance.*

Tolerance Tolerance to the behavioral (including reinforcing and appetite-suppressing) effects of stimulants has been demonstrated after high-dose, frequent, or continuous administration. There is significant cross-tolerance among various stimulants but not between stimulants and other drug groups, such as opioids.

Neurotoxicity Positron emission tomography (PET) scanning of chronic stimulant users (particularly amphetamine or methamphetamine users) suggests that stimulant use can lead to long-term decreases of dopamine synthesis, down-regulation of dopamine transporter function, and decreased cell membrane dopamine transporter density. While some of these changes do appear to reverse with abstinence, abnormal dopamine function can still be found for at least 3 years after stimulants were last used. Studies on cocaine and methylphenidate suggest that these drugs do not produce appreciable neurotoxicity. Cocaine has caused DNA synthesis inhibition and cell death of brain neurons in rodents, but the clinical relevance of these findings is unknown.

Summary Author: Christopher A. Cavacuiti
Laura M. Juliano • Sergi Ferré • Roland R. Griffiths

The Pharmacology of Caffeine

Caffeine is a nonselective A_1 and A_{2A} adenosine receptor antagonist that produces mild central nervous system stimulation. Caffeine is the most widely used mood-altering drug in the world. In the United States, 87% of children and adults regularly consume foods and beverages containing caffeine. In the United States, coffee is second only after oil in total value of all imports. While caffeine is not highly associated with any life-threatening illnesses, it is not completely innocuous. The physiologic and psychologic effects of caffeine can cause or exacerbate a variety of medical and psychiatric conditions. The ubiquity of caffeine use can lead to an under appreciation of it consequences.

DRUGS IN THE CLASS

Caffeine is the common name for 1,3,7-trimethylxanthine. More than 60 types of caffeine containing plants have been identified, including coffee, tea, cola, cacao, guarana, and yerba maté.

History
Cultivation of tea in China, coffee in Ethiopia, and cacao pod in South America date back thousands of years. Numerous failed attempts to eliminate or suppress the use of caffeine-containing foods on the basis of political, religious, economic, or medical grounds have been documented worldwide (including the United States, Arabia, Turkey, England, France, and Prussia).

Therapeutic Uses
As a mild central nervous system stimulant, caffeine is widely used to increase energy. As a respiratory stimulant, caffeine is used to treat apnea in neonates and infants. Caffeine is used as an analgesic adjuvant to treat various kinds of pain including headache. Because of its lipolytic and thermogenic effects, caffeine is commonly used in weight loss preparations and nutritional supplements.

Epidemiology
More than 85% of children and adults in the United States consume caffeine on a regular basis. Mean daily intake of caffeine for adult caffeine consumers has been estimated to be about 280 mg in the United States. The highest caffeine consumption (i.e., 336 mg per day) is among males aged 35 to 54 years.

PHARMACOKINETICS

Absorption and Distribution
Caffeine is rapidly and completely absorbed after oral administration, with peak levels reached in 30 to 45 minutes. Caffeine is readily distributed throughout the body, with concentrations in blood correlating with those in saliva, breast milk, amniotic fluid, fetal tissue, semen, and the brain.

Metabolism
The primary metabolic pathways involve the cytochrome P450 liver enzyme system. Caffeine metabolism is complex, with >25 metabolites identified in humans. Over 80% of caffeine is metabolized to the active

metabolite paraxanthine, suggesting that this metabolite needs to be considered in our understanding of the clinical pharmacology of caffeine.

Elimination

On average, caffeine half-life is 4 to 6 hours; however, there are wide individual differences in rates of caffeine elimination, with half-lives varying more than a 10-fold range in healthy adults. Drugs or conditions that affect CYP450 metabolism can significantly alter caffeine elimination.

MECHANISMS OF ACTION

The primary cellular site of action of caffeine is the adenosine receptor. At the CNS level, adenosine functions primarily as a CNS depressant. More specifically, adenosine inhibits both presynaptic and postsynaptic striatal dopaminergic neurotransmission. Caffeine is structurally similar to adenosine and acts as a competitive A_1 and A_{2A} adenosine receptor antagonist. Caffeine produces a variety of effects that are opposite to the effects of adenosine (e.g., central nervous stimulation, vasoconstriction).

While caffeine's motor-activating and reinforcing effects are believed to be due to increased striatal dopamine release as described above, the effects of caffeine on sleep do not seem to be dopamine dependent and are thought to be related to caffeine's antagonist activity at sleep-promoting adenosine receptors capacity in the brainstem, basal forebrain, and hypothalamic areas.

A number of mechanisms seem to play a role in the development of caffeine tolerance. Chronic caffeine exposure leads to the upregulation of A_1-A_{2A} receptors with a lower affinity for caffeine. Chronic caffeine exposure also leads to a significant increase in plasma and extracellular concentrations of adenosine.

PHYSIOLOGIC EFFECTS

Cardiovascular

At moderate dietary dose levels, caffeine produces increases in blood pressure. Caffeine tends to have no effect or to reduce heart rate in humans.

Gastrointestinal

Caffeine stimulates gastric acid secretions and is a colonic stimulant, with caffeinated coffee producing colonic motor activity similar to that produced by a meal.

Renal and Urinary

Caffeine is a diuretic, increasing urine volume 30% or more for several hours after caffeine ingestion. Caffeine also increases detrusor pressure on the bladder, which can lead to increased urinary frequency and urgency, particularly among those with preexisting detrusor instability.

Respiratory

Caffeine is a respiratory stimulant and a bronchodilator at high doses.

Skeletal Muscle

Caffeine is ergogenic across a variety of exercise situations, and in particular during prolonged exercise, with activity potentially mediated via multiple mechanisms, including effects on muscle contractility, increased fat burning, and decreased glycogen burning.

Hormonal

Caffeine increases plasma epinephrine, norepinephrine, renin, and free fatty acids, particularly in nontolerant individuals. It also increases adrenocorticotropic hormone and cortisol. Caffeine increases insulin levels in healthy subjects and increases postprandial glucose and insulin responses among patients with type 2 diabetes who are habitual coffee drinkers.

EFFECTS ON PHYSICAL HEALTH

Although caffeine is not associated with any life-threatening illnesses, there are some medical conditions that may be adversely affected by caffeine. There is also evidence that caffeine may have some protective effects against other diseases.

Adverse Health Effects

Caffeine can influence heart rate variability, increase arterial stiffness, and raise both systolic and diastolic blood pressure by about 10 Hg.

Both caffeinated and decaffeinated coffees contain lipids that raise total and low-density lipoprotein cholesterol.

Although some early case control studies reported positive associations between caffeine consumption and certain types of cancer including pancreatic, bladder, and ovarian cancer, more recent and carefully controlled studies have not provided convincing evidence that caffeine consumption increases the risk of cancer development.

Coffee has been shown to exacerbate gastroesophageal reflux; however, it is not clear if it is due to caffeine or other coffee constituents.

Caffeine is a general risk factor for urinary incontinence. Caffeine increases urinary calcium excretion. Thus, it has been suggested that caffeine may negatively affect overall calcium balance and increase the risk of osteoporosis.

Caffeine readily crosses the placenta barrier and is distributed to all fetal tissues including the central nervous system. Some recent studies suggest that maternal caffeine use increases the risk of spontaneous abortion in a dose-dependent fashion. A review of research on caffeine and pregnancy concluded that reproductive-aged women should consume no >300 mg caffeine per day.

Health Protective Effects

Caffeine consumption is associated with a reduced risk of Parkinson disease, liver disease, and type 2 diabetes. The potential mechanisms are unclear and may be due to coffee constituents other than caffeine.

EFFECTS ON HUMAN PERFORMANCE

A large number of studies have examined the effects of caffeine on human performance. The most consistent generality to emerge is that caffeine reliably increases performance on task performance that has been degraded by fatigue (e.g., under conditions of sleep deprivation or prolonged vigilance).

Caffeine can enhance performance during prolonged (>30 minutes) aerobic exercise, can reduce ratings of perceived exhaustion, and can improve speed or power output in simulated race conditions. The impact of caffeine on short-term, high-intensity exercise has been more difficult to demonstrate.

SUBJECTIVE EFFECTS

At normal dietary doses caffeine typically produces a profile of positive subjective effects, including increased well-being, happiness, energy, arousal, alertness, and sociability. Physical dependence also increases the positive mood effects of caffeine, likely through suppression of low-grade withdrawal symptoms. However, positive mood effects also occur among nonhabitual users.

Negative subjective effects, such as increased anxiety, nervousness, jitteriness, tense negative mood, and upset stomach, are generally dose dependent and are more commonly seen with acute doses >200 mg. Individuals with panic disorder and generalized anxiety disorder tend to be particularly sensitive to the anxiogenic effects of caffeine.

REINFORCING EFFECTS

Caffeine is the most widely self-administered mood-altering drug in the world and, historically, repeated efforts to restrict or eliminate consumption of caffeinated foods have been unsuccessful. Caffeine reinforcement has been demonstrated in humans and to a limited extent in animals. Avoidance of caffeine withdrawal symptoms clearly plays a central role in the reinforcing effects of caffeine among regular caffeine consumers.

CAFFEINE TOLERANCE

Tolerance has been clearly demonstrated in both animals and humans. Tolerance develops to caffeine's effects on sleep, diuresis, salivation, metabolic rate, and blood pressure. In some cases, the tolerance to such effects is incomplete.

CAFFEINE INTOXICATION

Reports of caffeine intoxication can be found in the medical literature dating back to the 1800s. Unlike many other drugs of dependence, but similar to nicotine, the high-dose intoxicating effects of caffeine are not usually sought out by users.

Caffeine intoxication is included as a diagnosis in the *DSM-IV-TR*. Common features of caffeine intoxication include restlessness, nervousness (anxiety), insomnia, gastrointestinal disturbance, tremors, tachycardia, and psychomotor agitation.

Epidemiology

There have been very few studies examining the incidence and prevalence of caffeine intoxication in the general population. A telephone survey found that 7% of current caffeine users met *DSM-IV* criteria for caffeine intoxication.

IDENTIFICATION AND MANAGEMENT OF INTOXICATION

Many features of caffeine intoxication overlap with other medical and psychiatric disorders. Caffeine intoxication should be considered as a differential diagnosis when assessing possible intoxication and withdrawal from other drugs, medication side effects, psychiatric disorders (e.g., anxiety disorders, mania, sleep disturbances), and somatic disorders (e.g., arrhythmia, hyperthyroidism).

ANXIETY AND CAFFEINE

Acute doses of caffeine generally >200 mg can increase anxiety ratings in both individuals with anxiety disorders and those without. Higher doses can precipitate panic attacks. Genetic polymorphisms in the A_{2A} receptor gene have been associated with caffeine-induced anxiety response. It appears that some but not all individuals with high anxiety levels will naturally avoid caffeine, and it is possible that some individuals may fail to recognize the role that caffeine plays in their anxiety symptoms. Caffeine cessation has been shown to produce improvements in anxiety in some patients, with some requiring no additional treatment. Clinicians should consider advising anxiety patients to eliminate caffeine to rule out caffeine as a contributor to anxiety symptoms.

SLEEP AND CAFFEINE

Caffeine increases wakefulness and reduces decrements in performance under conditions of sleep deprivation. Caffeine's effects on sleep appear to be determined by a variety of factors including dose, the time between caffeine ingestion and attempted sleep, and individual differences in sensitivity or tolerance to caffeine.

Caffeine-Induced Sleep Disorder

Caffeine-induced sleep disorder is a DSM-IV-TR diagnosis characterized by a prominent disturbance of sleep etiologically related to caffeine use. There is little information about the incidence or prevalence of caffeine-induced sleep disorder. Patients who complain of sleep problems should be advised to eliminate caffeine as a first line of treatment.

CAFFEINE WITHDRAWAL

Thirteen symptoms of caffeine withdrawal have been judged to be reliable across carefully controlled studies (Table 11.1).

Time Course of Withdrawal

Onset usually occurs 12 to 24 hours after terminating caffeine intake. Peak withdrawal intensity usually occurs 20 to 51 hours after abstinence and lasts for 2 to 9 days.

Dosing Parameters

Caffeine withdrawal occurs after abstinence from a dose as low as 100 mg per day. Caffeine withdrawal also occurs after relatively short-term exposure to daily caffeine, such that significant withdrawal can occur after only 3 consecutive days of 300 mg per day caffeine.

TABLE 11.1	Empirically Validated Signs and Symptoms Resulting from Caffeine Abstinence

- Headache
- Tiredness/fatigue
- Drowsiness/sleepiness
- Decreased energy/activeness
- Decreased alertness/attentiveness
- Decreased contentedness/well-being
- Irritability
- Depressed mood
- Difficulty concentrating
- Muggy/foggy/not clearheaded
- Flulike symptoms
- Nausea/vomiting
- Muscle pain/stiffness

Source: Juliano LM, Griffiths RR. A critical review of caffeine withdrawal: empirical validation of symptoms and signs, incidence, severity, and associated features. *Psychopharmacology (Berlin)* 2004;176:1–29.

CAFFEINE DEPENDENCE

The ICD-10 recognizes a diagnosis of substance dependence due to caffeine, whereas the *DSM-IV-TR* does not. The rationale for excluding caffeine dependence from *DSM-IV-TR* was that although caffeine withdrawal had been documented, there was no available database pertaining to other important features of substance dependence such as inability to stop use and use despite harm. More recently, a number of studies have identified individuals who report problematic caffeine consumption and fulfill *DSM-IV-TR* criteria for substance dependence on caffeine. Caffeine dependence has also been shown to be associated with a history of alcohol abuse or dependence.

HERITABILITY OF CAFFEINE USE

Genetic factors account for some of the individual variability in the use and effects of caffeine. Genetic variability in the adenosine A_{2A} receptor gene has been shown to be associated with levels of caffeine consumption as well as differential effects of caffeine on measures of sleep and anxiety. Twin studies have shown elevated concordance rates for identical twins for caffeine consumption, heavy caffeine consumption, coffee and tea intake, caffeine tolerance, caffeine withdrawal, and caffeine intoxication with heritabilities ranging between 34% and 77%. There is also evidence that a common genetic factor may underlie caffeine, tobacco and alcohol use.

ASSOCIATIONS BETWEEN CAFFEINE AND OTHER DRUGS

Cigarette smokers consume more caffeine than nonsmokers, and twin and co-occurrence studies suggest genetic links between caffeine use and smoking. Heavy use and clinical dependence on alcohol is associated with heavy use and clinical dependence on caffeine. Animal studies show that caffeine increases acquisition of cocaine self-administration and potentiates the stimulant and discriminative stimulus effects of cocaine.

CHAPTER 12

Summary Author: Christopher A. Cavacuiti
John A. Dani • Thomas R. Kosten • Neal L. Benowitz

The Pharmacology of Nicotine and Tobacco

Tobacco use is the leading cause of death in the United States, and it is projected to be responsible for 10% of all deaths globally by 2015. Its use causes approximately 440,000 deaths each year in the United States and produces >$75 billion in direct medical costs annually.

DRUGS IN THE CLASS

Nicotine is a naturally occurring alkaloid that serves as an insecticide in many plants. There are two stereoisomers of nicotine. The (S)-nicotine form is the active isomer that binds to nicotinic acetylcholine receptors (nAChRs) and is found in tobacco.

METHODS OF ABUSE

Nicotine and the reinforcing sensory stimulation associated with tobacco use are responsible for the compulsive use of tobacco in the form of cigarettes, bidis, cigars, pipes, snuff, and chewing tobacco.

POTENTIAL THERAPEUTIC USES

Nicotine and its analogues are also being investigated as potential therapeutic agents for ulcerative colitis, Parkinson disease, Alzheimer disease, attention deficit/hyperactivity disorder (ADHD), schizophrenia, anxiety, depression, obesity, sleep apnea, and Tourette syndrome.

HISTORICAL FEATURES

Native American tribes cultivated used tobacco for thousands of years before the arrival of Europeans. Tobacco was first exported to Europe in 1607. The World Health Organization estimates that one third of the global adult population smokes, and this number continues to rise. Tobacco use is one of the few causes of death that is increasing worldwide.

PHARMACOKINETICS

Absorption, Distribution, Metabolism, and Elimination

The absorption of nicotine depends on its pH. It is the unprotonated (alkaline) form of nicotine that is most readily absorbed. Below pH 6, smoke contains <1% unprotonated (free) nicotine. As the pH rises, so does the proportion of unprotonated nicotine. At pH 7.4, 30% of the nicotine is unprotonated. However, because alkaline smoke is irritating to the airways, it is harsh and difficult to inhale.

The smoke from cigars and pipes has an alkaline pH and is therefore irritating to airways, but the alkaline pH allows pipe and cigar smoke to be readily absorbed through oral mucosa eliminating the need for pipe and cigar smoke to be deeply inhaled. In contrast, smoke from cigarettes has an acidic pH and therefore causes less airway irritation. Despite the acidic pH of cigarette smoke, the nicotine is nonetheless rapidly absorbed because

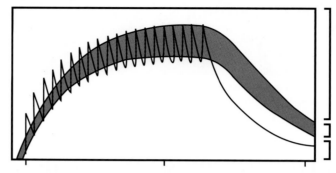

FIGURE 12.1   Assimilation of the plasma nicotine concentration throughout the day in relation to psychoactive effect.

of the huge surface area of the alveoli, and because once the nicotine containing aerosol droplets are mixed with the moist mucosa of the airways, the droplets are quickly buffered to a physiologic pH (~7.4), which facilitates transfer across cell membranes.

Inhaled nicotine avoids first-pass metabolism. It is quickly delivered from the large surface area of the alveoli to the arterial bloodstream and then to the tissues and the nicotinic receptors in the brain. Nicotine begins to reach the brain in approximately 20 seconds after inhalation. This initial rapid arrival of a large bolus of nicotine is believed to significantly contribute to nicotine reinforcement and the capacity of cigarettes to cause addiction.

Individual smokers seem to manipulate their nicotine intake to maintain a consistent level of nicotine from day to day. Smokers can control nicotine intake by altering their puff volume, frequency, intensity, and depth; this allows for very precise dose titration. Smokers also can increase smoke intake by blocking the ventilation holes of the filter with their fingers or their lips. Nicotine has a half-life of 2 hours or more with considerable accumulation of nicotine in the body tissues (including the brain) while smoking. During the day, nicotine accumulates over the hours that smokers are awake and persist for 6 to 8 hours after smoking ceases during sleep (Fig. 12.1).

Nicotine is extensively metabolized, primarily in the liver by CYP 2A6. The major metabolite (~80%) is cotinine. Nicotine and its metabolites are excreted in the urine.

Nicotine freely crosses the placenta and is found in breast milk.

Biochemical Assessment of Exposure to Nicotine and Tobacco

The 16-hour half-life of cotinine makes it useful as a plasma and salivary marker of nicotine intake. A cotinine value >14 ng/mL typically is taken to indicate smoking. Cotinine blood levels average about 250 to 300 ng/mL in regular smokers but range from 10 to 900 ng/mL.

While salivary and plasma cotinine are the most commonly used as biochemical markers of nicotine intake, other measures of smoking include expired carbon monoxide concentrations, blood carboxyhemoglobin concentrations, and plasma or salivary thiocyanate concentrations.

Drug Interactions with Nicotine and Tobacco

Smoking accelerates the metabolism of many drugs, particularly those metabolized by CYP1A2. Cigarettes appear to enhance the procoagulant effect of estrogens. For this reason, oral contraceptives are relatively contraindicated in women who smoke cigarettes. The stimulant actions of nicotine inhibit reductions in blood pressure and heart rate from beta-adrenergic blockers. Smoking results in less sedation from benzodiazepines and less analgesia from some opioids. Smoking also impairs the therapeutic effects of histamine H2-receptor antagonists using in treating peptic ulcers.

PHARMACOLOGIC ACTIONS CNS

Nicotine has a complex dose-response relationship. At lower doses (such as those achieved by smoking a cigarette), nicotine acts on the sympathetic nervous system to acutely increase blood pressure, heart rate, and cardiac output and to cause cutaneous vasoconstriction. At extremely high doses, nicotine causes hypotension and slowing of the heart rate, possibly via peripheral ganglionic blockade or vagal afferent nerve stimulation.

Psychoactive Effects

The primary CNS effects of nicotine in smokers are arousal, relaxation (particularly in stressful situations), and enhancement of mood, attention, and reaction time, with improvement in performance of some behavioral tasks. Some of this improvement results from the relief of withdrawal symptoms in addicted smokers, rather than as a direct enhancing effect.

Genetic Predisposition

Data from large twin registries suggest that about half of the total variance (range: 28%–84%) in smoking behavior can be attributed to genetic effects. Recent genome-wide association studies point to several genes that are promising signals for genetic determinants of nicotine dependence. Twin studies also support a model with common risk factors for both depression and cigarette smoking.

Psychiatric Comorbidity

Tobacco use is highly prevalent and more intense among psychiatric patients and among those who abuse other drugs. Rates of nicotine dependence are substantially higher among adults with ADHD (40%), schizophrenia (80%), and depression (55%) than in the general population (25%). These groups of patients have more difficulty in quitting compared with smokers without mental illness, often experiencing greater depression after stopping smoking than others.

Discrimination and Self-Administration

Animals will self-administer nicotine, but the environment, dose, and timing of the reinforcement schedule are more critical with nicotine than with other drugs of abuse such as cocaine. The tissue irritant effects of smoking may actually provide a form of "secondary reinforcement." Experienced smokers can use these effects to assess how much nicotine they are receiving when smoking Products that replicate the taste, flavor, throat, and chest sensations of cigarette smoking or the sensorimotor handling of a cigarette may reduce craving and some of the symptoms of nicotine withdrawal. Some of these products are being developed as smoking cessation aids.

Dependence, Tolerance, and Withdrawal

Studies suggest that the earlier the age at which use begins, the more difficult it is for the user to quit. In smokers who progress to chronic use, tolerance develops rapidly to the headache, dizziness, nausea, and dysphoria associated with the first cigarette. Conditioned cues (drug-associated memories) become established during the fine-tuned dosing of nicotine. Desiring a cigarette becomes associated with everyday events such as driving a car, finishing a meal, talking on the telephone, waking from sleep, and taking a break. A person who begins smoking a pack of cigarettes per day at age 17 would experience thousands of finely tuned doses of nicotine-conditioned internal emotional states and external cues by his or her mid-20s. The quantity and power of this conditioning is unique to cigarette smoking, and it is one of the reasons that smokers find cigarette smoking so difficult to quit.

There is a high rate of relapse among individuals who try to quit smoking. Population surveys consistently find that up to 75% of adults who smoke want to stop. About one third actually try to stop each year, but <3% succeed. Among persons who experience myocardial infarctions, laryngectomies, chronic obstructive pulmonary disease, and other serious medical sequelae of smoking, >50% revert to cigarette use within days or weeks after leaving the hospital.

Withdrawal

Tobacco use is sustained, in part, by the desire to prevent the symptoms of nicotine withdrawal. These symptoms vary, but include craving for nicotine, irritability and frustration or anger, anxiety, depression, difficulty concentrating, restlessness, and increased appetite. Performance measures such as reaction time and attention are impaired during withdrawal. The extinction of tobacco-associated conditioned cues requires months to years. There is an average weight gain of 3 to 4 kg during the first year after smoking cessation.

NEUROBIOLOGIC MECHANISMS OF ACTION

Acetylcholine (ACh) is the endogenous nAChR agonist. Nicotine is an exogenous agonist at nAChRs. Both ACh and nicotine stabilize the "open" conformation of the nAChR ion channel, which leads to a depolarization of cell membranes. The ubiquity and diversity of nAChRs allows them to play multiple, varied roles and to modulate the release of many neurotransmitters. The most widely observed synaptic role of nAChRs in the mammalian CNS is to influence neurotransmitter release. nAChR agonists such as nicotine boost the release of a variety of chemical messengers including epinephrine, norepinephrine, ACh, serotonin, GABA, glutamate, beta-endorphin, and dopamine. It is thought that increased dopamine levels in the reward center of the brain are primarily responsible for nicotine's addictive potential.

Several non-nicotinic chemicals in cigarette smoke (such as acetaldehyde and biogenic amines) reduce the activity of the enzymes monoamine oxidase A (MAO A) and monoamine oxidase B (MAO B). A main function of MAO is to metabolize catecholamines, including dopamine. Inhibition of MAO would be expected to result in higher brain levels of dopamine after exposure to nicotine. This MAO inhibition may play a role in making nicotine more rewarding and increase the likelihood of addiction. In addition, given that medications that inhibit MAO have antidepressant action, smoking-induced inhibition of monoamine oxidase might contribute to the perceived benefit of smoking by some depressed patients.

SYSTEMIC TOXICITY

Particulate and Gaseous Components of Tobacco Smoke

Tobacco smoke is composed of >500 gaseous compounds and about 3,500 particulate substances. Available evidence suggests it is not nicotine, but these other particulate and gaseous components of tobacco smoke that are primarily responsible for human morbidity and mortality.

Cardiovascular, Pulmonary, and Oncologic Toxicities

Smokers are exposed to about 4,000 different chemicals, including at least 50 known carcinogens. Oxidant chemicals are primarily responsible for endothelial dysfunction, platelet activation, thrombosis, and coronary vasoconstriction. Cigarette smoking causes an imbalance between proteolytic and antiproteolytic forces in the lung and heightens airway responsiveness.

Other Physiologic Effects and Toxicities

Cigarette smoking is associated with skin changes, including yellow staining of fingers, vasospasm and obliteration of small skin vessels, precancerous and squamous cell carcinomas on the lips and oral mucosa, and enhanced facial skin wrinkling.

Cigarette smoking in women is associated with lower levels of estrogen, earlier menopause, and increased risk of osteoporosis. In men, smoking may impair penile erection. Because the prevalence of erectile dysfunction in former smokers is no different from that in individuals who never smoked, erectile dysfunction is believed to improve with smoking cessation.

Smoking increases the risk of nuclear sclerosis, macular degeneration, and cataracts.

Nicotine causes both appetite suppression and an increase in metabolic rate. Smokers weigh an average 2.7 to 4.5 kg less than nonsmokers.

Nicotine increases lipolysis and releases free fatty acids. This could contribute to the increase in very low-density lipoprotein and low-density lipoprotein and the decrease in high-density lipoprotein seen in smokers.

Cigarette smoking is associated with the occurrence and delayed healing of peptic ulcers.

Tobacco and Pregnancy

Smoking during pregnancy nearly doubles the relative risk of having a low birthweight infant; the relative risks of spontaneous abortion and perinatal and neonatal mortality are increased by about one third.

Secondhand Smoke

Exposure to secondhand smoke (SHS) is causally associated with acute and chronic coronary heart disease, lung cancer, nasal sinus cancer, and eye and nasal irritation in adults. SHS is causally associated with asthma, chronic respiratory symptoms, and acute lower respiratory tract infections such as bronchitis and pneumonia in children. SHS also is causally associated with low birthweight and sudden infant death syndrome in infants.

More than 95% of SHS-exposed office workers exceeded the significant risk level for heart disease mortality and >60% exceeded the significant risk level for lung cancer mortality established by the Occupational Safety and Health Administration. The annual mortality attributable to SHS between 1995 and 1999 was estimated at 39,060 deaths.

Morbidity and Mortality

The cumulative result of these health effects is that each pack of cigarettes sold in the United States costs the nation an estimated $7.18 in medical care expenditures and lost productivity. Smoking is a leading cause of preventable death in the United States, accounting for an estimated 402,374 premature deaths annually between 1995 and 1999. On average, adult men and women smokers lost 13.2 and 14.5 years of life, respectively.

Tobacco and Other Addictions

There is a strong correlation between smoking and alcohol abuse. More severely dependent drinkers smoke more and are less likely to quit. Smoking and heavy drinking, in combination, are associated with substantially increased rates of oral and esophageal cancers.

Benefits of Cessation

The good news is that smoking cessation has benefits for smokers of all ages. The immediately decreased risk of cardiovascular death in those who stop smoking may reflect a decrease in blood coagulability, improved tissue oxygenation, and reduced predisposition to cardiac arrhythmias. Among former smokers, the reduced risk of death compared with continuing smokers begins shortly after quitting and continues for at least 10 to 15 years. After 10 to 15 years' abstinence, the risk of all-cause mortality returns nearly to that of persons who never smoked.

Summary Author: Christopher A. Cavacuiti
Sandra P. Welch

The Pharmacology of Cannabinoids

DRUGS IN THE CLASS

Tetrahydrocannabinol (THC), the major psychoactive ingredient in marijuana, first was isolated and purified in 1965. The term "cannabinoid" is now used for all compounds that are structurally related to THC. More than 400 chemicals are synthesized by the hemp plant, approximately 60 of which are cannabinoids. The first cannabinoid receptors were discovered in the 1980s, which in turn stimulated the search for endogenous ligands for cannabinoid receptors. Natural cannabinoid receptor ligands include arachidonoylethanolamide (also known as anandamide or AEA), 2-arachidonoylglycerol (2-AG), noladin ether, virodhamin, and N-arachidonoyldopamine. There are two known cannabinoid receptor subtypes, CB1 and CB2.

HISTORY

The use of cannabis dates back over 12,000 years. Cannabis use is believed to have started in central Asia and continued to flourish in Southeast Asia and India. The euphoric properties were discovered in India around 2000 BC. Cannabis was cultivated early in American history for its fiber. Recreational use of cannabis began to surge in the 1930s during the Prohibition Era. A dramatic increase in cannabis use was observed during the 1960s. Cannabis was placed in Schedule 1 of the Controlled Substances Act in 1970.

EPIDEMIOLOGY

Marijuana remains the nation's most commonly used illicit drug. The National Survey on Drug Use and Health 2006 report indicates that 44% of males and 35% of all females studied have used marijuana at least once in their life time.

According to the Drug Abuse Warning Network, marijuana reports were the second most frequently recorded major substance of abuse (excluding alcohol). There is increasing consumption in South America, and expanding markets in Western and Eastern Europe, as well as in Africa.

THERAPEUTIC USE

A minimum of 21 therapeutic potentials for cannabinoids are under investigation. The most intense interest has been directed toward the prevention of weight loss in wasting illnesses (such as AIDS), management of pain (especially neuropathic pain), prevention of emesis, control of glaucoma, and control of movement disorders. The use of smoked cannabis remains both politically and scientifically controversial although some studies of smoked cannabis are under way in the United States. The potential for development of alternative methods of drug delivery using either pure THC or one of the newer THC derivatives may obviate the problems and the controversial nature of the use of the smoked plant material.

Studies demonstrate that THC (in smoked form as well as other forms) significantly decreases neuropathic pain in HIV patients. Sativex (a 1:1 mixture of THC and cannabidiol) has been approved by Health Canada. It shows promise in treatment of numerous types of neurologic pain. The indicated use for Sativex at present is as an adjunct for neuropathic pain in multiple sclerosis patients and intractable pain in cancer patients.

In addition, synthetic THC (dronabinol, Marinol) is available, as is nabilone, a synthetic cannabinoid which mimics the main ingredient of marijuana (THC), but produces minimal euphoria. Nabilone is used therapeutically as an antiemetic, appetite stimulant, and as an adjunct analgesic for neuropathic pain. In Canada, the United States, the United Kingdom, and Mexico, nabilone is marketed as Cesamet. Both dronabinol and nabilone are labeled as Schedule III preparations.

Antiemetic Effect

Two oral formulations described previously, dronabinol (synthetic THC) (Marinol) and nabilone (Cesamet), are approved by the FDA for use in emesis refractory to conventional antiemetic therapy and as an appetite stimulant in patients with AIDS wasting or cancer.

Appetite Stimulation and Cachexia

The cannabinoid effect most commonly discussed is the effect on appetite. Smoked cannabis is well known to stimulate appetite. AIDS patients have lobbied to make cannabis available to those suffering from cachexia, the body wasting resulting from HIV infection.

Anticonvulsant Effect

Cannabis's therapeutic potential as an anticonvulsant was shown in the 1940s when children, poorly controlled on conventional anticonvulsant medication, were improved after the use of cannabis. Recently, cannabidiol (a natural component of cannabis with practically no THC-like psychoactivity) has been shown to have anticonvulsant effect in children who are refractory to other therapies.

Neurologic and Movement Disorders

There are numerous anecdotal reports that smoked cannabis is effective in relieving spasticity arising from multiple sclerosis and spinal cord injury. However, there have been few controlled studies comparing the effectiveness of either cannabis or THC with other therapies.

Analgesia

A variety of pharmacologic, anatomic, and electrophysiologic investigations indicate the CB1 receptor system plays a fundamental role in regulating pain. There is also increasing evidence that the CB2 receptor is a critical component of inflammatory pain. In addition, combination cannabinoid/opioid treatment produces effective antinociception with reduced risk of developing opioid tolerance or dependence.

Glaucoma

Although there is some variability among studies, most reveal that smoking cannabis lowers intraocular pressure to a significant degree. There is no evidence that cannabis or THC is more effective than other agents in controlling glaucoma or that it is effective in patients refractory to current therapies. One of the major drawbacks of cannabis is that it has to be smoked at relatively short intervals to depress intraocular pressure. There is now a topical preparation of cannabis, but its effectiveness remains controversial.

ABSORPTION AND METABOLISM

Preparations

The concentration of THC varies among the three most common forms of cannabis: marijuana, hashish, and hash oil. Marijuana is prepared from the dried flowering tops and leaves of the harvested plant. THC concentrations in marijuana leaves range from 0.5% to 5%. The flowering tops from unfertilized female plants may have THC concentrations of 7% to 14%. Hashish, dried cannabis resin and compressed flowers, has a 2% to 8% THC content. Hash oil, obtained by extracting THC from hashish (or marijuana) with an organic solvent, is a highly potent substance with between 15% and 50% THC concentration.

Kinetics

The most common route of administration is smoking marijuana as a hand-rolled "joint," the size of a cigarette or larger, often with tobacco added to assist burning. A typical joint contains between 0.5 and 1.0 g of cannabis varying in THC content between 5 and 150 mg (i.e., typically between 1% and 15%). The actual amount of THC delivered in the smoke has been estimated at 20% to 70%. Only a small amount of smoked cannabis (e.g., 2 to 3 mg of available THC) is required to produce a brief, pleasurable "high" for the occasional user. A water pipe known as a "bong" is a popular implement for all cannabis preparations because the water cools the hot smoke and loss of the drug through side stream smoke is decreased. Smokers generally inhale and hold their breath, which increases absorption of THC by the lungs.

Marijuana and hashish may also be taken orally via food products. However, the onset of the psychoactive effects is slow (about an hour) and absorption is erratic.

THC is metabolized to the active metabolite, 11-OH-THC, which is unlikely to contribute significantly to THC's pharmacologic effects because it is rapidly converted to conjugated 11-*nor*-9-carboxy-THC, which is inactive but serves as the primary urinary marker for detecting cannabis use. Because THC metabolites are lipid soluble, significant amounts of THC can be deposited in the fatty tissues of chronic THC users, which can lead to positive urine drug screens for weeks to months after THC use is discontinued.

PHARMACOLOGIC ACTIONS

Psychomotor Effects

Marijuana use leads to impaired judgment, perceptual distortions, slowed reaction time and information processing; impaired perceptual-motor coordination and motor performance; and impaired short-term memory, reduced attention, and slowed time perception. There is an additive effect of marijuana and alcohol on performance tasks such as driving.

Behavioral Effects

Some reviews warn that cannabis use may result in "amotivational symptoms," whereas others find no differences in motivation in cannabis users but do report a significant effect on general health and well being proposed to account for the motivational effects observed. Compared with light THC using controls, heavy users had significantly lower educational achievement, lower income, and a subjective self-assessment of impaired cognitive function, social life, and health. THC users also are at increased risk of quitting high school and have increased job turnover. The causal relationship between cannabis use and these behavioral effects is unclear. Most researchers have not been able to definitively isolate the effects of THC due to confounding variables such as individual characteristics and/or social surroundings. In addition, the effects of THC are difficult to analyze because many THC users have a history of polysubstance use.

Cognitive Effects

Marijuana use is associated with impairments in memory, attention, goal-directed activities, and integration of complex information. Cannabis users show persistent deficits in specific cognitive functions beyond the period of acute intoxication. The longer that cannabis is used, the more pronounced is the cognitive impairment.

MECHANISMS OF ACTION

The effects of THC are due to both peripheral and CNS activity. Behavioral effects are characterized at low doses as a mixture of depression and stimulation and, at higher doses, as predominantly CNS depression.

Neurobiology: Cannabinoid Receptors

Δ^9-THC is the prototypical cannabinoid and major psychoactive component in marijuana. The pharmacologic activity of Δ^9-THC is stereoselective, with the (–)-trans isomer having 6 to 100 times more potency than the (+)-trans isomer. Available evidence suggests that the main pharmacologic responses to Δ^9-THC, as well as the addictive properties of cannabinoids, are almost completely mediated by the CB1 (not the CB2) receptor.

Endocannabinoids

The behavioral effects of anandamide (the first endocannabinoid discovered) are comparable to those of other psychoactive cannabinoids, and cross-tolerance with other cannabinoids has been demonstrated.

ADDICTION LIABILITY

In animal studies, marijuana is self-administered and acts via reward neuroanatomy similar to those of other drugs of abuse. The self-administration of THC can be abolished by the administration of the CB1 antagonist

SR141716A. Thus, as with many other pharmacologic effects of THC, the abuse potential appears at this point to be mediated by CB1 receptor activation.

Interactions with Other Drugs of Abuse

The "Gateway drug theory" suggests that cannabis use increases the probability that users will eventually use "harder" drugs. While cannabis use typically precedes involvement with other drugs, there is no scientific evidence to suggest a neurobiological "gateway" effect of cannabis smoking. Such an effect may be due to the increased opportunity of cannabis users to associate with users of other types of drugs or the group peer pressure to use other drugs.

A combination of THC and alcohol in humans may result in increased levels of THC because of ethanol-induced increases in THC absorption resulting in enhanced subjective effects on mood. The chronic administration of THC may produce sensitization to the effects of amphetamine and heroin.

Tolerance

Tolerance has been demonstrated to develop to a variety to cannabinoid effects including antinociception, anticonvulsant activity, depression of locomotor activity, hypothermia, hypotension, corticosteroid release, and ataxia. The precise mechanism of the development of tolerance is unknown. However, studies have shown that chronic cannabinoid exposure leads to down-regulation of the CB1 receptor occurs in all CB1 receptor–containing brain regions.

Dependence

Both the DSM-IVTR and the World Health Organization recognize cannabis dependence. The risk of lifetime cannabis users becoming dependent on cannabis is approximately 9%.

Withdrawal

Marijuana abstinence includes effects that are typically the opposite of those produced by the drug, such as insomnia, anorexia, anxiety, irritability, depression, and tremor. The predominant abstinence symptoms are behavioral and affective symptoms. Relapse rates following cannabis withdrawal are higher than for many other drugs of abuse.

TOXICITY/ADVERSE EFFECTS

Intoxication

Marijuana users frequently report euphoria, hunger, and relaxation and less often, panic, anxiety, nausea, and dizziness. In rare instances, marijuana can increase paranoia and panic attacks at doses of 20 mg or higher. These effects are most often reported by naive users or patients receiving THC therapeutically who are unfamiliar with the drug's effects.

Psychopathology

Numerous large prospective, longitudinal studies in humans suggest that the use of cannabis increases the risk for schizophrenia, worsens symptoms, and is associated with a poorer prognosis. In addition, persons with a genetic vulnerability to psychoses, or having had previous psychotic episodes, as well as those who initiate cannabis use in early adolescence, are particularly prone to the development of schizophrenia. The use of cannabis has been shown to produce a nearly threefold increased risk of psychotic illnesses. The causal relationship between cannabis use and schizophrenia is unclear.

There is also a correlation between cannabis use and other affective disorders including depression and suicidal ideation. As with schizophrenia, the causal relationship between cannabis use and these affective disorders is unclear.

Effects on Major Organ Systems

Respiratory One of the major adverse health effect associated with marijuana smoking is damage to the respiratory system. Many of the same mutagens and carcinogens in nicotine cigarettes are found in marijuana smoke. However, clinical and epidemiologic evidence linking marijuana smoking to chronic obstructive pulmonary disease or respiratory cancer is equivocal.

Immunologic The existence of the CB2 receptor on cells of the immune system, bone, and in the CNS has led to the hypothesis that the cannabinoid system plays a significant role in immune modulation. Cannabinoids appear to cause immune suppression. Evidence suggests cannabinoids may decrease inflammation but could also be accompanied by an increased risk of viral infections. Of importance in humans was an observed increase in mortality of HIV-positive cannabis users.

Cardiovascular Both CB1 and CB2 receptors have been implicated in a number of cardiovascular processes, including vasodilation, cardiac protection, modulation of the baroreceptor reflex in the control of systolic blood pressure, and inhibition of endothelial inflammation and the progress of atherosclerosis. Marijuana increases heart rate and produces orthostatic hypotension. Endocannabinoids may regulate platelet function and possibly have a role in thrombogenesis.

Liver Considerable experimental evidence indicates that cannabinoid receptors play a crucial role in the pathogenesis of a variety of conditions related to liver diseases. Daily cannabis use is associated with liver steatosis and is a predictor of progressive liver fibrosis. Cannabis users metabolize and activate or inactivate drugs more slowly than normal.

*Endocrine*Virtually no hormonal system remains unaffected by activation of cannabinoid receptors. Effects of cannabinoids include inhibitory effects on pituitary lutenizing hormone, prolactin, and growth hormone and with little effect on the secretion of follicle-stimulating hormone. Cannabinoids have been shown to inhibit growth hormone secretion because of stimulation of somatostatin release. There are no data regarding the effect of cannabinoids on thyroid function in humans. THC induces ACTH and corticosterone secretion.

Reproductive Marijuana can disrupt the female reproductive system and induce galactorrhea. It is thought that endocannabinoids may play a role in the development and implantation of the embryo (by synchronizing the developmental stage of the embryo to the receptive stage for implantation in the uterus). Studies of smoking marijuana during pregnancy are unclear as to effects on the fetus because of "polypharmacy" (use of several drugs in combination) that is often observed with marijuana smokers. The lipid solubility of THC allows for rapid transit to the fats in breast milk, where it has been shown to accumulate and be passed to the newborn. In animal models, THC reduces the secretion of testosterone, and sperm production, motility, and viability, but effects in human males are not conclusive.

CHAPTER 14

Summary Author: Christopher A. Cavacuiti
Richard A. Glennon

The Pharmacology of Classical Hallucinogens and Related Designer Drugs

Hallucinogens are agents that, typically on ingestion of a single dose, consistently produce alterations in thought, mood, and perception; produce minimal autonomic side effects and craving; and fail to produce excessive stupor or central stimulation. This broad classification encompasses agents with varied chemical structures that can elicit varied pharmacologic effects.

The *classical* (aka *serotonergic* or *arylalkylamine*) *hallucinogens* are a subclass of the larger family of hallucinogens. Classical hallucinogens are a very large class of agents (numbering in the hundreds) that possess an arylalkylamine (i.e., indolealkylamine or phenylalkylamine) structure. In fact, classical hallucinogens are the single largest category of abusable drugs.

Not all arylalkylamines are hallucinogenic; some are devoid of this action, some are CNS stimulants, and yet others are empathogens with or without hallucinogenic character.

Different classical hallucinogens may not produce identical effects, but what they do have in common (with the exception of the harmala derivatives) is the ability to bind at 5-HT2A serotonin receptors.

Structural modification of arylalkylamines has resulted in the appearance of a variety of designer drugs on the clandestine market, and many, many more are theoretically possible. The most popular of the so-called designer drugs is methylenedioxymethamphetamine (MDMA). MDMA is not considered to be a classical hallucinogen or a CNS stimulant; it is usually referred to as an "empathogen" with some CNS stimulant properties.

HISTORICAL

Evidence suggests use of mescaline-containing plants >5,000 years ago, and mescaline was one of the first (classical) hallucinogens to be studied in depth because of its early identification and synthesis at the beginning of the 20th century. It was not until the 1940s that lysergic acid diethylamide (LSD) was accidentally discovered by Albert Hofmann, and its incredible potency realized. Interestingly, these two agents represent extremes in potency with LSD being >1,000 times more potent than mescaline. Popular interest in exploring these "mind-altering" substances or psychedelics for religious, artistic, and recreational purposes rose during the 1960s. Subsequently, clinical studies with hallucinogens became unpopular, and the Controlled Substances Act (1970) placed restrictions and prohibitions on human investigations with such substances. Since that time, few new human studies have been sanctioned, whereas, at the same time, the list of agents has grown exponentially. Now that human evaluations are once again being conducted, it is anticipated that the gap between the extensive amount of currently available animal data and the paucity of human studies will be bridged.

DRUGS IN THE CLASS

Classical hallucinogens, the indolealkylamines and the phenylalkylamines, are collectively referred to as *arylalkylamines*. Not all arylalkylamines are hallucinogenic and most of these agents have not been thoroughly investigated in humans. All have been shown to bind at 5-HT2 serotonin receptors and all (except certain β-carboline derivatives) have been demonstrated to behave as 5-HT2 receptor agonists or partial agonists.

Common drugs in the arylalkylamine class include LSD, mescaline (a constituent of the peyote cactus), 1-(2,5-dimethoxy-4-methylphenyl)-2-aminopropane (DOM), psilocybin (the active ingredient in various mushroom species), and harmaline. Certain so-called designer drugs (including 3,4-methylenedioxyamphetamine [MDA] and 3,4-methylenedioxymethamphetamine [MDMA], commonly known as ecstasy) are structurally related to these agents.

Indolealkylamines

N-Alkyltryptamines (Such as N,N-dimethyltryptamine (DMT), Psilocin, Psilocybin, and Constituents of "Shrooms")
DMT is considered the prototype of this subclass of agents and is the agent that has been most thoroughly investigated. DMT is a naturally occurring substance but is readily synthesized in the laboratory. Its actions are characterized by a rapid onset (typically <5 minutes) and short duration of action (about 30 minutes). Like some other members of this family, it is not orally active but generally is administered by inhalation, by smoking, and—less frequently—by injection.

Psilocin is 4-hydroxy DMT. Psilocin and its phosphate ester, psilocybin, are widely found in certain species of mushrooms and have given rise to the terms *shrooms* and *shrooming*.

α-Alkyltryptamines
In general, α-methyltryptamines, where they have been investigated, are somewhat more potent than their corresponding DMT counterparts. Otherwise, their structure–activity relationships (SARs) are similar.

Ergolines or Lysergamides (LSD, "Acid," "Blotter")
(+)LSD is perhaps the best known, and one of the most potent, of the classical hallucinogens. Although LSD itself is not naturally occurring, many related ergolines and synthetic precursors are found in nature. Its actions in humans can be divided into three major categories: perceptual (altered shapes and colors, heightened sense of hearing), psychic (depersonalization, visual hallucinations, alterations in mood and sense of time), and somatic (nausea, blurred vision, dizziness). In terms of overall principal effects, there seem to be few qualitative differences between those produced by LSD, psilocybin, and mescaline.

β-Carbolines (Harmaline, Harmine)
The β-carbolines are referred to as "harmala alkaloids." There have been very few studies with individual β-carbolines, especially under carefully controlled clinical settings. The most commonly occurring β-carbolines are harmine, harmaline, and tetrahydroharmine. Several are naturally occurring in South American plants; for example, β-carbolines are found in certain vines and lianas (e.g., *Banisteriopsis caapi*). In the Old World, β-carbolines are found as constituents of Syrian Rue (*Pegnum harmala*).

A number of traditional cultures have developed ceremonial harmala alkaloid concoctions and there is little question that these plant preparations are psychoactive. However, the mechanism of action of harmala alkaloids remains controversial. The plant preparations usually consist of admixtures in which indolealkylamines such as DMT or 5-OMe DMT sometimes have been identified. Some β-carbolines possess activity as monoamine oxidase (MAO) inhibitors, and it has been suggested that the MAO inhibitory effect of the β-carbolines simply potentiates the effect of any indolealkylamine hallucinogen present in the admixture by interfering with its metabolism. Over the past decade or so, β-carbolines have begun to make an appearance on the clandestine market, where they are often referred to as *fantasy-enhancing agents*.

Phenylalkylamines

Phenylethylamines (Mescaline, Peyote)
Phenylethylamines and phenylisopropylamines, collectively referred to as *phenylalkylamines*, represent the largest group of classical hallucinogens. Phenylethylamines and phenylisopropylamines are structurally very similar. Phenylisopropylamines are phenylethylamines that have been structurally altered through the introduction of an α-methyl group and by deletion or rearrangement of the position of its methoxy groups. These changes make phenylisopropylamines more lipophilic (enhancing onset of acting) and reduce susceptibility to metabolism (enhancing potency). Phenylethylamine hallucinogens typically produce behavioral effects that are similar to those of their corresponding phenylisopropylamines, but usually are severalfold less potent.

Certain hallucinogenic phenylisopropylamines are described as possessing some stimulant character, which can be minimized or altogether absent in the corresponding phenylethylamines. One of the best-recognized phenylethylamine hallucinogens is mescaline. It is a constituent of the peyote (and other) cactus. Because it is one of the oldest investigated hallucinogens, mescaline often serves as a standard and the potencies of other agents are compared with it (e.g., in terms of MU or mescaline units). Mescaline is a Schedule I substance under the federal Controlled Substances Act; however, the use of peyote in certain Native American religious practices is legally sanctioned.

Phenylisopropylamines (DMA, TMA, DOM, MDA) Numerous names and terminologies have been used to describe this large class of hallucinogens. One of the more common nomenclatures is that associated with the number and location of methoxy groups in the molecule. Analogues with two methoxy groups are called dimethoxy analogues (i.e., DMAs), whereas analogues with three methoxy groups are called trimethoxy analogues (TMAs). Replacement of the 4-methoxy group of 2,4,5-TMA with a methyl group results in DOM or 1-(2,5-dimethoxy-4-methylphenyl)-2-aminopropane. DOM represents the prototype member of this family of agents. 3,4-Methylenedioxyamphetamine (MDA) is structurally distinct from many of the other hallucinogenic phenylisopropylamines by virtue of lacking methoxy groups and possessing a methylenedioxy group instead. Where optical isomers of phenylisopropylamines have been examined, activity resides primarily with the $R(-)$ isomer. MDA has subjective effects similar to central stimulants (such as amphetamine and cocaine) as well as classical hallucinogens (such as LSD and mescaline).

Designer Drugs

Structure-activity relationship (SAR) is the study of how the chemical structure of a compound relates to its biological activity. It is known that adding or subtracting various chemical groups to a hallucinogenic compound will alter its biological effect in a fairly predictable manner. Clandestine chemists have utilized known SARs in order to create new designer drugs, or *controlled substance analogues*. These chemical modifications can alter the potency of hallucinogens as well as the ratio of hallucinogenic to stimulant effect.

Not all designer drugs result in actions that are entirely predictable. One of the most popular designer drugs is the MDA-derivative methylenedioxymethamphetamine also called MDMA or ecstasy. On the basis of established SAR, it might have been expected that MDMA would have more stimulant effect than MDA and less hallucinogenic action. What emerged was an agent that, in addition to its stimulant character, also produced an *empathogenic* effect (extroversion, heightened mood, heightened sense of confidence, and wellbeing) that would not be considered "hallucinogenic" in nature.

In recent times, agents such as MDA, p-methoxyamphetamine (PMA), p-methoxymethamphetamine (PMMA), and others have been represented and sold as MDMA on the illicit drug market. Several of these compounds have adverse cardiovascular effects associated. Some users are now using assay-based "test kits" that allow them to (at least to some extent) validate the authenticity of the substances they are using.

ABSORPTION AND METABOLISM

Few detailed studies have been conducted on the human metabolism of hallucinogenic agents. For many hallucinogens, their major route of metabolism is via monoamine oxidase (MAO) and cytochrome P450.

PHARMACOLOGIC ACTIONS

The effects of various hallucinogens are not necessarily identical, but they generally produce alterations in thought, mood, or perception. Stimulant and empathogenic effects are also well documented in the hallucinogen class of drugs.

MECHANISMS OF ACTION

Unfortunately, extensive human data, particularly data from well-controlled clinical studies with large subject populations, are available for only a few agents in this class.

Today, the classical hallucinogens are thought to produce their effect by acting as agonists at 5-HT2 receptors in the brain—the "5-HT2 hypothesis of classical hallucinogen action."

Although activation of 5-HT2A receptors seems to be responsible for the actions that the classical hallucinogens have in common, other neurochemical mechanisms might account for their differences. For example, LSD is a very promiscuous agent that binds with high affinity at many receptor populations for which most other classical hallucinogens show little to no affinity. Differences may also be due to the relative affinity of various hallucinogens for different 5-HT subtypes (e.g., 5-HT1A, h5-HT1D, 5-HT6).

ADDICTION LIABILITY

Classical hallucinogens are not generally considered to possess amphetamine-like or cocaine-like reinforcing properties on the basis of self-administration studies. There are a few exceptions, notably MDMA and MDA. MDMA is self-administered by nonhuman primates.

High-dose MDMA users, in particular, run a significant risk of persistent cognitive impairment and disturbances of affect and personality. MDMA has been shown to destroy brain serotonin neurons via reduction in the number of axon terminals. It has been suggested that reactive metabolites of MDA and MDMA, such as HHMA, or free radicals derived from MDMA, might play important roles in producing these neurotoxic effects. Another problem associated with MDMA use is its possible adverse cardiovascular actions. MDMA has been shown to induce fenfluramine-like proliferative actions on human cardiac valvular interstitial cells, which can lead to valvular heart disease. Furthermore, abuse of MDMA has been associated with the production of "serotonin syndrome." It is therefore prudent to screen for MDMA use when prescribing antidepressants (particularly MAO inhibitors).

While the use of MDMA and other hallucinogens can be fatal, it is appropriate to put the number of MDMA deaths in perspective: it has been stated that there are about 12 to 15 MDMA-associated deaths per year in the United Kingdom when it is estimated that 500,000 persons consume the drug every week. Another area of recent concern is the rise in other hallucinogens (such as PMA and PMMA) being sold as MDMA. The increasing number of deaths involving PMA or PMMA abuse is raising concern about these agents being substituted for MDMA.

Summary Author: Christopher A. Cavacuiti
Edward F. Domino • Shannon C. Miller

The Pharmacology of Dissociatives

DEFINITION (DRUGS IN THIS CLASS)

Dissociatives include an array of compounds sharing antagonist activity at the N-methyl D-aspartate (NMDA) receptor. The compounds noncompetitively block the effect of glutamic acid (a major excitatory neurotransmitter in the brain) at the NMDA receptor. The result is a clinical syndrome involving dissociation or disconnection of the brain from its external and internal environments. Dissociatives can be distinguished pharmacologically and clinically from true hallucinogens. Hallucinogens affect primarily the 5HT2a receptor instead of the NMDA receptor, and hallucinogens are associated with a somewhat different clinical syndrome of intoxication. With *hallucinogens*, visual hallucinations are the predominant symptom. With *dissociatives*, symptoms of dissociation and impaired reality testing predominate. In addition, many dissociatives have psychomimetic properties (meaning they induce a dreamlike and distorted "psychotic" state that resembles many but not all of the signs and symptoms of schizophrenia). Dissociatives such as phencyclidine (PCP) model both the positive (delusions, hallucinations) and the negative (blunted affect, ambivalence, asociality, autistic-like effects) symptoms of schizophrenia. Dextromethorphan (DXM) in large doses is readily metabolized to dextrorphan (DXO), a significant NMDA antagonist pharmacodynamically akin to PCP and ketamine.

SUBSTANCES INCLUDED IN THIS CLASS

Dissociatives include various arylcyclohexylamines, dizocilpine (MK-80l), and the gaseous anesthetic, nitrous oxide. In terms of arylcyclohexylamines, PCP and ketamine are the principal abused illicit compounds. DXM is the principal abused over-the-counter compound.

FORMULATION, METHODS OF USE AND ABUSE

Ketamine is commercially available as a sterile solution that is used for general anesthesia in both animals and humans as a Schedule III substance. It is used most often in children, who appear less susceptible than adults to emergent delirium. Ketamine is both synthesized in illegal labs and diverted from legitimate medical/veterinary sources. Ketamine is generally sold in powder form, which is insufflated by abusers. However, Ketamine may be abused by various routes and in different dose.

PCP is no longer available as a medical commercial preparation approved by the U.S. Food and Drug Administration (FDA). It is available in many illicit preparations in various forms and is used in a wide range of doses. It has many of the pharmacologic effects of ketamine, but is more potent, longer acting, and more likely to produce seizures. It is prepared illegally in various forms: powder, tablets, and liquid (salt in water, base in ether). The latter are typically sprayed onto plant leaves such as ginger, marijuana, mint, oregano, or parsley and then smoked.

Legal DXM preparations are administered orally. The usual antitussive dosage for adults is 10 to 20 mg every 4 hours. In doses of typically 300 to 1,800 mg (20–120 times the recommended dose), DXM produces PCP-like mental effect. Fortunately, DXM has a low toxicity even at high doses and DXM-related morbidity and mortality is rare. However, deaths have been reported. Moreover additional ingredients in over-the-counter DXM preparations make for additional hazards when taken in high doses. In addition, death from DXM-induced behavioral impairment has been reported—such as drowning while intoxicated and dissociating.

HISTORICAL FEATURES

Phencyclidine

The discovery of phencyclidine, or PCP, has been well documented by those involved with its therapeutic development. The drug was developed as an intravenous anesthetic. The anesthesia it produced was complicated by a prolonged emergence delirium; this quickly led to its demise as a clinically useful agent. However, it was rediscovered years later as a drug of abuse.

Ketamine

The desirable anesthetic properties of PCP were retained in the shorter-acting ketamine, which produced a much briefer emergence delirium. Ketamine was subsequently discovered by the drug abuse community; and has the perception among users as being medically safe to use as it is produced by pharmaceutical companies (for veterinary use).

Dextromethorphan

The history of DXM begins with the synthesis of methorphan in 1954 as an opioid analgesic. It was discovered that DXM (the D-isomer of methorphan) was primarily antitussive, whereas the L-isomer had more analgesic and narcotic-like properties. Compared with codeine as an antitussive, DXM was nearly equal. However, unlike codeine, DXM is fairly devoid of other opioid effects. DXM abuse has been a concern since at least the 1960s. DXM has become popular, particularly in children and adolescents, owing to this population incorrectly perceiving DXM as a "SMART" choice of drugs to abuse, because they perceive DXM as without "S"tigma, not costing much "M"oney to procure, having easy "A"ccess at local stores, devoid of medical "R"isks, and not included in routine employment or home-based drug "T"esting. In 1990, the FDA Drug Abuse Advisory Committee assessed DXM use by teenagers and recommended against placing the drug on the Controlled Drug Schedule but recommended more study of the problem.

Nitrous Oxide

Recreational use of nitrous oxide as a "laughing gas" has been well described since it first was discovered. In fact, it was first used as a recreational drug in 1799, 36 years before it was first used medically.

EPIDEMIOLOGY

PCP abuse appears to be more of a problem in large cities compared with the rest of the United States. According to Drug Abuse Warning Network data, since 1999, PCP-related emergency room visits have increased 109% (from 3,663 to 7,648).

Ketamine has often been considered as typically used with other drugs; however, sole use of ketamine has been reported. Although ketamine has often been self-administered by insufflation, emerging data suggest an increase in injection use of ketamine among youth.

DXM is considered one of the most commonly abused over-the-counter medications in the United States. The proportion of US students who reported having used DXM during the prior year for the expressed purpose of "getting high" was 4%, 5%, and 7% in grades 8, 10, and 12, respectively. There is an increasing trend of DXM abuse in older adults, and particularly in adolescents. The highest frequency of abuse was in 15- to 16-year-olds. Approximately 75% of DXM abuse cases reported to the California Poison Control System were ages 9 to 17 years old.

PHARMACOKINETICS

PCP half-life has been reported to vary from 7 to 46 hours. PCP is biotransformed (primarily via glucuronidation) in the liver to several metabolites and excreted in the urine. The clinical utility of acidification of the urine to remove PCP is no longer recommended because of the risk of increasing urinary myoglobin precipitation.

Ketamine is more lipophilic than PCP, which accounts for its rapid onset, short anesthetic duration of action, and shorter period of emergence delirium. As used in general anesthesia, an intravenous dose of 2.0 mg/ kg produces rapid induction. This dose produces an onset in 30 seconds, with the coma lasting for 8 to 10 minutes and emergence effects for 1–2 hours.

DXM is readily absorbed from the gut. Symptoms begin within 15 to 30 minutes of ingestion of intoxicating doses, with peak effects experienced in roughly 2.5 hours. Humans have a genetic polymorphism for the CYP2D6 biotransformation of DXM. Rapid metabolizers have a plasma elimination half-life of about 3.4 hours, and slow metabolizers (10%–15% of the population) may have half-lives exceeding 24 hours.

PHARMACODYNAMICS

PCP and Ketamine

Depending on the dose, patients who have taken arylcyclohexylamines such as PCP or ketamine present with widely different neurologic and psychiatric signs and symptoms. As the dose rises, one can observe patients becoming progressively more obtunded, with symptoms progressing from confusion and delirium, to psychosis; to semicoma and finally to coma and coma with seizures. The reverse pattern is seen when the patient is emerging from an arylcyclohexylamine-induced coma. Schizophrenic patients appear to be much more susceptible to a prolonged psychotic episode related to arylcyclohexylamine use. Long-term chronic effects may include dysphoria, reduced memory and cognition, apathy, and irritability. Although evidence supports the potential for tolerance and physical dependence, further research is needed.

DXM

DXM in clinical therapeutic doses produces relatively few side effects. These may include body rash, itching, nausea, and vomiting when combined with the other ingredients in cough preparations. DXM has significant serotonergic effects, and DXO has significant NMDA antagonist effects. Depending on dose, the drug can cause drowsiness, dizziness, altered vision, cardiovascular, and significant central nervous system effects that resemble PCP/ketamine intoxication.

DRUG–DRUG INTERACTIONS

Many other centrally acting drugs can produce a synergistic effect with dissociatives. Ketamine is biotransformed by CYP3A4 and increased levels occur with CYP3A4 inhibitors. Furthermore, DXM can induce a serotonin syndrome when taken with monoamine oxide inhibitors, selective serotonin reuptake inhibitors, or other serotonergically active substances. DXM is metabolized via CYP2D6 and thus DXM levels may be altered by medications that induce/inhibit CYP2D6.

NEUROBIOLOGY

Noncompetitive blockade of NMDA receptors appears to be the primary mechanism of action of these agents. It has also been hypothesized that dissociatives induce positive symptoms (delusions, hallucinations) via enhancing glutamate release, and negative symptoms (blunted affect, ambivalence, asociality, autistic-like effects) via NMDA antagonism.

Addiction Liability

Why these substances are reinforcing is difficult to understand except in the context of individuals who wish to experience the feelings of floating in space, dissociation, sensory isolation, mental distortions, and so forth that dissociatives provide. However, the fact that animals will self-administer PCP, ketamine, and DXM points to the fact that these agents do indeed have reinforcing effects. Ketamine in low doses is an effective antidepressant where effects last for 1–2 weeks, which may contribute to its addiction liability.

Toxicity/Adverse Effects

Dissociatives induce significant vesicular changes (termed Olney lesions) in rat brain posterior cingulate retrosplenial neurons. Not all species of animals evidence these changes. The relationship of such neurotoxicity to humans who use or abuse NMDA antagonists is as yet unclear. However, repeated high-dose administration of DXM during adolescence in rats may induce permanent deficits in cognitive function, providing concern in the setting of increased prevalence of DXM abuse in adolescents (a period of remarkable brain growth).

Intoxication and Overdose

Although a preliminary diagnosis of arylcyclohexylamine intoxication can be made on the basis of history, clinical signs, and symptoms, only a drug-positive blood or urine specimen will unequivocally establish it. Most clinical screening panels include PCP, but not the other agents discussed herein; thus, special requests may be required for specialized testing from a lab. Gas chromatography mass spectrometry is often still ideal for confirmation.

Psychotic manifestations of arylcyclohexylamine poisoning can be confused with catatonic schizophrenia, an acute toxic psychosis induced with other hallucinogens, and various acute organic brain syndromes. Arylcyclohexamine intoxication readily induces nystagmus, an organic brain syndrome, as well as cardiovascular and renal complications that are rarely if ever seen in psychiatric syndromes. The National Guideline Clearinghouse (www.guideline.gov) provides detailed guidelines for the management of DXM poisoning. A recent (2007) guideline entitled "Dextromethorphan poisoning: an evidence-based consensus guideline for out-of-hospital management" has also been published by Chyka and colleagues.

CHAPTER 16

Summary Author: Christopher A. Cavacuiti
Robert L. Balster

The Pharmacology of Inhalants

DEFINITION

Typically, abused inhalants are breathable chemicals that can be self-administered as gases or vapors. Drugs such as crack cocaine, which is aerosolized, as well as cannabis and tobacco, which are smoked, are consumed by inhalation but are not generally, or usefully, classified as inhalants.

History

The abuse of inhalants has a long history. Perhaps the best-known instances are the use of anesthetics for purposes of intoxication that began with their discovery >200 years ago. The euphoriant effects of nitrous oxide were noted by Sir Humphrey Davy, who synthesized the substance in 1798 and began calling it "laughing gas." While some inhalants (such as amyl nitrite) are regulated by the U.S. Food and Drug Administration and generally intended only available by prescription, many other inhalants are easily commercially available. In addition, many of these regulated solvents, fuels and anesthetics can be purchased via the internet.

Most of the inhalants that are used recreationally produce alcohol-like and depressant drug–like effects; other potential effects include hallucinations, tremor, and seizures. There have been discussions of strategies to prevent access to abused inhalants, to change their labeling, or to reformulate products to limit their abuse potential. These strategies needs to be viewed on a case-by-case basis to be certain that it will achieve the desired effect and not result in abusers seeking potentially more toxic products that almost certainly cannot be restricted (e.g., gasoline).

Epidemiology

Results of national surveys suggest that the prevalence of inhalant use is greatest among 12- to 17-year-olds compared with other age groups. The use of inhalants in this age group is only exceeded by alcohol, tobacco, and marihuana. About 1 in 10 youths used inhalants sometime in their life and 4.4% used them in the past year. Unlike other drugs of abuse, the prevalence of inhalant use actually decreases from 8th to 12th grade. However, it is incorrect to characterize this problem as a passing fad in youth. For about half of current users, duration of use exceeds 1 to 2 years, with about 10% using inhalants for 6 years or more. Inhalant use is also associated with other substance use disorders and may be an even stronger predictor of subsequent drug abuse problems than marijuana use.

DRUGS IN THE CLASS

Three subdivisions of abused inhalants are useful, as shown in Table 16.1. This subclassification is based on common pharmacological effects.

Volatile Alkyl Nitrites

The prototypic alkyl nitrite is amyl nitrite, used medically as a vasodilator for treatment of angina. Amyl nitrite is available as a volatile liquid in ampules that are broken open and the vapor inhaled. At one time, the ampules were available over the counter and abusers would "pop" them open—hence the street name "poppers." It seems likely that they are abused because of their ability to produce syncope secondary to venous pooling in the periphery and because of their effects on tumescence and smooth muscles, making them popular as aids to sexual activity.

TABLE 16.1	Pharmacologic Classification of Abused Inhalants	

Class	Examples	Sources
Volatile alkyl nitrites	Amyl nitrite	Antianginal medication ampules
	Butyl nitrite	Room odorizers
Nitrous oxide		Whipped creme chargers, cylinders for anesthesia, racing fuels, dairy industry foaming agent
Solvents, fuels, and anesthetics	Toluene	Adhesives, paint removers, and thinners (toluol), inks, nail polish and remover, industrial solvents and degreasers
	Xylene	Adhesives and printing inks, paints and varnishes, pesticides
	Trichloroethane	A solvent in water repellants, automotive cleaners, paints, adhesives and silicone lubricants, correction fluids, spray paints and paint removers, spot removers and other cleaning products
	Trichloroethylene	Correction fluids, stains and varnishes, paint removers
	Methylene chloride	A solvent in water repellants, automotive cleaners, primers and paints, adhesives and silicone lubricants, correction fluids, spray paints and paint removers, rust and spot removers, and other cleaning products
	Tetrachloroethylene	A solvent in water repellants, brake and carburetor cleaners, paints, adhesives and silicone lubricants, correction fluids, paint removers
	Difluoroethane, tetrafluoroethane, dichlorodifluoromethane	Compressed gas dusters for computers and other uses
	Butane, isopropane	Cigarette lighter fuel, aerosol propellant, bottled gas
	Ether, isoflurane	Anesthetics
	Ketones (MBK, MEK)	Solvents, adhesives

Nitrous Oxide

Most illicit use of nitrous oxide occurs when tanks of anesthetic quality nitrous oxide are diverted for illegitimate use. The tanks can be used to fill balloons for ready sale at concerts, raves, or parties. Reinforcing effects include euphoria ("laughing gas") and feelings of intoxication. When used as a legitimate anesthetic, concentrations of about 15% to 20% are used. When it is abused, many users breathe almost 100% nitrous oxide (e.g., from a balloon). This can lead to anoxia and nitrite-produced syncope, significant intoxication, and other acute psychologic effects.

Volatile Solvents, Fuels, and Anesthetics

This category includes a large collection of chemicals, which further research will likely reveal to have pharmacologic profiles, but the state of the science is insufficient at this point to propose a further subclassification. It has been hypothesized that many of these commercial chemicals share profiles of acute effects with subanesthetic concentrations of volatile anesthetics such as halothane, sevoflurane, and isoflurane.

ABSORPTION AND METABOLISM

The abused inhalants include compounds that are self-administered as gases, vapors, and aerosols. These three forms of inhalants have somewhat different absorption characteristics and require different methods of use (e.g., balloons for gases and bags or rags for volatile liquids).

Gases and vapors rapidly penetrate deep into the lung and, because of their high lipophilicity, are rapidly absorbed and distributed into arterial blood.

Elimination of inhalants is very rapid once the source is removed from the inspired air. For most of these chemicals, expired air is the major route of elimination. Most abused inhalants are metabolized to some extent, but this metabolism probably plays a greater role in determining their hepatic toxicity than their CNS effects.

Intoxication with inhalants is of shorter duration than with other drugs of abuse, with the result that many health care providers, as well as friends and family of users, rarely see an inhalant abuser who is grossly intoxicated.

MECHANISMS OF ACTION

The neuropharmacologic mechanisms by which inhalant intoxications occur are poorly understood. Although it is presumed that the abused solvents, fuels and anesthetics disrupt normal neural function, which systems are most affected and the mechanism by which such disruption occurs are not clear. Even the question of whether specific receptors are affected by these agents remains unresolved. The best current evidence is that acute solvent intoxication is probably associated with enhancement of GABAa and antagonism at N-methyl-D-aspartate (NMDA) receptors.

ADDICTION LIABILITY

All the vapors that have been tested produce clear, reversible, drug-like behavioral effects in animal studies. In addition, self-administration studies in rodents, primates, and humans have shown many inhalants to have reinforcing properties.

Tolerance and Dependence

Little is known about the development of tolerance to and dependence on inhalants, but in general they do not appear to be prominent features. In animal studies, abused inhalants do not readily produce a significant degree of tolerance to their behavioral effects. However, a mild withdrawal syndrome can be observed with some inhalants. Ethanol and barbiturates can suppress these withdrawal signs, suggesting a crossdependence within the depressant class.

Producing signs of dependence in animals requires near constant inhalant exposure. Thus, it is not surprising that physical dependence on inhalants is not seen often, if at all, in clinical settings.

Clinical Chemistry

Although few, if any, clinical facilities will routinely conduct tests for the presence of abused inhalants, such tests can be ordered through special services provided by commercial laboratories. Typically, these tests are performed on blood or urine. Because inhalants are eliminated so rapidly after acute exposure, such tests would be expected to have a high probability of producing false negatives.

TOXICITY/ADVERSE EFFECTS

Inhalants represent a wide and varied class of drugs and their toxicity differs depending on which of this broad array of chemicals and chemical mixtures is being abused. It is difficult for toxicologists to ascertain the specific etiology of any adverse health effects seen in inhalant users because

1. Inhalants are a diverse array of chemicals.
2. Few chronic users confine themselves to a single inhalant.
3. Many abused commercial inhalant products are complex mixtures.
4. Some adverse effects may be secondary to the lifestyles seen in solvent abusers, not the drug itself.

Acute Effects

Deaths related to the acute effects of inhalants are well documented. There are two primary sources: behavioral toxicity (accidents and injuries) and overdose. Overdose occurs when users lose consciousness while being continually exposed, allowing lethal concentrations to accumulate in the brain. At least some of the inhalants appear capable of producing acute cardiotoxicity, even in otherwise healthy young users.

Chronic Toxicity

Commonly damaged target organs included the nose and mouth area, lungs, brain, liver, and kidney. There also are physical dangers in using highly inflammable and explosive chemicals.

Neurotoxicity

Many, if not all, abused inhalants can be neurotoxic and components of some abused products are well-characterized neurotoxicants. Brain scanning, neurologic, and neuropsychologic assessment or autopsy reports of inhalant abusers show many types of neuropathologies, including loss of white matter, brain atrophy, and damage to specific neural pathways. It is not known what percentage of abusers have detectable brain damage or whether the inhalants alone were responsible for the observed effects.

Psychiatric Disorders

Recent reports suggest a very high rate of psychiatric disorders among inhalant abusers. For example, 70% of previous users of inhalants in one study met criteria for at least one lifetime mood, anxiety, or personality disorder and 38% experienced a mood or anxiety disorder in the past year. Females were more likely than males to have multiple comorbid psychiatric illness. Conduct disorder, mood disorders, and suicidality are also more prevalent among adolescent inhalant abusers.

Effects on Major Organ Systems

Many chronic solvent users develop irritation of the eyes, nose, and mouth and exhibit rhinitis, nose bleeding, conjunctivitis, and a localized facial rash. Inflammation of the lungs can result in coughing and may compromise respiration. Liver toxicity is a concern for many inhalants, especially those that undergo hepatic metabolism. Individuals with preexisting hepatitis or alcoholism are particularly vulnerable to inhalant-induced liver toxicity. Kidney damage also has been reported, in the form of glomerulonephritis, kidney stones, and renal tubular acidosis. There is also evidence that at least some inhalants are carcinogenic.

Fetal Solvent Syndrome

It has been estimated that as many as 12,000 women use inhalants while pregnant in the United States alone. The research on inhalant abuse and pregnancy suggests that decreased fertility and spontaneous abortions in some women may be related to inhalant abuse. Clinical reports of adverse effects in the offspring of solvent abusers include low birth weight, facial and other physical abnormalities, microcephaly, and delayed neurologic and physical maturation. Because certain features seen in these children resemble the fetal alcohol syndrome, a "fetal solvent syndrome" has been proposed.

Summary Author: Christopher A. Cavacuiti
Scott E. Lukas

The Pharmacology of Anabolic Androgenic Steroids

In terms of *steroids abuse*, the class of compounds that are being referred to are the *anabolic-androgenic steroids (AASs)*. These steroids must be distinguished from the *corticosteroids* and the *female gonadotrophic steroids*, neither of which are subject to abuse.

There is a long list of AASs that have been produced for both human and veterinary use.

DRUGS IN THE CLASS

The prototypic hormone, testosterone, is the standard to which all of the other AAS products are compared. In the 1940s, after chemists had succeeded in synthesizing testosterone, their efforts were directed toward separating its anabolic from its androgenic effects. Thus far, the androgenic component of these synthetics has never been completely separated from the anabolic effects; only the relative percentage of the two has been manipulated.

HISTORY OF STEROID USE

The introduction of AASs to the United States has been traced to the 1954 World Weightlifting Championships in Vienna, when the Soviet Union's coach informed the US coach that his team members were taking testosterone. In the ensuing years, the use of AAS by elite weight lifters and bodybuilders increased. The use of testosterone also spread to many other professional sports, especially those in which strength and body weight were important for success. Synthetic compounds gradually came to replace testosterone as the drugs of choice among athletes and body builders, primarily because of their higher ratio of anabolic versus androgenic effects and also because of their relative resistance to detection by laboratory tests. By the mid-1980s, 50% of the unannounced tests by the International Olympic committee were positive for AAS. Controversial use of AAS has tainted a large number of sporting events including Major League Baseball, US football, track and field, and professional cycling. The large majority of today's AAS users are not competitive athletes; a recent survey of AAS found that 78% were noncompetitive bodybuilders and not otherwise engaged in athletic events. Concern over the misuse of AAS by athletes and others led the U.S. Congress to enact the Anabolic Steroids Control Act, which effectively placed all of these compounds, including testosterone and its many analogues, in Schedule III of the federal Controlled Substances Act.

New-Generation "Performance Enhancers"

The advent of more sophisticated urine testing procedures for AAS, as well the desire by elite athletes for drugs that enhance element of performance beyond strength (such as endurance), has led to increased popularity of an entirely new generation of performance-enhancing drugs. These include other hormones such as human growth hormone (HGH or somatotropin), dehydroepiandrosterone (DHEA), erythropoietin ("Epo"), Continuous erythropoietin receptor activator (CERA), and thyroxine.

Production, Distribution, and Use

The major source of abused steroids is diversion from licit manufacture and distribution. Clandestine laboratory synthesis of these products is very rare. For both old- and new-generation performance enhancers, a number of "underground" guides as well as a variety of Web sites provide extensive information on, where to get them, doses to use and even recipes for adding them to training programs, and strategies to avoid doping detection.

While clandestine synthesis is rare, these products are ordered by mail from abroad, where safety standards for production are less stringent than in the United States. Many AAS products are also diverted from the domestic and international veterinary market, and the use of many of these drugs in humans has not been approved. Finally, the gray and black market for AAS has encouraged the development of a variety of inactive products that are falsely advertised as containing anabolic steroids.

At-risk Populations

It is now well established that athletes are not the only individuals to use and abuse AAS. While the rate of AAS abuse in the general US adult population remains low, much higher rates are seen in certain populations. Rates of use among individuals in fitness centers, for example, are much higher (~12.5%) than the general population.

Available evidence suggests that use among adolescent boys is higher than in the general population and is also continuing to rise. Over the past 5 to 6 years, AAS abuse among adolescent boys has risen from <2% to >3% and in certain populations of 15- to 19-year-old boys, nearly 10% reported using AAS. Compared with their nonusing counterparts, AAS-using adolescent boys are more likely to use marijuana, tobacco, and cocaine.

Women are also using these drugs, but all estimates indicate that the percentage is lower than in males. Among adolescent girls, a survey of 7,544 females in grades 9 to 12 found that 5.3% of the girls used AAS. Interestingly, these young women also engaged in a number of other unhealthy life choices including using tobacco, poor nutrition, marijuana use, diet pills, carrying weapons, and having sexual relations before the age of 13. AAS using females were also *less* likely to participate in team sports.

Both human and animal studies suggest that adolescents may be particularly sensitive to the effect of AAS on sexual and aggressive behavior. There is also concern that adolescent AAS use (particularly in males) can lead to neural "rewiring" that sets the tone for lifelong aggressive and violent tendencies. Adolescent use of steroids may also lead to stunted growth through premature closure of epiphyseal plates. This in direct contradiction to the belief of many adolescents who believe steroid use will help them grow taller.

THERAPEUTIC USE AND MISUSE

Therapeutic Use

Available evidence suggests most AAS is diverted from legitimate sources, rather than synthesized in clandestine labs. Being able to distinguish appropriate from inappropriate use may help stem the tide of AAS diversion.

The most common reason for therapeutic AAS use is when the testicles fail to produce sufficient endogenous AAS. However, the doses that are prescribed are much lower than those used by bodybuilders. The equivalent of 75 to 100 mg per week of testosterone suffices as replacement, but weight lifters and bodybuilders have reportedly used weekly doses of 1,000 to 2,100 mg.

Misuse

AASs are abused by a variety of populations: (a) athletes who use them to improve performance, (b) aesthetes who use them solely to improve appearance and perhaps gain some weight, and (c) the fighting elite who use them to enhance aggression and fighting skills. Patterns of AAS use and AAS abuse treatment plans may differ depending on the particular population.

Athletes Athletes use AASs to improve their performance. Perhaps one of the greatest mistakes a clinician makes in dealing with an athlete is attempting to dissuade their use on the grounds that the drugs cannot improve performance. In fact, this is not true. Available evidence suggests that AAS can improve performance in a variety of ways, including increases muscle capacity, reduce body fat, increase strength and endurance, improved recovery from injury. Furthermore, many athletes report that AAS-assisted training allows the user to increase both the frequency and the intensity of workouts—factors that also contribute to performance.

AASs are used by athletes in three basic patterns: "stacking," "pyramiding," and "cycling." *Stacking* is the practice of using multiple products at the same time. *Cycling* refers to the practice of using different combinations over a period to avoid the development of tolerance or loss of effectiveness. *Pyramiding* involves starting with a low dose and then gradually increasing the dose until peak levels are achieved a number of weeks before competition. A survey of bodybuilders and weightlifters revealed that they use an average 3.1 agents, engage in cycles that last 5 to 10 weeks in length, and use doses that peak at 5 to 29 times greater than physiologic replacement doses.

Aesthetes Another group of users is composed of young men and women who use these drugs primarily to increase their weight or to improve their self-perceived physical appearance. A survey of 6th to 12th grade Canadians revealed that 2.8% of the respondents had used these drugs over the past year. A disturbing trend was that 29.4% of these students reported that they injected the drugs and 29.2% of these reported that they shared needles with friends.

Fighting Elite This group includes bouncers at bars, security personnel, and even law enforcement officers; these individuals seek to increase their strength and aggressiveness in order to "better" perform their job. Very little research has been done on this population of AAS users.

Personality Profiles

Compared with controls, AAS users score higher on measures of paranoia, schizoid, antisocial, borderline, histrionic, narcissistic, and passive-aggressive personality profiles. Longitudinal studies suggest that many of these abnormal personality traits developed *after* the AAS use began, suggesting that such disturbances are secondary to AAS use.

There appears to be both a pathologic self-perception of body image (body dysmorphism) and a very narrow (stereotypic) view of what a male body should look like among AAS users. The term *reverse anorexia nervosa* has been coined by this group to describe symptoms association with muscle dysmorphia or a pathological preoccupation with muscularity. As with other forms of body dysmorphism like anorexia nervosa, muscle dysmorphia is associated with a greater incidence of suicide attempts, higher frequency of substance abuse, and poorer quality of life.

ADVERSE EFFECTS

Figure 17.1 depicts some of the more commonly identified effects and side effects of AAS use in humans.

ADDICTION LIABILITY

The addiction liability of AAS is difficult to study. Addiction liability generally refers to the direct reinforcing effects of the drug itself. Yet in the case of AAS abuse, many of reinforcing effects do not come from the drug. Rather, the reinforcement comes from the social and psychological rewards that follow when one "performs" better or "looks" better.

Demonstrating tolerance and physical dependence on these agents has also proved to be elusive because there are limitations in the doses that can ethically be given to human subjects in controlled trials.

Reward

The studies on reward with AAS use are contradictory. On the one hand, there are studies of healthy non-AAS users feeling euphoric, full of energy, and having increased sexual arousal after being given an AAS. On the other hand, other studies have found that humans cannot tell whether they have been given an active AAS or placebo.

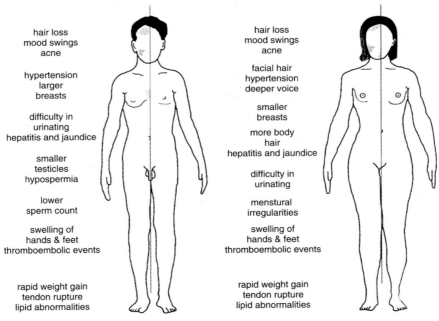

FIGURE 17.1   Side effects of anabolic-androgenic steroids.

A variety of other studies also suggest that reinforcing effect of AAS use is not a direct "drug-reward" effect:

1. Unlike many other addictive drugs, steroids lack a well-defined pattern of self-administration in animals.
2. The common "pattern of use" with steroids in humans (i.e., taken or injected once per week as part of an exercise program) is also different than for most other drugs of abuse.
3. Many users of black market steroids have claimed to have experienced significant improvements in their performance and/or appearance. Yet when these products have been tested, they were found to be devoid of steroids or any other active ingredients.

Tolerance

Although the clinical trial evidence supporting tolerance development is not strong, a study of beliefs among AAS using weight lifters showed that 20% of those surveyed believe that tolerance develops, and >80% believe that dependence develops.

Dependence

Although evidence of physical dependence on AAS has not been widespread, there are a few detailed reports of clear signs of withdrawal when their use was abruptly stopped. In a survey of weight lifters, 84% reported experiencing withdrawal effects. The most frequently reported symptoms were craving for more steroids (52%), fatigue (43%), depressed mood state (41%), restlessness (29%), anorexia (24%), insomnia (20%), decreased libido (20%), and headaches (20%).

Given the disproportionately high use of other drugs among AAS users, the possibility of polydrug abuse/dependence should also always be considered when dealing with AAS abusers.

Diagnostic Classifications

It is apparent from the historical literature that AAS users have met formal criteria for dependence in the American Psychiatric Association's *DSM-IV*.

Research comparing AAS using weight lifters with their nonusing counterparts suggests that a disproportionate number of AAS users suffer from reverse anorexia nervosa (a belief than one is small and weak, when one is actually large and strong).

ABSORPTION AND METABOLISM

AASs are taken either orally or injected deep into the muscle; there is no intravenous formulation, nor is there a smokable product. About half of an oral dose of testosterone is metabolized via the first-pass effect, so very large oral doses are needed. These high doses can put significant strain on the liver, causing drug-induced hepatitis and jaundice.

MECHANISMS OF ACTION

About 95% of the testosterone in males is synthesized in the testes, whereas the remaining 5% comes from the adrenals. About half of the circulating testosterone is tightly bound to sex hormone–binding globulin, and the other half is lightly bound to albumin, from which it freely dissociates and from whence it can diffuse passively into target cells. In skeletal muscle, testosterone causes new myofilaments to form, which in turn causes myofibrils to divide. It is also believed that AASs cross-react with glucocorticoid receptors, creating an "anticatabolic" effect on protein.

Others have suggested that AAS may function indirectly by allowing AAS users to work out harder and longer. Postulated mechanism includes AAS blockage of the fatigue effect of cortisol or AAS-induced enhancement of aggressiveness and motivation at the CNS level.

The increase in body weight, especially during the first weeks of use, is almost certainly attributed to the stimulation of mineralocorticoid receptors, resulting in sodium and, ultimately, water retention as well as increasing amounts of circulating estrogen that has been aromatized from testosterone. This effect gives the muscles, particularly the deltoid, a "puffy" appearance.

The increase in red blood cell production is probably the major reason that long-distance athletes (such as runners and cyclists) may use these drugs because endurance, rather than bulk muscle mass, is an asset.

FUTURE VISTAS

Many antidoping experts speculate that the next frontier in improved human performance will come not from new drugs, but rather from performance-enhancing genetics or "gene doping." This practice is defined by the World Anti-Doping Agency (WADA) as "the nontherapeutic use of genes, genetic elements and/or cells that have the capacity to enhance athletic performance." While no documented cases of human gene doping have yet occurred, WADA has already begun to set gene doping standards for future events.

CHAPTER

18

Summary Author: Thea Weisdorf
Aleksandra Zgierska • Michael F. Fleming

Screening and Brief Intervention

One in five of primary care adult patients reports problems related to substance use. Often these problems, especially alcohol use disorders, are closely associated with serious medical complications, such as memory loss, hypertension, liver disease, and others. Screening and brief intervention (SBI) and when appropriate, a referral to an addiction treatment program (SBIRT) is a promising solution for for decreasing negative outcomes associated with alcohol and drug use.

Brief intervention (BI) is a time-limited, client-centered counseling designed to reduce substance use. Its duration ranges from 5 to 20 minutes. Multiple BI sessions are more effective than a single contact. BI's approach is based on a harm reduction model as opposed to an abstinence-based one. The treatment goal is to reduce negative, substance use-related consequences. SBI is one of the most popular clinical "tools" utilized by primary care providers and can be viewed as a part of the provider's responsibilities along with ordering tests, prescribing medications, etc.

NATIONAL RECOMMENDATIONS ON THE IMPLEMENTATION OF SUBSTANCE ABUSE SCREENING AND TREATMENT IN MEDICAL CARE SETTINGS

The U.S. Preventative Services Task Force (USPSTF) recommends routine SBI to reduce tobacco and alcohol "misuse" by adults, in primary care settings, including pregnant women; it also recommends that clinicians provide tobacco cessation interventions for tobacco users. The USPSTF concludes that there is insufficient evidence to recommend routine SBI for alcohol and tobacco use among children and adolescents, and for drug use.

Many other health care organizations have adopted policies for their members to implement SBI for alcohol, tobacco, and other drug use. The National Institute on Alcohol Abuse and Alcoholism (NIAAA), National Institute on Drug Abuse (NIDA), Substance Abuse and Mental Health Services Administration (SAMHSA), and the National Quality Forum (NQF) have endorsed recommendations to implement SBI in general and mental health care settings. Adoption of new billing codes for structured screening and BI delivery reflects these national trends and policies.

CLINICAL GUIDELINES

Screening for At-Risk Drinking, Alcohol Abuse, and Alcohol Dependence

- *Prescreening question* about *any* alcohol use—"Do you sometimes drink beer, wine, or other alcoholic beverages?"
- *Screening* about the frequency of heavy drinking, defined as five or more drinks per day for men up to age 65, and four or more drinks per day for women and men older than 65—"How many times in the past year have you had 5 (4) drinks…?"
- Other screening options: for example, CAGE and AUDIT surveys.
- If *negative* screen, follow with individually tailored advice to maintain alcohol consumption below the "at-risk" drinking" limits.

- If positive screen, must determine the patient's weekly alcohol consumption (two questions: "On average, how many days a week do you have an alcoholic drink?" and "On a typical drinking day, how many drinks do you have?") and ask about drinking related harms to determine the presence or the absence of alcohol abuse or dependence (DSM-IV criteria).

Brief Intervention ("Advice and Assist") for At-Risk Drinking and Persons Who Meet Criteria for Alcohol Abuse or Dependence

After screening is completed, clinician should provide the patient with a non-judgmental *assessment* of his or her drinking and its consequences as well as clear advice (*recommendations*).

The next step is to assess the patient's *readiness to change* and negotiate a patient-specific *treatment goal*. Even if abstinence is an ideal goal, cutting down may reduce the drinking-related harms. For those who meet criteria for alcohol dependence and those with specific comorbid medical or psychiatric problems, abstinence should be advised as a primary treatment goal. If the patient is willing to change, the clinician should discuss a *treatment plan* to achieve the patient's goals. Alcohol-dependent patients can be referred and encouraged to see an addiction specialist and attend a mutual self-help group such as AA. They should also be assessed for the need for medically managed treatment, such as detoxification and pharmacotherapy, and for comorbid mental health disorders. All patients should be provided with educational materials and scheduled for follow-up appointments.

Follow-Up Sessions

At follow up, patient progress should be documented. Former "at-risk drinkers" should be rescreened at least annually. Patients who are alcohol dependent need careful monitoring for follow-through with an alcohol treatments program, self-help groups, and treatment of coexisting medical and mental health conditions. Those who do not meet their treatment goals should be supported with empathy, restated willingness to help, acknowledgement that change is difficult, and close follow-up; the patient's diagnosis and treatment goals should be reevaluated during each follow-up visit.

For patients not willing to change, the clinician should restate the drinking-related health concerns, reaffirm a willingness to help when the patient is ready, and encourage the patient to reflect about perceived "benefits" of continued drinking versus decreasing or stopping drinking, and barriers to change.

CURRENT EVIDENCE ON SCREENING AND BRIEF INTERVENTIONS: A BRIEF SUMMARY

Screening and Brief Intervention for Unhealthy Alcohol Use (At-Risk Use through Dependence)

In primary care settings, SBI for alcohol problems in adults is a clinically effective and cost-effective service with economic savings similar to screening for colorectal cancer, hypertension or visual acuity, and to influenza and pneumococcal immunizations. Limited evidence suggests that SBI can reduce morbidity and mortality in problem drinkers.

The evidence for SBI in trauma settings is not as strong as for a primary care setting. In emergency department (ED) settings, there is limited and conflicting research whether SBI can reduce drinking and result in fewer subsequent ED visits among at-risk drinkers. Evidence on the effectiveness of alcohol SBI in general inpatient settings is inconclusive. Of note, the majority of general medical inpatients, identified as "positive" by screening, have alcohol dependence.

There is insufficient evidence on SBI efficacy in adolescents and in different cultural groups. Primary care clinicians delivering the intervention yield the largest effect. There has been growing support for different ways of SBI delivery (e.g., via mail, phone, or web based). The optimal interval for SBI "booster sessions" is unknown.

Screening and Brief Intervention for Illicit Drug Use and Prescription Opioid Misuse

A single item has been validated in primary care to screen for drug use: "How many times in the past year have you used an illegal drug or used a prescription medication for nonmedical reasons?" Answering "one or more" represents a positive screen.

Current evidence is insufficient to assess the balance of benefits and harms of screening adolescents, adults, and pregnant women for illicit drug use. To date, there is only limited research evaluating the efficacy of SBI for illicit drug use and disorders, with strongest evidence existing for cannabis use and cannabis use disorders.

There is no current literature on the efficacy of SBI for prescription opioid-related use disorders.

SUMMARY

SBI is now on the forefront of our efforts to reduce tobacco- and alcohol-related harms. The implementation of SBI in all clinical settings has become a high priority for federal and other funding initiatives and health care systems. Much work still needs to be done from evidence and research perspectives.

The evidence for the use of SBI for adolescents in general clinical settings is weak. The utility of SBI for illicit and prescription drug use disorders in is unclear. More research is needed on on the impact of SBI on mortality and the use of SBI for hospitalized patients; it is of particular importance as many of them are alcohol dependent. There is no evidence on the use of SBI in dual diagnosis settings.

SCREENING AND BRIEF INTERVENTION FOR PREGNANT WOMEN

ALCOHOL

Introduction

Alcohol has harmful effects on the fetus and can be responsible for lifelong consequences such as the fetal alcohol syndrome (FAS). In addition, alcohol consumption has been associated with more subtle developmental problems such as moderate intellectual and behavioral deficits – symptoms similar to FAS but less severe and much more common. The US Surgeon General states that no level of alcohol consumption by pregnant women can be considered safe and women who may be / are pregnant or are considering pregnancy should abstain from alcohol.

Screening

The goal of screening is to identify women who are pregnant or are considering pregnancy and are using alcohol, and, then, to advise them to abstain. Of note, many women will reduce their alcohol use as soon as they become aware of their pregnancy, and so, their "current" use may not be an accurate reflection of their prior consumption. In addition, because of fear and stigma associated with alcohol use during pregnancy, women may underreport their alcohol consumption.

Screening instruments developed for general populations may perform less well in women, especially in women of childbearing age. There are several screening instruments developed specifically for pregnant women, for example, **T-ACE** (based on the CAGE survey), TWEAK, and NET. T-ACE and TWEAK are the best-performing brief screening questionnaires among pregnant women.

Brief Intervention

Results of the Trial for Early Alcohol Treatment (Project TrEAT), support the hypothesis that SBI, conducted in primary care among pregnant women and women of childbearing age with unhealthy alcohol use, is effective in reducing alcohol consumption, including heavy drinking.

Limited studies (for example, by Chang et al.) provide encouraging evidence on the benefits of SBI in pregnancy, indicating that SBI can help eliminate or at least reduce women's prenatal drinking, minimize fetal risk and maximize pregnancy outcomes (e.g., improved birth weight, reduced fetal death). There is some evidence that SBI may be particularly effective in reducing drinking among women who drink more heavily, and when a partner participated in the intervention.

OTHER DRUGS

Introduction

Drug use is associated with medical complications in pregnant women, such as placental abruption, chorioamnionitis, placental insufficiency, spontaneous abortion, postpartum hemorrhage, and preeclampsia. Drug use alone or in association with alcohol can also have significant impact on the fetus.

Screening

Chasnoff et al. demonstrated that the 4Ps Plus, a five-item instrument, was a reliable measure with good sensitivity and specificity for substance use (alcohol, marijuana, heroin, cocaine, and methamphetamines) during pregnancy. The questionnaire asks about *P*ast substance use, use during *P*regnancy, and use by *P*arents and *P*artners. The result is positive if questions about use during or before pregnancy are affirmative.

Brief Intervention

There is insufficient evidence to determine the benefits and harms of screening for illicit drug use among pregnant women. Confidentiality of the clinician–patient relationship may be challenged in states where the law requires physicians to report illicit drug use by pregnant women, and where law defines this use as criminal behavior. Thus, physicians should be aware of their state's law regarding the reporting of substance use during pregnancy before considering a drug use-targeted SBI.

CONCLUSION AND RECOMMENDATIONS

Alcohol

The current recommendation for pregnant women, women who might be pregnant, and women who are trying to conceive is to abstain from alcohol. For breastfeeding mothers, recommendations are to avoid consumption of alcohol or not to nurse for at least 2 hours per drink after drinking. These women should be screened using validated tools such as T-ACE and TWEAK. Women found to be positive by screening should receive a BI.

Pregnancy itself, or assessment of alcohol use, may lead women to decrease or stop drinking. BI can decrease risky use in young women (pregnant or not). SBI effects may be limited to women who drink the largest amounts. Partner involvement may have beneficial effects. BIs should include specific feedback on consequences of drinking on the fetus and infant as well as medical complications related to alcohol use during pregnancy and identification of risky situations. Reporting issues should be discussed.

Other Drugs

There is currently insufficient evidence to determine the benefits and harms of routine screening for illicit drug use among pregnant women. When drug use is known, though, physicians should give feedback on consequences of use as well as advice to abstain. The four Ps Plus is a validated instrument used for screening among pregnant women. Screening can be affected by the specific context of pregnancy and the potential legal consequences.

Trauma Centers, Hospitals, Emergency Departments

Compared to those in the general population, individuals with substance use disorders are overrepresented among patients presenting to EDs and among those hospitalized for general medical conditions or for traumatic injuries. Alcohol is the major risk factor for virtually all categories of fatal and nonfatal injury, including traffic accidents, burns and fire, drowning, air traffic injury, occupational injury, homicide, suicide, and domestic violence. Although currently evidence is insufficient to recommend routine screening for drug use, trauma centers, hospitals, and EDs are ideal places for clinicians to implement SBIRT for substance use disorders.

CASE FINDING AND SCREENING

Routine clinical information alone will identify many patients with alcohol and drug problems, such as falling down the stairs when intoxicated, delirium tremens, or a gunshot wound sustained in a "crack house." When this information is not readily available, clinical "case finding" has its limitations.

Screening instruments such as the CAGE, "Brief MAST" or "AUDIT" questionnaires have their limitations in busy trauma service. Single questions such as "When was the last time you had more than five drinks (four drinks for women) in 1 day?" represents a "quick screen" and can lead to further questioning if positive.

Several biochemical markers may suggest the presence of an alcohol use disorder, but none are sensitive or specific enough for routine screening. There are no biochemical markers useful as screening tests for drug use.

Mandatory toxicology testing can be useful first-line screening among acutely ill patients. There are limitations to the sensitivity, specificity, and predictive value of toxicology as a marker for alcohol or drug use disorders among inpatients. Interpretation of toxicology results can be challenging because they often detect only recent use and sometimes it is difficult to distinguish between licit and illicit drug use.

Another useful method of obtaining information about the patient's drug use is by obtaining prescription records directly from pharmacies or statewide electronic databases.

CLINICAL ASSESSMENT

A clinical assessment that suggests alcohol or drug abuse or dependence is of immediate clinical importance, as treatment to prevent or manage a withdrawal syndrome may be indicated. Patients with a history of excessive drinking (≥8 or more drinks per day), withdrawal symptoms early in the hospitalization, a high admission blood alcohol concentration (>150 mg/dL), or a concurrent acute medical illness may be at particularly high risk for severe alcohol withdrawal syndrome (AWS). A history of licit or illicit use of sedative should alert the medical staff for a potentially life-threatening sedative withdrawal syndrome.

INITIAL MANAGEMENT OF WITHDRAWAL SYNDROMES

- Parenteral thiamine should be administered to all patients with or at risk for alcohol withdrawal to prevent the development of Wernicke encephalopathy which can occur if certain alcohol-dependent patients receive glucose-containing intravenous fluids.
- Long-acting benzodiazepines are recommended first-line therapy to prevent and treat AWS.
- In sedative dependence, withdrawal can occur within the first 24 hours after admission (short-acting benzodiazepines) or may be delayed for several days (barbiturates or long-acting benzodiazepines).
- Opiate withdrawal is most commonly treated with clonidine (primary agent) and benzodiazepines (for agitation, insomnia), and other symptomatic care (for diarrhea, abdominal cramps, etc.). Long-acting opioids (i.e., buprenorphine, methadone) can also be used to assist assessment and treatment.

INTERVENTION AND DISCHARGE PLANNING

Hospitalized patients with substance use disorders are good candidates for an intervention to prevent future problems because

- They are in a controlled environment.
- They are acutely ill; especially if their illness can be linked to substance use, it may increase the patient's motivation to change ("teachable moment").
- They have the attention of their families as well.

There are conflicting reports about the effectiveness of SBIs in ED settings. Many factors may contribute to such conflicting findings, including insurance issues and difficulties in organizing treatment plans and referrals. It is generally left to the individual treating physician, who may well feel as though doing "something" is better than doing "nothing."

IMPLEMENTATION OF SCREENING AND BRIEF INTERVENTION IN CLINICAL SETTINGS USING QUALITY IMPROVEMENT PRINCIPLES

SUMMARY

The application of the Greenhalgh model to the VA's experience in implementing SBI was outlined in the section and demonstrated important aspects for other health care systems wishing to implement SBI. Some of the essential aspects included a quality improvement infrastructure, an EMR, data systems available for monitoring, feedback and performance measurements. Flexibility in implementation, commitment of necessary resources, attention to provider's educational needs and feedback were also deemed essential for successful implementation of SBI.

Screening for Alcohol and Other Drug Use Disorders in the Elderly

By 2019, it is estimated that one in five Americans will be over the age of 65. Alcoholism is present in 6% to 11% of older persons admitted to hospital. It is estimated to be the third most common psychiatric disorder among elderly persons with twice as many men as women affected. Many older alcoholics admitted to hospitals are not diagnosed.

About one third of older alcoholics are classified as late onset, meaning they first present beyond the age of 65. Elders are more likely to be widowed, retired, and socially isolated.

PATHOPHYSIOLOGY

Elders have proportionally more body fat and less water than younger individuals, and therefore achieve relatively higher blood alcohol concentrations with ingestion of lower quantities of alcohol. The elderly commonly use other pharmacological agents, which also increase risks when combined with alcohol. There are several factors leading to low detection rates of alcoholism in elderly:

- Underdiagnosis by health care providers
- Less socialization, less awareness by peers of drinking behaviors
- Family unwillingness to report
- Institutionalized persons not included in community surveys
- Less job or legal pressure to initiate treatment
- Patient unaccepting of diagnosis

Alcohol can be an etiologic or exacerbating factor to several of the diseases common in elders such as depression, delirium, chronic fatigue, seizures, repeated infections, hypertension, malnutrition, peripheral neuropathy, sexual dysfunction, and cardiomyopathy. Screening tools that can be used for the geriatric population include the following:

Tool	Sensitivity	Specificity
MAST	1.0	0.83
UMAST	0.96	0.86
GMAST (short version)	0.94	0.78
Cyr/Wartman	0.52	0.76
CAGE (one of four considered positive screen)	0.91	0.48
ARPS short version	0.92	0.51

The use of lab tests to aid in the diagnosis is of limited utility.

Impact of Alcohol Use Disorders on Health

Consequences of alcohol use in the elderly can be more severe than in the younger populations. Neurocognitive impairment is worsened by alcohol use; other health realities of aging, such as hip fractures, make manifestations of alcohol use disorders more severe.

Intervention

Brief office or urgent care/ED BI is effective in this age group as in others. The nonlabeling approach is more readily accepted by this cohort. In addition, this age group is more concerned specifi cally with the ability to live independently than with job or legal issues. No evidence exists to support differential benefit of an elderly-specific treatment.

SUMMARY

The diagnosis of alcohol and other drug use disorders is often missed as a result of lack of appropriate screening, underreporting, age bias, and misattribution of alcohol-related health issues to either aging or other diseases common in elders. Appropriate screening tools exist and are useful. BI and standard treatment strategies are effective. The health yield of sobriety is huge as alcoholism is even more dangerous when it occurs in older persons. Alcohol recovery rates are at least as favorable in elders as in younger populations.

CHAPTER 19

Summary Author: Thea Weisdorf
Elizabeth A. Warner • Neil Sharma

Laboratory Diagnosis

Laboratory testing can play a key role in the diagnosis and evaluation of substance abuse and dependence. Testing can include direct identification and measurement of suspected drugs of abuse in body fluids or tissues or can indirectly measure consequences of substance use. The accurate interpretation of laboratory findings requires knowledge of the type of test performed, the limits of detection, and the recognition of the possibility of false-positive and false-negative tests.

When suggested by clinical findings, laboratory testing can assist in the initial diagnosis of a substance use disorder and can identify substances associated with overdoses or trauma. Laboratory tests also are used both to monitor abstinence in treatment programs and to monitor treatment adherence (e.g., in methadone treatment programs).

APPROACH TO DRUG TESTING

Interpretation of Test Results
Skill is required in the interpretation of the resulting data and should be interpreted in the clinical context. The clinician should know

- Which drugs are detected by the tests
- How long the drug is detectable after use
- Which substances can give either false-positive or false-negative results

Body Fluids for Testing
The most commonly used sources for clinical drug testing include urine and blood. Other sources are oral fluid, sweat, hair, and meconium (the latter to screen for prenatal exposure to drugs in the neonate).

Urine

- Most common source for screening as it can be collected easily and noninvasively
- Large quantity is available and drugs are often present in high concentrations.
- Can be easily adulterated or substituted
- Validity of specimen can be improved with temperature, pH, specific gravity, and creatinine parameters.

Blood

- More helpful for recent ingestions
- Less likely to be adulterated or substituted
- Drugs generally present in blood much shorter time
- Poor venous access in injection drug users
- Venipuncture requires training, is invasive, and involves risk of infection to blood taker

Oral Fluid

- Noninvasive, easy to collect, directly observed collection
- Adulteration less likely than with urine

- Measurements of drug concentrations closely estimate circulating concentrations; good for recent drug use
- Disadvantages include shorter period of time in oral fluid than urine
- Measurements can be contaminated by recent smoking or ingested drugs

Sweat

- Patches applied to absorb sweat
- Can identify drug excretion over an extended period
- Quantification of drug levels is difficult since it is not usually possible to measure total amount of sweat secreted

Hair

- More applicable in a forensic or research study environment than in the clinical or workplace setting
- Can be collected easily and noninvasively
- Adulteration and substitution less likely
- Pigmented hair has higher concentration of drugs than nonpigmented hair
- UV light and hair coloring decrease concentrations of drugs
- More labor-intensive preparation to extract the drug
- Sensitive assays required since concentrations of drugs are low
- Not helpful in assessing acute intoxication
- Can provide a history of the pattern of substance use over a longer time span

Collection Procedures

Universal precautions, timing of the collection, and proper labeling are essential. Chain of custody regulations not used routinely for clinical purposes, but used for workplace testing and legal situations.

Specimen Validity Testing

Testing for urine specimen validity is required in federal workplace testing. In clinical settings, validity testing is not required. For federal workplace testing, extensive guidelines mandate that all specimens be tested for creatinine concentration and pH. The temperature of recently collected urine should approximate body temperature (90°F–100°F) within 4 minutes of collection. Testing for potential adulteration is also required in federal workplace testing. Examples of in vivo adulteration include pills, capsules, or "tea" that is ingested before giving a urine specimen. In vitro adulterants include common household products, such as bleach, vinegar, table salt, and baking soda, as well as commercially available kits, such as "Urine Luck." A number of commercially available urine specimen validity dipsticks are available for testing in clinical or nonregulated settings.

Laboratory Methods

The initial procedure for drug testing usually is a screening urine immunoassay. Immunoassays are inexpensive, easily automated, and yield rapid results. In these tests, an antibody reacts to a portion of the drug or its metabolite. A major limitation of immunoassays is cross-reactivity, which can yield false-positive results. Examples of compounds that may cause false-positive results in urine immunoassays are shown in Table 19.1.

Because of the serious consequences that may ensue after a positive urine screen, positive tests on immunoassay can be confirmed with a second analytic procedure to verify the results. The second procedure should be independent of the initial test and should use a different technique and chemical principle from that of the initial test in order to insure reliability and accuracy.

Chromatography is most commonly used as a confirmatory test. Gas chromatography with mass spectroscopy (GC/MS) can identify and quantify extremely small amounts of drugs or metabolites and as such is the "gold standard" for confirming positive immunoassays. GC/MS is required in workplace or forensic testing before reporting the test positive.

Cutoff

A cutoff is a defined concentration of an analyte in a specimen at or above which the test result is reported as positive and below which it is reported negative. For screening tests, if a test result is reported as negative, generally no further testing is done. If a specimen is reported as positive, a confirmatory test may be ordered. Lower cutoff levels are associated with a higher sensitivity and with longer detection times. Table 19.2 lists approximate duration of detection time from the time of last use, using commonly used cutoffs.

TABLE 19.1	Compounds that May Cause False-Positive Results in Urine Immunoassays
Amphetamine/methamphetamine	
Benzphetamine (Didrex)	Haloperidol
Bupropion	Metoclopramide
Chloroquinez	Risperidone
Chlorpromazine	Sertraline
Ephedrine	Thioridazine
Fenfluramine	Verapamil
Labetalol	Marijuana
Mexiletine	Efavirenz
N-acetyl procainamide	Pantoprozole
Phentermine	Quinaprine
Phenylephrine	Methadone
Phenylpropanolamine	Quetiapine
Propranolol	Opiates
Pseudoephedrine	Gatifloxacin
Quinacrine	Levofloxacin
Ranitidine	Ofloxacin
Selegiline	Papaverine
Trazodone	Rifampicin
Tyramine	Poppy seeds
Vicks inhaler	Phencyclidine
Barbiturate	Dextromethorphan
Phenytoin	Diphenhydramine
Benzodiazepines	Thioridazine
Oxaprozin	Venlafaxine
Sertraline	Propoxyphene
LSD	Cyclobenzaprine
Amitriptyline	Diphenylhydramine
Chlorpromazine	Doxylamine
Doxepin	Imipramine
Fluoxetine	Methadone

On-Site Testing

Point of care or on-site testing refers to tests that are performed outside of the laboratory. Commercially available immunoassay kits are available to test urine or oral fluid for commonly abused drugs. These tests are performed at the time of specimen collection. The assays are rapid and easy to perform and require little training. However, the interpretation of these tests is somewhat subjective. Cutoffs are not standardized and may be different than those suggested by the Substance Abuse and Mental Health Services Administration (SAMHSA). Point-of-care tests are more expensive than tests performed in large numbers by laboratories.

TABLE 19.2	Approximate Detection Time Using Screening Urine Immunoassays (with Commonly Used "Cut-Offs")
Drug	**Duration of detection^a (approximate)**
Amphetamine	1–3
Methamphetamine	3 d
Barbiturate	
Short acting	1–4 d
Long acting	Several weeks
Cocaine	3 d
Marijuana	
Single joint (using 50 ng/mL cutoff)	2 d
Heavy use (using 20 ng/mL cutoff)	Up to 27 d
Opioids	
Heroin, codeine, morphine	1–2 d
Methadone (using a specific assay for methadone)	2–3 d
PCP	7 d

^{a}The duration of detection is variable and depends on dose, route of administration, pattern of use, laboratory cutoff, and individual metabolism.

Federal Regulations

The SAMHSA, an operational division of the U.S. Department of Health and Human Services, oversees drug testing of federal workers. The U.S. Department of Transportation (DOT) requires drug and alcohol testing of safety-sensitive transportation employees. Both agencies have developed extensive guidelines for specimen collection, chain-of-custody procedures, and specimen validation. The federal guidelines for federal workplace and DOT drug testing limit drug testing to five substances (amphetamines, cannabinoids, cocaine, opiates, phencyclidine [PCP]) and establish cutoff values for screening and confirmatory testing of these substances.

Clinical Laboratories

Clinical laboratories perform drug and alcohol testing for diagnostic purposes. These specimens are not subject to the same collection and testing requirements used in federal workplace testing. Many clinical laboratories will use the same cutoffs as those required in the workplace.

DRUG-SPECIFIC TESTS

Alcohol

Tests that are widely used to monitor recent alcohol ingestion include gamma-glutamyl-transferase (GGT), aspartate amino transferase (AST), and erythrocyte mean cell volume (MCV). GGT is the most sensitive marker of alcohol abuse (elevated in ~75% of persons with diagnosed alcohol dependence). But GGT is not specific for alcohol use disorders and is elevated in patients with fatty liver and other liver diseases. Thus, the GGT is not generally useful for universal screening.

With abstinence, the MCV will fall, but may take approximately 3 months to see improvement after abstinence given the life span of 120 days of the red blood cell. Several other non–alcohol-related conditions can cause an increase in the MCV, including chronic liver disease, hypothyroidism, folate deficiency, and megaloblastic disorders. Also, the MCV is not very sensitive for detecting heavy drinking.

Carbohydrate-deficient transferrin (CDT) is a less commonly used marker for heavy alcohol use. One must drink four to seven standard drinks (50–80 g of alcohol) per day for a week is required to increase CDT levels. CDT as well can be elevated in non–alcohol-related diseases.

Serum aminotransferases, AST, and alanine amino transferase (ALT) may be elevated in patients with alcohol use disorders (but less sensitive as markers than the GGT). AST is usually more elevated than ALT in alcohol-related liver disease.

There have also been a number of promising markers for alcohol abuse proposed (FAEE, WBAA, and others), but currently their clinical use is limited by short half-lives, technical difficulties, and cost. It must be kept in mind that the sensitivity and specificity of any of these markers are affected by the pretest probability when being used as a screening tool, resulting in more false positives in populations with low pretest probabilities. Also, there are poor dose-response relationships between markers and usage; thus, the markers are not suitable for direct quantification of alcohol consumption.

Acute Alcohol Intoxication

Blood alcohol concentration detects alcohol use with the preceding few hours. Testing for alcohol levels in blood can be done using enzymatic analysis or GC. While GC is considered the gold standard for measuring ethanol in forensic laboratories, many clinical laboratories use enzymatic methods.

Less invasive means of detecting the blood alcohol concentration include analysis of alcohol in the exhaled air. Breath alcohol testing is usually done in traffic law enforcement and DOT testing.

In order to allow clearance of any ethanol that may be in the mouth, a 15-minute waiting period is required before a breath test is performed. The concentration of ethanol is most accurately measured when the subject takes a deep breath, with the measurement taken in the last third of the breath.

Oral fluid can also be used to estimate serum ethanol concentrations. The U.S. DOT has approved on-site oral fluid tests for alcohol screening of safety-sensitive employees in the transportation industry.

Urine testing for alcohol provides a qualitative marker of recent alcohol ingestion. The presence of alcohol in the urine suggests alcohol intake within the preceding 8 hours, but this is variable due to the length of time the urine has been in the bladder. Ethanol glucoronide (Etg), a metabolite of alcohol, can be detected in the urine for 22 to 31 hours after drinking and has been used as a marker to monitor abstinence. Etg testing is highly sensitive but has less reliable specificity (i.e., reacts to commercial products such as mouthwash) and therefore is not endorsed by SAMHSA to use it to monitor abstinence where legal or disciplinary actions can result from a positive test result.

Amphetamines

Amphetamines are a group of stimulants that include amphetamine, methamphetamine, "Ecstasy" (3,4-methylenedioxymethamphetamine or MDMA) or 3,4-methylenedioxymethamphetamine (MDA), and "Eve," which is 3,4-methylenedioxy-N-ethylamphetamine (MDEA). One should not routinely assume that MDMA would be detected on an amphetamine immunoassay since different screening tests for amphetamines have different degrees of selectivity. Routine GC/MS amphetamine assays can distinguish methamphetamine from amphetamine (but not between the *l*-isomers and *d*-isomers of the chemical).

Amphetamines have the most false-positive results of the frequently tested drugs of abuse. Substances such as the decongestants phenylpropanolamine, pseudoephedrine, and l-methamphetamine (found in Vicks nasal inhaler), and certain appetite suppressants have been found to cause positive results.

Urine pH influences the excretion of amphetamines. At high pH levels, there is a marked reduction in amphetamine and methamphetamine excretion. Individuals have been known to ingest large quantities of bicarbonate to reduce the amount of amphetamines excreted in the urine. The duration of detection of amphetamine in the urine by immunoassay is variable but generally accepted to be 1 to 3 days.

Barbiturates

Barbiturates, which are central nervous system depressants, are divided into three categories: ultrashort-acting (thiopental) used in anesthesia; short-acting (pentobarbital, secobarbital, and amobarbital) which are the most widely abused; and the long-acting (phenobarbital), used therapeutically as anticonvulsants and have low abuse potential. Most urine immunoassays are directed toward the parent compound, secobarbital. The duration of detection after barbiturate use is variable and depends on dose, but short-acting barbiturates can be detected from 1 to 4 days after use, while long-acting barbiturates can be detected for several weeks after use.

Benzodiazepines

The interpretation of urine immunoassays for benzodiazepines is complicated by the multiple drugs available, their variable potencies (allowing a large dose range), and their diverse metabolites, which may show poor cross-reactivity with commonly used immunoassays. Urine specimens usually contain little of the parent benzodiazepine.

The cutoff for benzodiazepines immunoassays usually is either 200 or 300 ng/mL, which can detect high doses but may not detect a therapeutic dose. The high-potency benzodiazepines, such as triazolam, are more difficult to detect in immunoassays because they are prescribed in low doses. The benzodiazepine antagonist, flumazenil, is not detected on a benzodiazepine immunoassay.

False-positive results on immunoassays have been reported with substances such as sertraline and tolmetin.

Cocaine

Screening urine immunoassays measure benzoylegonine, the major urinary cocaine metabolite, commonly using a cutoff of 300 ng/mL. The detection of cocaine in the urine is variable and depends on the amount of drug ingested. The usual detection time after cocaine use is 2 to 3 days. Immunoassays for benzoylecgonine are quite specific, and false-positives results with other drugs have not been reported. Immunoassays and GC/MS do not differentiate cocaine hydrochloride from crack cocaine.

Lysergic Acid Diethylamide

At a cutoff of 0.5 ng/mL, urine immunoassays detect LSD for 2 to 5 days after use. There is about a 4% false-positive testing on immunoassay with multiple drugs, including amitriptyline, chlorpromazine, doxepin, fluoxetine, haloperidol, metoclopramide, risperidone, sertraline, thioridazine, and verapamil. Therefore, caution must be exercised in interpreting these tests.

Marijuana

The primary psychoactive component of the marijuana plant is tetrahydrocannabinol (THC). THC has a highly lipophilic nature and is stored in fat tissues and slowly released. Urine screening tests for marijuana typically use cutoffs of 20, 50, or 100 ng/mL. The federally mandated cutoff for workplace testing is 50 ng/mL. The detection time for marijuana is variable and depends on the amount ingested, whether the person is a chronic or an occasional user, and the sensitivity of the assay. The mean detection time of a single marijuana cigarette is <2 days using a 50 ng/mL cutoff.

A positive test is helpful in identifying past marijuana use, but it does not correlate with level of impairment. There has been some debate about the degree to which passive exposure to marijuana smoke influences drug screens. Using extreme conditions, urine specimens of individuals passively exposed to high concentrations of marijuana smoke did test positive with immunoassays. However, on quantitative GC/MS individual with more realistic exposure to marijuana smoke generally are below the cutoffs used in federal workplace or clinical testing.

Opiates and Opioids

Opiates include morphine, codeine, and heroin. Opioid is a more comprehensive term that includes all agonists and antagonists with morphine-like activity. Currently available opiate immunoassays are targeted to detect morphine and have little or no cross-reactivity with synthetic opioids such as fentanyl, propoxyphene, buprenorphine, or methadone and variable cross-reactivity with hydrocodone, hydromorphone, and oxycodone. There are currently available immunoassays specific for oxycodone or buprenorphine. The opioids meperidine, fentanyl, and pentazocine also are not detected in routine urine opiate drug screens.

Both heroin and codeine are metabolized to morphine. Heroin first metabolizes into 6-monoacetylmorphine (6-MAM). 6-MAM is the specific byproduct of heroin metabolism and not a metabolite of morphine, codeine, poppy seeds, or other synthetic opioids. However, 6-MAM is rapidly eliminated and usually detected in the urine for <8 hours after heroin use. Poppy seeds contain small quantities of codeine and morphine, and ingestion of them can result in positive urine opiate screens for 48 hours at a cutoff of 300 ng/mL.

Methadone

Most drug testing for methadone is done to assess compliance with methadone maintenance treatment. Methadone requires a specific opiate drug test. Screening immunoassays have little cross-reactivity with other opioids. Using a cutoff of 300 ng/mL, these screening tests detect methadone in the urine for 2 to 3 days after use. If there is concern that an individual may be spiking a urine specimen with methadone, further testing can be done to detect the presence of the major methadone metabolite.

Phencyclidine

PCP testing in drug screening programs for federal employees is required. Using a cutoff value of 25 ng/dL, urine immunoassay results are positive for approximately 7 days after a single dose and for up to 21 days after chronic use. Saliva levels of PCP are higher than blood levels and PCP may be more stable in saliva than blood. These two factors make saliva a promising tool in the detection of PCP.

Club Drugs

Newer generation tests of amphetamine immunoassays have improved cross-reactivity to MDMA and MDA than before. Ketamine and gamma-hydroxybutyrate (GHB) are not detected by routine urine drug tests and require specialized testing.

Ethical Considerations

Very few guidelines on drug testing for clinical purposes have been developed. Drug testing is commonly ordered under the general "consent to treatment" without specific informed consent, as a diagnostic test to guide treatment. The U.S. Preventive Services Task Force (USPSTF) endorses drug testing in clinical situations in which "there is reasonable suspicion of substance abuse" and recommends obtaining informed consent prior to testing. Likewise does the American Academy of Pediatrics (AAP) in recommending that adolescents should be tested with informed consent. Urine drug testing can be helpful in identifying a patient's possible cause of illness and guide decisions on appropriate pharmacotherapy. Urine drug testing is also helpful in the management of patients on chronic opioid therapy, both to assess adherence with prescribed therapy and to detect drug abuse.

CONCLUSIONS

Laboratory testing in the evaluation of patients with known or suspected substance use disorders, when performed in appropriate clinical setting, can assist in making an accurate diagnosis. However, there are limitations of any test. For alcohol, breath and blood are useful for recent ingestion, but none of the markers for chronic alcohol abuse are ideal screening tests. For other drugs, urine testing can identify recent drug use but does not confirm drug dependence.

Laboratory testing in the clinical setting is intended to guide diagnosis and treatment planning and does not follow the stringent requirements of workplace or forensic testing.

Summary Author: Thea Weisdorf
Theodore V. Parran, Jr. • Richard A. McCormick • John S. Cacciola

Assessment

ASSESSMENT IN MANAGING PATIENTS WITH SUBSTANCE USE DISORDERS

Individual patient assessment is a basic clinical skill and one of the foundations of quality patient care. Patient assessment can be an extremely complex clinical or research evaluation involving a multidisciplinary team.

Addiction is a brain disease that, when active, affects the behavioral control areas. Thus, signs and symptoms of active addictive disease are primarily behavioral. Addictive disease typically affects all domains of life (self-image, self-respect, interpersonal relationships, vocations and hobbies, financial status, legal standing, employment or school performance, and finally physical health).

NEEDS OF DIFFERENT ASSESSORS

Different clinicians have different clinical decision-making needs when it comes to the initial assessment of substance use disorders, and these different clinicians can be generally divided into four groups: primary care clinicians, addiction medicine or psychiatry specialists, substance use disorders treatment programs, and substance use disorder researchers.

The primary care provider needs to perform a reasonably brief patient assessment to verify the diagnosis, stage the severity of the disease from the perspectives of psychosocial morbidity/end-organ damage/physical dependence, stage the patient's readiness for behavior change, and screen for important medical or psychiatric comorbidities.

The addiction medicine or psychiatry specialist will likewise assess the severity of the addictive disease and stage of readiness for behavior change, as well as provide expert evaluation for medical withdrawal or detoxification needs. Further evaluation for co-occurring psychiatric disorders, evaluation of prior attempts at treatment, pattern of remissions and relapses, and the potential role for pharmacotherapy should also be part of this specialist assessment.

The substance use disorders treatment program will emphasize prior treatment experiences, identification and management of co-occurring medical and psychiatric conditions, family issues and the therapeutic milieu, and past relapse patterns.

The substance use disorder research organization's emphasis tends to be on quantitative evaluation of the degree of accumulated morbidity in the patient's life, patient-centered research into treatment matching efforts, identification and exploration of patient characteristics that predict response to treatment.

TASKS OF THE ASSESSMENT PROCESS

Assessment of substance use disorders within the context of the rest of the patient's life circumstances is a process that should be utilized when evaluating every patient. The tools used may change depending upon the clinical situation, the skill and resources available to the clinician, and the specific characteristics of patient presentation, but the basic areas to be assessed remain fairly constant (Table 20.1).

When assessment is viewed from the perspective of timing, one recognizes that since 1990, the addiction treatment field has worked to improve the *pretreatment* assessment of alcoholism and other addictions in order to provide better treatment decisions. More recently, concepts such as *intratreatment* and *posttreatment assessment* have come into favor, encouraging ongoing assessment at transition points in the treatment process. This permits the continued adaptation of the treatment plan, a key criterion for most treatment program accreditation reviews.

TABLE 20.1	Major Areas for Addiction Assessment

1. Diagnostic criteria
2. Presence and level of intoxication
3. Suicidal or homicidal ideation
4. Physiologic dependence and withdrawal potential
5. Level of addiction-associated morbidity
6. Medical comorbidities
7. Psychiatric comorbidities
8. Legal issues
9. Readiness for behavior change
10. Prior treatment successes and relapse patterns

SOURCES OF ASSESSMENT INFORMATION

The assessment process is able to gather information from many different sources of one's life, which is relevant in the life of a patient affected by addictive disease, such as the interpersonal, interpersonal, vocational and hobbies, financial, legal, educational, and of course physical. Sources that are commonly utilized in assessing addictive disease include patient history, physical exam, laboratory and toxicology results, family interview, medical-legal history questioning, educational and occupational interview, and readiness for behavior change evaluation.

It is important to interview patients in ways that avoid defensiveness about their behaviors resulting from their addiction. Patient self-report reliability is improved by using a consistent series of questions that progress from general and open-ended to specific information gathered in a more closed-ended question form and by utilizing the family or significant other interview whenever possible.

A psychiatric screening interview and a specific screening for suicidal or homicidal ideation are necessary in this population. Also, assessing for abuse is necessary owing to the high rates of interpersonal violence in patients with chemical dependence. Even the cultural background, spiritual inclination, and belief system that the patient holds regarding substance use disorders can be essential areas of assessment.

ASSESSMENT TOOLS

A thorough assessment should evaluate each area of patient function that is necessary for the needs of the clinician performing or requesting the assessment. In addition, the assessment tool used should be reliable, reproducible, and verifiable.

Some of the tools (AUDIT, and AUDIT-C, DAST, CAGE) are primarily *screening tools*, but the assessment process is a clear and direct extension of the screening and diagnosis process. Further information on many of these tools, and other assessment options, can be found online at *niaaa.nih.gov/publications, drugabuse.gov*, or *samsha.gov*.

Often, the first step in conducting an addiction assessment is to establish degree of risk associated with the current level of acute intoxication or withdrawal. The CIWA-Ar is a brief 10-item scale that can be administered in <5 minutes. It quantifies the severity of the alcohol withdrawal syndrome by rating ten common alcohol withdrawal symptoms and can be clinically useful in monitoring progress over time.

The AUDIT (Alcohol Use Disorders Identification Test) was developed to identify hazardous use, harmful use, and dependence on alcohol in primary care. The 10-item questionnaire includes three questions on consumption and seven on the impact of alcohol use. The AUDIT has been shown to have good sensitivity and specificity in medical and general populations. It has also been shown to be useful for screening patients with major psychiatric disorders and as an assessment instrument for patients seeking alcohol treatment.

Similar instruments, such as the Drug Abuse Screening Test (DAST), a 20-item questionnaire, screen for abuse of drugs other than alcohol.

The Psychoactive Substance Use Disorders module of the Structured Clinical Interview for *DSM-IV* (SCID) is a semistructured diagnostic interview that establishes *DSM-IV* Axis I diagnoses for substance use disorders. It is widely used and considered the "gold standard" for establishing diagnoses in research applications.

The Addiction Severity Index (ASI) Drug/Alcohol Use section provides a reliable measure of lifetime use and use within the past 30 days. The ASI has been widely used in both clinical and research applications. The ASI sections can be readministered to assess progress over time.

Self-report instruments also provide a broadened assessment of the consequences of use. The Drinker Inventory of Consequences (DrInc) measures the adverse consequences of alcohol abuse in five domains: physical, social, impulsive, interpersonal, and intrapersonal. This is a 50-item test and takes only about 10 minutes to complete. There is a similar companion instrument, the Inventory of Drug Use Consequences (InDUC).

In that many patients with substance use disorders present with *psychiatric comorbidities*, these psychiatric illnesses require concomitant or sequential treatment. The SCID has modules for each of the other major syndrome groups: anxiety disorders, affective disorders, and psychotic disorders. Administration of the full SCID can take 2 hours or more depending on the patient's complexity.

Short self-report instruments are commonly used such as the Beck Depression Inventory and the Beck Anxiety Inventory. Both are relatively short instruments that take about 10 minutes to administer and can be readministered over time to monitor progress. The South Oaks Gambling Screen (SOGS) has been demonstrated to reliably identify substance abusers with problem or pathological gambling.

It is important to assess the *motivational level* of the patient. Widely used are the Stages of Change Readiness and Treatment Eagerness Scale (SOCRATES) and the University of Rhode Island Change Assessment (URICA). Both are relatively short, easy to administer, and have been used successfully with a wide range of patients, including the severely mentally ill, substance-abusing patients.

More comprehensive assessments measuring *resistance to treatment* are measured by the Recovery Attitude and Treatment Evaluator (RAATE) instrument, which has both a semistructured clinical interview option and a self-report version.

Assessment instruments can be valuable aids in constructing a *relapse prevention* plan. The Inventory of drinking situations is a 100-item self-report instrument that allows a patient to assess his or her tendency to drink in a variety of situations that can be categorized as urges and temptations.

It is also useful to understand the *coping skills* that the patient possesses. The Coping Response Inventory (CRI) is one such relatively short self-report tool to accomplish this.

Adherence to treatment remains a major impediment to recovery. Self-efficacy and expectations about the effect of alcohol and drugs have been demonstrated to be related to adherence. Self-efficacy for alcohol-related situations can be measured using the Situational Confidence Questionnaire (SCQ), a short self-report questionnaire.

SELECTING THE RIGHT ASSESSMENT TOOL

Assessment is a necessary part of the evaluation of patients with addictive disease and is a critical bridge between screening and diagnosis and treatment planning. The setting in which the assessment is done largely determines which assessment tool(s) will be employed. The following settings exemplify this.

Primary Care Office Setting

Screening tools such as the CAGE, AUDIT, DAST, and s-MAST provide assessment information about patterns of use, adverse consequences of use, and other important information, such as prior success or failure with abstinence, prior treatment experience etc.

Addiction Physician Setting

In general, the addiction medicine or psychiatry physician needs when approaching the assessment process require much more in-depth evaluation and use of more formal tools for staging the addictive disease. These have been outlined above and should also include aforementioned screening tools for depression and anxiety. Here as well, review of prior treatments, length and characteristics of remissions, relapses, and current supports and resources available is essential. Evaluation for acute and postacute withdrawal issues is necessary as well.

Addiction Treatment Program Setting

Here, a formalized addiction assessment process is incorporated. These may include previously mentioned structured interviews such as the ASI or the SCID.

SUMMARY

Quality assessment permits the development of a comprehensive problem list and a thorough treatment plan. Assessment of all the various domains of life affected by addictive disease as well as medical and psychiatric comorbidities, detoxification needs, prior treatment, relapse patterns, readiness for change, and treatment resistance are all critical areas of focus. Repeating the use of some of the aforementioned quantitative tools can measure improved functioning and decreased morbidity.

CHAPTER 21

Summary Author: Thea Weisdorf
Andrew J. Treno • Paul J. Gruenewald • Harold D. Holder • Lillian G. Remer

Environmental Approaches to Prevention

Alcohol-involved problems are a serious public health issue. The prevention of these problems is a major need in contemporary America. Estimates of the extent of alcohol involvement in trauma include 39% of traffic-crash fatalities, 47% of homicides, 29% of suicides, 30% to 40% for fatal recreational injuries, and 10% to 25% for home injuries. There are an estimated 17,000 persons who die each year in alcohol-related traffic crashes and some 2.7 million violent victimization events involving alcohol each year. Alcohol involvement in violence-related injuries has been estimated as 28% to 43%, with a large percentage of violence occurring among young people between the ages of 15 and 20. Alcohol consumption is also a major problem in the US work force, linked to increased medical costs, worker's compensation claims, sick leave/absenteeism, accidents, early retirement, and loss of productivity.

Treatment alone is not an adequate response to major public health problems. Prevention and reduction of alcohol-related problems can have both short- and long-term value. Limiting factors to prevention successes to date have multiple etiologies. Today, prevention researchers recognize that alcohol-related problems result from the interaction between individuals and their larger environment, which encompasses social, cultural, economic, and political factors. Some of these environmental factors can be easily changed. This chapter is divided into three sections. The first section provides a brief summary of the environmental perspectives on the reduction of alcohol and other drug problems. The second section describes several examples of major demonstration projects developed in keeping with this perspective. The third section discusses how environment-based studies provide the core scientific research needed to develop adequate theoretical models of the ecologies of drinking and related problems.

ENVIRONMENTAL STRATEGIES

Environmental approaches to the reduction of alcohol and drug problems can be contrasted with more traditional approaches in a number of ways. First, environmental approaches often include changing formal institutions (e.g., reducing hours and days of sale of alcohol) but may also include attempts to change informal systems (e.g., breaking up markets for illegal drugs). Second, these approaches differ in their use of the media. Traditional approaches target individuals, whereas environmental approaches typically target policymakers or "gatekeepers," such as state legislators, law enforcement agencies, or even parents within families. Environmental interventions can also use media to increase public awareness or to influence social norms. A third important distinction between environmental and traditional approaches to prevention is their orientation toward persons at risk. Rather than targeting individuals at risk directly, the environmental approach targets the broader alcohol and drug environment. Fourth and finally, traditional approaches attempt to reduce the individual demand for drugs, whereas environmental approaches seek to reduce supply of a substance or the risks associated with its use.

Environmental prevention programs generally target acute problems such as motor vehicle crashes, injuries, violence and drug-related crime, rather than chronic medical conditions, such as alcohol dependence or liver cirrhosis. Environmental prevention efforts rarely focus on reduced use; rather they attempt to reduce the harm resulting from use. It follows that while environmental prevention programs may reduce harms related to alcohol and drug abuse (such as motor vehicle crashes and AIDS transmission), they may not change the chronic problems that result from prolonged use (such as heart and liver disease).

The importance of the focus on acute problems relates to the social costs of alcohol and drug abuse in terms of years of life lost owing to acute harm. The immediate short-term burden that acute alcohol and drug problems place on the health care and enforcement systems renders them more costly to society than many other major health problems. Acute problems are so costly because they are distributed so widely in the population of substance abusers. Thus, the term "prevention paradox" is employed, which refers to the observation that while high-risk individuals produce more problems on an individual basis, lower risk individuals produce more problems on an aggregate basis. A focus on high- and low-risk individuals therefore makes sense, which is the main advantage of employing environmental strategies.

DOMAINS OF ENVIRONMENTAL PREVENTION

Environmental prevention programs act in three domains: the physical, the social, and the economic. Prevention programs may alter physical access by affecting proximity to sources of alcohol, drugs, and tobacco (i.e., eliminating the sale of tobacco through vending machines). They may alter social access by affecting the social networks that encourage and enable distribution of these substances (i.e., free access during on-campus celebrations). Prevention programs may alter economic access by increasing the real costs of these substances and changing the economic geography of availability.

STRUCTURE OF ENVIRONMENTAL PREVENTION

In environmental prevention, the relationships between physical, social, and economic contexts of human behavior become very important. Individual use of drugs and alcohol produces problems (i.e., drinking may lead to drinking and driving). The environment creates a stage on which human activities play themselves out to produce problems. There are four ways in which the alcohol environment can affect problems related to drinking and drug use.

Direct Effects on Substance use

The most obvious way in which environmental prevention activities reduce problems related to alcohol and drugs is to alter the behaviors of drinkers and drug users. Demographic, economic, and physical restrictions on availability can reduce use and problems. For example, increasing the minimum legal drinking age to 21 has been linked to a 13% reduction in the number of high school seniors reporting drinking.

Price increases are clearly associated with declines in alcohol consumption, with heavy and youth drinkers being particularly sensitive to price changes. Also, increases and decreases in the physical availability of alcohol have been linked to increases and decreases in alcohol sales, suggesting that a 10% reduction in outlet densities would be associated with a 3% reduction in alcohol sales.

Other ways in which the environment may directly affect drinking behaviors include the introduction of responsible beverage service programs (decreased use), local enforcement of underage sales laws (reduction in use), privatization of alcohol monopolies, which yield lower prices, greater numbers of outlets, and increased sales (all resulting in increased use).

Indirect Effects on Problems

Studies have clearly demonstrated the potential impact of environmental change on problem outcomes such as traffic crashes. For example, raising the legal drinking age to 21 has been linked to a 20% reduction in single-vehicle night time crashes among youth drivers. Also, higher alcohol prices have been linked to lower rates of traffic deaths and cirrhosis mortality. Yet another example is mandated server-training policies which have been linked to reductions in alcohol-involved crashes.

Direct Effects on Problems

Environmental prevention efforts can directly affect problem outcomes and provide alternative paths to prevention. Aspects of the psychological, social, economic, and physical environments apparently unrelated to alcohol and drug use can confound research efforts to evaluate any prevention activity, but they also can become an important part of environmental prevention. Most environmental prevention studies recognize that multiple environmental supports must be incorporated in the prevention of problem outcomes. One example showed that a combination of media campaigns, enforcement of speed and DUI limits, and community awareness reduced fatal motor vehicle crashes by as much as 25%.

Effects on Relationships Between Substance Use and Problem Outcomes

The social, economic, and physical environments determine the nature of problems experienced by individuals. Researchers found strong indications that environmental contexts focus problems in ways that can be taken advantage of in future preventive intervention programs. In the case of alcohol-related traffic crashes, the location of alcohol outlets along different types of roadways affects drinking, driving, and crashing. Within low traffic flow areas of communities (i.e., downtown areas), greater numbers of alcohol outlets do not lead to significantly greater numbers of alcohol-related crashes. Conversely, within high traffic flow areas of communities (i.e., along highways), greater numbers of alcohol outlets lead to substantively greater numbers of alcohol-related crashes. Similar observations are beginning to emerge in studies of violence related to alcohol outlets and problems related to illegal drug markets. Disrupting the geographic link between location of sales and location of users leads to reduced drug sales and problems.

ENVIRONMENTAL STRATEGIES AND ALCOHOL POLICY

"Policy" usually refers to structural change, as through a regulation, law, or enforcement priority. As suggested by this chapter, communities have begun to go beyond policy to affect the drinking environment itself as an approach to reducing alcohol-involved problems. National as well as state, region, or provincial laws often establish the base for local policies, including legal drinking ages, regulation of alcohol outlets, the legal blood alcohol level for driving after drinking, advertising restrictions, and service to obviously intoxicated persons and underage persons. Environmental interventions are politically feasible because they do not target specific subgroups in a discriminatory manner. In general, they are cost effective because they do not require case finding, service provision, or cost maintenance. It would appear as if there are three basic policy strategies used to reduce alcohol-related problems.

The first class of interventions reduces alcohol availability by limiting the times and days that alcohol outlets may sell or serve alcohol (i.e., control of days and hours of legal sales) or by reducing the number of outlets that provide opportunities for such purchases (i.e., outlet density restrictions or state-controlled monopoly).

A second group of interventions operate through the application of specific penalties to either consumers or providers either by establishing liability for second parties for serving alcohol to persons of specific statuses (minimum legal drinking age) or to levels of intoxication (dram shop liability) or by punishing persons for consuming alcohol in specific amounts conjoint to specific activities (DUI enforcement).

A third approach focuses on altering the alcohol environment through training of providers (server training). While having the advantage of being the least politically controversial, it would seem the least effective largely owing to high turnover rates in the hospitality industry, low levels of monitoring of servers, and competitive economic pressures to overserve patrons and to sell to minors.

EFFICACY TRIALS

Based upon the promising results found from basic policy studies, several important community-based environmental preventive intervention studies were undertaken. These projects went beyond the scientific evidence to test whether environmental prevention efforts could be effective at the community level in preventing three harmful outcomes related to alcohol: drinking and driving, underage access and use, and violence related to alcohol.

These studies were the Saving Lives Project (six communities in Massachusetts) designed to reduce alcohol-impaired driving and related problems; the Communities Mobilizing for Change on Alcohol Project (15 communities in Minnesota and western Wisconsin) designed to reduce access to alcohol among youth under the legal drinking age of 21; the Community Trials Project, a five-component community-level intervention conducted in three experimental communities matched to three controls, whose goal was to reduce alcohol-related harm among all persons in the three experimental communities; and the Sacramento Neighborhood Alcohol Prevention Project whose goal was to implement and evaluate neighborhood-level interventions intended to reduce youth and young-adult access to alcohol, risky drinking, and associated problems, particularly in low-income ethnically diverse neighborhoods. In all of the above Projects, environmental preventive interventions were associated with reductions in the harmful outcomes related to alcohol outlined above.

International Contexts

In addition to these successful US environmental prevention programs, several other important efforts have been fielded throughout the world. Notable environmental strategies have been implemented and tested in Australia, Sweden, Brazil, Finland, Denmark, Italy, Israel, New Zealand, and Canada.

EMERGENCE OF ECOLOGIC RESEARCH

Despite the demonstrated effectiveness of environmentally based preventive interventions, much empirical research and efficacy testing remains to be done. We have moved from demonstrating that environmental interventions are effective to considering which are the most effective. Yet the mechanisms that make them work are not understood. Without a convincing theoretical statement of plausible mechanisms that relate observed environmental measures to outcomes and without accompanying empirical tests of these mechanisms, the causal processes that support these correlations remain unknown. The ultimate goal here is to state and test strong social ecologic theories about alcohol-related problems such as drinking and drunken driving, intimate partner violence and alcohol parental alcohol use and child abuse and neglect, and the relationships of community policy and enforcement activities to underage drinking.

ENVIRONMENTAL STRATEGIES AND DRUG POLICY

Environmental strategies for the reduction of harm related to the use of illicit drugs are in their infancy when compared to alcohol prevention programs. Much of what is conceived as "environmental" is instead only "enforcement" when considering illegal substances. Ideally the equivalent actions with regard to alcohol (arrests for drunken driving) are intended to reduce this illegal activity by deterring driving after drinking. Arrests make enforcement an environmental prevention activity. In the arena of illegal drug sales, it is difficult to ascribe such preventive benefits to enforcement outside of the greater costs incurred by users through the disruption of drug supply networks. In a similar manner, greater costs for drugs may arise through the "War on Drugs" and other interdiction activities. However, the effectiveness of such strategies has been shown to be very limited.

Other prevention strategies with regard to illegal drug use are oriented to individuals or families, not the environment of drug use. The majority of these efforts are programs to educate young people to resist use, to help moderate the dire consequences of disrupted families on youth use, and more general media campaigns to encourage users to stop and discourage nonusers from beginning to use drugs. Strikingly, there is little literature on environmental prevention per se.

CHAPTER

22

Summary Author: Ashok Krishnamurthy
William L. White

Addiction Medicine in America: Its Birth and Early History (1750–1935) with a Modern Postscript

THE BIRTH OF ADDICTION MEDICINE

The recent recognition of addiction medicine as a medical specialty obscures the fact that American physicians have been involved in the treatment of severe and persistent alcohol- and other drug-related problems for more than two centuries.

The roots of addiction medicine began not in a young America but in the ancient civilizations of Africa and Europe.

The earliest intimations of the concept of addiction and its treatment reflect the fleeting observations of individuals rather than an organized cultural response to alcohol and other drug problems.

The earliest American medical responses to alcoholism emerged within the systems of medicine practiced by Native American tribes.

Alcohol-related problems rose dramatically in Native America as alcohol became increasingly used as a tool of economic, political, and sexual exploitation in the 18th and early 19th centuries.

Native American healers used botanical agents to suppress cravings for alcohol (hop tea), to induce an aversion to alcohol (the root of the trumpet vine), and to facilitate personal transformation within sobriety-based cultural and religious revitalization movements.

Addiction was not a noted problem in American until increased alcohol consumption, a shift in preference from fermented to more potent forms of distilled alcohol, and the emergence of a pattern of socially disruptive "frontier drinking" emerged in the late 1800s.

In 1774, the philanthropist and social reformer Anthony Benezet published a treatise, *Mighty Destroyer Displayed*, which recast alcohol from its status as a gift from God to that of a "bewitching poison."

Benezet's warning was followed by a series of publications by Dr. Benjamin Rush—his 1784 pamphlet, *Inquiry into the Effects of Ardent Spirits on the Human Mind and Body*, was the first American treatise on alcoholism. Rush catalogued the symptoms of acute and chronic drunkenness, described the progressiveness of these symptoms, and suggested that chronic drunkenness was a "disease induced by a vice." Rush was the first prominent physician to claim that many confirmed drunkards could be restored to full health through proper medical treatment.

Between 1774 and 1829, America "discovered" addiction through the collective observations of her physicians, clergy, and social activists. There was an emerging view that chronic drunkenness was a problem with biologic roots and consequences and thus the province of the physician.

These earliest pioneers declared that chronic intoxication was a diseased state, and they articulated the major elements of an addiction disease concept: biologic predisposition, drug toxicity, pharmacologic tolerance, disease progression, morbid appetite (craving), loss of volitional control of alcohol/drug intake, and the pathophysiologic consequences of sustained alcohol and opiate ingestion.

Addiction medicine emerged in the shift from treating medical consequences of alcohol addiction to treating the addiction itself.

Early Professionalization and Medical Advancements (1830–1900)

One of the most significant milestones in the history of addiction medicine was the 1849 publication of Magnus Huss's text, *Chronic Alcoholism*. After an extensive review of the chronic effects of intoxication, Huss declared:

> *These symptoms are formed in such a particular way that they form a disease group in themselves and thus merit being designated and described as a definite disease... It is this group of symptoms which I wish to designate by the name Alcoholismus chronicus.*

Huss's text stands as the landmark addiction medicine text of the mid-19th century. It contributed a clinical term—*alcoholism*—that came into increasing medical and public popularity in the transition between the 19th and 20th centuries.

In 1870, Dr. Joseph Parrish led the creation of the American Association for the Cure of Inebriety (AACI), which brought together the heads of America's most prominent inebriate homes and asylums. The AACI bylaws posited that

1. *Intemperance is a disease.*
2. *It is curable in the same sense that other diseases are.*
3. *Its primary cause is a constitutional susceptibility to the alcoholic impression.*
4. *This constitutional tendency may be either inherited or acquired.*

The AACI held regular meetings to exchange ideas and published the first specialized medical journal on addiction—the *Journal of Inebriety*.

American physicians specializing in addiction began releasing texts on the nature of addiction and their treatment methods in the 1860s: Dr. Albert Day's *Methomania: A Treatise on Alcoholic Poisoning* and Dr. W. Marcet's *On Chronic Alcoholic Intoxication*. The production of such literature virtually exploded in the 1880s and 1890s.

The central organizing concept of 19th-century addiction medicine specialists was that of *inebriety*. Addiction medicine texts were often organized under such headings as *alcoholic inebriety, opium inebriety, cocaine inebriety,* and *ether inebriety*. Inebriety specialists talked eloquently about the need to individualize treatment and, by the 1880s, had begun to recognize and study the problem of posttreatment relapse.

Understanding of the potential physiologic foundations and consequences of addiction increased during the last two decades of the 19th century. *Carl Wernicke's 1881 discovery of a psychosis with polyneuritis that resulted from chronic alcoholism and Sergei Korsakoff's 1887 description of an alcoholism-induced psychosis characterized by confusion, memory impairment, confabulation, hallucinations, and stereotyped and superficial speech both underscored the potential organic basis of alcoholic behavior.*

Demedicalization and the Collapse of Addiction Treatment (1900–1935)

Between 1900 and 1920, addiction treatment institutions closed in great numbers in the wake of a weakened infrastructure of the field, rising therapeutic pessimism, economic austerity triggered by unexpected depressions, and a major shift in national policy. The country turned its gaze to state and national prohibition laws as the solution to alcohol and other drug-related problems.

As inebriate homes and asylums and the private addiction cure institutes closed in tandem with the spread of local and state prohibition laws, alcoholics were relegated to other institutions.

These included the "foul wards" of large city hospitals, the back wards of aging state psychiatric asylums, and the local psychopathic hospital.

Wealthy alcoholics/addicts sought discrete detoxification in a new genre of private hospital or sanitarium established for this purpose.

Alcohol-related problems decreased dramatically in the early 1920s but rose to preprohibition levels by the late 1920s. The 18th Amendment to the U.S. Constitution transferred cultural ownership of alcohol problems from physicians to law enforcement authorities. A similar process was underway with drugs other than alcohol, but it took two decades for this shift in approach to fully emerge.

Early 20th-century addiction texts by physicians such as George Pettey and Ernest Bishop boldly proclaimed that narcotic addiction was a disease. *The medical treatment of narcotic addicts was dramatically altered by passage of the Harrison Anti-Narcotic Act of 1914. This federal act designated physicians and pharmacists as the gatekeepers for the distribution of opiates and cocaine.*

The Harrison Act, in effect if not intent, *transferred responsibility for the care of addicts from physicians to criminal syndicates and the criminal justice system by threatening physicians with both loss of license and incarceration* if they provided maintenance rather than rapid detoxification of addicts.

Physician culpability in the problem of narcotic addiction made it difficult for the AMA to oppose this government infringement in medical practice. In 1919, the AMA passed a resolution opposing ambulatory treatment, in effect opposing narcotic maintenance as treatment.

The influence of psychiatry on the characterization and treatment of addiction increased in tandem with the decline of a specialized field of addiction medicine.

Few institutional resources existed for the treatment of alcoholism and narcotic addiction during the 1920s and early 1930s, but the growing visibility of these problems began to generate new proposals for their management.

The opening of the California Narcotics Hospital at Spadra in 1928 marked the beginning of state support for addiction treatment.

Drs. Arthur B. Light and Edward G. Torrance conducted research on opiate addicts at the Philadelphia General Hospital; they demonstrated that withdrawal from opiates is not life threatening and usually not dangerous—a finding that was misused by policy makers to withhold medical care for addicts.

In 1928, the Bureau of Social Hygiene published Charles Terry and Mildred Pellens' work, *The Opium Problem*. In this important report, Terry and Pellens *made a strong argument in favor of addiction maintenance as the most appropriate treatment for addicts who are not able to sustain abstinence.* Their views were viciously attacked, and it would only be years later that the study *would be recognized as one of the best treatises on opiate addiction ever written.*

THE REBIRTH OF ADDICTION TREATMENT (1935–1970)

The modern alcoholism movement was ignited by the founding of Alcoholics Anonymous (1935). Two goals of this movement were to encourage local hospitals to detoxify alcoholics and to encourage local communities to establish posthospitalization alcoholism rehabilitation centers.

This movement spawned new institutional resources for the treatment of alcoholism from the mid-1940s through the 1960s, including "AA wards" in local hospitals, model outpatient alcoholism clinics developed in Connecticut and Georgia, and a model community–based residential model.

A mid-20th-century reform movement advocating medical rather than penal treatment of the opiate addict also helped spawn the rebirth of addiction medicine. This began with the founding of state-sponsored addiction treatment hospitals (e.g., Spadra Hospital in California) and led to the creation of two U.S. Public Health Hospitals within the Bureau of Prisons—one in Lexington, Kentucky (1935), the other in Fort Worth, Texas (1938).

Three replicable models of treatment emerged: ex-addict–directed therapeutic communities, methadone maintenance pioneered by Drs. Vincent Dole and Marie Nyswander, and outpatient drug-free counseling.

State and federal funding for alcoholism and addiction treatment slowly increased from the late 1940s through the 1960s and was followed by landmark legislation in the early 1970s *that created the NIAAA and the National Institute on Drug Abuse (NIDA)*—the beginning of the federal, state, and local community partnership *that has been the foundation of modern addiction treatment.*

National Institute on Alcohol Abuse and Alcoholism (NIAAA) and NIDA also made heavy investments in research that led to dramatic breakthroughs in understanding the neurobiology of addiction that encouraged more medicalized approaches to severe alcohol and other drug problems.

ADDICTION MEDICINE COMES OF AGE (1970–2008)

Two professional associations have significantly advanced the reemergence of addiction medicine as a clinical specialty of medical practice: the American Society of Addiction Medicine (ASAM) and the American Academy of Addiction Psychiatry (AAAP).

The ASAM can trace its roots to the establishment of the creation of a New York City Medical Committee on Alcoholism in 1951 by the National Council on Alcoholism, the 1954 founding of the New York State Medical Society on Alcoholism under the leadership of Dr. Ruth Fox, and the movement of this group in 1967 to establish itself as a national organization—the American Medical Society on Alcoholism (AMSA).

AMSA was later evolved into the American Medical Society on Alcoholism and Other Drug Dependencies and then into the ASAM.

ASAM's achievements include the following:

- Advocating the AMA's addition of addiction medicine to its list of designated specialties (achieved in June 1990)
- Offering a certification and recertification process for addiction medicine specialists based on the early work of the California Society of Addiction Medicine
- Hosting its annual addiction medicine conference
- Publishing its widely utilized patient placement criteria
- Development of the *Principles of Addiction Medicine*
- Publishing first the *Journal of Addictive Diseases* and presently the *Journal of Addiction Medicine*

The AAAP (formerly the American Academy of Psychiatrists in Alcoholism and the Addictions) was established in 1985 with the goal of elevating the quality of clinical practice in addiction psychiatry.
The AAAP's contributions include

- Advocating that the American Board of Psychiatry and Neurology grant addiction medicine a subspecialty status
- Administering an addiction psychiatry certification and recertification process
- Hosting an annual conference on addiction psychiatry
- Publishing the *American Journal on Addictions*
- Promoting fellowships in addiction psychiatry

Several additional initiatives have advanced addiction-related medical education. The NIAAA and the NIDA created the Career Teacher Program (1971–1981) that develop addiction-related curricula for the training of physicians in 59 US medical schools.

In 1976, Career Teachers and others involved in addiction-related medical education and research established the Association of Medical Education and Research in Substance Abuse (AMERSA). AMERSA draws its members primarily from American medical school faculty, hosts an annual meeting, and publishes the journal *Substance Abuse*.

In 2008, there are >14,400 physicians working within a network of 13,200 specialized addiction treatment programs in the United States who help care for the >1.9 million individuals and families admitted for treatment each year.

Summary Author: Ashok Krishnamurthy
Mark J. Willenbring

Treatment of Heavy Drinking and Alcohol Use Disorders

BACKGROUND

Only about one in eight persons who develop alcohol dependence ever seek or receive treatment in an addiction treatment center.

In addition, most treatment offered lasts a few weeks for a disorder that often lasts years. This limits the population level impact of treatment and means that many people suffer needlessly.

DEVELOPMENT OF MODERN APPROACHES TO TREATMENT

Modern behavioral treatment approaches grew initially out of the success of Alcoholics Anonymous (AA) on the one hand and the growth of academic psychiatry and psychology after World War II on the other.

The Minnesota Model of treatment was initially conceived by a psychologist and a physician working at Willmar State Hospital in Minnesota in the 1950s.

Key features of the Minnesota Model of treatment are

1. Use of both professional staff (some of whom may be recovering from alcohol dependence)
2. Patient and family education
3. Strong linkage to AA
4. Requirement of abstinence from all addictive substances other than tobacco and caffeine
5. Belief that alcoholism is a primary, progressive disease that cannot be cured

The model was initially provided only in 28-day programs in hospitals or residential facilities but is now provided in outpatient settings as well.

Twelve-step facilitation is a manualized version of the Minnesota Model that has been adapted for an individual outpatient approach.

The concepts of group therapy and therapeutic community were first proposed in the mid-1940s, with subsequent development and spread in the 1950s and 1960s.

Albert Ellis developed the first type of cognitive-behavior therapy, Rational-Emotive Therapy, in the mid-1950s, and Aaron Beck developed cognitive therapy for depression in the 1960s.

Specific therapies for alcohol dependence based on these earlier psychologic theories include

- Therapeutic communities
- Aversion therapy
- Cognitive-behavior therapy
- Skills training
- Community reinforcement
- Contingency management

Over the same period, pharmacotherapy for alcohol dependence was attempted with many new psychiatric medications as they were discovered or developed.

Disulfiram was approved for use as a deterrent or aversive agent in 1949. It took 46 years for the next medication, **naltrexone**, to be approved for treatment of alcohol dependence in 1995. More recently, **acamprosate** and **topiramate** have been shown to be effective.

While there has been considerable progress toward enlightened, humane, and effective treatment, many obstacles still remain:

- In >90% of community programs (not including the Veterans Affairs health care system), group counseling and referral to AA provided by counselors with minimal education are the only modalities offered.
- *In most cases, there is no physician involvement in treatment other than treating withdrawal.*
- Treatment is time limited, focused on inducing and maintaining remission, and offers little except repetition for patients who do not respond.
- Because of the lack of integration of addiction treatment programs with medical and psychiatric treatment, few programs are able to identify and treat coexisting mental and physical disorders in their patients, even though these are very common in a treatment-seeking population.
- In many community programs, supervision is minimal and therapeutic discussions often consist of casual talk unrelated to therapy rather than formal counseling.
- Very few community treatment programs offer currently available pharmacotherapy or even educate their patients about it.

How Should Treatment Outcome be Determined?

Until relatively recently, total, continuous, permanent abstinence was considered by most to be the only goal of treatment and the only measure of outcome.

Reasons for this are complex, but include the strongly held belief of AA members and Minnesota Model treatment providers that anything less than a commitment to total lifetime abstinence would result in failure. Additionally, abstinence was easier for researchers to measure and verify.

On the other hand, some researchers believed that drinking (including heavy drinking) was a learned behavior, and that it might therefore be possible for patients to learn new ways of (moderate) drinking.

Whether abstinence or reduced drinking should be the goal remains a matter of contention. Reduced drinking as a goal is often called *harm reduction*. This term is an unfortunate one that describes a pragmatic public drug policy most interested in results, as opposed to a more idealistic one focused more on intention.

In the case of clinical care, the term is used to describe a pragmatic approach when abstinence cannot be obtained.

The research community has developed increasingly sophisticated ways to measure outcome, in three broad categories:

- **Drinking Behavior Models:**
  - Generally measures the amount of self-reported drinking (rather than the harm associated with drinking)
  - *Most often determined by taking the individual through a structured process of retrospective self report; the most commonly used instrument for this is the Timeline Follow-Back.*
  - Retrospective self-report is still the standard approach in treatment trials, because it is the easiest to measure reliably across studies and most research supports its validity and reliability.
- **Diagnostic Criteria Models:**
  - Full Remission (recovery) is defined as no longer meeting any of the seven criteria of dependence.
  - Partial remission means meeting one or two dependence criteria, but not enough to qualify for the dependence diagnosis.
  - Nonremission is continuing to meet full diagnostic criteria.
  - The clinical utility and predictive validity of these categories are not fully established.
  - Drinking quantity and frequency are not included in the diagnosis.
- **Life function Models:**
  - Measures the impact of drinking on multiple life areas such as occupational achievement, social function, and psychologic and physical health

THE SPECTRUM OF HEAVY DRINKING AND ALCOHOL USE DISORDERS

In the United States, a single alcohol serving is defined as the amount of ethanol in 1.5 oz (45 mL) of 80 proof spirits, 12 oz of beer, or 5 oz of table wine, each containing about 14 g of absolute ethanol. *Because actual alcohol levels in beer and wine vary, these amounts are meant to be approximate.*

The National Institute of Alcohol Abuse and Alcoholism of the National Institutes of Health recommends that men *drink no >4 alcohol servings per day* and *14 servings per week* and that women *drink no >3 servings per day* and *7 servings per week.*

Drinking within these limits is considered "low-risk" drinking. *Lower limits or abstinence may be indicated in the presence of coexisting medical or psychiatric disorders, in older people, or when medication interactions are a concern.*

Women who are pregnant or at risk of becoming pregnant are advised to abstain.

Drinking more than the recommended daily limit constitutes a "Heavy drinking day," and "heavy drinking" is defined as drinking in excess of the maximum limits on a regular basis, such as exceeding the daily limits weekly or more often.

"At-risk drinking" is heavy drinking in the absence of meeting any criteria for an alcohol use disorder.

About 70% of the US adult populations report either being abstinent or engaging in low-risk drinking in any given year. About 21% are at-risk drinkers. Nine percent have an alcohol use disorder (5% abuse and 4% alcohol dependence).

As a health risk factor, at-risk drinking is analogous to high blood pressure or hyperlipidemia before end-organ damage.

Most heavy drinking occurs between the ages of 18 and 25, which is also when the prevalence of alcohol use disorders peaks. Importantly, *>40% of daily or near daily heavy drinkers do not meet any criteria for alcohol use disorder.* Similarly, *only 20% to 40% of people with alcoholic liver cirrhosis also have alcohol dependence.*

Finally, not all alcohol-related harms occur in people who have alcohol use disorders, in part because there are twice as many at-risk drinkers as there are people with alcohol use disorders. Trauma, in particular, may occur because of a single occasion of heavy drinking, or in someone who only drinks to excess occasionally.

Diagnostic criteria for alcohol dependence can be grouped as

1. Impaired control
2. Increased salience
3. Physiologic adaptation

Drinking must also be causing clinically significant impairment or distress. Thus, heavy drinking itself is not considered an alcohol use disorder, even if it results in physical harm.

The Spectrum of Drinking, Disorders, and Treatment

The goal of treatment depends on the nature, extent, and severity of the disorder. Coexisting conditions or circumstances are also important determinants of the therapeutic approach and methods used.

Abstainers and low-risk drinkers require health promotion, such as education about the recommended maximum limits adjusted for that person's individual situation.

The goal for at-risk drinkers is to reduce consumption, preferably below recommended maximum limits, to reduce risk of future harm.

At-risk drinkers (and possibly those with mild dependence) respond well to facilitated self-change and brief counseling by physicians in primary care—which produces a 25% overall reduction in drinking 1 year later, and a greater decrease in heavy drinking

For individuals with more than minimal levels of dependence, however, more intensive forms of treatment are needed. Brief counseling alone is not effective with dependent drinkers in general.

Treatment of abuse without dependence or of frequent heavy drinking resulting in end-organ damage when alcohol use disorder criteria are not met is not well developed.

Recent epidemiologic studies have found that in persons who have abuse but do not qualify for dependence, about 90% qualify for abuse because of physically hazardous use, mostly drunk driving.

Other abuse criteria (role failure, interpersonal problems, and legal problems) are typically met only in individuals who also meet criteria for dependence, and are associated with greater severity of alcohol use disorder.

New research has demonstrated that *72% of US adults with a lifetime diagnosis of dependence have a single episode, lasting on average 3 to 4 years.*

People with mild to moderate dependence and relatively little comorbidity are unlikely to seek treatment in addiction treatment programs.

Treatment with oral naltrexone plus brief behavioral support by health care clinicians is at least as effective as state of-the-art outpatient addiction therapy in these cases.

About two thirds of individuals who develop dependence do so in adolescence or young adulthood—however, only about half of them go on to a chronic course: those who do are more likely to have a family history of alcohol dependence, antisocial personality traits, and/or to have started drinking in early adolescence.

Most people who meet dependence criteria do not have a chronic course and most recover without professional treatment or even attendance at mutual help groups.

Most people, on recognizing a problem, attempt to change alone or with informal help, and the majority are eventually successful, albeit after several years of active dependence.

More research is needed on early intervention in the course of illness for those at high risk for chronicity.

Another 40% of dependent persons have midlife onset of moderate severity dependence, and those who do are more likely to have coexisting psychopathology.

For those who do not respond to self-change efforts and nonintensive or brief treatment, referral to specialty addiction treatment is needed.

For individuals with severe and persistent or recurrent alcohol dependence, commonalities include

- Very early onset
- Coexisting substance use disorders
- Mental and physical disorders
- Social disabilities
- Antisocial personality disorder
- Family history of alcohol dependence
- Most likely to seek and receive treatment (voluntary or involuntary)

Even though most of this group has a chronic or recurrent course, addiction treatment programs typically offer treatment for only a few weeks or months. Furthermore, few programs are staffed to address the serious comorbidities present, so they are ignored or dealt with through referral to other agencies.

Studies of heavy drinkers with severe medical complications such as liver cirrhosis suggest that addressing drinking using a care management approach in the context of general medical care is effective at reducing drinking and inducing abstinence and decreasing mortality.

Treatment programs suffer from insufficient funds, resulting in poorly trained and underpaid staff and excessive turnover.

Current major needs are as follows:

1. Provide earlier identification and appropriate treatment to a much broader spectrum of individuals who drink heavily or who have alcohol dependence than is currently the case.
2. Early intervention strategies for youth who begin drinking in early adolescence and who are at high risk for later development of severe chronic dependence are needed.
3. Better understanding of the factors driving change in heavy drinkers and how to facilitate that change both in addiction treatment and in other settings
4. Early identification and treatment of heavy drinking and dependence in primary care and general mental health care

TYPES OF TREATMENT AND TREATMENT EFFECTIVENESS

The best way to match the type and intensity of treatment to the individual needs of a patient with alcohol dependence remains unclear.

No systematic outcome advantage has been demonstrated for residential or intensive day program treatment compared with once or twice weekly outpatient treatment.

No behavioral treatment has been shown to be better than others that are conceptually distinct and use different behavioral techniques.

About 10% of people with alcohol dependence have a severe chronic form of the disorder, yet most treatment programs offer only a few weeks or months of treatment.

In practical terms, the addiction treatment offered or available likely depends on

1. Patient preference
2. Availability
3. Access
4. Coercion

5. Urgent needs (imminent withdrawal or suicide risk)
6. Clinician orientation (rather than on scientific evidence)

The outcome of treatment varies according to the diagnosis or stage of illness.

At-risk drinkers who are identified and offered education and brief motivational counseling on average reduce drinking about 25% over the following year.

Treatment outcome for dependence is remarkably similar across studies and treatment modalities, both behavioral and pharmacologic. About one-third remain in remission for a year, about 45% show improvement but not full remission, and about one-quarter show no response.

What Causes and Maintains Change in Drinking Behavior?

Help seeking is strongly associated with increased odds of achieving recovery.
Help seekers are

1. Older
2. Have more severe dependence
3. Have more coexisting mental and physical disorders
4. Have less social support
5. More likely to have the relapsing form of the illness

For those who do seek help, both professional treatment and twelve-step participation are associated with increased likelihood of recovery, especially abstinent recovery.

In people who have been treated for alcohol dependence, recovery is in turn strongly associated with improved mortality.

Integrating the Evidence and Personalizing Practice

Although differences among different behavioral techniques tend to be minor, the quality of behavioral treatment is important.

Empathic and skillful therapy is more effective than confrontation and education.

It is important to offer a variety of treatment options, because patients are likely to vary in their preferences.

Unless someone is unable to abstain from living in the community, there is no systematic advantage of residential versus outpatient treatment.

Available medications offer small but clinically important benefit in early recovery and therefore patients should routinely be offered the opportunity to use them. As with behavioral treatments, however, there is no consensus that any one medication is better than another, or that there is a specific sequence in which they should be used.

A social network supportive of abstinence is at least as important as whatever treatment occurs in determining outcome.

For any given diagnosis (e.g., at-risk drinking versus dependence), there is not yet a way to identify patient characteristics that reliably predict differential response to different treatments.

CHAPTER 24

Summary Author: Ashok Krishnamurthy
Andrea G. Barthwell • Lawrence S. Brown, Jr.

The Treatment of Drug Addiction: An Overview

GOALS OF DRUG ADDICTION TREATMENT

Drug addiction is a complex disorder that can involve virtually every aspect of an individual's functioning—in the family, at work, and in the community.

Treatment of drug abuse and addiction is delivered in many different settings, using a variety of behavioral and pharmacologic approaches.

In the United States, >11,000 specialized drug treatment facilities provide rehabilitation, counseling, behavioral therapy, medication, case management, and other types of services to persons with drug use disorders. Care of individuals with substance use disorders includes

- Assessing needs
- Providing treatment for intoxication and withdrawal
- Developing, with appropriate support, the treatment plan that may consist of referrals to psychosocial care (Table 24.1)

TREATMENT SETTINGS

Decisions regarding the site of care should be based on

- Patient's ability to cooperate with and benefit from treatment offered
- Ability to refrain from illicit use of substances
- Need to avoid high-risk behaviors
- Need for structure and support

Patients move from one level of care to another based on these factors and an assessment of their ability to benefit from a different level of care.

While some hospitals have inpatient Addiction Medicine Consultation Services with specialty-trained clinicians, other hospitals limit their management of addiction to basic detoxification and referral.

Detoxification

Detoxification refers not only to the *attenuation of the physiologic and psychologic features of withdrawal syndromes but also to the process of interrupting the momentum of compulsive use in persons diagnosed with substance dependence.*

It can be delivered in ambulatory settings with and without extended on-site monitoring. In residential or inpatient settings, it is delivered under clinically managed, medically monitored, or medically managed conditions.

Hospital Settings

Hospitalization is appropriate for patients whose assessed need cannot be treated safely in an outpatient or emergency department setting due to

1. Acute intoxication
2. Severe or medically complicated withdrawal potential

TABLE 24.1 Principles of Effective Treatment

1. No single treatment is appropriate for all individuals.	Matching treatment settings, interventions, and services to each individual's particular problems and needs is critical to his or her ultimate success in returning to productive functioning in the family, workplace, and society.
2. Treatment needs to be readily available.	Because individuals who are addicted to drugs may be uncertain about entering treatment, taking advantage of opportunities when they are ready for treatment is crucial. Potential treatment applicants can be lost if treatment is not immediately available or is not readily accessible.
3. Effective treatment attends to multiple needs of the individual.	To be effective, treatment must address the individual's drug use and any associated medical, psychologic, social, vocational, and legal problems.
4. An individual's treatment and services plan must be assessed continually and modified as necessary to ensure that the plan meets the person's changing needs.	A patient may require varying combinations of services and treatment components during the course of treatment and recovery. In addition to counseling or psychotherapy, a patient at times may require medication, other medical services, family therapy, parenting instruction, vocational rehabilitation, and social and legal services. It is critical that the treatment approach be appropriate to the individual's age, gender, race/ethnicity, and culture.
5. Remaining in treatment for an adequate period is critical for treatment effectiveness.	The appropriate duration for an individual depends on his or her problems and needs. Research indicates that, for most patients, the threshold of significant improvement is reached at about 3 mo in treatment. After this threshold is reached, additional treatment can produce further progress toward recovery. Because people often leave treatment prematurely, programs should include strategies to engage and keep patients in treatment.
6. Counseling (individual and group) and other behavioral therapies are critical components of effective treatment.	In therapy, patients address issues of motivation, build skills to resist drug use, replace drug-using activities with constructive and rewarding non–drug-using activities, and improve their problem-solving abilities. Behavioral therapy also facilitates interpersonal relationships and the individual's ability to function in the family and community.
7. Medications are an important element of treatment for many patients, especially when combined with counseling and other behavioral therapies.	Methadone and levo-alpha-acetylmethadol are very effective in helping individuals addicted to heroin and other opiates stabilize their lives and reduce their illicit drug use. Naltrexone is an effective medication for some opiate-dependent patients and some patients with co-occurring alcohol dependence. For persons addicted to nicotine, a nicotine replacement product (such as patches or gum) or an oral medication (such as bupropion) can be an effective component of treatment. For patients with co-occurring mental disorders, both behavioral treatments and medications can be critically important.
8. Addicted or drug-abusing individuals with co-occurring mental disorders should have both disorders treated in an integrated way.	Because addictive disorders and mental disorders often occur in the same individual, patients presenting for either condition should be assessed and treated for the co-occurrence of the other type of disorder.

(Continued)

TABLE 24.1	Principles of Effective Treatment *(Continued)*
9. Medical detoxification is only the first stage of addiction treatment and by itself does little to change long-term drug use.	Medical detoxification safely manages the acute physical symptoms of withdrawal associated with stopping drug use. Although detoxification alone is rarely sufficient to help addicts achieve long-term abstinence, for some individuals it is a strongly indicated precursor to effective addiction treatment.
10. Treatment does not need to be voluntary to be effective.	Strong motivation can facilitate the treatment process. Sanctions or enticements in the family, employment setting, or criminal justice system can increase significantly both entry into treatment and retention in treatment, as well as the success of treatment interventions.
11. Possible drug use during treatment must be monitored continuously.	Lapses to drug use can occur during treatment. The objective monitoring of a patient's drug and alcohol use during treatment, as through urinalysis or other tests, can help the patient withstand urges to use drugs. Such monitoring also can provide early evidence of drug use so that the individual's treatment plan can be adjusted. Feedback to patients who test positive for illicit drug use is an important element of monitoring.
12. Treatment programs should provide assessment for HIV/AIDS, hepatitis B and C, tuberculosis, and other infectious diseases, and counseling to help patients modify or change behaviors that place themselves or others at risk for infection.	Counseling can help patients avoid high-risk behaviors. Counseling also can help those who are already infected manage their illnesses.
13. Recovery from drug addiction can be a long-term process and frequently requires multiple episodes of treatment. As with other chronic illnesses, relapses to drug use can occur during or after successful treatment episodes.	Addicted individuals may require prolonged treatment and multiple episodes of treatment to achieve long-term abstinence and fully restore functioning. Participation in self-help support programs during and following treatment often is helpful in maintaining abstinence.

Source: From National Institute on Drug Abuse. *Principles of drug addiction treatment: a research-based guide.* Rockville, MD: NIDA (NIH Publication No. 99-4180); 1999:1–3.

3. Co-occurring medical or psychiatric conditions that complicate detoxification or impair treatment
4. Failure of engagement in treatment at a lower level of care
5. Life- or limb-threatening medical conditions that would require hospitalization
6. Psychiatric disorders that make the patient an imminent threat to self or others
7. Failure to respond to care at any level such that the patient endangers others or poses a self-threat

Partial Hospital Programs and Intensive Outpatient

Partial hospitalization is considered for patients who require intensive care but have a reasonable chance of making progress on treatment goals in the intertreatment interval, including maintenance of abstinence.

- Often provided to individuals whose treatment is hospital or residential initiated
- Who still require frequent and concentrated contact with treatment professionals to monitor their behavior and manage their risk of relapse
- -Often have a history of relapse after completion of treatment
- Are returning to a high-risk environment
- And need to develop support for their recovery-focused efforts beyond the treatment system

The difference between partial hospital programs and intensive outpatient is seen in intensity, number of hours per day, setting of the program, and structure of the program.

Outpatient Programs

- Treatment varies in the type and intensity.
- Costs less than residential or inpatient treatment
- Is more suitable for:
  - Individuals who have insight into their disease
  - Patients who have a high degree of predicted compliance
  - Those with low symptomatology
  - Those who live in areas with high resource availability and use
  - Those with supportive structure in his or her home environment

High rates of attrition can be problematic, particularly in the early phase.

Outcomes are highly correlated with time in treatment, and as a result, retention should be one focus of treatment, along with self-efficacy regarding adherence to the abstinence plan.

In many outpatient programs, as in much of treatment in general, group counseling is emphasized.

Most alcohol abuse and dependence is treated outside of the hospital after medical complications associated with detoxification are addressed.

Similarly, cocaine, nicotine, and marijuana abuse/dependence are also generally treated on an outpatient basis (as long as the focus on reduced substance use can be maintained and there are no other reasons for hospitalization).

RESIDENTIAL PROGRAMS, INCLUDING THERAPEUTIC COMMUNITY

Residential programs

- Provide care 24 hours a day.
- Generally conducted in nonhospital settings.
- Generally provided to patients who do not meet the clinical criteria for hospitalization.
- Short-term programs provide intensive but relatively brief residential treatment based on a modified twelve-step approach.
- Duration of treatment should be determined by the clinical response to therapy.
- Duration of treatment also varies on the length of time necessary for the patient to meet specific criteria predictive of success.

Reduced health care coverage for addiction treatment has resulted in a diminished number of these programs, and the average length of stay under managed care review is much shorter than in early programs.

One residential treatment model is the therapeutic community (TC). TCs are residential programs with planned lengths of stay from 6 to 12 months. TCs focus on the "resocialization" of the individual and use the program's entire "community"—including other residents, staff, and the social context—as active components of treatment.

Addiction is viewed in the context of an individual's social and psychologic deficits, so treatment focuses on developing personal accountability and responsibility and socially productive lives. Treatment is highly structured and can at times be confrontational, with activities designed to help residents examine damaging beliefs, self-concepts, and patterns of behavior, and to adopt new, more harmonious and constructive ways to interact with others.

Compared with patients in other forms of drug treatment, the typical TC resident has more chronicity and criminal involvement.

Retention lengths predict outcomes on abstinence with abstinence success rates of 90% for graduates of 2-year programs and 25% for dropouts of the same programs completing <1 year.

Community Residential Rehabilitation

Community residential rehabilitation facilities include "halfway houses" or "sober living facilities," with the former providing more structure and supervision.

Individuals referred to these settings are generally deemed to be at risk for relapse without such support.

This setting is offered to the individual whose environmental risk is great or those needing a number of services after primary treatment to address deficits in vocation, employment, and social supports.

Case Management

Case management is a collaborative process that assesses, plans, implements, coordinates, monitors, and evaluates the options and services to meet an individual's health needs.

Case management is provided to individuals whose social situation and complex needs would impair their ability to adhere to a prescribed treatment plan and follow-up care.

Aftercare Programs

Aftercare generally follows an episode of care and is focused on maintenance of gains made in treatment over a prescribed period. The patient's affiliation with a twelve-step program is encouraged and the transition to self-efficacy is monitored.

Treatment in the Physician's Office, Including Screening and Brief Interventions

Brief interventions include assessment, feedback, and responsibility for change, advice, and menu of options provided using empathic listening and encouraged self-efficacy.

Criminal Justice Settings for Mandated Treatment, Including Drug Courts

Research has shown that combining criminal justice sanctions with drug treatment can be effective in decreasing drug use and related crime.

Individuals under legal coercion tend to stay in treatment for a longer period and do as well as or better than others not under legal pressure.

Often, drug-addicted persons encounter the criminal justice system earlier than other health or social systems.

Addiction treatment may be delivered before, during, after, or in lieu of incarceration.

Prison-Based Treatment Programs

A number of treatment options exist for those that are incarcerated.

- Didactic drug education classes
- Self-help programs
- Treatment based on TC or residential milieu therapy models

TC models have been studied extensively and found to be quite effective in reducing drug use and recidivism to criminal behavior.

Those in treatment are generally segregated from the general prison population, so that the "prison culture" does not overwhelm progress toward recovery.

Treatment gains can be lost if inmates are returned to the general prison population after treatment. Research shows that relapse to drug use and recidivism to crime are significantly lower if the drug offender continues treatment after returning to the community.

Community-Based Treatment for Criminal Justice Populations

Several criminal justice alternatives to incarceration have been tried with offenders who have drug disorders, including limited diversion programs, pretrial release conditional on entry into treatment, and conditional probation with sanctions.

Drug courts mandate and arrange for drug addiction treatment, actively monitor progress in treatment, and arrange other services for drug-involved offenders.

TREATMENT SERVICES

Clinical Monitoring

As with the treatment of other medical disorders and irrespective of the therapeutic approach chosen, clinical monitoring is extremely important in achieving successful clinical options.

Because of the limitations of self-report in the initial assessment and during clinical monitoring, clinical drug testing represents an important tool for addiction medicine specialists.

When used in concert with a good history, physical examination, and biologic markers, clinical drug testing facilitates screening, assessment, diagnosis, and clinical monitoring of a substance use disorder in the hands of an experienced practitioner.

Managing Intoxication and Withdrawal

Intoxication and withdrawal can be life threatening without appropriate, if not emergent intervention.

The therapeutic response is contingent on the substance used, the presence or absence of evidence of a compromised cardiopulmonary system, and the underlying health status of the patient.

Pharmacotherapy is the cornerstone for patients suffering from either intoxication or withdrawal.

Effective treatment for intoxication requires a hospital setting, whereas withdrawal can be treated in either an inpatient or outpatient setting.

Detoxification is a commonly used approach in responding to patients with clinical signs of intoxication or withdrawal.

- Under the care of a physician, individuals are systematically withdrawn from addicting drugs.
- Can be done in an inpatient or outpatient setting
- Is intended to reduce or eliminate the medical consequences of withdrawal/pain of withdrawal/acute increase in craving
- *Is a precursor to treatment*
- Is not designed to address the psychologic, social, and behavioral problems associated with addiction
- Is most useful when it incorporates formal processes of assessment and referral to subsequent addiction treatment

Behavioral Therapy

Behavioral therapies are particularly important for the treatment of substance use disorders for which pharmacologic treatments are inefficacious.

These therapies attempt to arrest compulsive substance use through modification of behaviors, feelings, social functioning, and thoughts.

Because no form of psychotherapy has proven superior to another for all patients, successful referral to services is more important than physician determination of the most appropriate approach.

Failure to refer to adjunctive psychotherapy is associated with reduced efficacy of known effective pharmacotherapy because medications frequently address only part of the substance dependence syndrome.

Cognitive-Behavioral Therapy

Cognitive-behavioral therapy is based on the theory that learning processes play a critical role in the development of maladaptive patterns of behavior.

Cognitive-behavioral therapy targets two processes, dysfunctional thoughts and maladaptive behaviors.

Relapse prevention is a hallmark cognitive–behavioral intervention used in addiction treatment.

Relapse prevention encompasses several cognitive-behavioral strategies that facilitate abstinence as well as provide help for persons who experience relapse. The goal of relapse prevention is to help addicted individuals learn to identify and correct problematic behaviors.

A central element of this treatment is anticipating the problems patients are likely to meet and helping them develop effective coping strategies.

Research indicates that the skills individuals learn through relapse prevention therapy remain after the completion of treatment.

Motivational Enhancement Therapy

Motivational enhancement therapy is a patient-centered counseling approach that attempts to initiate behavior change by helping patients resolve their ambivalence about engaging in treatment and stopping drug use.

This approach employs strategies to evoke rapid and internally motivated change in the client, rather than guiding the client stepwise through the recovery process.

Motivational interviewing principles are used to strengthen motivation and build a plan for change. Coping strategies for high-risk situations are suggested and discussed with the client.

Community Reinforcement Approach Plus Vouchers

Community reinforcement approach is an intensive outpatient therapy for the treatment of cocaine addiction.

The treatment has dual goals: to achieve cocaine abstinence long enough for patients to learn new life skills that will help sustain abstinence and to reduce alcohol consumption for patients, whose drinking is associated with cocaine use.

Voucher-Based Reinforcement Therapy in Methadone Maintenance Treatment

Voucher-based reinforcement therapy helps patients achieve and maintain abstinence from illegal drugs by providing them with a voucher each time they provide a drug-free urine sample.

The voucher has monetary value and can be exchanged for goods and services consistent with the goals of treatment.

Initially, the voucher values are low, but their value increases with the number of consecutive drug-free urine specimens the individual provides. Cocaine- or heroin-positive urine specimens reset the value of the vouchers to the initial low value.

Studies show that patients receiving vouchers for drug-free urine samples achieved significantly more weeks of abstinence and significantly more weeks of sustained abstinence than patients who were given vouchers independent of urine toxicology results.

Day Treatment with Abstinence Contingencies and Vouchers

This approach was developed to treat crack addiction among homeless persons.

Psychodynamic Therapy/Interpersonal Therapy

Individualized counseling focuses directly on reducing or stopping the patient's illicit drug use.

It also addresses related areas of impaired functioning—such as employment status, illegal activity, and family/social relations—as well as the content and structure of the patient's recovery program.

In studies that compare opiate-dependent patients receiving **methadone** alone with those receiving **methadone** coupled with counseling, *individuals who received* **methadone** *alone showed minimal improvement in reducing opiate use.*

In another study with cocaine-dependent patients, individualized drug counseling, together with group counseling, was quite effective in reducing cocaine use.

Treatment of the Adolescent with Multidimensional Family Therapy

Multidimensional family therapy is an outpatient, family-based, drug treatment approach for adolescents.

It approaches adolescent drug use in terms of a network of influences (individual, family, peer, and community) and suggests that reducing unwanted behavior and increasing desirable behavior occur in multiple ways in different settings. Treatment includes individual and family sessions held in the clinic, in the home, or with family members at the family court, school, or other community locations.

Teens acquire skills in communicating their thoughts and feelings to deal better with life stressors and vocational skills. Parallel sessions are held with family members.

Multisystemic Therapy

Multisystemic therapy addresses the factors associated with serious antisocial behavior in children and adolescents who use drugs.

These factors include characteristics of

- The adolescent (e.g., favorable attitudes toward drug use)
- The family (poor discipline, family conflict, or parental drug abuse)
- Peers (positive attitudes toward drug use)
- School (dropout, poor performance)
- -Neighborhood (criminal subculture)

Multisystemic therapy significantly reduces adolescent drug use during treatment and for at least 6 months after treatment.

PHARMACOLOGIC THERAPIES

Opioid Agonist Treatment

Opioid agonist treatment usually is conducted in outpatient treatment settings, such as **methadone** maintenance treatment (MMT) programs or the physician's office.

They employ long-acting synthetic opiate medications such as **methadone** or **buprenorphine**, taken orally for a sustained period at a dose sufficient to prevent opiate withdrawal, block the effects of illicit opiate use, and decrease opiate craving.

Patients stabilized on MMT can hold jobs, avoid the crime and violence of the drug culture, and reduce their exposure to HIV by stopping or decreasing injection drug use and drug-related high-risk sexual behaviors.

Patients stabilized on opiate agonists can engage more readily in counseling and other behavioral interventions that are essential to recovery and rehabilitation.

Narcotic Antagonist Treatment Using Naltrexone

Treatment of opiate-dependent patients with **naltrexone** usually is conducted in outpatient settings, although initiation of the medication often begins after medical detoxification in a residential setting.

Naltrexone is a long-acting synthetic opiate antagonist with few side effects that is taken orally, either daily or three times per week, for a sustained period.

Candidates for therapy with **naltrexone** *must be medically detoxified and opiate-free for several days* before the drug can be given, *to avoid precipitating the opiate abstinence syndrome.*

Naltrexone, when used properly, completely blocks the effects of self-administered opiates, including euphoria.

The theory behind this treatment is that the repeated lack of the desired opiate effects, as well as the perceived futility of using the opiate, will gradually extinguish the habit of opiate addiction.

Naltrexone itself has no subjective effects or potential for abuse and is not addicting. Patient noncompliance is a common problem; therefore, a favorable treatment outcome requires that there also be a positive therapeutic relationship, effective counseling or therapy, and careful monitoring of medication compliance.

CHAPTER 25

Summary Author: Ashok Krishnamurthy
A. Thomas McLellan • James R. McKay

Integrating Evidence-Based Components into a Functional Continuum of Addiction Care

INTRODUCTION

Problems in Delivery of Effective Addiction Treatment

Addictive disorders—here defined as any *substance use disorder meeting DSM-IVR criteria for abuse or dependence*—occur in approximately 10% to 15% of the adult population.

They result in dramatic costs to society such as lost productivity, social disorder, and excessive health care utilization.

It is disturbing and potentially dangerous to public health and safety *that <15% of those who meet diagnostic criteria for a substance use disorder receive any kind of addiction treatment.*

Among those who do enter treatment, >80% receive outpatient care, usually in a nonprofit community-based specialty treatment program that is not affiliated with any part of the larger health care system.

Perhaps for these reasons, studies of state treatment systems indicate that the modal duration of outpatient treatment is only one to three visits; *<30% remain actively engaged in outpatient care by 60 days.*

The great majority of outpatient addiction treatment programs provide only group counseling and referral to Alcoholics Anonymous (AA).

Studies have shown that the quality of addiction treatment is frequently worse than quality of general health care.

PART 1—THE CONCEPTUAL, ORGANIZATIONAL, AND FINANCIAL INFRASTRUCTURE OF CONTEMPORARY ADDICTION TREATMENT

Conceptual Issues

Although the concept of addiction as a chronic illness has been attractive in research and even clinical circles, this conceptual shift has so far not led to much change in the way addictions have been treated, insured, or evaluated.

Organization, Management, and Financing Issues

Conceptual confusion regarding the nature of addiction has confused the content of treatment interventions, insurance benefits, provider credentialing, and outcome evaluation methods.

PART 2—WHAT MIGHT AN APPROPRIATE CONTINUUM OF ADDICTION CARE LOOK LIKE?

Development of a Continuum of Care in Mainstream Health

Taking other chronic illnesses as a model, it seems reasonable to think of clinical stages linked conceptually and organizationally toward the overall goal of promoting patient self-management of their addiction.

Each stage of care within the continuum would have specific clinical goals, but achieving the goals of the early stages would prepare the patient for advancement to succeeding stages of care.

Within each stage of care, various treatment components (medications, behavioral therapies, other interventions) would be evaluated with regard to their ability to affect the symptom and function goals appropriate to the particular stage of care of the patient.

PART 3—EVIDENCE-BASED CLINICAL PRACTICES WITHIN AND ACROSS THE CONTINUUM OF ADDICTION TREATMENT

Screening, Brief Interventions, and Brief Treatments

There are many studies showing significant prevalence of alcohol and other substance use disorders in emergency room populations, trauma centers, primary mental health centers, and school health settings.

Brief intervention (i.e., educational and motivational interventions lasting <10 minutes) and brief treatment (similar interventions of two to five sessions) studies within these populations *have generally shown significant reductions in substance use, lasting at least 6 to 12 months.*

The content of brief intervention settings varies depending on the severity of an individual's problems. It includes several common elements known by their acronym *FRAMES: feedback, responsibility, advice, menu of strategies, empathy, and self-efficacy.*

There is also evidence that primary care physicians can often improve the outcomes and reduce the substantial costs of treating common, chronic illnesses such as diabetes, hypertension, asthma, several types of cancer, and sleep—simply by *identifying and managing their co-occurring substance use problems.*

Goals within the Screening, Brief Interventions, and Brief Treatment Stage The goals of this stage of the substance abuse treatment continuum are to reach individuals whose substance use may be below that considered abuse or dependence, but whose use is nonetheless too frequent or too serious for their medical health.

Once identified, the power of the medical teaching moment as well as the motivational interviewing helps patients understand that their substance use may be a problem and that they are capable of changing their substance use.

In those cases in which the patient cannot reduce and control substance use, referral to a specialty care treatment program is warranted.

Behavioral Therapies Studies of brief interventions as a treatment intervention have shown posttreatment outcomes that are not different from those seen among individuals with more extensive treatments.

Because of their brevity, they have been particularly attractive to primary care physicians dealing with alcohol-dependent individuals in family medicine or emergency medical settings.

Family Involvement Family-oriented "interventions" designed to confront individuals who are in denial about their substance use problems and peer support interventions such as Al-Anon to assist families of substance-dependent individuals to deal with the associated problems of addiction generally lead to improvements in family functioning *but little change in the substance user.*

Medications There are now several medications available for primary care physicians to use in office-based treatment of substance use problems. These medications will be reviewed elsewhere.

Detoxification Stage of Treatment

Goals of Detoxification Detoxification is a relatively brief, explicitly medical procedure, usually provided in a hospital setting and designed to stabilize the physical and emotional effects of recent termination of heavy alcohol or drug use.

This stage of treatment is designed for people who *experience frank withdrawal symptoms* or *significant physiologic or emotional instability* after a period of prolonged abuse of drugs.

Significant physiologic withdrawal is not present in all cases—even those with the more serious forms of addiction.

However, alcohol, opioid, and sedative/tranquilizer dependence may produce a characteristic rebound physiologic withdrawal syndrome 8 to 30 hours after the last dose of the drug.

Users of amphetamine, cocaine, and even marijuana can also experience substantial emotional and physiologic symptoms and often require a period of stabilizing treatment.

The purpose of the detoxification stage of treatment is not to produce cure or lasting sobriety, but rather to prepare an unstable patient to do well in the subsequent rehabilitation phase of treatment.

Detoxification is rarely effective in helping patients achieve lasting recovery, particularly patients with more severe or protracted histories of substance dependence.

Medications There have been significant advances in the use of medications to reduce the dangers and alleviate the suffering associated with the withdrawal and stabilization of physiologic and emotional problems attendant to the cessation of heavy substance use. These are reviewed elsewhere.

Behavioral Therapies Because detoxification is a typically short (3–5 days) medical procedure and because patients' attention and concentration may be compromised for much of this period, extended therapies within this context are not typically possible.

However, the same brief interventions and brief therapies described in the Screening and Brief Interventions stage of care are also possible and sensible in this context.

Residential Recovery–Oriented Stage of Treatment

Residential rehabilitation or "recovery"-oriented treatment is appropriate for patients who are no longer suffering from the acute physiologic or emotional effects of recent substance abuse.

Recovery-oriented treatments are provided in outpatient and **methadone** maintenance settings as well as residential settings.

Outpatient programs account for about 80% of all treatment programs

Residential treatment is qualitatively different in that it offers protected and secluded care to enable patients to regain personal health and social functioning as well as control over their substance use urges.

"Recovery" and Rehabilitation Although continuation of abstinence from alcohol and other drugs of abuse is widely considered *necessary* for achieving recovery, abstinence by itself is not *sufficient* to assure the equally desirable qualities of improved personal health and independent social function.

Goals of Recovery-Oriented Treatments Patients suitable for residential rehabilitation treatments usually also have significant problems in medical and mental health, family and social relationships, and sometimes legal and employment problems that may have resulted from or led to their substance use problems.

Residential recovery-oriented treatments for addiction have the following goals:

- Maintain physiologic and emotional improvements initiated during detoxification; enhance and sustain reductions in alcohol and drug use.
- Teach, model, and support behaviors that lead to improved personal health, family and social function, and reduced threats to public health and public safety.
- Motivate behavioral and lifestyle changes that are incompatible with substance use.

Medications In the context of the broad goals of this stage of the continuum of substance abuse treatment, other medications, beyond those designed to control alcohol and other substance use, may also be helpful in effecting recovery goals.

There is a large and important literature sample that examines the use of medications to reduce psychiatric problems among addicted individuals.

Finally, there is increasing evidence that the prescription of *appropriate* psychotropic medications can alter that prognosis.

Behavioral Therapies Several of the behavioral therapies and interventions discussed in the next section may also be appropriate for use in residential settings, but have rarely been studied in that context. Two that seem particularly pertinent to the goals of residential care are described here and also in the section that follows.

Twelve-Step Facilitation Therapy (TSF)

It is designed to assist in

- Engaging patients into accepting their inability to control their substance use
- Acknowledging the effects of their substance use on their lives and the lives of their loved ones
- Ultimately taking steps to deal with the problems through the 12 steps and 12 traditions of AA

TSF is typically delivered as a time-limited (12- to 15-session) intervention, either as an individual treatment or in groups.

TSF is a highly structured intervention whose sessions begin with a review of the patient's recovery week, including any Twelve-Step meetings attended, episodes of substance, and urges to drink or use drugs.

One aspect of TSF that clearly separates it from other therapies is its active promotion of spirituality as a key to lasting recovery.

The evidence for effectiveness of TSF was first shown in the large, multisite National Institute on Alcohol Abuse and Alcoholism Project MATCH study of alcohol-dependent patients.

Individual Drug Counseling The drug-dependence field has employed a structured form of individual counseling employing many of the same practical elements, but not a formal spiritual component.

Individual counseling is discussed here briefly because it is widely used within recovery-oriented residential settings and because it has shown benefits in helping patients to adjust and improve during that stage of care.

Linking Patients to AA or Other Mutual-Help Groups Most AA groups now accept individuals with a range of addiction problems.

Research studies done to date have generally found that *only about 25% to 35% of those who attend one meeting of AA go on to active participation.*

There are now many controlled trials and field studies of AA showing that participation in posttreatment self-help groups is related to better outcome among cocaine- or alcohol-dependent individuals.

Intensive/Traditional Outpatient Stage of Treatment

Outpatient treatment is designed to provide continuing support for the behavioral changes achieved during detoxification or residential treatment and to support personal changes in health and social function while monitoring early threats to relapse.

Goals of Intensive/Outpatient Treatments Outpatient treatments share many of the goals and therapeutic components of more intensive, residential recovery-oriented treatment.

In general, the medications, therapies, and services that have been applied and studied in the rehabilitation/recovery phase of treatment can also be applied in the outpatient phase of treatment.

Specifically, outpatient treatments for addiction have the following three goals:

- Maintain physiologic and emotional improvements initiated during detoxification or residential treatments.
- Maintain abstinence from alcohol and other drugs.
- Motivate and support behavioral and lifestyle changes that are incompatible with substance use.

Medications Because at least half of substance-dependent patients in treatment suffer from co-occurring problems of depression, anxiety, or phobia, standard psychotropic medications can be important in the achievement and maintenance of improved mental health.

It is important to note that psychotropic and antiaddiction medications may not control the targeted substance use or mental health problems when used in the context of a primary care setting.

More severely dependent patients or those with more psychiatric problems may do poorly in outpatient treatment without medications for their symptoms.

Behavioral Therapies With the exceptions of individual drug counseling and linkage to AA, most evidence-based behavioral therapies are not widely used during this stage of the addiction continuum.

Interventions designed to engage family and to change previous peer relationships may be particularly important at this stage of the continuum as the patient attempts to develop and sustain a new recovery-oriented lifestyle within the home setting.

Cognitive Behavioral Therapy The therapy is based on the findings that biased or inaccurate thoughts and beliefs, coupled with poor coping skills, lead to a greater risk for relapse.

The therapy is usually individual (but also group) delivered in 8 to 16 weekly sessions.

Change in thinking about and reactions to relapse-provoking situations and improvements in coping abilities require practice and time.

CBT may be the most studied of all the therapies in addiction due perhaps to the very carefully developed manuals developed to train and guide the provision of the therapy.

Studies of CBT with cocaine-dependent patients have shown general acceptance by patients (attendance at >50% of planned sessions) and better posttreatment rates of abstinence than patients given no therapy or group counseling alone. Similarly, CBT has also been associated with generally good engagement and posttreatment outcomes among alcohol-dependent patients.

Twelve-Step Facilitation Therapy Many studies have confirmed the effectiveness of this therapy versus usual care.

Individual Drug Counseling In almost all studies, patients who have received this form of counseling had better during and posttreatment outcomes, with those who attended a greater frequency of sessions typically showing the best results.

Importantly, there are very few studies that have shown positive effects from *group* drug counseling. Indeed, in one large trial among cocaine-dependent patients, it was only individual counseling and not group counseling that was associated with improved outcomes. This is important in that *group* drug counseling is by far the most prevalent component of treatment in the national treatment system.

Other Interventions and Services

Voucher-Based Reinforcement of Abstinence Voucher-based reinforcement of abstinence retained more patients in treatment, produced more abstinent patients, longer periods of abstinence, and greater improvements in personal function than the standard counseling approach.

Clinical Case Management and Wraparound Services Studies have documented that "wraparound services" such as primary medical care, housing, employment training, psychiatric care, and parenting assistance for these addiction-related problems can be effective adjuncts to standard addiction-focused care.

Family Involvement

Marital, Family, and Couples Therapies In a recent review of controlled studies of this type with alcohol-dependent patients, marital and family therapy, and particularly behavioral couples therapy, were significantly more effective than individual treatments at inducing and sustaining abstinence, improving relationship functioning, and reducing domestic violence and emotional problems of children.

Similar reductions in substance use and partner violence have also been seen in controlled trials of marital, family, or couples therapy with opiate- and cocaine-dependent patients.

Behavioral Couples Therapy Behavioral couples therapy treats the substance-abusing patient with his or her spouse to arrange a daily "sobriety contract" in which the patient states his or her intent not to drink or use drugs, and the spouse expresses support for the patient's efforts to stay abstinent.

Findings show that behavioral couples therapy produces more abstinence and better relationship function than typical individual-based treatment and also reduces social costs and domestic violence.

CRAFT CRAFT is based on a combination of standard functional analysis of behavior combined with principles of reinforcement. The therapy was developed to teach and promote the practice of these principles by members of a household.

Specifically, families who learn the CRAFT intervention are taught skills for modifying a loved one's alcohol or drug-using behavior and for enhancing treatment engagement.

The Continuing Care Stage of Treatment The term continuing care has been used to indicate the stage of treatment that follows an initial episode of more intensive care, usually inpatient/residential or intensive outpatient.

Continuing care is provided in a variety of formats and modalities:

- Group counseling
- Individual therapy
- Telephone
- Counseling
- Brief checkups
- Self-help meetings

These interventions are usually 3 months or longer in duration, with some interventions lasting as long as 2 years.

The results of recent reviews indicate that continuing care interventions were more likely to produce positive treatment effects when they

- Had a longer planned duration
- Made more active efforts to deliver treatment to patients
- Provided incentives to clients or practitioners for continued participation

Most continuing care is still AA or another mutual help group and most insurance programs and public substance abuse benefit designs do not reimburse care at this stage.

Substance-dependent patients who complete detoxification, residential, and/or outpatient treatment stages *without* engaging into continuing care are at great risk of relapse.

Goals of Continuing Care Care at this stage of the continuum is generally less formalized, involves less contact in specialty care settings, and is more dedicated to monitoring for early signs of relapse while simultaneously supporting engagement in AA and any parts of a lifestyle that provide insurance against relapse.

Continuing care has the following goals:

- Maintain physiologic and emotional improvements initiated during residential or outpatient treatments.
- Monitor progress in recovery and possible relapse and intervene where appropriate on signs of relapse.
- Continue to teach and foster more effective coping behaviors and self-care.
- Support healthy relationships and behaviors that are incompatible with substance use and promote recovery.

Behavioral Therapies All the behavioral therapies discussed under the residential and outpatient stages of the continuum are as likely to be useful in this stage of treatment.

Types or Modalities of Continuing Care

Participation in AA/Narcotics Anonymous/Cocaine Anonymous *AA remains the most prevalent form of continuing care for individuals who are actively participating in outpatient treatment, or who have completed residential treatment.*

Individuals who frequently attend AA and other self-help programs usually do better than those who do not.

Office-Based Therapy Although office-based therapy is formal treatment and is reimbursed under many insurance plans, this type of care is not part of the specialty addiction treatment spectrum.

Telephone Continuing Care Consistent with a "disease management" perspective, several groups have shown that extended therapeutic contact provided via the telephone can have positive effects.

Recovery Management Check-ups Another approach to the long-term management of substance use disorders is to provide brief "checkups" on a regular basis, with referral to treatment if necessary.

Scott, Dennis, and colleagues from Chestnut Health Systems have developed such a protocol, which they refer to as "Recovery Management Checkups" (RMC).

Specifically, RMC patients were less likely to meet criteria for needing treatment in five or more quarters than patients in the control condition (23% vs. 32%).

Extended Medical Monitoring Continuing care for substance use disorders and co-occurring medical problems can be provided through primary care practices.

The integrated care model, referred to as "Integrated Outpatient Care" or IOT, provided monthly clinic visits with a nurse practitioner or physician.

Integrated care models produce much higher rates of extended participation in both medical and addiction treatment over the 2-year follow-up than standard care.

IOT also produced better substance use outcomes. At the end of the 2-year follow-up, 74% of IOT patients were abstinent versus only 47% of those in standard care.

CHAPTER 26

Summary Author: Ashok Krishnamurthy
John W. Finney • Rudolf H. Moos • Paula L. Wilbourne

Effects of Treatment Setting, Duration, and Amount on Patient Outcomes

TREATMENT SETTINGS

Only about 10% of substance use disorder (SUD) patients in the United States receive residential treatment and only 1% receive inpatient treatment where presumably medical or psychiatric care also is readily available.

Rather than debating inpatient versus outpatient therapy, what should be the more pressing issue is whether certain types of patients benefit more from an initial phase of inpatient/residential treatment before continuing outpatient care than from outpatient treatment alone.

Rationales for Inpatient/Residential and Outpatient Treatment

Five rationales for initial inpatient/residential SUD treatment settings:

1. Such settings provide a *respite* for patients, removing them from unstructured and unsupportive environments that perpetuate their addiction.
2. Such settings may allow patients to receive more treatment because treatment is more *intensive* and patients may be less likely to drop out of treatment.
3. Such settings provide *medical/psychiatric care* and other *comprehensive services* not otherwise available to these patients.
4. Inpatient treatment prepares a patient better to *engage* in continuing outpatient treatment.
5. Such treatment settings suggest to patients that their problems are *more severe* and that resolving them is more paramount than would be the case if treatment were offered in an outpatient setting.

Arguments in favor of outpatient treatment:

1. Provides an opportunity for *more accurate assessments of the antecedents of substance use* and for testing *coping skills in real-life situations*
2. *Greater generalization of learning* should take place in outpatient settings.
3. Might *mobilize help in the patient's natural environment* (e.g., from a family physician or self-help groups), to a greater extent than does inpatient or residential treatment
4. Results in a *more successful transition to continuing care*

Who Benefits from Inpatient/Residential Treatment?

Considerable evidence suggests that *more impaired patients benefit more from an initial episode of inpatient or residential treatment than from outpatient treatment alone.*

At least six studies have found that patients with greater alcohol or drug use severity at treatment intake who receive an initial episode of inpatient or residential treatment experience better outcomes than those receiving only outpatient treatment.

The American Society of Addiction Medicine (ASAM) Placement Criteria and Matching Patients to Treatment attempt to match patients to five levels of care:

1. Early intervention
2. Outpatient treatment

3. Intensive outpatient/partial hospitalization treatment
4. Residential/inpatient treatment
5. Medically managed intensive inpatient treatment

Placement decisions are based on a patient's standing on six dimensions:

1. Acute intoxication or withdrawal potential
2. Biomedical conditions and complications
3. Emotional/behavioral conditions or complications
4. Treatment acceptance/resistance
5. Relapse/continued use potential
6. Recovery/living environment

Research is still needed to validate the specific placement assessments and algorithms used in the ASAM system. There is not yet a precise, empirically supported guideline for allocating patients to different levels of care.

DURATION AND AMOUNT OF TREATMENT

The tendency in the United States has been toward shorter episodes of treatment, given reduced insurance coverage for SUD care.

Evidence suggests that brief motivational interventions are best directed toward persons who are ambivalent about changing the substance use behavior.

Length of Stay in Inpatient/Residential Treatment

Several recent randomized trials also have found no, or only isolated (i.e., on a few outcomes) beneficial effects for longer inpatient/residential alcohol or substance abuse treatment. These findings suggest it is not useful to assign unselected clients to longer stays in residential or inpatient treatment.

In contrast, many naturalistic studies of substance abuse treatment have found longer stays in treatment to be associated with better outcomes, even a reduction in premature mortality. The fact that individuals in naturalistic studies have better outcomes with longer treatment suggests that many clients may be able to determine whether or not they will benefit from longer treatment.

In select populations, longer episodes of inpatient and residential care, extended care, community residential care, and care in therapeutic communities have been associated with

- Better substance use outcomes
- Psychosocial functioning
- Lower readmission rates for subsequent inpatient care
- Lower readmissions for SUD patients concurrent mental health disorders

It may be that beneficial effects of longer stays in inpatient/residential treatment *apply only to more impaired patients with fewer social resources.*

Continuing Outpatient Care

Most SUD treatment providers recommend additional outpatient treatment to maintain or enhance the therapeutic gains achieved during inpatient/residential or intensive or initial outpatient (e.g., day hospital) treatment.

Studies and reviews of treatment intensity, length of stay, and outpatient care suggest that an effective strategy may be to provide *lower intensity addiction treatment over a longer duration*—that is, treatment spread out at a lower rate over a longer period.

More extended treatment may improve patient outcomes because it provides patients with ongoing support and the potential to discuss and resolve problems before the occurrence of a full-blown relapse.

Brief interventions may be most effective for relatively healthy patients who have intact community support systems.

Patients who have severe substance dependence, concomitant psychiatric disorders, or insufficient social resources appear to be appropriate candidates for longer treatment and intensive monitoring.

IMPLICATIONS FOR POLICYMAKERS AND SERVICE PROVIDERS

The advent of managed care in the United States in the 1990s brought an increasing emphasis on outpatient treatment so that in 2005, 89% of the individuals in treatment for alcohol and other drug use disorders were seen in less expensive outpatient settings.

An important agenda over the next decade will be to validate specific placement criteria for allocating individuals to different settings of care and to determine appropriate durations and intensities of care for different types of individuals.

Most providers today follow those recommendations in the spirit of the ASAM placement and matching criteria:

1. Provide outpatient treatment for those individuals who have sufficient social resources and no serious medical/psychiatric impairment
2. Use less costly intensive outpatient treatment options for patients who have failed with brief interventions or for whom a more intensive intervention seems warranted, but who do not need the structured environment of a residential setting.
3. Retain residential options for those with few social resources or a living environment that is a serious impediment to recovery.
4. Reserve inpatient treatment options for individuals with serious medical/psychiatric conditions.
5. Have longer term treatment options available for clients who desire them.
6. Use active methods of engagement at the start of treatment (e.g., motivational interventions) and when clients transition to continuing care (e.g., "contracting, prompting, and reinforcement").

CHAPTER 27

Summary Author: John Young
David Mee-Lee • Gerald D. Shulman

The ASAM Placement Criteria and Matching Patients to Treatment

The Patient Placement Criteria for the Treatment of Substance-Related Disorders of the American Society of Addiction Medicine (ASAM PPC) was designed to help clinicians and payers use and fund levels of care in a rational, cost-effective, and therapeutic manner. The use of the ASAM criteria can assist patients in accessing a much broader continuum of care and menu of services than is typically available. The continuing development and refinement of the criteria represent a shift from

- Unidimensional to multidimensional assessment
- Program-driven to clinically driven treatment
- Fixed length of service to variable length of service
- A limited number of discrete levels of care to a continuum of care

The first edition of the PPC was published by ASAM in 1991. A second edition was developed in 1996, ASAM PPC-2, and in 2001, a revision of PPC-2 was published, ASAM PPC-2R.

SELECTING AN APPROPRIATE TREATMENT

Individualized, assessment-driven treatment represents an ideal approach to care whereby problems are identified and prioritized in the context of the patient's severity of illness, interference with treatment or recovery, and level of function. Treatment services are then matched to the patient's needs over a continuum of care. Assessment of treatment response influences future treatment recommendations and length of treatment.

Outcomes-driven treatment adds the element of measurement of outcomes and modification of the treatment plan in real time (Fig. 27.1).

No single treatment is appropriate for all individuals at all times.

The Concept of "Unbundling"

At present, most addiction treatment services are "bundled," with several different services packaged together and paid for as a unit. Today, however, there is increasing recognition that clinical services can be provided separately from environmental supports. Indeed, many managed care companies and public treatment systems are suggesting that treatment modality and intensity be "unbundled" from the treatment setting. In this way, any type of clinical service can be delivered in any setting. With unbundling, the type and intensity of treatment are then based on the patient's needs and not on limitations imposed by the treatment setting; there would no longer be "programs," but rather a constellation of services to meet the needs of each patient.

A transition to unbundled treatment would require systemic changes in state program licensure and public funding and insurance reimbursement. To assist clinicians and programs to advance this approach, the ASAM PPC-2R criteria proposed a future directions matrix. Although it requires empirical validation, the *Matrix for Matching Multidimensional Risk with Type and Intensity of Services* is designed to assist the user to determine the level of risk using a five-point risk rating scale in each dimension, the needed services, and the appropriate level of care.

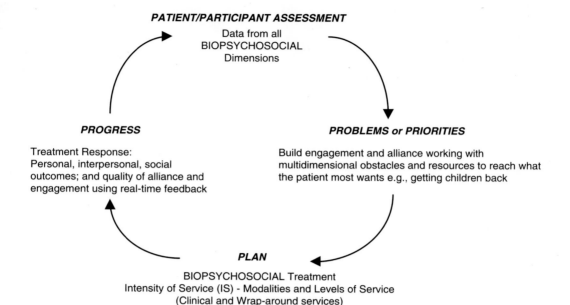

FIGURE 27.1   Individualized, outcomes-driven treatment.

UNDERSTANDING THE ASAM PATIENT PLACEMENT CRITERIA

Four features characterize the ASAM Patient Placement Criteria:

1. Comprehensive, individualized treatment planning
2. Ready access to services
3. Attention to multiple treatment needs
4. Ongoing reassessment and modification of the plan

The criteria advocate for a system in which treatment is readily available, because patients may be lost. By expanding the criteria to incorporate more use of outpatient care, especially for those in early stages of readiness to change, the ASAM criteria have helped to reduce waiting lists for residential treatment and thus have improved access to care.

The criteria are based on a philosophy that effective treatment attends to multiple needs of each individual—medical, psychologic, social, vocational, legal, and environmental—and not just his or her alcohol or drug use. To engage the patient in a collaborative therapeutic alliance, the assessment is in the service of what the patient wants. It serves to identify obstacles and resources, liabilities and strengths within each of the assessment dimensions (Fig. 27.2).

Principles Guiding the Criteria

Goals of Treatment   The goals of intervention and treatment determine the methods, intensity, frequency, and types of services provided. The health care professional's decision to prescribe a type of service and subsequent discharge of a patient from a level of care are based on how that treatment and its duration will influence the resolution of the dysfunction and improve the patient's prognosis. Thus, treatment may extend beyond simple resolution of symptoms or behaviors to the achievement of overall healthier functioning—the difference between abstinence alone and recovery.

Individualized Treatment Plan   The treatment plan is individualized in consultation with the patient; such a plan should be based on the patient's goals for treatment, a comprehensive biopsychosocial assessment of the patient, and, when possible, an evaluation of the family.

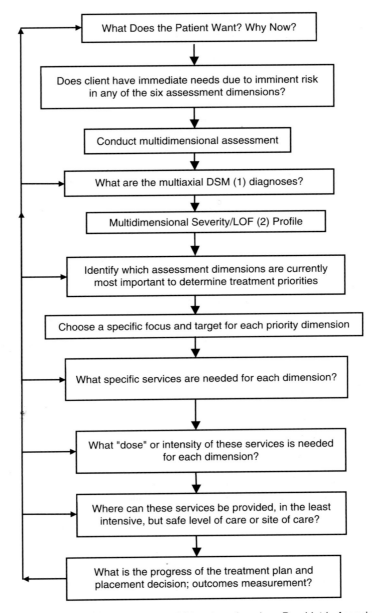

What Does the Patient Want? Why Now?

Does client have immediate needs due to imminent risk in any of the six assessment dimensions?

Conduct multidimensional assessment

What are the multiaxial DSM (1) diagnoses?

Multidimensional Severity/LOF (2) Profile

Identify which assessment dimensions are currently most important to determine treatment priorities

Choose a specific focus and target for each priority dimension

What specific services are needed for each dimension?

What "dose" or intensity of these services is needed for each dimension?

Where can these services be provided, in the least intensive, but safe level of care or site of care?

What is the progress of the treatment plan and placement decision; outcomes measurement?

(1) = Diagnostic and Statistical Manual of Mental Disorders, American Psychiatric Association
(2) = Level of Function

FIGURE 27.2 Decision tree to match assessment and treatment/placement assignment.

The plan should be written to facilitate measurement of progress. As with other disease processes, length of service should be linked directly to the patient's response to treatment rather than a predetermined time frame based on the length of the treatment program or on reimbursement.

Choice of Treatment Levels The preferred level of care is the least intensive level that meets treatment objectives, while providing safety and security for the patient. Although the levels of care are presented as discrete levels, in reality, they represent points along a continuum of treatment services through which the patient might progress in a variety of ways, depending on his or her needs and response.

For patients who have been previously treated and have relapsed, the choice of the current level of care should be based on an assessment of the patient's history and current functioning, not automatic placement in a more intensive level of care. Such placement by policy assumes that relapse after treatment indicates that the previous level of care was of insufficient intensity. In fact, poorly matched services may have been the problem.

Continuum of Care To provide the most clinically appropriate and cost-effective treatment system, a continuum of care must be available, offered by either a single provider or multiple providers. Such a continuum is distinguished by a philosophical congruence among the various providers of care and a seamless transfer of the patient between levels of care (including timely transfer of the clinical record). It is most helpful if providers envision admitting a patient into the continuum *through*, rather than *to*, their program.

Progress Through the Levels of Care As a patient moves through treatment in any level of care, his or her progress should be continually assessed to ensure that treatment is addressing the patient's changing needs. In the process of patient assessment, certain problems and priorities are identified as justifying admission to a particular level of care. The resolution of those problems and priorities determines when a patient can be treated at a different level of care or discharged from treatment. The appearance of new problems may require services that can be effectively provided at the same level of care or that require a more or less intensive level of care.

Length of Stay The patient's progress toward achieving his or her treatment plan goals and objectives determines length of stay or service. While more convenient and predictable for the provider, fixed length of stay programs are less effective for individuals.

Clinical Versus Reimbursement Considerations The ASAM criteria are intended as a clinical guideline for making the most appropriate placement recommendation for an individual patient, not as a reimbursement guideline. If the criteria only covered the levels of care commonly reimbursable by private insurance carriers, they would not address many of the resources of the public sector and, thus, would tacitly endorse limitations on a complete continuum of care.

Treatment Failure Two incorrect assumptions are associated with the concept of "treatment failure." The first is that the disorder is acute rather than chronic, so that the only criterion for success is total and complete cure and elimination of the problem. Such expectations are recognized as inappropriate in the treatment of other chronic disorders, such as diabetes or hypertension. The second assumption is that responsibility for treatment "failure" always rests with the patient (as in, "The patient was not ready"). However, poor treatment outcomes also may be related to a provider's failure to provide services tailored to the patient's needs.

Some benefit managers require that a patient "fails" at one level of care as a prerequisite for approving admission to a more intensive level of care (e.g., "failure" in outpatient treatment as a prerequisite for admission to inpatient treatment). In fact, such a requirement is no more rational than requiring all breast cancer patients to first have a lumpectomy as a requirement for a mastectomy. Such a strategy potentially puts the patient at risk because it delays care at a more appropriate level of treatment and potentially increases health care costs if restricting the appropriate level of treatment allows the addiction disorder to progress.

Should a patient use alcohol or other drugs during treatment, the immediate response should be to revise the treatment plan rather than automatically change the level of care or discharge the patient. Some benefit managers require that a patient be "motivated for sobriety" as a requirement for admission to a program; given the characteristic symptoms of denial and lack of readiness to change of addiction disorders, the only requirement should be that the patient is willing to enter treatment. Clinicians can then facilitate the patient's self-change process.

ASSESSMENT DIMENSIONS

The ASAM criteria contain descriptions of treatment programs at each level of care, including the setting, staffing, support systems, therapies, assessments, documentation, and treatment plan reviews typically found at that level.

The criteria identify six assessment areas (dimensions) as the most important in formulating an individualized treatment plan and in making subsequent patient placement decisions. Table 27.1 outlines the six dimensions and the assessment and treatment planning focus of each dimension.

TABLE 27.1	ASAM Criteria Assessement Dimensions
Assessment dimensions	**Assessment and treatment planning focus**
1. Acute intoxication and/or withdrawal potential	Assessment for intoxication or withdrawal management. Detoxification in a variety of levels of care and preparation for continued addiction services.
2. Biomedical conditions and complications	Assess and treat co-occurring physical health conditions or complications. Treatment provided within the level of care or through coordination of physical health services.
3. Emotional, behavioral, or cognitive conditions and complications	Assess and treat co-occurring diagnostic or subdiagnostic mental health conditions or complications. Treatment provided within the level of care or through coordination of mental health services.
4. Readiness to change	Assess stage of readiness to change. If not ready to commit to full recovery, engage into treatment using motivational enhancement strategies. If ready for recovery, consolidate and expand action for change.
5. Relapse, continued use, or continued problem potential	Assess readiness for relapse prevention services and teach where appropriate. Identify previous periods of sobriety or wellness and what worked to achieve this. If still at early stages of change, focus on raising consciousness of consequences of continued use or continued problems as part of motivational enhancement strategies.
6. Recovery environment	Assess need for specific individualized family or significant other, housing, financial, vocational, educational, legal, transportation, childcare services. Identify any supports and assets in any or all of the areas.

There is an increased focus on recovery and strength-based, person-centered assessments and services. A strength-based assessment addresses not only a patient's needs, obstacles, and liabilities but also his or her strengths, assets, resources, and supports to promote recovery.

LEVELS OF CARE

The ASAM criteria conceptualize treatment as a continuum marked by five basic levels of care:

Level 0.5: Early intervention
Level I: Outpatient services
Level II: Intensive outpatient/partial hospitalization services
Level III: Residential/inpatient services
Level IV: Medically managed intensive inpatient services

Within each level, a decimal from 0.1 to 0.9 expresses gradations of intensity within the existing levels of care; for example, a II.1 level of care provides a benchmark for intensity at the minimum description of Level II care. Table 27.2 provides more detail on each of the levels of care.

PLACEMENT DILEMMAS

Co-Occurring Disorders

The ASAM PPC-2R incorporates criteria that address the large subset of individuals who present for treatment with Axis I substance-related disorders and co-occurring Axis I/Axis II mental disorders. Table 27.3 summarizes what kinds of patients with co-occurring disorders are best treated in three kinds of programs: addiction only

TABLE 27.2 ASAM Criteria Levels of Care

ASAM PPC-2R level of detoxification service for adults	Level	(Note: There are no separate detoxification services for adolescents)
Ambulatory detoxification without extended onsite monitoring	I-D	Mild withdrawal with daily or less than daily outpatient supervision; likely to complete detoxification and to continue treatment or recovery.
Ambulatory detoxification with extended onsite monitoring	II-D	Moderate withdrawal with all-day detoxification support and supervision; at night, has supportive family or living situation; likely to complete detoxification.
Clinically managed residential detoxification	III.2-D	Minimal to moderate withdrawal but needs 24-h support to complete detoxification and increase likelihood of continuing treatment or recovery.
Medically monitored inpatient detoxification	III.7-D	Severe withdrawal and needs 24-h nursing care and physician visits as necessary; unlikely to complete detoxification without medical, nursing monitoring.
Medically managed inpatient detoxification	IV-D	Severe, unstable withdrawal and needs 24-h nursing care and daily physician visits to modify detoxification regimen and manage medical instability.
ASAM PPC-2R Levels of Care	**Level**	**Same levels of care for adolescents except Level III.3**
Early intervention	0.5	Assessment and education for at risk individuals who do not meet diagnostic criteria for substance-related disorder.
Outpatient services	I	<9 h of service per week (adults); <6 h/wk (adolescents) for recovery or motivational enhancement therapies/strategies.
Intensive outpatient	II.1	Nine or more hours of service per week (adults); six or more hours per week (adolescents) in a structured program to treat multidimensional instability.
Partial hospitalization	II.5	Twenty or more hours of service per week in a structured program for multidimensional instability not requiring 24-h care
Clinically managed low-intensity residential	III.1	24-h structure with available trained personnel with emphasis on reentry to the community; at least 5 h of clinical service per week
Clinically managed medium-intensity residential	III.3	24-h care with trained counselors to stabilize multidimensional imminent danger. Less intense milieu and group treatment for those with cognitive or other impairments unable to use full active milieu or therapeutic community.
Clinically managed high-intensity residential	III.5	24-h care with trained counselors to stabilize multidimensional imminent danger and prepare for outpatient treatment. Able to tolerate and use full active milieu or therapeutic community.
Medically monitored intensive inpatient	III.7	24-h nursing care with physician availability for significant problems in Dimensions 1, 2, or 3. 16 h/d counselor ability.
Medically managed intensive inpatient	IV	24-h nursing care and daily physician care for severe, unstable problems in Dimensions 1, 2, or 3. Counseling available to engage the patient in treatment.

(Continued)

TABLE 27.2	**ASAM Criteria Levels of Care (*Continued*)**		
ASAM PPC-2R Levels of Care	**Level**	**Same levels of care for adolescents except Level III.3**	
Opioid maintenance therapy	OMT	Daily or several times weekly opioid medication and counseling available to maintain multidimensional stability for those with opioid dependence.	

ASAM, American Society of Addiction; PPC, Patient Placement Criteria.

services, dual diagnosis capable, and dual diagnosis enhanced. Because co-occurring disorders are so prevalent, the ASAM criteria encourage all programs to be at least dual diagnosis capable (Table 27.4).

Assessment of Imminent Danger

Residential treatment has often been used for patients with chronic relapse problems, those with poor recovery environments or homelessness, and to "break through denial." In the ASAM PPC, residential treatment is reserved for stabilization of those in imminent danger. Such patients need a residential program that offers clinical staff and services 24 hours per day to respond to the patient's issues that pose the imminent danger (i.e., there is a strong probability that behaviors such as continued drug or alcohol use will occur, that such behaviors will present a significant risk of adverse consequences to the individual or others, and that such adverse events will occur in the very near future).

Mandated Level of Care or Length of Service

In some cases, an individual is referred for treatment at a specific level of care or for a specific length of service (e.g., an offender in the criminal justice system may be given a choice of a prison term or a fixed length of stay

TABLE 27.3	**Matching Patients with Co-Occurring Disorders to Services**
Patients	**Services**
Addiction only patients: Individuals who exhibit substance abuse or dependence problems without co-occurring mental health problems or diagnosable Axis I or II disorders	Addiction only services: Services directed toward the amelioration of substance-related disorders without services for the treatment of co-occurring mental health problems or diagnosable disorders. Such services are clinically inappropriate for dually diagnosed individuals.
Patients with co-occurring MH problems of mild to moderate severity: Individuals who exhibit (a) subthreshold diagnostic (i.e., traits, symptoms) Axis I or II disorders or (b) diagnosable but stable Axis I or II disorders (i.e., bipolar disorder but compliant with and stable on lithium).	Dual diagnosis capable: Primary focus on substance use disorders but capable of treating patients with subthreshold or diagnosable but stable Axis I or II disorders. Psychiatric services available onsite or by consultation; at least some staff members are competent to understand and identify signs and symptoms of acute psychiatric conditions.
Patients with co-occurring mental health problems of moderate to high severity: Individuals who exhibit moderate to severe diagnosable Axis I or II disorders, who are not stable and require mental health as well as addiction treatment.	Dual diagnosis enhanced: Psychiatric services available onsite or closely coordinated; all staff cross-trained in addiction and mental health and are competent to understand and identify signs and symptoms of acute psychiatric conditions and treat mental health problems along with the substance use disorders. Treatment for both mental health and substance abuse disorders is integrated. This service is most similar to a traditional "dual diagnosis" program.

TABLE 27.4   Application of the ASAM Criteria to Clinical Presentations

Use of the *ASAM Patient Placement Criteria* in treatment planning involves much more than simply a decision about level of care. The assessment dimensions and the broad continuum of care surveyed by the ASAM dimensions provide an opportunity to focus treatment, consistent with a disease management approach. The following vignettes, which represent segments of comprehensive assessments, are designed to illustrate some of the more common problems encountered in determining severity of illness, developing treatment plans, and making placement decisions. Each vignette illustrates an initial response, a discussion, and a revised response.

Case 1: Mr. A

Mr. A is a 58-year-old male who meets diagnostic criteria (DSM-IV-TR) for "Alcohol Dependence with Physiological Dependence." In terms of Dimension 1, he is currently in mild withdrawal from alcohol (Clinical Institute Withdrawal Assessment of Alcohol Scale, Revised, CIWA-Ar, score of 7) with a history of no more than moderate severity withdrawal. However, he stopped drinking only 2 h ago. Mr. A is hypertensive by history, not well controlled with medication even when sober, and current blood pressure is 140/100. Severity in Dimensions 3 through 6 is low.

Initial Response

Based on only mild withdrawal severity in Dimension 1, Mr. A is referred for Level I-D detoxification, ambulatory detoxification without extended on-site monitoring. For his Dimension 2 problem, he is referred back to his primary care physician for review of his hypertension.

Discussion

Given that Mr. A is withdrawing from alcohol, a sedative drug, the resultant autonomic arousal will create an increase in blood pressure. His current blood pressure reading is only 2 h since his last drink and insufficient time has elapsed for the full withdrawal syndrome to have developed. It can be assumed that the autonomic arousal could markedly increase his blood pressure, and because his baseline blood pressure is already elevated, the interaction between Dimensions 1 and 2 increases his overall severity.

Revised Response

Because of the high severity resulting from the interaction between Dimensions 1 and 2, Mr. A should be treated in Level III.7-D medically monitored inpatient detoxification service. An alternative might be referral to a Level II-D ambulatory detoxification with extended on-site monitoring if the patient enters treatment early in the week and could be observed for a number of days or if the II-D service operates 7 d/wk.

Case 2: Ms. P

A 16-year-old woman is brought to the emergency department of an acute care hospital with a report that, in the course of an argument with her parents, she has thrown a chair. Her parents suspect drug intoxication is the cause and report that she has been staying out unusually late at night and mixing with "the wrong crowd." They report a great deal of family discord, anger, and frustration, particularly directed by the young woman toward her father. Ms. P has no history of psychiatric or addiction treatment.

The parents both are present in the emergency department, although Ms. P was brought in by the police after her mother called for help. An emergency physician and a nurse from the psychiatric unit jointly evaluate Ms. P; they agree that she needs to be hospitalized in view of the animosity at home, her violent behavior, and the possibility that she is using an unknown drug.

Following the ASAM assessment dimensions, they organize the clinical information as follows:

Dimension 1: acute intoxication and/or withdrawal potential: Although she was intoxicated at the time of the chair-throwing incident, Ms. P is no longer intoxicated and has not been using alcohol or other drugs in sufficient quantities or for a long enough period to suggest the possibility of a withdrawal syndrome.

Dimension 2: biomedical conditions and complications: Ms. P is not taking any medications, is physically healthy, and has no current complaints.

Dimension 3: emotional, behavioral, or cognitive conditions and complications: Ms. P has complex problems with anger management, as evidenced by the chair-throwing incident, but is not impulsive at present if separated from her parents, especially her father.

(Continued)

TABLE 27.4	Application of the ASAM Criteria to Clinical Presentations (*Continued*)

Dimension 4: readiness to change: Ms. P is willing to talk to a therapist, blames her parents for being overbearing and not trusting her, and agrees to come into treatment but does not want to be at home with her father.

Dimension 5: relapse, continued use, or continued problem potential: The team concludes that Ms. P is likely to engage in drug use if released. They believe that, if she returns home immediately, there may be a reoccurrence of the fighting and, possibly, violence.

Dimension 6: recovery environment: Ms. P's parents are frustrated and angry as well. They are mistrustful of their daughter and want her hospitalized to provide a break in the family fighting.

Initial Response

Based on Ms. P's recent history of violent acting out, the emergency physician and the psychiatric nurse recommend that she be admitted to the hospital's psychiatric unit, at least for the night.

Discussion

Ms. P's acting out occurred when she was intoxicated, which she no longer is. The major conflict appears to be a family issue, particularly between Ms. P and her father. There is no indication of a severe or imminently dangerous biomedical, emotional, behavioral, or cognitive problem that requires the resources of a medically managed intensive inpatient setting.

Revised Response

The initial goal is to separate Ms. P from her father, which might be done by arranging for Ms. P to stay with a relative or family friend overnight, or by having Ms. P and her mother stay at a motel for the night. Based on the available information, Ms. P's behavior and conflict with her parents may reflect normal adolescent struggles rather than psychopathology. To address this, outpatient family counseling should be considered. Given the information available, there is also nothing indicating that Ms. P suffers from a diagnosable substance use disorder.

In crisis or mandated treatment situations, clinicians often come under pressure from family or referral agencies to provide a certain level of care. However, when the essential information is organized according to the ASAM dimensions, the patient's real severity and needs are more easily identified. This leads to a more appropriate clinical plan and avoids wasteful use of resources by focusing on the services needed to meet the patient's individual needs.

ASAM, American Society of Addiction Medicine.

in a treatment center). Such mandated referrals may not be based on clinical considerations and thus may be inconsistent with a placement decision arrived at through the ASAM criteria. In such a case, the provider should make reasonable attempts to have the order amended to reflect the assessed clinical level or length of service.

If the court order or other mandate cannot be amended, the individual may be continuing treatment at a level of care or for a length of stay greater than is clinically indicated. The resident's readiness for discharge or transfer and the staff's attempts to implement a clinically appropriate placement should be noted in the clinical record, and the treatment plan should be updated in a manner that provides the resident with the opportunity to continue the recovery process at the same level of care.

Logistical Impediments

Logistic problems present major challenges in rural and frontier areas because of large distances and few treatment resources or personnel. Underserved inner-city areas with lower socioeconomic and disadvantaged people may also lack the resources for people to easily access services. When logistic considerations are an impediment to the indicated services (e.g., lack of available transportation is a barrier to a patient's access to an indicated outpatient program), an outpatient service combined with unsupervised/minimally supervised housing may be an appropriate treatment intervention.

Need for a Safe Environment

When a patient lives in an environment that is so toxic as to preclude recovery efforts (as through victimization or exposure to an active addict) and a Level I or II outpatient service is indicated, the patient may need referral to a safe place to live while in treatment, as well as to treatment itself. One example might be combining a women's shelter with a Level II.1 or II.5 treatment program.

Assuring Individualized Treatment

There are at least three efficient ways to determine whether a program is providing truly individualized treatment.

1. Take 10 closed clinical case records and compare the treatment plans. If the reviewer cannot clearly distinguish patients by their treatment plans, the treatment is not individualized.
2. Review the progress notes and determine whether they relate back to the objectives or strategies in the treatment plan.
3. For programs that receive reimbursement from multiple payers, compare lengths of service by sources of payment. If the lengths of stay correspond to payer type, then the program is payment-driven rather than offering individualized treatment.

Summary Author: Christopher A. Cavacuiti
Peter D. Friedmann • Karran A. Phillips • Richard Saitz • Jeffrey H. Samet

Linking Addiction Treatment with Other Medical and Psychiatric Treatment Systems

Persons with substance use problems are at substantial risk for coexisting medical and mental health problems. Similarly, patients in addictive disorder treatment commonly experience medical and psychiatric problems, which can distract from recovery and increase relapse risk. Yet providers operate in distinct systems of care, each with its own —often exclusive—focus. As a result, substance-using patients with psychiatric or medical illnesses sometimes are bounced between systems—told that they must be abstinent before they can receive treatment for their psychiatric and medical problems or that they are too sick (medically or psychiatrically) to get into an addiction treatment program—resulting in a clinical "Catch-22."

Patients who present with complex, interrelated, comorbid problems make apparent the disconnect between these parallel yet typically separate systems of care. Linkages across the separate medical, mental health, and addictive disorder disciplines will be needed to improve the quality of care delivered to patients with addictive disorders.

BENEFITS OF LINKED SERVICES

From a patient's perspective, the potential for improved overall care is the motivating force for linkage of systems (Table 28.1). Examples of improved quality of care from such linkages include the potential for improved pain control in a patient receiving substance abuse treatment services, proper attribution of side effects of medications (versus substance use or withdrawal), and better access to detoxification and treatment for patients in the medical system. A pragmatic patient benefit is the provision of convenient, comprehensive, and coordinated care. Finally, linking services also may decrease stigma, as all providers would acknowledge and support the patient's recovery efforts.

From the perspective of the primary care provider and the mental health clinician, possible benefits of linkage include early identification of and relapse prevention for substance use disorders, increased consideration of alcohol and drug problems in the formulation of differential diagnoses, better access to addictive disorder treatment services, enhanced patient adherence to appointments and medications, and improved addictive disorder training and experience for personnel. From an addiction treatment provider's perspective, stronger linkages could yield improved outcomes of addictive disorder treatment. Ready availability of needed medical and mental health services also would allow addictive disorder professionals to do what they do best: focus on the core substance use issues. Exposure to examples of successful treatment could reduce stigma on the part of medical and mental health professionals toward addictive disorders and enhance their appreciation of the value of addictive disorder treatment. Addictive disorder providers could learn about the medical and mental health complications of addictions and enhance their appreciation of clients' conditions, health care needs, and prevention approaches. The linkage of services could provide an opportunity to affect other behavior-related issues, such as sexually transmitted diseases (including human immunodeficiency virus [HIV]) and smoking.

From a societal perspective, stronger linkages might lower long-term costs, including savings from reduced HIV incidence and other health-related sequelae of averted substance use, reduced incarceration and other

TABLE 28.1	**Treatment with Other Medical Psychiatric Services**

From the patient's perspective

- Structured format
- Improves overall quality of care
- Facilitates access to addictive disorders treatment for patients in medical care settings
- Enhances access to primary medical care for patients receiving addictive disorder treatment
- Improves patient well-being in terms of addictive disorder severity and medical problems
- Provides care that may be easier to access
- Increases the patient's satisfaction with his or her health care

From the primary care provider's perspective

- Promotes screening of all patients for alcohol problems
- Facilitates inclusion of alcohol and drug causes when considering a differential diagnosis
- Allows more achievable access to the addictive disorder treatment system
- Supports the prevention of relapse to alcohol and drug abuse
- Encourages other mental health services for primary care patients
- Enhances adherence with appointments and medical regimens
- Provides addictive disorder training opportunities for personnel

From the addiction treatment provider's perspective

- Improves addictive disorder treatment outcomes
- Reduces stigma about addictive disorder issues among medical providers
- Provides training opportunities about addictive disorder–related medical problems
- Promotes healthier behaviors
- Enhances medical providers' appreciation of the value of addictive disorder treatment
- Creates support for reimbursement parity for addictive disorder services
- Develops ongoing quality improvement efforts within addictive disorder programs

From a societal perspective

- Reduces costs of health care, criminal justice, and loss of productivity
- Reduces duplication of services and administrative costs
- Improves health outcomes of specific populations

criminal justice expenditures, and increased productivity. Other benefits could include reduced duplication of services across these systems and improved health outcomes for specific populations burdened with the substantial morbidity associated with alcohol or drug use disorders.

BARRIERS TO OPTIMAL LINKAGE

Many barriers impede better linkage of services. One well-documented problem has been the perspective of many medical practitioners that addressing alcohol and drug abuse issues is not providing medical care and thus is outside their purview.

Clinicians in practice generally report having received minimal training in substance use disorders, and they screen inadequately for preclinical cases. Because they neither find patients with less severe addictive disorders nor follow up those who have had success in treatment, most physicians have experienced few successes; in effect, only patients who do poorly and develop severe medical and psychosocial problems are "visible." This biases the spectrum of medical providers' clinical experience and further discourages physician involvement.

Payment and Service Linkage Issues

In our current health care system, payment for addiction treatment and mental health care has been limited compared with payments for other medical services. The refusal of reimbursement serves as a disincentive for physicians to screen and document alcohol use, and the opportunity for intervention is missed despite an estimated health savings of 3.81 US dollars for every 1.00 US dollar spent on screening and intervention.

Moreover, many managed behavioral health plans have separated the financing of care for mental and addictive disorders from that for the rest of the patient's ailments. Such plans have reduced the utilization of services for addictive disorders. Separate systems could foster the continuation of episodic, poorly coordinated care for substance-abusing patients.

Current systems of payment often do not cover addictive disorder services provided by primary care physicians; financial reimbursements generally are taken from separate budgets, and the financial benefits of averted medical complications occur late. Consequently, the cost of treatment for an addictive disorder that prevents subsequent HIV infection may be appreciated as a treatment expense, rather than as a savings of future medical care costs. Another financial disincentive to linked services is the perception that costs of such care may be limitless. The fear of the cost of appropriate addictive disorder services persists, despite analyses that document the limited effect even a worst case scenario would have on health care expenditures.

However, in 2008, the Paul Wellstone Mental Health and Addiction Equity Act of 2007 (HR 1424) was signed into law; it seeks to improve health for all Americans by granting greater access to mental health and addiction treatment and prohibiting health insurers from placing discriminatory restrictions on treatment.

Concerns About Confidentiality and Stigma

Practical difficulties interfere with obtaining timely two-way written releases of information. Addictive disorder information must be specified in information releases to be shared and is often kept separate from the standard medical record. Though the protection of patient confidentiality is noble, in some cases, it can impede integrated care.

Stigma remains a fundamental barrier in the treatment of any patient with alcohol or drug abuse. In addition to effects on patient behavior, such as limiting recognition of needs and readiness to accept services, stigma might result in medical clinicians' disinclination toward spending time addressing drug and alcohol issues or a perception of diminished stature of substance abuse treatment providers.

MODELS OF LINKED SERVICES

Alcohol- and drug-abusing patients use services in inefficient ways (e.g., emergency department [ED] presentations rather than outpatient clinic visits), and they do not receive care in the continuous, longitudinal, and comprehensive manner that is often essential for the high-quality management of any chronic disease. Two basic models have been proposed to bring the system of care for patients with substance use disorders closer to a primary care or chronic disease management model (Table 28.2). One model uses a centralized approach in which treatment of addictive disorders, primary medical care, and mental health services are colocated at a single site. A second model uses a distributive approach to facilitate effective patient referrals to services at different sites.

Centralized Models

This fully integrated, "one-stop shopping" model has been best described in primary care medical clinics and in addictive disorder treatment programs. In addition to overcoming the substantial political, bureaucratic, attitudinal, and financial barriers that separate addicted persons from needed services, centralized delivery overcomes the problems of geographic separation, patient disorganization, and poor motivation that inhibit patients with addictive disorders from keeping outside appointments. In 1999, Willenbring and Olson reported favorable results for a model of integrated alcohol treatment in a primary care clinic for poorly motivated, medically ill alcoholics. Their model included at least monthly visits, outreach to patients who missed appointments, clinic notes that cued the primary care provider to monitor alcohol intake at each visit, provider-delivered brief advice that emphasized reducing the harm from alcohol use and cutting down rather than strict abstinence, verbal and graphic feedback of improvement and deterioration in biologic markers such as gamma-glutamyl transferase (GGT), and on-site mental health services as needed. During 2 years of follow-up, patients in the integrated clinic had improved alcohol treatment outcomes (including greater abstinence), improved outpatient visit adherence, and lower mortality compared with similar patients referred to traditional alcohol dependence treatment and ambulatory medical care. Less resource-intensive intervention models developed for problem drinkers in primary care also have proved feasible, with some models successfully incorporating behavioral health personnel into primary care practices. However, if these efforts are to be generalized to primary care settings as they exist today, substantial training of clinicians will be required, as physicians often estimate their competence in

TABLE 28.2	Distributive Integrated Service Models

Centralized models

- Addiction treatment and pharmacotherapy in primary medical care and mental health services sites
- Addiction providers located in group HMOs, private practices, or clinics
- Behavioral medicine and primary medical provider offices co-located in shared space
- Addiction treatment delivered at public health clinics (e.g., sexually transmitted infections, HIV or tuberculosis care)
- Addiction treatment delivered in a general hospital with proximate medical and mental health clinics
- Addiction treatment and primary care services co-located in a community mental health setting
- Addiction-trained nurse practitioner or physician available in a primary care practice to prescribe and monitor naltrexone, to prescribe and monitor buprenorphine, and to initiate and manage detoxification
- Addiction and mental health specialty teams present in medical care sites (e.g., consult teams in EDs or hospitals)
- Smoking cessation counseling and pharmacotherapy delivered as part of primary care
- Brief interventions and advice for unhealthy substance use in doctor's offices, EDs, and hospitals
- Primary medical care and mental health services delivered at addiction treatment sites
- Medical and mental health providers or clinic located at a methadone treatment program
- Co-located primary care and addiction care
- An integrated alcohol and medical clinic
- An addiction medicine physician with medical and psychiatric skills
- A multiservice community agency with a central location

Distributive

- Health maintenance organizations or preferred provider organizations with defined, yet decentralized, referral networks
- Addiction triage and referral, or central intake and assessment centers that perform medical and mental health assessments and referral for multiple addiction treatment programs
- Community-based case management
- Evaluation at addiction treatment sites with external referral for ongoing medical and mental health care
- Defined networks of providers with facilitated communication and financial/contractual links and systems
- Informal links between clinicians or agencies facilitated by releases of information, transportation, and case management
- A multiservice community agency with a single owner but several locations

alcohol-related behavior change lower than in other health-related behavior change such as smoking cessation, stress, exercise, and weight management.

Though general practitioners have frequently participated in the management of illicit drug dependence disorders elsewhere in the world, this has only recently occurred in the United States with the enactment of legislation permitting office-based treatment of opioid dependence. Sublingual buprenorphine and a combination of buprenorphine and naloxone have been used for this purpose in the United States since 2003. In a 12-week randomized trial of opiate-dependent patients treated with buprenorphine maintenance, there was higher retention in the primary care setting than in a drug treatment program. In addition to achieving positive treatment outcomes, office-based buprenorphine has been well received by patients; several studies have found that buprenorphine works as well as methadone for patients with opiate addiction of mild to moderate severity.

Centralized models of primary medical and mental health care in addiction treatment settings may also improve addicted patients' access to these services. Among patients with substance abuse–related medical conditions, integrated care models compared to independent care models have shown significant decreases in hospitalization rates, inpatient days, and emergency room use. Similarly, on-site delivery of primary care to methadone maintenance patients and long-term residential patients has been shown to reduce subsequent ED and hospital use. Other work suggests that integration of addictive disorder treatment and community mental health services reduces relapse and improves social stability for patients dually diagnosed with addictive disorders and mental illness. Centralizing primary medical care, substance dependence treatment, and psychiatric services has also proved an effective way to manage concomitant medical conditions such as hepatitis C and tuberculosis.

Distributive Models

Successful referral is the central task of the distributive model, but the substantial interorganizational distance between addiction treatment programs and mainstream health care presents great barriers. Because substance-abusing populations can have disorganized lifestyles and poor motivation, contemporary distributive models typically use case management to facilitate referrals.

In addiction treatment programs, distributive arrangements are commonly used to link patients to medical and mental health services. Distributive arrangements range, for example, from an addictive disorder treatment unit that contracts with a local group practice to provide physical examinations and routine medical care to its patients to one that makes ad hoc referrals to a local community mental health center. This model requires no rearrangement of existing health care delivery systems; however, it does require efforts (and therefore costs) to assure that linkage is facilitated.

Case management can facilitate these referrals: a study of public addiction treatment programs found that contracted referral with case management increased medical services utilization two- to threefold over ad hoc referrals. More recent work has emphasized the importance of transportation assistance to increase the delivery of needed services.

The distributive model predominates in the United States. Though it can be less effective than the centralized model in linking substance-abusing patients to needed services, its relatively low cost, flexibility, and adaptability (especially to integration of secondary and tertiary care services) suggest that the distributive model, with further refinements, is likely to remain the method of coordinated services in the near future.

Vulnerable Populations

Integrated models may be most germane and show the most benefit to vulnerable populations including HIV-infected, homeless, and incarcerated individuals. They have been found to promote delivery of HIV-related care, medication adherence, and outpatient medical services. An analysis of data gathered from New York State Medicaid claims found that regular drug abuse and medical care reduced hospitalizations by approximately 25% among HIV-positive and HIV-negative patients with drug abuse diagnoses.

Homeless individuals have high rates of social instability, comorbidity, and chronic drug use, which make them ideally suited for systems of integrated care. A retrospective medical record review of homeless and housed patients enrolled in office-based opioid treatment over 12 months found that homeless patients receiving buprenorphine/naloxone fared comparably to housed with regard to such measures as treatment failure, utilization of counseling, and participation in mutual help groups.

Despite the high prevalence of substance use disorders in correctional settings, a survey of the medical directors of all 50 states and the federal prison system demonstrated that among respondents who had jurisdiction over 88% of US prisoners, only 8% referred opiate-dependent inmates to methadone programs upon release. Efforts to close the gap between the high prevalence of substance use disorders in incarcerated individuals and the limited treatment options available should include improved treatment matching and linkage of services both during and after incarceration.

Summary Author: Christopher A. Cavacuiti
David Y-W Lee • Hong Wang

Alternative Therapies for Alcohol and Drug Addiction

HERBAL REMEDIES WITH ANTIADDICTIVE POTENTIALS

During the 19th century, China saw a huge increase in recreational opium use. At its peak, half the Chinese population (nearly that of the US population today) were addicted to opium. To combat this huge problem, a variety of Chinese herbal remedies were developed for treating opium addiction or relieving the withdrawal syndrome.

The Chinese remedies developed during this time were often combinations of more than a dozen herbs. Many traditional Chinese medical practitioners today continue to use combination of medicinal plants for the treatment of substance use disorders and other ailments. It is believed that using these plants in combination can produce synergistic effects that improve efficacy and lower toxicity.

Few of these traditional Chinese remedies have been investigated scientifically. Of those remedies that have been studied, YGT (also known as NPI-025) is probably the traditional medicine that has been studied the most thoroughly. It consists of five herbs: Qiang Huo, Gou Teng, Chun Xiong, Fu Zi, and Yan Hu Suo. These are among the most frequently used herbs for substance abuse treatment in China. Discussed below are some of the bioactivity studies related to two of the herbs in YGT—Yan Hu Suo and Gou Teng.

Yan Hu Suo (*Corydalis yanhusuo*)

Corydalis yanhusuo, one of the five Chinese medicinal plants in YGT, is noted to contain significant levels of the bioactive compound *l*-tetrahydropalmatine (*l*-THP). *l*-THP has both D1 receptor agonist and D2 receptor antagonist actions. Preliminary studies with other D1 agonist/D2 antagonist drugs have suggested that this class of drugs may reduce cocaine self-administration. This is very exciting, given that there are currently no effective pharmacotherapies for cocaine or methamphetamine addiction.

Gou Teng (*Uncaria rhynchophylla*)

Uncaria rhynchophylla is an important traditional Chinese medicine used in the treatment of pain, infantile convulsions, headaches, dizziness, hypertension, and rheumatoid arthritis. Of the dozen compounds extracted from this herb, two major alkaloids (rhynchophylline and isorhynchophylline) have binding activity for dopamine receptors and may have "antiaddictive" properties.

TRANSCUTANEOUS ELECTRICAL ACUPUNCTURE STIMULATION

Studies suggest that acupuncture (especially when combined with electrical stimulation) may be effective in relieving opioid withdrawal. A number of studies suggest that acupuncture can increase levels of endogenous opioids (endorphins), which may explain why acupuncture alleviates pain and controls withdrawal. While acupuncture has shown promising results, one of its major drawbacks is that treatments are generally required several times a day. Portable electrical stimulators, such as the Han's Acupoint Nerve Stimulator (HANS), may offer a solution to this problem, since they allow patients treat themselves by using acupoint stimulation without a needle.

OPIATE DETOXIFICATION WITH TRANSCUTANEOUS ELECTRICAL ACUPUNCTURE STIMULATION

Transcutaneous electrical acupuncture stimulation (TEAS) has been reported to reduce both subjective symptoms of withdrawal such as anxiety and objective signs of withdrawal such as tachycardia. Several studies have compared patients detoxified using conventional treatments such as Buprenorphine (BPN) or Methadone (MTD) with patients detoxified using conventional treatment plus Han's Acupoint Nerve Stimulation (HANS). In these studies, the patients treated with conventional treatment plus HANS required lower doses of conventional (BPN/MTD) treatment and also required fewer days of treatment.

PREVENTION OF CRAVING AND RELAPSE TO OPIATE ABUSE

Electrical acupuncture has been shown to reduce craving. In a study of patients recovering from heroin addiction, those treated with low-frequency HANS reported lower craving scores on a visual analog scale (VAS) than those treated with high-frequency HANS or mock (low-intensity) HANS. Many studies have confirmed that drug withdrawal and drug cravings can be triggers for relapse. By reducing withdrawal and cravings, it is theorized that HANS may also decrease the risk of relapse, and indeed, preliminary studies suggest using HANS for relapse prevention do indeed suggest that it may be helpful.

ACUPUNCTURE AND ALCOHOL ABUSE

The literature on acupuncture and alcohol abuse is conflicting. Some studies have provided positive results, whereas others have not.

CONCLUSION

Clinicians continue to face ongoing challenges when treating drug dependence. Alternative therapies such as acupuncture and traditional medicines have the potential to widen our range of available substance use disorder treatments.

Traditional medicines have been used in China and elsewhere for >2,000 years. Many plants contain bioactive compounds, and it is estimated that roughly one half of current pharmaceuticals originally were procured from plants. It is therefore reasonable to assume that traditional herbal remedies and the active isolates from these plants may potentially be useful in the treatment of substance use disorders.

Though alternative therapies may provide new treatments for existing drug treatments, rigorous studies to evaluate both the risks and the benefits of such treatments are needed.

CHAPTER 30

Summary Author: John Young
Alex Wodak

The Harm Reduction Approach to Prevention and Treatment

Harm reduction policies and programs, spanning prevention and treatment, aim to decrease the adverse health, social, and economic consequences of legal and illegal psychoactive drugs without *necessarily* diminishing drug consumption.

DEFINING HARM REDUCTION

The term harm reduction is used with a bewildering variety of interpretations; the ambiguity of the term adds to the confusion of an area already complicated by emotional fervor. The essence of harm reduction is a paramount focus on pragmatically reducing adverse consequences of drug use, whereas any impact on drug consumption is regarded as a lower priority.

The notion that the best should never be allowed to be the enemy of the good is the essence of harm reduction. Adopting and then ensuring delivery of achievable but suboptimal objectives are far more effective in public policy than aiming for utopian objectives and then failing to achieve them.

A more expanded view of harm reduction emphasizes the maximization of the potential benefits of psychoactive substances as an aim additional to minimizing potential harms. Accordingly, emphasis is given to more judicious use of dependence-producing medications. For example, the common practice of suboptimal prescription of opioids in the management of cancer and chronic nonmalignant pain often results in considerable distress from inadequate pain relief. Excessive fear of inducing drug dependence despite a cancer patient's limited life expectancy is often a significant factor in the decision to prescribe subtherapeutic doses of analgesics. Similarly, the evidence that medicinal use of cannabis is relatively safe and has many worthwhile benefits is growing, yet availability of medicinal cannabis is still limited.

Though harm reduction approaches are not intended primarily to reduce consumption of drugs, this is often an unintended long-term result. For example, many drug users who have attended needle syringe programs for some time canvass the idea of achieving abstinence and request referral to drug treatment.

MISCONCEPTIONS ABOUT HARM REDUCTION

The commonest misconception regarding harm reduction is that this approach and efforts to promote abstinence from psychoactive drugs are mutually exclusive options. In some ways, abstinence from drugs is the most complete form of harm minimization. Harm reduction reminds clinicians of the supreme importance of keeping drug users alive and avoiding irreversible damage.

Harm reduction is also often misconstrued as rejecting the role of drug law enforcement; on the contrary, harm reduction usually involves a far closer partnership between law enforcement and health. Police in many countries have become convinced of the importance of allowing needle syringe and methadone programs to function without undue law enforcement interference in order to ensure that the significant community benefits of these programs, including reducing crime, are not jeopardized. Some senior police also recognize that harm reduction may reduce official corruption that so often accompanies largely unsuccessful attempts to control the supply of drugs through reliance on drug law enforcement.

Harm reduction can even be seen to include attempts to reduce the harm resulting from drug law enforcement: a study carried out in 89 large cities in the United States found that the higher the numbers of per capita drug arrests, police employees, and corrections expenditures in a particular city, the higher the HIV seroprevalence among injecting drug users.

EXAMPLES OF HARM REDUCTION APPROACHES

Applications of harm reduction to alcohol in licensed premises are diverse and include the replacement of glasses with shatterproof drinking containers and the provision of heavy furniture bolted to the floor. Fortification of flour with thiamine virtually eliminates the Wernicke-Korsakoff syndrome, a form of brain damage strongly associated with severe alcohol dependence. The application of harm reduction to tobacco is more controversial, but nicotine replacement therapy to help smokers quit is analogous to the use of methadone to help heroin users quit. The lack of an effective substitution pharmacotherapy for stimulant (amphetamine, cocaine) injectors is a major problem in many countries where stimulants are the most commonly injected drug.

Needle syringe programs and opiate substitution treatment with methadone or buprenorphine are often considered the epitome of harm reduction. The evidence that both these interventions are effective, safe, and cost-effective is now very compelling and widely accepted.

HIV among injecting drug users can be easily controlled by the early and vigorous implementation of a comprehensive "harm reduction package" consisting of education, needle syringe programs, drug treatment, and community development of drug users. Needle syringe programs usually provide a great deal of practical education and also serve as important entry points for drug treatment and provision of other basic services.

Opiate substitution treatment is the most frequently evaluated intervention in all of medicine: abundant, consistent, and compelling evidence supports the effectiveness of methadone maintenance treatment in reducing HIV among injecting drug users and the achievement of multiple other important benefits including substantially reducing drug overdose deaths, crime, and illicit drug use. Social functioning is improved during substitution treatment; it also ensures that antiretroviral treatment achieves similar results for injecting drug users as it does for other groups at high risk of HIV.

Drug treatment is a critical part of the harm reduction package. In harm reduction settings, patients undergoing drug treatment often are encouraged to negotiate treatment goals and parameters with clinicians. Cycles of remission and relapse are regarded as part of the natural history of drug dependence rather than as a reflection of poor motivation or defective character. Drug treatment in a harm reduction framework is regarded as similar to the management of many relapsing and remitting chronic medical conditions rather than as an offshoot of law enforcement; retention in treatment is stressed and correlated with favorable outcomes.

Not all drug users accept or benefit from pharmacotherapies, so nonpharmacologic treatments should also be provided. Though the emphasis of drug treatment from an HIV control perspective is always appropriately focused on injecting drug users, it is also important to offer assistance to people who consume drugs without injecting, such as those who smoke or snort drugs. This includes responding effectively to factors that increase the likelihood of drug users undertaking a transition to injecting: lack of assistance for people who have developed drug problems but do not inject can provide a perverse incentive to begin injecting in order to get help.

Harm reduction should include efforts to improve the basic social conditions of injecting drug users including their general health, housing, welfare, and employment.

SPECIAL POPULATIONS

From a public health perspective of HIV control, some "bridge populations" of injecting drug users require particular attention; these include men who have sex with men, sex workers, users with severe mental illness, prison inmates, and those from indigenous and other minority backgrounds.

Medically supervised injecting centers are particularly effective at attracting severely disadvantaged injecting drug users in proximity to major drug markets. These centers provide many worthwhile benefits including reducing fatal and nonfatal overdoses and improving neighborhood amenity without producing significant unintended consequences such as increasing crime.

Understanding and responding to the needs of drug users from disadvantaged groups improve service design and use. Community development of injecting drug users helps to ensure that this population becomes part of the solution. Involving injecting drug users in the design and implementation of HIV prevention strategies increases their effectiveness.

Harm reduction is needed not only in community settings but also in so-called "closed settings" such as detention centers, jails, and prisons. Reliance on drug law enforcement to control illicit drugs inevitably means that many injecting drug users spend long periods of their drug injecting careers in correctional institutions; however, with so little to lose, high-risk drug injecting often continues in closed settings. Once behind bars, the risk of acquiring HIV infection is further increased by multiple factors including the large number of injecting equipment–sharing partners, the severely degraded condition of needles and syringes, the lack of HIV prevention strategies found in community settings, and the mixing of diverse demographic and geographic groups.

OFFICIAL RESPONSES TO HARM REDUCTION

Harm reduction has been explicitly accepted as the national drug policy in a number of developed countries, including Australia, Canada, and France.

There is strong and growing support for harm reduction at the national level. Needle syringe programs and opioid substitution programs are now provided in >60 countries, with numerous countries reporting substantial unmet demand for methadone treatment.

All 25 members of the European Union now provide needle syringe programs and methadone or buprenorphine maintenance treatment. Needle syringe programs and/or opiate substitution programs are becoming established, or expanding, in central Europe, China, India, Vietnam, Malaysia, Taiwan, and Indonesia. Iran has become a world leader in implementation and expansion of harm reduction to control HIV among injecting drug users.

Support for harm reduction is also strong at the international level. The largest section of the United Nations Office on Drugs and Crime (UNODC) is now harm reduction, employing more staff providing harm reduction than any other organization in the world. Harm reduction is now supported by virtually all of the United Nations organizations with responsibility for illicit drugs including UNAIDS, UNICEF, and the World Bank; in 2004, the World Health Organization (WHO) included methadone and buprenorphine in its List of Essential Medicines. Many other international organizations support harm reduction, including the International Red Cross.

The United States maintains a ban on federal government funding for needle syringe programs.

OUTCOMES OF HARM REDUCTION APPROACHES

Reviews of the evidence for needle syringe programs have concluded that these programs are effective in reducing HIV infections and are unaccompanied by serious unintended negative consequences, including increased use of illicit drugs. A study of data from 103 cities around the world showed that cities with needle syringe programs had an average annual decrease in HIV of 18.6%, compared with an average annual *increase* of 8.1% in cities without such programs. The mean annual increase in seroprevalence, weighted according to the number of subjects sampled, was 3.6% in cities without and 0.2% in cities with needle syringe programs. Though a standard methodology for measurement of HIV seroprevalence between and within cities was not used, it is difficult to envisage any systematic design flaw capable of producing these results.

Cost-effectiveness analyses have estimated that needle syringe programs in the United States can generally prevent an HIV infection for between $4,000 and $12,000. Using conservative assumptions drawn from published studies, it was estimated that between 4,000 and 10,000 HIV infections could have been prevented in the United States if needle syringe programs had been implemented; these infections will ultimately cost up to half a billion US dollars in HIV/AIDS treatment costs.

Compelling evidence supporting the effectiveness of methadone treatment against a range of important outcomes is drawn from a large literature. Methadone treatment has been demonstrated to reduce deaths from drug overdose, total mortality, morbidity, HIV risk behavior, HIV seroprevalence, HIV seroincidence, unemployment rates, and crime. Methadone treatment costs much less than other treatment modalities, incarceration, or no treatment. In general, retention in drug treatment is closely linked to satisfactory outcomes, and methadone programs are far more successful than other treatment modalities in attracting and retaining large numbers of drug users.

No country that has started harm reduction has ever regretted doing so and then terminated their harm reduction programs.

ALTERNATIVES TO HARM REDUCTION

Demand Reduction

Demand reduction typically involves a broad range of educational measures including mass and school campaigns and programs directed at established drug users and high-risk groups. Treatment of drug users is also classified as a form of demand reduction.

Some measures intended to reduce demand also reduce supply and vice versa. For example, methadone treatment might be regarded as simply reducing demand for street drugs in a relatively small number of heroin-dependent individuals. However, those seeking entry to methadone maintenance programs are usually severely dependent and probably include many of the heaviest consumers in the community; removing these individuals from the heroin market could have a significant effect on demand. As many of these users also are likely to traffic in drugs, their entry into treatment may also temporarily disrupt the heroin supply system.

Supply Reduction

Supply reduction involves attempts to reduce crop production, drug production, transport from countries of origin to countries of destination (interdiction), entry to the country of destination (customs), distribution (police) at wholesale and retail levels, and financial surveillance. Supply reduction forms the core of traditional international drug policy and usually receives the overwhelming majority of government expenditure in response to illicit drugs.

Outcomes of Alternative Approaches

The deterioration in the global illicit drug situation has occurred despite progressive strengthening of illicit drug law enforcement over several decades. Illicit drug use was a problem in only a few developed countries a generation ago; in 2004, the number of injecting drug users in the world was estimated to be 13.2 million, and the global turnover of the illicit drug trade was recently estimated to be US$ 322 billion.

This inexorable deterioration of the global illicit drug situation has been accompanied by increasingly serious consequences of illicit drug use. Soon after the AIDS epidemic was first recognized in the early 1980s, it was evident that HIV had spread alarmingly among and from populations of injecting drug users. HIV has irrevocably changed the nature and perception of injecting drug use. Hepatitis C is now recognized to be globally more prevalent among injecting drug users than HIV. Multidrug-resistant TB has appeared as a significant health problem in some countries and is now recognized to be closely associated with uncontrolled HIV epidemics in injecting drug users.

Demand Reduction Approaches

There is little evidence of significant and sustained reduction in demand from mass audience, school-based, or specially targeted educational campaigns.

Demand for illicit substances appears to be greater in populations with high levels of youth unemployment, poor housing, limited educational opportunities, poor health services, and neglected, crime-ridden neighborhoods. It is difficult to assess the role of these factors in stimulating demand for drugs, but lack of data should not be taken as evidence that they are unimportant.

Supply Reduction Approaches

A substantial literature documents the relative ineffectiveness of supply reduction and predicts continuing failure. The experience of most countries has been that drug production has increased almost every year apart from occasional reductions in production caused by bad weather in growing areas. Illicit drug use is spreading to more and more countries around the world. The range of drugs used has increased. Many countries have experienced an exponential growth in drug-related crime and deaths. The response to the national and international deterioration of the illicit drug situation has been an ever-increasing emphasis on attempts to restrict the supply of illicit drugs. International collaboration has increased. More funds have been allocated to attempts to reduce drug cultivation and production. Penalties for drug trafficking or drug use have been increased. Drug squads have been expanded. The number of prison inmates serving sentences for drug-related offenses has increased. Financial surveillance has been intensified.

Estimates of the allocation of government expenditure in response to illicit drugs have shown consistently that drug law enforcement is very generously funded while health and social interventions are generally funded parsimoniously. An impressive study commissioned by the U.S. Army and carried out by the RAND Corporation evaluated the return on a $1 investment in a variety of measures designed to reduce the societal cost of cocaine. The return was 15 cents for crop reduction and eradication in South America, 32 cents for interdicting transport of cocaine between South America and the United States, 52 cents for US customs and police, and $7.46 for drug treatment of cocaine users.

Finally, the alarming possibility exists that supply reduction may have inadvertently exacerbated health problems. Emphasis on supply reduction and public health goals may be inimical. Antiopium policies adopted in Hong Kong, Thailand, and Laos were followed by the disappearance of opium smoking—which was replaced by heroin injecting.

CHAPTER 31

Summary Author: Christopher A. Cavacuiti
Dennis McCarty • Victor A. Capoccia • David H. Gustafson

Quality Improvement for Addiction Treatment

Outcomes from addiction treatment services compare favorably with treatments for other chronic conditions (such as hypertension, diabetes, and asthma). However, addiction treatment faces a number of challenges that other chronic illnesses do not:

1. The impact of addiction (e.g., family dysfunction, crime, unemployment) is more visible (and less socially acceptable) than the impact of other chronic illnesses.
2. Effective treatment interventions for hypertension, diabetes, and asthma have been in use for much longer and are generally deemed to be effective by the public and by the medical profession. In contrast, the treatment of addiction is commonly (though mistakenly) viewed as a hopeless endeavor.
3. Unlike other chronic illnesses, there is a persistent expectation that patients with diagnosed drug and alcohol disorders will remain symptom-free (i.e., without substance use) after their treatment ends.

INSTITUTE OF MEDICINE REPORTS

The Institute of Medicine (IOM) within the National Academy of Sciences advises health care providers and policy makers on how to redesign health systems in order to improve quality of care. Six dimensions of quality have been identified by the IOM: Care should be safe, effective, patient centered, timely, efficient, and equitable. The IOM has noted in its reports that evidence-based treatments are not used routinely for alcohol, drug, and mental health disorders. In addition, they note that this substandard care leads to greater expense and suffering. The IOM explicitly recommends that alcohol, drug, and mental health treatment systems emphasize the six dimensions of quality of care and that public agencies and other payers promote the development of process and outcome measures that track quality of care.

Furthermore, the IOM has noted that health policy and reimbursement processes have more impact on patient outcomes than variation in individual practitioner knowledge or behavior. In other words, improved outcomes will come more readily from improving the system than by trying to improve the skills of the practitioners.

DEFINING AND MEASURING QUALITY TREATMENT AND OUTCOMES

Public expectations, demands for accountability from payers and policy makers, and a strong desire from within the field of addiction medicine to improve performance drive efforts to define and measure effective treatments and treatment outcomes. Below are some of the important systems and agencies measuring addiction treatment quality.

National Outcome Measures and the State Outcomes Measurement and Management System

The Substance Abuse and Mental Health Services Administration (SAMHSA) is implementing a national system to measure state performance related to treatment and prevention of alcohol, drug, and mental health disorders. This system is called the State Outcomes Measurement and Management System (SOMMS), and it is designed to increase the accountability of state systems and participating treatment services.

In order to allow for estimates of cost effectiveness, states must provide outcome data as well as economic data. These reports are required as a condition of federal funding. In terms of outcomes, states must report on the following National Outcome Measures (NOMs) at client admission and discharge:

- Abstinence from alcohol and other drugs
- Employment/education
- Crime and criminal justice
- Stability in housing
- Access capacity
- Retention

Washington Circle Measures

According the Washington Circle (WC) Web site: "WC is a group of national experts in substance abuse policy, research and performance management who seek to improve the quality and effectiveness of prevention and treatment services through the use of performance measurement systems."

National Quality Forum

The National Quality Forum (NQF) is a Congressionally chartered membership organization charged with using empirically based consensus process to define and disseminate standards and measures for the health care system. A summary of the NQF's evidence-based treatment recommendations for alcohol, tobacco, and drug use disorders can be found in Table 31.1.

ACCREDITATION FOR TREATMENT PROGRAMS

In the United States, the Joint Commission on Accreditation of Health Care Organizations (JCAHO), the Commission on Accreditation of Rehabilitation Facilities (CARF), and the Council on Accreditation for Children and Family Services (COA) are the primary entities that provide accreditation for alcohol and drug treatment programs. However, the 2006 National Survey of Substance Abuse Treatment Services (N-SSATS) notes that less than half of the facilities reported accreditation from JCAHO (22%), CARF (18%), or COA (4%).

Accreditation Process

Accreditation requires an organization to conduct an extensive internal analysis of its performance. The standards are aimed at minimum at promoting patient safety and optimally at improving patient outcomes. Surveyors identify strengths and the need for improvement and then present a recommendation to the accrediting body for multiyear, limited, conditional, or denial of accreditation.

Accreditation for Opioid Treatment Programs

The accreditation process for opioid treatment programs is more rigorous and more ubiquitous than for other types of addiction treatment programs. Federal regulations require that all opioid treatment programs receive certification from a national accreditation organization or a state agency documenting that the treatment program meets regulatory standards and will comply with the standards. The CARF and the JCAHO are approved to provide national accreditation.

BUILDING SYSTEM CAPACITY TO DELIVER EFFECTIVE TREATMENTS

According to a 15-year follow-up of >400 programs, fewer than 10% offered medication-assisted treatment, and fewer than half offered psychosocially based interventions supported by empirical research. Barriers to more effective care include high turnover, low use of technology, and minimal presence of medical expertise.

Network for the Improvement of Addiction Treatment (NIATx)

Participating NIATx programs form a learning community that share best practices in an effort to reduce time to admission, decrease no-shows, enhance retention in care, and increase admissions. NIATx uses five key process-improvement principles to facilitate organizational change.

TABLE 31.1	**Summary of NQF Standards for the Treatment of Substance Use Disorders**

Domain No. 1: Identification of Substance Use Conditions

Screening and Case Finding
Patients should be screened for substance use disorder (SUDs) during new patient encounters and at least annually.
Health care providers should employ a systematic screening method to identify patients who use drugs.

Diagnosis and Assessment
Patients who have a positive screen should receive further assessment.
Patients with a diagnosed SUD should receive a multidimensional, biopsychosocial assessment.

Domain No. 2: Initiation and Engagement in Treatment

Brief Intervention
All patients identified with tobacco use and/ or excess alcohol use should receive brief motivational counseling.

Promoting Engagement in Treatment for Substance Use Illness
Health care providers should systematically promote engagement in SUD treatment.

Withdrawal Management
Supportive pharmacotherapy should be available and provided.
Assess withdrawal symptoms and risk of serious adverse consequences.
Withdrawal management alone does not constitute treatment for dependence.

Domain No. 3: Therapeutic Interventions to Treat Substance Use Illness

Psychosocial Interventions
Empirically validated psychosocial treatment interventions should be initiated for all SUD patients.

Pharmacotherapy
Pharmacotherapy should be offered and available to all adult patients with diagnosed opioid, alcohol, and nicotine dependence. Pharmacotherapy, if prescribed, should be provided in addition to and directly linked with psychosocial treatment/support.

Domain No. 4: Continuing Care Management of Substance Use

Patients should be offered long-term, coordinated management of their SUD and any coexisting conditions. Care should be monitored and adapted on an ongoing basis.

1. *Understand the Customer*: Focus groups and interviews with clients can help increase understanding of treatment experiences. For example, a NIATx review of walk-through reports (in which simulated patients "walk through" the admissions process) revealed that many clients are faced with conflicting and incorrect information regarding the intake process, as well as redundant and burdensome intake forms, unanswered telephone lines, and unreturned voice mail.

2. *Fix Key Problems*: Agency change requires active support from the highest levels of the organization. Change is most likely to be successful when it meets the needs of both the patient and the program. For example, a NIATx program found that reducing the delay from first contact to admission from 4 days to 1 day led to a substantial increase in both treatment admissions and program revenue.

3. *Pick a Powerful Change Leader*: Not every counselor or employee has the skill or desire to lead change. It is important, therefore, to choose "change leaders" carefully. Change leaders should be supportive of the improvements that need to be made and have the respect of peers, staff and leaders throughout the organization.

4. *Seek Outside Ideas and Encouragement*: NIATx encourages members get ideas on best practices from other NIATx participants and from other industries.

5. *Use Rapid PDSA Cycles*: PDSA (Plan, Do, Study Act) cycles are a central component of process improvement. First (PLAN), the problem must be defined, needs must be assessed, and a decision must be made about what change is required. Second (DO), the change must be implemented. A key facet is that the test is for a limited time and limited number of patients. Initially, it is a feasibility test. Third (STUDY), a few simple measures are collected and analyzed to see if the change led to the desired outcome. Fourth (ACT), based on the planning, doing, and studying, the change team decides what to do next. If the change was helpful, it may be expanded. Change teams also learn from changes that are not improvements. They modify and try again using an iterative process.

Strengthening Treatment Access and Retention-State Implementation (STAR-SI): the NIATx State Initiative

In the STAR-SI, the participating state agencies create incentives and provide support mechanisms to promote statewide adoption of NIATx principles and results.

Advancing Recovery

This is one of the most recent facets of the NIATx model. The aim of the Advancing Recovery program is to utilize the NIATx model to facilitate system changes that promote implementation of evidence-based practices.

CHAPTER 32

Summary Author: Christopher A. Cavacuiti
Nady el-Guebaly • Vladimir Poznyak • Juana Maria Tomás-Rosselló

International Perspectives on Addiction Management

Historically, international efforts to control use of psychoactive substances have focused on reducing the worldwide supply. International efforts to decrease the demand for drugs and to share best practices in terms of treatment and harm reduction are more recent and are gaining momentum. There are a number of international medical organizations committed to demand reduction, including the United Nations (UN), the World Health Organization (WHO), the United Nations Office on Drugs and Crime (UNODC), the World Medical Association (WMA), the World Psychiatric Association (WPA), and the International Society of Addiction Medicine (ISAM).

WORLDWIDE PREVALENCE OF PSYCHOACTIVE SUBSTANCE USE

Worldwide psychoactive substance use is highly prevalent, and large segments of the world population are exposed to the effects of dependence-producing substances. Alcohol is the most widely used psychoactive substance worldwide, and about 2 billion people use alcohol beverages around the world. Currently, there are >1 billion people in the world who smoke tobacco and around 200 million people using drugs considered "illicit" in the United States. According to WHO estimates, in 2000, the number of people with alcohol dependence or harmful use of alcohol worldwide reached 76.4 million, and number of people with drug use disorders was 15.3 million.

Of the 200 million people worldwide who use "illicit" drugs, cannabis (162 million) represents the first, and amphetamine-type stimulants or ATS (35 million) the second most widely used substances, followed by opiates (16 million) and cocaine (13 million). It is estimated that 25 million people, equivalent to 0.6% of the world population aged 15 to 64, are drug dependent. It is also estimated that there are 13.1 million Injection Drug Users (IDUs) worldwide and that >10% of all HIV infections worldwide are due to the use of contaminated drug-injecting equipment.

HISTORICAL SYNOPSIS OF INTERNATIONAL DRUG TREATIES

A number of international drug treaties provide the legal basis for the present international drug control system that is aimed at ensuring the availability of narcotic and psychotropic substances for medical and scientific purposes while preventing their diversion into illicit channels.

Several elements of these Conventions/Treaties are particularly relevant to the practice of addiction medicine. In the Conventions of the International Narcotics Control Board (INCB), signatory countries are required to

- Take all practicable measures for the prevention, identification, treatment, and rehabilitation of persons involved in drug abuse.
- Promote the training of personnel involved in delivering these interventions.
- Promote measures that reduce the harm associated with drug use including reductions in the "sharing of hypodermic needles among injecting drug abusers."

- Treatment programs that include "drug substitution and maintenance treatment" do not breach current treaties provided that these programs adhere to "established national sound medical practice."
- Treatment and rehabilitation may be provided either as an alternative or an addition to criminal conviction or punishment.

SELECTED ACTIVITIES OF THE UNODC

The UN has had drug control functions since its inception, having inherited them from the League of Nations. UNODC's mandate includes reporting on national and global demand for illicit drugs, sharing of best practices, and supporting Member States in developing strategies and activities for the reduction of demand for illicit drugs.

Progress Toward Reaching a Balance Between Supply and Demand Reduction

As reported by Member States to the UNODC through the Biennial Reports Questionnaire, although treatment and rehabilitation interventions are being expanded, they are still well below the amount and quality that are needed. Historically, there have been significant barriers between what is known in terms of evidence-based approaches to addiction and what has been available to community treatment agencies and the clients they serve. For instance, opioid dependence detoxification remains the most common reported approach despite evidence of its lack of effectiveness as a stand-alone intervention, while the intervention with the most solid evidence base—pharmacologic maintenance—remains rather infrequently used in most regions.

Key UNODC Initiatives Related to Addiction Medicine

1. *Youthnet*: The UNODC supports the Global Youth Network (aka "Youthnet": *www.unodc.org/youthnet*) for the prevention of drug abuse among youth. Youthnet provides information, resources, training, and funding to >500 youth groups around the world. Unfortunately, many prevention programs around the world, while well intentioned, implement activities that do not have the backing of scientific evidence.
2. *Treatnet*, the "International Network of Drug Dependence Treatment and Rehabilitation Resource Centres" *(www.unodc.org/treatnet)* has focused on and developed good-practice documents on four key topics: community-based treatment, treatment in prison settings, treatment and HIV/AIDS prevention and care, and sustained recovery management.
3. *Global Assessment Programme (GAP)*: GAP develops drug epidemiologic surveillance and evaluation systems. The aim of GAP is to use these data to design and implement more effective responses to national/global drug abuse problems.
4. *UNAIDS*: The UNODC is a cosponsor of the Joint United Nations Programme on HIV/AIDS (UNAIDS). UNODC advocates that evidence-informed, comprehensive, and large-scale interventions for IDUs be an integral part of national HIV/AIDS frameworks.

Key WHO Initiatives Related to Addiction Medicine

The WHO is the UN specialized agency on health. The WHO is a public health–focused organization. It is focused on the public health consequences of psychoactive substances, irrespective of their legal status.

1. *Global Burden of Disease (GBD) Study*: This WHO conducted study provided a better understanding of the impact of psychoactive substance use on population health. The GBD provided mortality estimates and estimates of disease burden expressed in Disability Adjusted Life Years (DALYs) lost. Tobacco, alcohol, and illicit drug use were among the leading preventable risk factors to health, responsible for 8.9% of the total disease burden if taken together.
2. *Prevention and Treatment of Tobacco Dependence*: The WHO advocates for the six most effective tobacco control policies: (a) raising taxes and prices, (b) banning advertising, (c) protecting people from secondhand smoke, (d) warning everyone about the dangers of tobacco, (e) offering help to people who want to quit, and (f) monitoring the epidemic and prevention policies.
3. *Prevention and Treatment of Alcohol and Other Drug Dependence*: The WHO sponsored the randomized controlled trial of screening and brief interventions for alcohol through the AUDIT instrument and later both alcohol and drug use implemented in the framework of the WHO ASSIST (Alcohol Screening and Substance Involvement Screening Test) project. The latter project was conducted in several countries, and demonstrated that screening for drug use and providing brief interventions was effective in reducing cannabis, opioid,

and stimulant use. The WHO has also been a strong advocate of the "addiction as a disease" approach to substance use disorders. The WHO asserts that substance dependence "is not a failure of will or of strength of character but a medical disorder that could affect any human being" and "a complex disorder with biological mechanisms affecting the brain and its capacity to control substance use." The public health relevance and importance of drug dependence treatment, including opioid agonist pharmacotherapy, is increasingly recognized by the WHO and others.

4. *Treatment Systems for Substance Use Disorders*: The WHO has indentified the following "priority areas" in treating substance use disorders and other mental health issues: (a) provision of treatment in primary health care; (b) making pharmacotherapy available; (c) providing care in the community; (d) educating the public; (e) involving communities, families, and consumers; (f) establishing national policies, programs, and legislation; (g) developing human resources; (h) linking with other sectors; (i) monitoring community mental health; and (j) supporting more research.

THE EVOLVING ROLE OF INTERNATIONAL MEDICAL ASSOCIATIONS

The founding of medical associations created opportunities for addressing issues of global concern by medical professionals. The WMA has several position statements in relation to the use of substances, and the WPA currently includes a Section of Addiction Psychiatry. The ISAM was founded in the late 1990s. Currently, the ISAM has a membership spanning 98 countries from all continents. The ISAM committed itself to advance the knowledge about addiction seen as a treatable disease, advocate for the major role physicians worldwide have to play in its management as well as enhance the credibility of their role, and, last, develop educational activities including consensus guidelines.

The Advocacy Role

International medical associations help bolster the perception of addiction as a treatable disease by disseminating information about empirically based treatment practices. International medical associations can also advocate for care providers as well as patients. The stigma associated with addiction often runs off on addiction care providers. Medical associations like ISAM can help battle the stigma that exists both in the general public and the medical profession.

International Dissemination of Information

ISAM has held meetings throughout the world in order to better disseminate information as well as to overcome the barriers of distance and travel costs and network with practitioners worldwide.

International Accreditation of Specialists

The development of a medical field with specialized expertise must be accompanied by an accreditation process. Since 2005, an International Certification in Addiction Medicine with an international editorial board has been held with applicants from six countries and 40 certificants so far (www.isamweb.org).

Reaching out to Colleagues from Developing Countries

ISAM has made a number of efforts to reach out to colleagues from Developing Countries including (a) a differential fee structure, (b) organizing meetings in different countries and continents, (c) maximizing electronic outreach, and (d) collaborating with the WHO and NIDA in providing fellowships to colleagues from developing nations.

Impact of Culture on Medical Practice

Policies addressing the use of various drugs including alcohol and tobacco vary from country to country. The management of opioid dependence may, arguably, arouse the most polarizing divide among national drug policies. The support or denial of the need for opioid maintenance therapy varies widely from country to country (and even from region to region within countries). Organizations like ISAM must strive to promote empirically based practices while at the same time accounting for local culture and economic resources.

CHAPTER

33

Summary Author: Thea Weisdorf
Martha J. Wunsch • Carol Boyd • Mary G. McMasters

Nonmedical Use of Prescription Medications

The rapid growth of inappropriate use of scheduled prescription medications presents serious public health concerns and unique medical and policy issues when compared with the abuse of illegal drugs such as heroin or cocaine. There has been a remarkable increase in the number of persons who report they are new abusers of scheduled prescription medications, most notable over the past 5 to 10 years. The four-scheduled drug classes most often involved are stimulants, sedative-hypnotics, sedative-anxiolytics, and opioid analgesic medications. This chapter presents an overview of what is known about the new phenomenon of nonmedical use of prescription medications (NUPM) and consequences such as poisoning and overdose deaths. Finally, this chapter will introduce some strategies for prevention when prescribing these medications and identification and management of individuals who are using these prescription medications in nonmedical ways.

DEFINITIONS

The National Institute on Drug Abuse (NIDA) defines abuse of prescription drugs as "any intentional use of a medication with intoxicating properties outside of a physician's prescription for a bona fide medical condition, excluding accidental misuse." Prescription drug abuse, according to NIDA, includes taking a medication prescribed for someone else, even if it is taken for an appropriate medical condition. The federal Drug Enforcement Administration's (DEA) definition of abuse is similar with an emphasis on the social inappropriateness of the act. Both the American Society of Addiction Medicine (ASAM) and the American Psychiatric Association (APA) use *DSM-IV TR* criteria to define abuse and addiction, emphasizing physical and psychosocial consequences but there is little emphasis addressing problematic or nonmedical uses of prescription medications.

Nonmedical Use of Prescription Medications

In this chapter, NUPM refers to the use of a scheduled, prescription medication without the prescribing clinician's knowledge. Examples of this include:

- Sharing or selling prescription with someone else
- Changing the amount or timing of the dosage without the prescribing physician's knowledge
- Using a medication prescribed for someone else including a friend or family member
- Snorting or injecting your own medication to achieve euphoria
- Procuring of scheduled medications via theft, duplicitous doctor shopping, or illegal drug dealing

PREVALENCE

All national studies over the past 15 years have shown an increase in reports of the NUPM. Prescription pain medication is the drug class most often used nonmedically among the general population.

NUPM: Prescription Opioids

The reported prevalence of NUPM, in the case of opioids, varies from almost none to nearly half of patients studied. This discrepancy is based on the validity of such reports, including a lack of agreement in the definitions, loosely defined behavioral criteria and results of urine toxicology tests. Among primary care patients, NUPM is reported to occur in one quarter to one third of patients. Among patients coming for addiction treatment, opioid addiction is reported to occur more often among women, individuals from rural areas, and among patients prescribed opioids for the treatment of chronic pain. Reviews of many studies have shown that rates of addiction, dependence, aberrant use of medication, abuse, misuse, and problematic opioid use vary widely, occurring up to 50% of the time. Reports show that extended-release and immediate-release oxycodone and hydrocodone were the most widely abused prescription opioids in the United States, and individuals who abused prescription opioids were more likely to live in rural, suburban, and small- to medium-sized urban areas.

NUPM: Benzodiazepine Medications

Much less is known about the prevalence and incidence of NUPM in this class of medications. Physicians should be aware that patients and non-patients use sedative hypnotics and tranquilizers for a variety of reasons. If there is non-medical use, patients are at higher risk for substance abuse and addiction to other medications and substances as well.

NONMEDICAL USE BETWEEN ADOLESCENT AND YOUNG ADULTS

NUPM is of particular concern among youth, especially given the understanding that earlier onset of alcohol, tobacco, and marijuana use is associated with development of substance abuse and addiction in adulthood.

Prevalence

Young adults suffer from the highest prevalence of NUPM, with an estimated 5% reporting such use of a scheduled pain medication in the past month. The National Survey on Drug Use and Health (NSDUH) 2006 reported prescription opioid analgesics surpassing marijuana as the most commonly used drug for new initiates each year.

The nonmedical use of stimulants appears to be most prevalent among young adults aged 18 to 25 (Fig. 33.1).

Motivation for Adolescent/Youth Adult Misuse

In one web-based survey of Midwestern 10- to 18-year-olds, youth endorsed many reasons for NUPM. These young people reported using stimulants to study, focus, and lose weight; pain medication to relieve pain; and

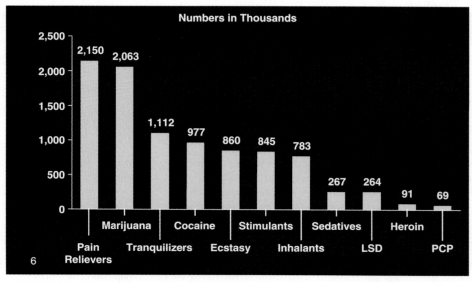

FIGURE 33.1 Past year initiates for specific illicit drugs among persons age 12 or older: 2006.

tranquilizers and sedative hypnotics for anxiety or as sleep aids. In other words, youth used these medications for the treatment of symptoms for which these medication were often prescribed.

Sources of Prescription Medications

Controlled prescription medications used nonmedically are most often obtained from friends and family. Other sources include doctor shopping, theft from pharmacies, online purchases, and stealing from friends or family members for whom they have been prescribed. Purchase from "street sources" was less common. Although most surveys report relatively little use of the Internet as a source for NUPM, there is a proliferation of prescription web sites that sell and ship primarily prescription Schedule IV and III medications. These sites change name and location often.

Methods of obtaining medication vary by age and gender. Younger students in middle and high school are more likely to get medication from family or friends. Male college student are more likely to obtain diverted medications from peers, but family members remain the source of sedative hypnotic, sleeping, and pain medications for college age women. Adolescents may take bottles of medications from their parents' medicine cabinets to parties to distribute for recreational use; a practice described as "pharming." In these settings, medications are often used in combination with over-the-counter medications, such as dextromethorphan and pseudoephedrine, and alcohol.

SOCIAL, LEGAL, AND MEDICAL CONSEQUENCES

Legal consequences of NUPM and diversion may include arrest for prescription forgery, theft, and trafficking of these medications for illegal purposes. The increase in NUPM has been accompanied by an increased number of deaths from overdose where these medications are identified on toxicology. Poisoning, which include overdoses involving illicit drugs, alcohol, and medications, is the leading cause of injury death for individuals' aged 35 to 44 years, and prescription opioid-related overdose deaths have increased at alarming rates in portions of the United States. At the same time that heroin poisonings increased by 12.4% from 1999 to 2002, the number of prescription opioid poisonings in the United States increased by 91.2%.

Methadone prescribed for analgesic use, often in tablet form, accounts for more inadvertent deaths than methadone prescribed for agonist maintenance treatment, usually dispensed in liquid form. In U.S. medical examiner cases when methadone was identified on toxicology, it was more likely to have been diverted from physician prescription than diverted from an opioid treatment program. Often, multiple prescription medications (opiates, benzodiazepines, antidepressants), illicit drugs, and alcohol are found on toxicology, making precise determination of the cause of death difficult. Attribution to suicide or unintentional death may also be difficult to ascertain.

STRATEGIES FOR IDENTIFICATION OF NUPM

Whether or not there is a diagnosis of abuse or addiction, patients prescribed medications and using nonmedically are not easily identified. Although many screening tools have been developed for use among chronic pain patients, there are no accepted and validated screening assessments to identify nonmedical use of other prescribed medications. Nonetheless, some of the strategies used to assess for problematic opioid use may be helpful in such scenarios.

Urine drug screens can be used to identify specific prescribed medications, thus differentiating the prescribed from nonprescribed and helping the physician identify NUPM. Universal precautions, as described by Heit and Gourlay, although not empirically validated for use other than with the patient prescribed opioids, may be used to identify and minimize NUPM. This is outlined in Table 33.1.

Prescription Monitoring Programs

In response to concerns about misuse, abuse, and diversion, and in an effort to assure continued access for patients to medications, state and federal governments have implemented systems to monitor the prescription and distribution of controlled substances. Prescription Monitoring Programs (PMPs), both computerized and noncomputerized, monitor prescribing practices of controlled substances in an attempt to decrease diversion of prescription medications. There are few studies evaluating the efficacy of specific state PMPs in decreasing NUPM.

Designed and directed by state agencies, the most common goals of these programs are education, delivery of information, execution of public health initiatives, early intervention and prevention of diversion, investigation and enforcement of abuse, and protection of confidentiality. The use of computer technology allows

TABLE 33.1	Universal Precautions

1. **Make a Diagnosis with Appropriate Differential**
   Identify any treatable causes for pain, where they exist, and direct therapy to the pain generator.
   Address any comorbid conditions, including substance use disorders and other psychiatric illness.

2. **Psychologic Assessment Including Risk of Addictive Disorders**
   Inquire about personal and family history of substance misuse.
   Discuss patient-centered urine drug testing with all patients regardless of what medications they are currently taking.
   Assess patients using illicit or unprescribed licit drugs and offer or refer for further assessment for possible substance use disorders.

3. **Informed Consent**
   Discuss with and answer any questions the patient may have about the proposed treatment plan including anticipated benefits and foreseeable risks.
   Explore specific issues of addiction, physical dependence, and tolerance at the patient's level of understanding.

4. **Treatment Agreement**
   Clarify expectations and obligations of both the patient and the treating practitioner either verbally or in writing.

5. **Preintervention and Postintervention Assessment of Pain Level and Function**
   Conduct an ongoing assessment after initiation of treatment and document success in meeting clinical goals to support the continuation of any mode of therapy.

6. **Appropriate Trial of Opioid Therapy: Adjunctive Medication**
   Assure that pharmacologic regimens are individualized and based on subjective, as well as objective, clinical findings.

7. **Reassessment of Pain Score and Level of Function**
   Assess the patient and use corroborative support from family or other knowledgeable third parties to help document continued therapy.

8. **Regularly Assess the "Four As" of Pain Medicine**
   Document how analgesia, activity, adverse effects, and aberrant behavior and affect to support pharmacologic options.

9. **Periodically Review Pain Diagnosis and Comorbid Conditions, including Addictive Disorders**
   Assess for evolution of underlying illnesses evolve and shift treatment focus as needed.

10. **Documentation**
    Carefully and completely record initial and follow-up evaluations to support the best interest of all parties.

Source: Created from Gourlay DL, Heit HA, Almahrezi A. Universal precautions in pain medicine: a rational approach to the treatment of chronic pain. *Pain Med.* 2005;6(2):107–112.

prescribing physicians access to the database immediately, sometimes while a patient is undergoing evaluation in the practitioner's office. The PMP is one mechanism the physician can use to decrease diversion by determining when a patient is receiving prescriptions from multiple providers. Additionally, the PMP can be utilized to check for appropriate use of other psychoactive prescribed medications.

ADDICTION TREATMENT: PRESCRIPTION MEDICATIONS

There are many circumstances under which concern arises about misuse, abuse of, or addiction to prescription medications. The addiction clinician must work tirelessly to design effective intervention or treatment plans. Concerning behaviors include using medications for euphoric effects, diversion of prescribed medications, concomitant use of alcohol, and marijuana or other illicit drugs, overtaking prescribed medication or combining medications. A patient may lose access to medications despite the fact that, in the patient's opinion, this nonmedical use was justified. They may not agree that use of alcohol or illicit drugs, in addition to their medications, is a problem. Some may obtain prescription medications illicitly because they no longer have a "legitimate prescription." Patients may engage in doctor shopping or may attempt to secure prescriptions from emergency rooms. Others will buy medications "on the street" or borrow or steal from family members or friends. A careful history, including information from family members and others who support the patients, should be combined with urine drug screens to formulate a diagnosis.

When there is an untreated diagnosis of addiction to either prescription or illicit drugs, it is difficult to effectively treat a chronic pain disorder with opioids, an anxiety disorder with benzodiazepines or an attention disorder with stimulants. Stabilization of the addiction diagnosis is essential, and in some cases includes the treatment of withdrawal.

Treatment for patients abusing or addicted to prescriptions medications varies little from the actual treatment for each corresponding drug class. Medication-assisted treatment with methadone or buprenorphine may be indicated in cases of opioid abuse or addiction; stabilization with a cross-tolerant long-acting medication, such as phenobarbital, or a long-acting benzodiazepine such as diazepam may be needed for benzodiazepine abuse or addiction. Those patients abusing or addicted to stimulants will benefit from strategies used in the treatment of the cocaine- or methamphetamine-addicted patient, including contingency management, peer support, and intensive counseling. As is common in addiction, the diagnoses of depression and anxiety often requires concurrent treatment. In summary, the treatment modalities employed for any patient with addiction should be employed in the patient abusing and addicted to prescription medications.

After addiction problems and psychiatric comorbid conditions are stabilized, these patients will require collaborative treatment with medical providers for the treatment of chronic pain, anxiety, depression, or attention disorders. Ideally, the clinical setting for treatment is one in which there is multidisciplinary collaboration between addiction medicine and other clinicians, all of whom aware of the potential for misuse, abuse, and diversion of controlled substances.

SUMMARY

In summary, nonmedical use of prescription medications, including misuse, abuse, diversion, and addiction, is increasing in the United States. Prescribers should use a consistent and nondiscriminatory approach with patients prescribed medications with potential for abuse, with the understanding that identification of patients at risk can be difficult. The use of precautions, clear documentation, and utilization of state PMPs may be helpful to the clinician. When concern about misuse, abuse, and addiction occurs, physicians must determine the circumstances that have led to the problematic use of a prescribed medication. When indicated, treatment of NUPM should balance medical considerations of comorbid conditions with abuse and addiction. Patients abusing prescription medication will need treatment for withdrawal, stabilization, treatment of addiction, and reassessment of the contributing medical conditions that necessitated prescription of controlled medications.

34

Summary Author: Thea Weisdorf
Joan E. Zweben

Special Issues in Treatment: Women

Within the past decade, treatment providers have devoted increasing attention to defining and addressing the unique needs of women. This chapter discusses treatment issues specific to women, including the relationship of drug and alcohol use problems to psychiatric and medical conditions, and reviews new findings on gender-specific treatment.

EPIDEMIOLOGY

Gender Differences in Alcohol and Other Drug Use

Several large-scale epidemiologic studies document gender differences in the use of alcohol and almost all other drugs, with higher rates found in men. However, more recent studies are showing a smaller gender difference for all age groups except adolescents aged 12 to 17. With these young people, the gap virtually disappeared for alcohol, marijuana, cocaine, and cigarettes. Stimulants such as cocaine and methamphetamine have a particular appeal for women. Their use is associated with loss of appetite and desirable weight loss, and the stimulating effects are often initially perceived as alerting and beneficial with the many work and household tasks that confront them.

Common Psychiatric Disorders in Women with Addictive Disorders

Most adults in treatment for addictive disorders have at least one coexisting psychiatric disorder, but the pattern differs for women. Prominent studies have found that women were more likely to have an affective disorder than men (with the exception of mania, for which rates were the same). One study showed lifetime prevalence for a major depressive episode of 21.3% and a 12-month prevalence of 12.9% for women, compared with 12.7% and 7.7% for men. Women also had a higher lifetime and 12-month prevalence of three or more disorders.

MEDICAL CONSIDERATIONS

Alcohol

The influence of alcohol on women's health has been much more carefully studied than other drugs. Although women are less likely than men to drink heavily or even moderately, when they do so, they are more vulnerable to alcohol-related liver damage, cardiovascular disease, and brain damage. One study following a large number of adults over 12 years found that women developed alcohol-related liver disease at approximately half the consumption levels of men. Negative consequences occur at lower levels of consumption and after much shorter periods of drinking. This is referred to as the "telescoped course" in women.

Researchers have explored the mechanisms by which women achieve higher blood alcohol concentrations than men after drinking equivalent amounts of alcohol, even when doses are adjusted for body weight. Women tend to have lower levels of alcohol dehydrogenase and lower volumes of distribution, leading to an increased effect of alcohol from an equivalent exposure in a man. The relationship between drinking and breast cancer risk has been also studied since the 1980s. Alcohol consumption raises breast cancer risk even after adjustment for age, family history, and other known dietary and reproductive risk factors. The increased risk appears to be modest and dose related, and the form of alcohol appears to be irrelevant.

Prenatal Alcohol Exposure

Drinking during pregnancy remains a serious concern. Fetal alcohol syndrome (FAS) is a set of birth defects considered the single leading nonhereditary cause of mental retardation. The growth deficiency and characteristic set of facial traits tend to become more normal over time, but the alcohol-induced damage to the developing brain is enduring. These mental impairments include deficits in general intellectual functioning and specific difficulties with learning, memory, attention, and problem solving, in addition to manifestations in psychosocial arenas. The impairments are dose related and may be evident in children without the distinguishing physical features of FAS. Several terms have been developed to describe alcohol-related conditions including *alcohol-related birth defects* (referring to alcohol-related physical abnormalities of the skeleton and certain organ systems) that occur in the absence of the characteristic growth deficiency and facial characteristics of FAS and *alcohol-related neurodevelopmental disorder*, referring to the mental impairments in the absence of FAS. The effects of lower levels of alcohol exposure prenatally are still unclear and thus the prevailing belief that there is no demonstrated safe level of alcohol consumption during pregnancy.

Drugs

The evidence of gender differences in the effects of drug use is not as extensive at this time as it is for alcohol. Several studies suggest that some women may have greater vulnerability to the effects of cocaine relative to men. Mechanisms including female steroid hormones, estrogen, menstrual cycle phase, and differences in receptor function have all been suggested.

Methadone is considered the gold standard maintenance treatment for opioid-dependent pregnant women. It is important that the dose be adequate. Higher doses are not associated with increased risks of neonatal abstinence. Likewise, women who are stable on methadone should not be discouraged from breastfeeding.

Buprenorphine is not currently approved by the U.S. Food and Drug Administration for use in pregnancy. It, along with methadone, is category C in pregnancy. The Maternal Opioid Treatment Human Experimental Research project is a double-blind, double-dummy, flexible-dosing, parallel-group clinical trial. It seeks to develop guidelines based on risk-benefit ratios. It is important to use buprenorphine alone rather than in combination with naloxone so that there is no prenatal exposure to naloxone. Buprenorphine does provide the potential option to expand treatment access in rural areas and other circumstances where methadone is unavailable or unacceptable to the pregnant patient. The overall goal is to reduce early treatment dropout in pregnant women, as it is well known that participation in treatment is associated with better maternal and neonatal outcomes.

Domestic Violence

A large number of women are treated in hospital emergency departments for violence-related injuries, usually inflicted by an intimate partner. Women who have been battered report that their general health is fair or poor and that they have needed medical care that they have not received. Chronic headaches, hearing, vision, and concentration problems can reflect neurologic damage, and a host of other stress-related symptoms can manifest. Therefore, psychosocial treatment efforts must integrate good medical care to be fully comprehensive.

HIV/AIDS

Women are compromising a larger proportion of AIDS cases than ever before, with 27% of new AIDS cases in girls and women over the age of 13 reported in 2005 (compared to <5% in 1985). HIV/AIDS is the leading cause of death for African American women aged 25 to 34. Heterosexual sex with a man with HIV is the most common mode of transmission, followed by sharing injection drug works used by someone with HIV. Similar patterns of increase are also beginning to be apparent in the distribution of reported hepatitis C cases. The condom remains the major method to reduce sexual transmission of HIV; however, women are not always in a position of power to insist that the condom be worn. Addicted women are at an additional disadvantage in attempting to practice safer sex. These women may also fear emotional or physical abuse if they insist on safe sex.

For the HIV-infected women, managing caretaking responsibilities often is an issue added to the physical and psychiatric burdens of the disease. They struggle with how to address their health issues and their possible deaths with their children. Women who have given birth to HIV-positive children have an added layer of anxiety and guilt. All of these women require as much support and counseling as possible.

PSYCHIATRIC DISORDERS

The need for treatment interventions that are sensitive to gender differences has brought increasing attention to co-occurring disorders and their effects on addicted women. It is preferable to address multiple disorders with an integrated approach. It has become more widely accepted in the addiction treatment community that psychotropic medications are compatible with recovery, especially when prescribed by physicians knowledgeable about addiction. In this section, we review the most common psychiatric disorders found in women with substance abuse problems; anxiety disorders (especially posttraumatic stress disorder [PTSD]), mood disorders, eating disorders, and borderline personality disorders.

Anxiety Disorders

As a group, anxiety disorders constitute the most common psychiatric disorders among women, with a total lifetime prevalence of 30.5% and a 12-month prevalence of 22.6%. The experience of anxiety is characterized by sensations of nervousness, tension, apprehension, and the fear that arises from the anticipation of internal or external danger. These feelings constitute important survival signals, so the task is to distinguish what is normal and appropriate from states that require intervention. Women in early recovery will experience heightened distress as they try to cope with situations on which they previously relied on alcohol and other drugs, and also as they more clearly see the impact of their self-destructive behaviors. However, overwhelming anxiety is debilitating, it interferes with new learning, and it contributes to relapse. Psychosocial strategies are beneficial for the management of anxiety regardless of whether it is normal or excessive. Fortunately, the first-line medications for anxiety and panic disorders are no longer the benzodiazepines, but the selective serotonin reuptake inhibitors. When anxiety symptoms do not resolve with abstinence, a variety of psychosocial interventions can be used, selected to address the tasks specific to the woman's stage of recovery.

Benzodiazepines, commonly prescribed for anxiety disorders, can be problematic for those with a personal or family history of addiction. Nonreinforcing alternatives, such as sedating antidepressants or buspirone (BuSpar) for anxiety or trazodone (Desyrel) for insomnia, are recommended. Anticonvulsants, antihypertensives, or the newer atypical neuroleptic medications can also be used.

Of all the anxiety disorders, PTSD is the most difficult and complex to manage. The relationship between female gender and PTSD is robust across patient populations. Rape and sexual molestation were the most frequently reported "most upsetting event" with childhood parental neglect and childhood physical abuse reported more frequently by women. A lifetime history of at least one other disorder was present in 79% of women with PTSD, and more than one third of the women with PTSD failed to recover from their PTSD. Participants in addiction treatment have much higher rates of traumatic experiences and PTSD than the general population. Treatment providers must equip themselves to meet these complex needs so as to avoid common outcomes such as early dropout, and increased difficulty in obtaining positive outcomes from treatment.

Mood Disorders

In assessing for depression, it is important to rule out the direct effects of alcohol, illicit drugs, or medications, as well as general medical conditions, such as hypothyroidism, that can lower mood. This is especially true in the identification of mood disorders in pregnant women, as these women tend to do worse on drug use outcomes than with other disorders.

Negative mood states that are the direct result of alcohol or illicit drugs generally clear within 2 to 3 weeks, with symptoms of longer duration suggesting an independent mood disorder. A sad or depressed mood is only one of many signs and symptoms of a clinically significant depression and may not be the most prominent feature. Other indications include disturbances in emotional, cognitive, behavioral, or somatic regulations. The mood disturbance itself can include apathy, anxiety, or irritability along with, or instead of, sadness. Not all clinically depressed patients feel sad, and many who feel sad are not clinically depressed. Women may have a markedly reduced interest in, or capacity for pleasure or enjoyment, making it difficult for them to experience rewards in recovery or to invest in new social relationships with others who do not drink or use drugs.

Eating Disorders

Eating disorders are more prevalent among substance-abusing women than in the general population, with bulimia being more common than anorexia. Stimulants and over-the-counter diet preparations are particularly appealing to women seeking to lose or control weight.

There are many possible relationships between substance use and eating disorders. Some patients report that heroin is appealing because it facilitates vomiting. Stimulants are attractive because they make women feel capable, energetic, and suppress the appetite. Alcohol can be used to suppress the panic associated with bingeing and vomiting or to quash the shame that follows an episode.

Because secrecy is a feature of both disorders, careful inquiry is important during the initial assessment, and observation by staff members in necessary throughout treatment. A thorough medical evaluation should assess possible problems and be part of a plan for nutritional stabilization, including strategies to stop aberrant eating behaviors, as well as medication planning and discharge planning that actively addresses both disorders. Selective serotonin reuptake inhibitors have been shown to be beneficial in treating bulimia, but not restrictive anorexia. Both cognitive-behavioral approaches and psychotherapy are well supported by evidence to assist in the management of eating disorders.

Borderline Personality Disorder

Misdiagnosis of borderline personality disorder is quite common, because of confusion of borderline characteristics with the behaviors exhibited during active alcohol and drug use and early recovery. An accurate diagnosis is crucial because borderline patients are viewed in many settings as difficult and unrewarding to treat.

Persistent characteristics of borderline personality disorder include unstable mood and self-image, unstable, intense, interpersonal relationships; extremes of overidealization and devaluation, and marked shifts from baseline to impulsive outbursts, anxiety states, or other extreme moods. Women constitute about 75% of those with the diagnosis, which is estimated at 2% of the general population. Literature strongly suggests a relationship between borderline pathology and childhood physical and sexual abuse. Histories of childhood sexual abuse and a family history of substance use disorder are associated with longer time to remission of borderline personality disorder.

In summary, the prevalence of co-occurring disorders in women underlines the importance of offering psychiatric services. In addition to education about addiction, programs should include material on co-occurring mental health disorders and how they can influence relapse and recovery.

According to the large National Epidemiologic Survey on Alcohol and Related Conditions, women are also at greater risk of avoidant, dependent, and paranoid personality disorders. Little focus on specific treatment interventions for this group of women has been undertaken.

SPECIAL POPULATIONS

Variations in cultural groups and sexual orientation play important roles in addiction treatment. The use of alcohol and other drugs may be taboo for women, so recognition of their use or seeking treatment may be impossible. Those from patriarchal cultures can face strong taboos about disclosing family secrets especially around interpersonal violence. Many women also fear institutions such as the police, social services, and mental health agencies. Much more work in the area of cultural sensitivity, education, and prevention need to be done to make an impact on these women's lives.

Lesbians are another subgroup of women at particular risk. This is, in part, because of the supposed extensive use of alcohol and drugs as part of the culture. Historically, gay bars were seen as gathering places and safe arenas for self-expression. Clearly, socializing patterns built around bars and drug sharing increase the risk of addiction. Even when problems are recognized, gay women can avoid treatment if they fear discrimination.

ADDITIONAL TREATMENT ISSUES

Women tend to seek help in medical or mental health settings, aiding in the improvement in the diagnosis and treatment of women with substance abuse disorders. Barriers clearly exist, including lack of pregnancy services, lack of childcare, fears of loss of custody, and inadequate services for women with co-occurring disorders. Treatment retention has been shown to improve with inclusion of children in residential treatment and other key factors.

Management and Retention Issues

The finding that women have high rates of three or more disorders has consequences for treatment. Work by Brown and colleagues supports the hypothesis that the most immediate or threatening problems will be what a woman focuses on first, and she selects her treatment modalities accordingly. Thus, women with addictive disorders who are in domestic violence situations are relatively resistant to addressing their alcohol and drug use. They are preoccupied with achieving greater safety and see their alcohol and other drug problems as secondary. Treatment providers need to be willing to start by addressing those problems the woman is most ready to change while cultivating readiness in other areas.

It is generally agreed by providers that women-only programs or activities are an important aspect of effective treatment, particularly those associated with pregnancy and parenting. Women-only programs also were more likely to assist with housing transportation, job training, and practical skills training. These programs also were more likely to be funded through the Medicaid system instead of fees or private insurance.

It appears that gender-specific treatment is also associated with higher rates of continuing care. There is also reason to think that women-only groups tend to foster greater interaction, emotional and behavioral expression and more variability in style than mixed-gender groups.

Physical and Sexual Abuse and Domestic Violence

Co-occurring psychopathology typically is associated with less favorable addiction treatment outcomes. Yet abused clients were more likely than their nonabused counterparts to participate in counseling and just as likely to complete treatment and remain drug-free during and up to 6 months after treatment.

Trauma-related difficulties can impair parenting in a variety of ways. Women with histories of childhood trauma can have attachment problems that impact their own parenting. They often lack appropriate role models, leading to reliance on physical punishment, difficulties setting appropriate boundaries, and neglect. Current alcohol and other drug use will exacerbate these vulnerabilities.

It has been noted that children with battered mothers experience posttraumatic stress reactions themselves. Preschool children are more vulnerable to the effects of domestic violence than older children. The extensive variety and complexity of children's reactions to domestic violence argues for routine assessment and case management for these families.

Treatment Culture

Women clients and treatment providers have noted that the male-dominated treatment culture characteristic of some programs is not conducive to meeting women's needs. An emphasis on harsh confrontation is particularly problematic in populations with a high frequency of traumatic experiences. Women with severe psychiatric disorders can decompensate and leave treatment if confrontation is too intense.

Both the National Institute on Drug Abuse and the Center for Substance Abuse Treatment have funded specialized research and treatment demonstration programs focused on women, and these programs have enhanced the development of provider groups committed to improving women's treatment. Provider groups serving women also emphasize the importance of female leadership at all levels to serve as role models.

Women and the Criminal Justice System

Women constitute the fastest-growing segment of the criminal justice population nationally and yet have the fewest appropriate social services available to them. Women today are more likely than men to serve time in prison for drug offenses. Half the women reported committing their crimes while under the influence of drugs or alcohol, and about 40% reported using drugs daily before arrest. Incarcerated women were overwhelmingly confronted with obstacles such as absent parents, poor education, poverty, drug accessibility, and minimal social resources. Additionally, many were victims of childhood sexual or physical abuse and traumatic experiences as adults. They had high rates of depression and other psychiatric disorders, as well as suffering from low self-esteem, addiction, and shame. Many women's situations made it difficult to reduce the risk of HIV infection. One study found HIV infection rates of 7.5% in incarcerated women, several times higher than found in the community.

One third of incarcerated women reported that a parent or guardian had abused drugs or alcohol. Prison-based treatment is growing rapidly, and specialized programs for women are integral to this. Community-based services after treatment in prison significantly increase the percentage of offenders who remain drug free 18 months after release. Drug courts and diversion initiatives have also shown success in reducing recidivism, likely in proportion to their access to psychiatric and social services.

CONCLUSIONS

Biomedical effects of gender differences are far better understood for alcohol than for the illicit drugs. Research and treatment funding incentives over the past 20 years have provided a much better understanding of women's treatment needs and preferences. Removing barriers, such as lack of transportation and childcare services, increase women's participation in treatment. Treatment for women must be comprehensive. Attention to the children's physical, social and emotional is necessary to reduce the negative effects of their parents' addictive disorders. Programs need to be capable of addressing co-occurring mood and anxiety disorders. Finally, women report that women-only groups and other activities and role models at all levels of decision-making are important to them.

CHAPTER **35**

Summary Author: Thea Weisdorf
Fred C. Blow • Kristen L. Barry

Treatment of Older Adults

Many of the medical and psychiatric disorders experienced in aging are influenced by lifestyle choices and behaviors such as the consumption of alcohol and use/misuse of medications/drug. Older adults are more vulnerable to the effects of alcohol and medications. They may seek health care for a variety of conditions that are not immediately associated with increased alcohol consumption and medication use/misuse. These include greater risk for harmful drug interactions, injury, depression, memory problems, liver disease, cardiovascular disease, cognitive changes, and sleep problems. Therefore, systemic screening, brief interventions, and referrals to appropriate treatments for problems related to alcohol and prescription drug use are particularly relevant to providing high-quality health care to this population. At-risk and problem drinking are the largest classes of substance use problems seen in older adults. However, with the aging of the "Baby Boom" generation, with the leading edge at age 62, it is anticipated that clinicians will see a greater use of illicit drugs. Of note is the 45 to 64 year age group who had somewhat higher rates of nonmedical prescription drug abuse than today's elderly (National Epidemiologic Survey on Alcohol and Related Conditions).

SCOPE OF THE PROBLEM IN OLDER ADULTHOOD

Little attention has been paid to the intersection of the fields of gerontology/geriatrics and alcohol studies. Specific treatment and intervention strategies for older adults who are alcohol dependent or hazardous drinkers are only beginning to be disseminated.

The prevalence estimates of problem drinking in older adults have ranged from 1% to 15%. These rates vary widely because of differing definitions and sample methodologies. Older adults are at higher risk for inappropriate use of medications than younger groups. Combined difficulties with alcohol and medication misuse may affect up to 19% of older Americans. Factors such as previous or coexisting drug, alcohol, or mental health problems, old age, and being female also increase vulnerability for misusing prescribed medications. Despite the high prevalence of alcohol problems, most elderly patients with alcohol problems go unidentified by health care personnel. Signs and symptoms of potential problems related to alcohol use in older adults are shown in Table 35.1.

Most research conducted on substance use and misuse in older adults has focused on drinking and alcohol abuse. The rates of illegal drug abuse in the current elderly cohort are thought to be very low. The potential for abuse of psychoactive drugs is a growing concern with midlife and older adults. Nicotine dependence remains prevalent across age groups including older adults.

Substance Abuse/Dependence Diagnostic Classification for Older Adults

There are concerns that the *DSM-IV* criteria for classifying alcohol-related problems may not apply to older adults with substance use problems because older adults may not experience some of the legal, social, or psychological consequences specified in the criteria and often seen in younger adults with abuse/dependence. Additionally, increased sensitivity to alcohol in the elderly can make it difficult to assess for "tolerance." The criteria related to physical and emotional consequences of alcohol use may be especially important. See Table 35.2.

Issues Unique to Older Adults

In addressing alcohol problems or prescription medication misuse in later life, the use of nonjudgmental, motivational approaches can be a key to successfully engaging these patients in care. Because of historical and cultural factors that lead to stigma, older adults who drink at risk levels can find it particularly difficult to identify their

TABLE 35.1	Signs and Symptoms of Potential Alcohol Problems in Older Adults: Time to Ask Questions	
Mental/cognitive/relationship changes	**Physical health**	**Alcohol and medication**
Anxiety	Poor hygiene	Increased alcohol tolerance
Depression	Falls, bruises	Unusual medication response
Social isolation	Poor nutrition	
Excessive mood swings	Incontinence	
Disorientation	Sleep problems	
Memory loss		
New decision-making problems		
Idiopathic seizures		

Adapted from Barry KL, Oslin D, Blow FC. *Alcohol problems in older adults: prevention and management.* New York, NY: Springer Publishing; 2001.

own risky drinking. In working with patients who do not recognize that their level of alcohol consumption can lead to problems, brief education regarding changes in metabolism with aging, the interactions between alcohol and specific medications (e.g., sedatives), the potential for falls and the relationship between alcohol and some medical problems (e.g., hypertension) can be helpful.

Co-occurring Disorders in Older Adulthood

Rates of psychiatric illness in older adults with substance use disorders range from 21% to 66%. Depression and co-occurring risk drinking in older adults are associated with increased suicidality and greater inpatient and outpatient service utilization. In addition, illnesses, bereavement, job loss, and retirement can all be issues that can affect depressed feelings and alcohol use in this age group.

Most older adults who are experiencing problems related to their alcohol consumption do not meet *DSM-IV* criteria for alcohol abuse or dependence. However, drinking even small amounts of alcohol can increase risks

TABLE 35.2	Substance Abuse/Dependence Criteria Considerations in Diagnosing Older Adults

1. Tolerance: older adults may have problems with even low levels of intake because of their increased sensitivity to alcohol and higher blood alcohol levels.
2. Withdrawal: many adults with late-onset alcohol use disorders do not develop symptoms of physiologic dependence.
3. Taking larger amounts or over a longer period: self-monitoring is more difficult with increased cognitive impairment and that can interfere with an individual's ability to recall if he or she is drinking more than was intended.
4. Unsuccessful efforts to cut down or control use: this issue is similar for individuals across the lifespan.
5. Spending much time to obtain and use alcohol: because the negative consequences of alcohol can occur at relatively low levels, older adults may not report this behavior.
6. Giving up activities because of use: older adult may decrease their activity level for a variety of reasons making detection of problems by others more difficult.
7. Continuing use despite physical or psychologic problems: some older adults may not know or understand that some of the problems they are experiencing can be related to their use of alcohol or drugs/medications.

Modified from Barry KL, Oslin D, Blow FC. *Alcohol problems in older adults: prevention and management.* New York, NY: Springer Publishing; 2001; Blow FC. *Substance abuse among older adults.* Rockville, MD: U.S. Department of Health and Human Services, Public Health Service, Substance Abuse and Mental Health Services Administration, Center for Substance Abuse Treatment; Treatment Improvement Protocol (TIP) Series; 1998.

for developing problems in older adults, particularly when coupled with the use of some OTC or prescription medications.

At-risk and problem drinking among the elderly is likely to exacerbate existing depressive disorders. Drinking, leading to a major depressive disorder may aggravate Subsyndromal depression. Depressed alcohol-dependent patients have been shown to have a more complicated clinical course of depression with an increased risk of suicide and more social dysfunction than nondepressed alcoholics. Moreover, they were shown to seek treatment more often. Relapse rates for those who were alcohol dependent, however, did not appear to be influenced by the presence of depression.

Alcohol Use Guidelines for Older Adults

The National Institute on Alcohol Abuse and Alcoholism (NIAAA) and the CSAT Treatment Improvement Protocol on older adults recommend that persons, male or female, aged 65 and older consume no more than one standard drink per day or seven standard drinks per week. In addition, older adults should consume no more than four standard drinks on any drinking day. These drinking limit recommendations are consistent with data regarding the relationship between heavy consumption and alcohol-related problems within this age group. These recommendations are also consistent with the current evidence for a beneficial health effect of low-risk drinking.

Screening and Detection of Alcohol Problems in Older Adults

Screening can be done as part of routine mental and physical health care and updated annually, before the older adult begins taking any new medications, or in response to problems that may be alcohol- or medication related. OTC use often remains unevaluated in clinical settings and the use of some OTC preparations can be problematic with alcohol or prescription medication.

Screening for alcohol-related problems is not always standardized and not all standardized instruments have good reliability and validity with older adults. The four widely used screening instruments in older adults are the Michigan Alcoholism Screening Test-Geriatric (MAST-G) and the shortened version, the SMAST-G, the CAGE, and the Alcohol Use Disorders Identification Test (AUDIT). The MAST-G and the SMAST-G were developed specifically for older adults.

The MAST-G is a 24-item scale with good sensitivity and specificity in older adults. The SMAST-G is a validated shortened form containing 10 items (Table 35.3).

TABLE 35.3 Short Michigan Alcoholism Screening Test—Geriatric Version (SMAST-G)	YES (1)	NO (0)
1. When talking with others, do you ever underestimate how much you actually drink?	_____	_____
2. After a few drinks, have you sometimes not eaten or been able to skip a meal because you did not feel hungry?	_____	_____
3. Does having a few drinks help decrease your shakiness or tremors?	_____	_____
4. Does alcohol sometimes make it hard for you to remember parts of the day or night?	_____	_____
5. Do you usually take a drink to relax or calm your nerves?	_____	_____
6. Do you drink to take your mind off your problems?	_____	_____
7. Have you ever increased your drinking after experiencing a loss in your life?	_____	_____
8. Has a doctor or nurse ever said they were worried or concerned about your drinking?	_____	_____
9. Have you ever made rules to manage your drinking?	_____	_____
10. When you feel lonely, does having a drink help?	_____	_____
TOTAL S-MAST-G SCORE (0–10)	_____	

Scoring: 2 or more "yes" responses indicative of alcohol problem.
For further information, contact Frederic C. Blow, PhD, at the University of Michigan Department of Psychiatry, 4250 Plymouth Road, Box 5765, Ann Arbor, MI 48109; (734) 761-2210.
©The Regents of the University of Michigan, 1991.

TABLE 35.4	**Alcohol Use Disorders Identification Test-C Alcohol Screening**	
1. How often did you have a drink containing alcohol in the past year?		
• Never		(0 points)
If you answered "never," score questions 2 and 3 as zero.		
• Monthly or less		(1 point)
• Two to four times per month		(2 points)
• Two to three times per week		(3 points)
• Four or more times a week		(4 points)
How many drinks did you have on a typical day when you were drinking in the past year?		
• 1 or 2		(0 points)
• 3 or 4		(1 point)
• 5 or 6		(2 points)
• 7–9		(3 points)
• 10 or more		(4 points)
How often did you have six or more drinks on one occasion in the past year?		
• Never		(0 points)
• Less than monthly		(1 point)
• Monthly		(2 points)
• Weekly		(3 points)
• Daily or almost daily		(4 points)

The Alcohol Use Disorders Identification Test-C is scored on a scale of 0–12 (scores of 0 reflect no alcohol use). A score of 3 or more in older adults is considered positive and suggests the need for further evaluation. Generally, the higher the AUDIT-C score, the more likely it is that the patient's drinking is affecting his/her health and safety Dawson DA, Grant BF, Stinson FS, et al. Effectiveness of the derived Alcohol Use Disorders Identification Test (AUDIT-C) in screening for alcohol use disorders and risk drinking in the US general population. *Alcohol Clin Exp Res.* 2005;29(5):844–854.

The CAGE questionnaire contains four items regarding alcohol use: **C**ut down, **A**nnoyed, **G**uilty, and **E**ye-Opener (see previous sections on Alcohol Screening). Two positive responses are considered a positive screen and indicate that further assessment is warranted. The sensitivity and specificity of the CAGE varies but is less sensitive with older adults (see Table 35.4). As an example, older adults rarely need a drink upon wakening (eye-opener) or they may consume alcohol at a level they used when younger and not believe they need to cut down.

The AUDIT is well validated in adults under 65 in primary care settings and has had initial validation in a study of older adults. A copy of this tool can be found at: *http://www.niaaa.nih.gov/NR/rdonlyres/287137A9-62BF-4EDE-A752-4A351C57A0B8/0/Audit.pdf.* The AUDIT-C (the first three questions: quantity, frequency, binge) had psychometric properties similar to the full AUDIT.

BROAD-BASED ASSESSMENT OF SUBSTANCE USE PROBLEMS

To assess dependence, questions should be asked about alcohol or drug-related problems, a history of failed attempts to stop or cut back, or withdrawal symptoms such as tremors. Medication assessments include questions about prescriptions, particularly antidepressants, benzodiazepines, opioid pain medications, OTC medications, and herbal remedies. For older adults with positive screens, assessments are needed to confirm the problem, to characterize the dimensions of the problem, and to develop individualized treatment plans. The application of the *DSM* criteria can be difficult in older adult populations because the symptoms of other medical diseases and psychiatric disorders overlap to a considerable extent with substance use–related disorders.

Substance Abuse Assessment Instruments

The use of validated substance abuse assessment instruments can be of great help to clinicians. Structured assessment interviews possess the desired qualities of quantifiability, reliability, validity, standardization, and recordability.

Two structured assessment instruments have been developed: the Structured Clinical Interview for *DSM-III-R* (SCID) and the Diagnostic Interview Schedule (DIS) for *DSM-IV*. The SCID takes approximately

30 minutes to administer the 35 questions that probe for alcohol abuse or dependence. The DIS is a highly structured interview that can be used by nonclinicians and assesses both current and past symptoms and is available in a computerized version. The DIS is generally used for research rather than for clinical administration.

BRIEF ALCOHOL INTERVENTIONS WITH OLDER ADULTS

The majority of clinical trials have shown the efficacy of brief alcohol interventions as an initial approach to at-risk and problem drinkers in primary care settings. Brief interventions are characterized by five or fewer sessions of durations of a few minutes to an hour. Brief interventions can often motivate patients to seek and engage in additional treatment as needed. It can provide immediate attention to individuals at risk and prevent or minimize potential consequences in a cost-effective, efficient way.

Effectiveness of Brief Alcohol Interventions with Older At-Risk Drinkers

There had been little attention given to brief intervention research in older adults until recently. Two recent randomized clinical brief intervention trials have shown that older adults can be engaged in brief intervention protocols; that the protocols are acceptable in this population, and there is a substantial reduction in drinking among the at-risk drinkers receiving the interventions compared with a control group.

BRIEF INTERVENTION CONTENT AND STEPS

The important aspects of brief interventions include screening, feedback on behavior, motivation to change, strategies for change, a behavioral agreement, and follow-up to determine if more intensive steps are needed. The following steps are often included in a brief intervention for older adults:

1. Identifying future goals—this helps to set the context for the BI and provides increased motivation for change.
2. Customizing feedback in the form of a health profile on screening questions relating to drinking patterns and other health habits.
3. Introducing the concept of standard drinks and alcohol content of various beverages.
4. Discussing the types of drinkers and where the patient's drinking pattern fits into the population norms for their age group.
5. Reasons for drinking, weighing the pros and cons of drinking, and reasons to cut down or quit drinking.
6. Considering changing quitting or cutting down on drinking. Maintaining independence, physical health, and mental capacity can be key motivators in this age group.
7. Sensible drinking limits and strategies for cutting down on drinking. Strategies that are useful in this age group include developing social opportunities that do not involve alcohol, pursuing hobbies and interests from earlier in life, etc.
8. Drinking agreement. Negotiated drinking limits that are signed by the patient and the intervener.
9. Coping with risky situations. Social isolation, boredom, and negative family interactions can present special problems in this age group.
10. Summarizing the session.

Brief interventions generally include some educational information on the adverse effects of alcohol in older adults and the warning signs of alcohol problems and impairments.

SBIRT Model

SBIRT (Screening, Brief Intervention, Referral to Treatment) is a comprehensive model for addressing alcohol and drug use in medical settings. It employs the results of randomized clinical trials and best evidence-based practices to provide a framework for early detection, focused motivational enhancement, and targeted encouragement to seek needed substance abuse treatment. It can be applied to both younger and older adults. The model has been tested and incorporated most often into emergency care settings but has been expanded to primary care.

FORMAL SUBSTANCE ABUSE TREATMENT IN OLDER ADULTHOOD

There have been few systematic studies of formal alcoholism treatment outcome for older adults. Because traditional residential alcoholism treatment programs provide services to very few older individuals, sample sizes for treatment outcome studies have often been inadequate.

Pharmacologic treatments are seldom used in the long-term treatment of older alcohol-dependent adults. Until recently, disulfiram was the only medication approved by the U.S. FDA for treating alcohol dependence, and it was seldom used for older adults because of concerns regarding potential side effects. In multicenter, double-blind, placebo-controlled evaluation of veterans, naltrexone, an opioid antagonist was found to have no significant differences in percentage of days drinking and drinks per day at 52-week follow-up. Another 12-week double-blind, placebo-controlled trial study showed no significant differences between the groups in abstinence, but half as many subjects in the treatment group lapsed into significant drinking compared to the control group.

There are no studies to date of the efficacy or safety of acamprosate, another promising agent in the treatment of alcohol dependence, in older adults.

Psychosocial Interventions with Older Adults

It is not surprising that older adults seem to do best in programs that offer age-appropriate care with providers who are knowledgeable about aging issues. Most of the treatment outcome research on older adults with substance use disorders has focused on compliance with treatment program expectations. These results have shown that age-specific programming improved treatment completion and resulted in higher rates of attendance at group meetings compared to mixed age treatment.

Age of onset of alcohol problems has been a major focus of research for elderly treatment compliance studies. Those classified as late onset problem drinkers were significantly more likely to complete treatment. Some studies have shown that drinking relapses during treatment were unrelated to age of onset and that onset age did not contribute to variance in program completion, but was related to meeting attendance rate. One study suggested that elderly alcoholics might respond better to individual-focused interventions rather than traditional mixed-age, group-oriented treatment.

Limitations of Treatment Outcome Research

Existing studies have an inherent selectivity bias and provide no information on treatment dropouts or on short- or long-term treatment outcomes, as they focus mainly on factors related to completion of a program. Issues such as sampling (studies involve mainly male subjects), age cut-offs (vary widely in different studies), and the use of relatively unstructured techniques for assessing alcohol-related symptoms and consequences can limit the generalizability of previous studies. Furthermore, most studies have not addressed other relevant domains that may be positively affected by treatment, such as physical and mental health status, and psychologic distress.

Relapse Prevention

Psychologic factors such as social isolation, loneliness, loss and grief, and depression can become antecedents to alcohol use and relapse for older adults. Older adults report using alcohol to alleviate negative emotional states. Comorbid medical conditions such as pain also put older adults at higher risk for relapse.

A Group Treatment Approach to Substance Abuse Relapse Prevention

Relapse prevention requires planning for the potential psychosocial and physical health factors that place them at risk for relapse.

The Substance Abuse and Mental Health Services Administration published a manual entitled *Substance Abuse Relapse Prevention for Older Adults: A Group Treatment Approach*. This manual details a relapse prevention method using cognitive-behavioral and self-management treatment techniques adapted specifically for use with older adults in a counselor-led group treatment setting. The goals of this approach are to engage and support clients as they receive skill training and to analyze, understand, and control the day-to-day factors that have led clients to abuse substances.

CONCLUSION

The results of research on screening, brief interventions, brief treatments and formal treatment for older adults indicate that a nonconfrontational, respectful approach as that used in brief interventions and elder-specific treatment is the most acceptable and generally effective approach with older adults who are experiencing physical or mental health difficulties related to alcohol or medications.

CHAPTER 36

Summary Author: Thea Weisdorf
Joseph J. Westermeyer

Cultural Issues in Addiction Medicine

Addictive disorders vary widely across nations and cultural groups. Clinicians who appreciate the interaction of culture and addiction may enhance their clinical effectiveness. Cultural factors can increase the risk of addiction and undermine patients' and clinicians' efforts at recovery. Similarly, an appreciation of cultural factors influencing patients and their social networks can enhance treatment outcomes.

DEFINITIONS RELATED TO SUBSTANCE USE AND ABUSE

Several concepts related to culture are helpful in guiding the addiction specialist in understanding the role of culture in contributing to, as well as alleviating addictive disorders (Table 36.1).

CULTURE AND PATTERNS OF SUBSTANCE USE AND ABUSE

Cultures prescribe or proscribe the use of various psychoactive substances. For example, the Jewish and the Roman Catholic religions require the use of alcoholic beverage at specific ceremonies (e.g., Passover dinner, Catholic mass). On the other hand, cultures and ethnic groups associated with Islam forbid alcohol drinking. A review of individual ethnic patterns of substance use and abuse in the United States may be helpful to the clinician who is unfamiliar with trends outside of his or her own community or ethnic group, but these "stereotypes" may be misleading for the following reasons:

- Within any major group, there are considerable differences among subgroups.
- Rates of substance abuse may change with the generations since immigration.
- Sociocultural changes within ethnic groups can affect the pattern of substance use and abuse over time.

Clinicians must conduct individual assessments for each new patient, while avoiding stereotyping. Failure to do so will result in both missed diagnosis (in patients from groups with low rates of substance abuse) and overdiagnosis (in patients from groups with high rates of substance abuse).

CULTURAL ASPECTS OF CLINICAL ASSESSMENT

The first step in conducting a cultural history consists of asking the patient about the ethnic origins of his or her parents and grandparents. This would include their place of birth, national origin, language learned at home, migrations, roles and affiliations in the ethnic community and in the community at large, educational experiences, and marital history.

The second step consists of assessing the parent's overall enculturation of the patient in his or her ethnic groups of origin. Of note here, parental substance abuse can disrupt a health identity formation and undermine cultural competence.

Adoption or foster home placement can affect ethnic affiliation and identity, especially if the new parents differ in their ethnic origins from the biologic parents. The developing child's enculturation can affect the use of psychoactive substances. During late adolescence or early adulthood, the patient may have chosen to relocate away from the family/community of origin to go to college or to marry cross-culturally, for example. Learning to live in another culture can involve stressors that may precipitate excessive substance use.

TABLE 36.1	Definition of Culture-Related Terms with Utility in Understanding, Assessing, and Treating Substance Use Disorders
Term	**Definition**
Culture	The sum total of a people's way of life, including their geography, topography, climate, work and recreation, technology and economic production, political organization, law and law enforcement, family organization and function, child raising and education, life cycle patterns and age-sex roles, language and communication, clothing, beliefs and norms, customs and ceremonies, recreation and "time out" from social roles, and diet and health care
Ethnicity	Groups within a culture that share their own unique cultural attributes, which may include national origin, language, shared ancestors, religion, traditions, clothing, and/or beliefs or norms
Subculture	Groups within a culture that share major sociocultural characteristics, such as occupation, identity, or values. Examples include professional groups, guilds or unions, political parties, recovery organizations, commercial groups, or recreational associations. Subcultures depend on the majority culture for their existence; they are not freestanding and cannot sustain themselves.
Cultural competence	The ability to function effectively within a culture. Such competence depends on the ability to communicate with others, earn a living, function within family and community groups, avoid interpersonal or legal problems insofar as possible, and develop an identity consistent with cultural expectations.
Clinical cultural competence	The ability of a clinician to interact effectively with people from cultures different from that of the clinician; this ability is fostered by (a) awareness of one's own cultural world view, (b) positive attitudes toward cultural differences, (c) knowledge regarding the range of cultural practices and world views, and (d) skill in evaluating and treating patients from cultures different from the clinician's own culture.
Norm	Behaviors within a culture that possess positive or negative valance; norms typically exist with any behavior that is viewed in a judgmental way or has moral overtones.
Ideal norm	These norms describe the manner in which a person should behave.
Behavior norm	These norms describe the manner in which the people in a group actually do behave, regardless of the expressed ideal norm.
Identity	An individual's view of himself or herself based on group affiliations
Enculturation	Training of children to become culturally competent—a process sometimes also termed "ensocialization."
Acculturation	A process by which two adjacent cultural groups adapt certain aspects of one another's culture; also applied to migrants into a new culture, who must acquire attitudes, knowledge, and skill of the new culture to function as an adult.

SUBSTANCE-SPECIFIC HISTORY

- *Observations of role models:* What substances did the parenting adults use in the home or outside the home?
- *Socialization into psychoactive substance use:* Who first taught or guided the patient's use of psychoactive substances? Did this occur in the home or outside with peer groups?
- *Early experience with substance use:* Who determined the substances, occasions for use, dose, and patterns of use? How did use assist coping in the family, in school, etc.?
- *Linkage with other developmental tasks:* Was the patient learning other developmental tasks at the same time?

ADDICTION AND PATIENTS' CULTURAL FUNCTION

The relationship between psychoactive substances and social performance is a complex one. Psychoactive substance use may foster social coping, at least initially. Nonproblematic use of psychoactive substances can be a manifestation of successful enculturation (e.g., nonproblematic use of alcohol in the United States). Over time, addiction generally undermines cultural performance.

Loss of social coping and competence during the course of substance use disorder is a common feature of addiction in all cultures. Examples of competence loss include the following:

1. Marital status: i.e., divorce
2. Employment status: i.e., jobs of brief duration, longer periods of unemployment, etc.
3. Housing: i.e., living with friends who abuse substances, homelessness, etc.
4. Community participation: i.e., alienation and isolation from events, activities, etc.
5. Friends: i.e., most friends use substances heavily.
6. Legal: i.e., breaking laws related to DUI, drug possession, etc.
7. Financial: i.e., inability to pay bills, bankruptcy, etc.

The addiction subculture may comprise a welcome identity group to a person who is estranged from family and other groups. Thus, the young person who has failed to achieve social competence in their community of origin may drift toward the identity proffered by a drug subculture.

CULTURE, TREATMENT, AND RECOVERY

Addiction and the Intimate Social Network
Social network reconstruction can compose a potent means of intervening in the addiction process and then providing support during recovery. A key element involves elimination of active substance abusers from the network, with retention of those committed to the patient's ultimate recovery.

Cultural Recovery in Addictive Disorders
A number of strategies have proven useful in social network reconstruction during recovery:

- Joining a recovery group whose members are also looking for new associates (e.g., Alcoholics Anonymous)
- Joining a group that shares similar interests
- Joining a charitable organization or a social group with a charitable purpose
- Volunteering at a health care facility, a school, or similar facility
- Returning to a group or organization from the past, such as an ethnic association or church group
- Going back to school or taking a job that leads to new contacts

These strategies will lead to affiliation with new people and groups, affording the recovering person a new lease on life. They replace the groups associated with psychoactive substance use in the person's previous life.

Often, a more difficult task lies in building bridges back to relatives and family members. These people have probably been hurt or alienated by the addiction-related behaviors of the past. Frequently, they have come to distrust the recovering person. He/she should expect a long period of rebuilding the lost trust. If the recovering person undergoes a series of slips or recurrences—common in the early months of recovery—this can reaffirm the family's worse fears. Fortunately, for those involved in Twelve-Step work, several of the steps prepare the recovering person for making amends to family members and former friends who have suffered from the consequences of addiction.

Culture-Specific Treatment
Therapies specific to particular cultures, ethnic groups, nationalities, and religions can contribute to recovery from substance use disorders.

Some of these interventions are ceremonial in nature, such as a healing ceremony, or religious ritual.

Pharmacotherapies can also play pharmacocultural roles during rehabilitation. For example, clinicians can provide disulfiram to recovering alcohol-dependent patients who will be exposed to alcohol use in their home communities. Taking disulfiram can be an acceptable excuse for not participating in a group-drinking activity instead of being viewed as a rejection of a friendly, cultural event.

Some culture-related groups may not specifically address addiction, but can nonetheless support recovery.

CONCLUSIONS

Disparity between ideal and behavioral norms, as it applies to substance use, can result in outcomes that are costly to many individuals as well as the society and culture at large.

Clinicians can increase their effectiveness by understanding the cultural elements that the patient brings to the clinic. This task begins with understanding the patient's enculturation from childhood to young adulthood and possible subsequent acculturation experiences. Current and past cultural affiliations can be helpful in devising a successful recovery plan. Assessing the patient's intimate social network is an important first step. Cultural resources and traditions can serve clinicians and patients in the challenging process of recovery.

Summary Author: Thea Weisdorf
Mary E. Larimer • Jason R. Kilmer • Ursula Whiteside

College Student Drinking

PREVALENCE AND CONSEQUENCES

Peak lifetime alcohol use generally occurs in an individual's late teens and early 20s. The prevalence of heavy episodic (or binge) drinking (defined as reaching a blood alcohol level of 0.08 or higher, usually by consuming five or more drinks for men, four or more for women, in a 24-hour period) and the detrimental consequences resulting from this type of drinking have led major governmental health organizations to classify college student binge drinking as a major public health problem.

Drinking Rates and Disorders among College Students

Approximately 85% of college students have consumed alcohol, and 73% have been drunk at least once in their lives. Five percent of students report drinking daily, while 40% have engaged in binge drinking in the past 2 weeks. Estimated prevalence of alcohol abuse and dependence varies; however, approximately 18% of college students met criteria for an alcohol use disorder.

Alcohol-Related Problems and Consequences

An estimated 1,700 unintentional college student deaths per year involve alcohol. College-specific, drinking-related consequences range from the more extreme (death, injury, assault, sexual abuse, unsafe sex, health problems, suicide, and drunk driving) to the less problematic but still life-interfering (academic problems, vandalism, property damage, police involvement).

Damage to Self Damage to self includes mild impairments such as nausea, vomiting, and hangovers. Higher levels of drinking are associated with poorer academic records, alcohol-related health problems and legal offences (driving under the influence, or arrests for an alcohol-related offence).

Damage to Others Damage to others includes being affected by alcohol-related automobile accidents, vandalism and litter, noise, fighting, public urination and vomiting. It is estimated that approximately half a million college students annually are unintentionally injured because of drinking—with approximately 97,000 students experiencing alcohol-related sexual assault or date rapes.

Damage to Institution Damage to institution includes problems such as violence, vandalism, and property damage. It has been estimated that somewhere between 50% and 80% of violence occurring on campuses is alcohol related.

Risk Factors Related to College Student Drinking

Certain factors put some college students at particularly high risk for heavy drinking and related problems. Identified risk factors include demographic and environmental influences, cognitive and motivational factors, and affective factors, among others.

Demographics
Sex and Ethnicity

- On average, college men drink more often, consume larger quantities of alcohol, and are more likely to engage in binge drinking than are college women.
- College males are more likely to meet criteria for an alcohol use disorder and experience more alcohol-related problems.
- White college students are most likely to engage in binge drinking.
- Like Native American/Alaskan Native students, white students experience more problems related to binge drinking.
- African American students are least likely to engage in binge drinking.
- Asian American and African American students are less likely to experience alcohol-related problems.
- Hispanic/Latino students fall in the middle of these groups.

Athletics

- For both males and females, involvement in athletics at the high school or college level is related to more frequent drinking and other risk behaviors.

Membership in the Fraternity/Sorority (Greek) System

- Members of the Greek system consume alcohol at greater frequencies and quantities than their non-Greek peers.
- Greek organization members also experience greater alcohol-related problems than non-Greek members.
- Greek membership (for males) was found to be the highest risk factor (of 17 others) for heavy episodic drinking.
- There can be great variability in drinking rates within the Greek system.

Drinking Expectancies

- Alcohol expectancies are the set of beliefs, positive and negative, one carries about the effects of alcohol consumption.
- Positive expectancies have been shown to predict drinking as well as differentiate between problem and nonproblem college student drinking.
- Among adolescents, positive alcohol expectancies have been found to be a more successful predictor of problem drinking than family history of alcohol problems.

Drinking Motives

- Drinking motives, or reasons for drinking, not surprisingly predict alcohol use behaviors.
- Conformity, enhancement, social, and coping reasons are the most cited drinking motives.

Social Norms and Misperceptions

- Perceptions of what is "normal behavior" for a group of individuals, or social norms, are known to influence behavior.
- College students overestimate the rates at which other college students drink, the amount other college students drink, and the extent to which other students support heavy drinking.
- These overestimations were found to be the strongest predictors of college student drinking.

Environmental Risk and Protective Factors

- The cost of alcohol in and surrounding the campus environment can be related to alcohol use and increases in total cost can reduce consumption (i.e., limits on "Happy hour").
- Rates of college student drinking are impacted by high-risk specific events associated with increased consumption of alcohol (i.e., birthdays, graduations, holidays, etc.).
- Drinking games have been identified as a risk factor for "problematic" drinking and associated with heavy drinking (binge) episodes.
- Involvement with athletics and the culture surrounding collegiate sporting events is associated with risk for higher rates of drinking and for consequences associated with alcohol consumption.
- Protective factors against high-risk drinking on campuses include, but are not limited to, substance-free housing and Twelve-Step recovery groups.

College Drinking Prevention Strategies

The NIAAA's Task Force on College Drinking developed a four-tier prevention strategy to address the serious concerns of college student's drinking. Tier I represents interventions with the strongest evidence of efficacy, and Tier IV, the weakest or ineffective interventions, with Tiers II and III in between. The following interventions are outlined with their respective efficacies designated as tiers I, II, or III.

Cognitive-Behavioral Skills–Based Interventions   This intervention has considerable support in the college drinking prevention literature and is designated as tier I intervention. These interventions combine CBT skills training (such as identifying and planning for or avoiding risky situations using protective behavioral strategies such as drink spacing, counting drinks, and limit setting to reduce intoxication, discussing myths about alcohol's effects, and communicating assertively about drinking decisions) with norms clarification (correcting misperceptions about drinking norms, exploring assumptions that everybody drinks), using motivational interviewing style to reduce resistance and promote change.

A second cognitive–behavioral intervention designated as tier I was expectancy challenge interventions. These interventions, aimed at changing students' positive expectations for alcohol intoxication and are delivered by two methods. The first method is experiential—the alcohol placebo effect is directly applied to demonstrate how one's expectations about drinking influence his or her experience. Typically, students who are told they are drinking alcohol but actually receive a nonalcoholic drink, or placebo, still show the social effects associated with drinking (i.e., they become more social, talkative). The second method is didactic, wherein students are educated about this phenomenon (e.g., Discussion of alcohol myths, such as "I can't be outgoing at a party without alcohol" and placebo effects).

The simple behavioral approach of self-monitoring or self-assessment of alcohol use and/or consequences has also been found to show efficacy in college drinking prevention.

Brief Motivational Interventions   Brief motivational interventions (BMIs), typically incorporating assessment and personalized feedback regarding alcohol use, norms, and consequences, are viewed as efficacious in reducing and preventing excessive alcohol use and related harm in college populations. A manual for the BASICS intervention (Brief Alcohol Screening and Intervention for College Students) has been developed and provides the strongest evidence in support of efficacy. It includes a comprehensive assessment followed by a 1-hour personalized feedback interview. The interview is structured around a review of graphic feedback generated from the assessment. These interventions may work to hasten the natural developmental process out of high-risk drinking (as the effects of BMIs weaken over time, especially by 12-month follow-up). This strategy has been successfully implemented in a variety of settings, including campus health clinics and fraternity social organizations.

Feedback-Only Interventions   As effective and evidential as the BMIs are, they are costly and difficult to offer to college students, since they require trained providers to deliver them. New research is looking at more cost-effective methods for reaching a broader audience of students, using minimal intervention strategies such as provision of written, mailed, or Internet motivational feedback. Early results have been encouraging showing that these interventions were associated with reductions in alcohol use. Though some studies showed the effect was greater for in-person motivational feedback, mailed/computerized interventions alone were associated with significant reductions in drinking.

Environmental Interventions   Although less empirical evidence support prevention efforts that target the college environment, such efforts are emerging as important components of an overall prevention strategy. The five subcategories of strategic interventions within the environmental change category are

1. Promoting alcohol-free options
2. Creating an environment that supports health-promoting norms
3. Limiting alcohol availability on- and off-campus
4. Restricting alcohol promotion and marketing on- and off-campus
5. Developing and enforcing policies and laws surrounding alcohol consumption

Suggestions are made for environmental changes to reduce the risk of specific events such as spring break, for example, inviting parents to visit campus during spring break, providing alternative activities, etc.

Issues surrounding enforcement of policy are also of great importance. Some studies suggest (though results are inconsistent) that more laws restricting underage drinking and laws governing the volume of sales are associated with lower levels of drinking.

The use of a campus-community coalition can be beneficial. This coalition typically assembles key stakeholders from both settings who can collaborate together in efforts to reduce problems on campus and in the surrounding area.

CONCLUSIONS AND FUTURE DIRECTIONS

Alcohol use on college campuses is an important health, safety, liability, and risk management issue, and advances have been made in identifying effective strategies to reduce alcohol consumption and associated consequences.

Alcohol use does not occur in a vacuum. Research suggests that 34% of college students also report use of an illicit drug in the past year. Efforts to prevent or intervene with alcohol will necessarily need to consider these related behaviors.

Also related to the context of student alcohol use are co-occurring mental health problems. There is a documented greater than fivefold increase in students prescribed psychotropic medication on college campuses over a recent 10-year period. Given success with brief interventions targeting depression and targeting alcohol, future research must consider strategies to address the overlap of mental health issues and substance use.

Research indicates that BMIs utilizing assessment and in-person feedback, as well as cognitive-behavioral skills–based interventions are efficacious in reducing alcohol use in colleges. There is a need to integrate these services into points of contact for the students (i.e., residences, Greek social organizations, student services, etc.) and a need for reliable and valid screening strategies to be employed to assess the student's alcohol problems, if present.

Given the success of mailed and computerized feedback, the widespread implementation of a program of screening and brief feedback intervention is now feasible on many college campuses.

College student alcohol use and associated consequences are not unique problems on any one campus. As colleges and universities move toward developing campus-community coalitions and getting involved in statewide coalitions, efforts to impact college student health become more than the responsibility of the individual campus.

CHAPTER 38

Summary Author: Thea Weisdorf
Jon E. Grant • Brian L. Odlaug • Marc N. Potenza

Pathologic Gambling: Clinical Characteristics and Treatment

Pathologic gambling is a psychiatric disorder characterized by persistent and recurrent maladaptive patterns of gambling behavior, which is associated with impaired functioning, reduced quality of life, and high rates of bankruptcy, divorce, and incarceration. Pathologic gambling is currently classified in *DSM-IV-TR* as an "impulse control disorder not elsewhere classified." The diagnosis requires that a person meet five of the possible ten criteria listed for the disorder (Table 38.1). The term problem gambling has been used to describe forms of disordered gambling. Problem gambling, like problem drinking, is not an officially recognized disorder by the American Psychiatric Association.

There remains controversy about whether pathologic gambling is better understood as a compulsive disorder or an addictive disorder. This is probably so because pathologic gambling is often resistant to treatment. It remains unclear whether the treatment approaches of traditional addiction treatment (group, Twelve-Step, relapse prevention, etc.) are superior, inferior, equivalent, or need to be combined with those of psychiatric treatments (medication, cognitive-behavioral therapy [CBT], psychotherapy). However, evidence supports significant phenomenological, clinical, epidemiologic and biologic links with substance use disorders.

TABLE 38.1 **Diagnostic Criteria for Pathologic Gambling**

A. Persistent and recurrent maladaptive gambling behavior as indicated by five (or more) of the following:
1. Is preoccupied with gambling (e.g., preoccupied with reliving past gambling experiences, handicapping or planning the next venture, or thinking of ways to get money with which to gamble)
2. Needs to gamble with increasing amounts of money in order to achieve the desired excitement
3. Has repeated unsuccessful efforts to control, cut back, or stop gambling
4. Is restless or irritable when attempting to cut down or stop gambling
5. Gambles as a way of escaping from problems or of relieving a dysphoric mood (e.g., feelings of helplessness, guilt, anxiety, depression)
6. After losing money gambling, often returns another day to get even ("chasing" one's losses)
7. Lies to family members, therapist, or others to conceal the extent of involvement with gambling
8. Has committed illegal acts such as forgery, fraud, theft, or embezzlement to finance gambling
9. Has jeopardized or lost a significant relationship, job, or educational or career opportunity because of gambling
10. Relies on other to provide money to relieve a desperate financial situation caused by gambling
B. The gambling behavior is not better accounted for by a Manic Episode.

Note: Reprinted from the American Psychiatric Association. *Diagnostic and Statistical Manual of Mental Disorders*, 4th ed (Text revision). Washington, DC: American Psychiatric Association; 2000, with permission.

EPIDEMIOLOGY

A range of prevalence estimates have been reported for pathologic gambling depending upon the time frame of the study and the instruments used to diagnose the disorder. A meta-analysis of 120 prevalence estimate surveys completed in North America from the late 1970s to the late 1990s found that the lifetime estimate of pathologic gambling was 1.6% and of problem gambling was 3.85%, for a combined rate of 5.45% for some kind of disordered gambling.

There has been an accelerated proliferation of gambling venues during the past decade, particularly with Native American casinos and riverboat gambling. With increased opportunities to gamble, it is likely that we can expect greater rates of pathologic gambling in the future.

Clinical Characteristics

Although prospective studies are largely lacking, pathologic gambling appears to follow a trajectory similar to that of substance dependence, with high rates in adolescent and young adult groups, lower rates in older adults, and periods of abstinence and relapse.

Significant clinical differences have been observed in men and women with pathologic gambling. Men are more likely to be single and living alone as compared to women with the disorder. Male pathologic gamblers are also more likely to have sought treatment for substance abuse, have higher rates of antisocial personality traits, and have marital consequences related to their gambling. Women, who constitute approximately 32% of pathologic gamblers in the United States, seem to progress more quickly to a pathologic state than do men.

The types of gambling preferred by men tend to be different from those preferred by women. Men with pathologic gambling have higher rates of "strategic" forms of gambling, including sports betting, video poker, and blackjack. Women have higher rates of "nonstrategic" gambling, such as slot machines or bingo. Both men and women report that advertisements trigger their urges to gamble, but women report that gambling acts as an escape from stress or depression.

Functional Impairment, Quality of Life, and Legal Difficulties

Individuals with pathologic gambling suffer significant impairment in their ability to function socially and occupationally. Work-related problems such as absenteeism, poor performance, and job loss are common. It is also frequently associated with marital problems and diminished intimacy and trust within the family. Financial difficulties often exacerbate personal and family problems.

Not surprisingly, individuals with pathologic gambling report poor quality of life. Pathologic gambling is also associated with greater health problems and increased use of medical services. Possible reasons for these issues include the sedentary nature of gambling, reduced leisure and exercise time, reduced sleep, increased stress, and increased nicotine and alcohol consumption.

Suicidal ideation and suicide attempt/completion are other concerns brought on by pathologic gambling. Large numbers of gamblers report having suicidal ideation related to their gambling losses and between 17% and 24% of Gamblers Anonymous participants have attempted suicide owing to gambling.

Many individuals with pathologic gambling have faced legal difficulties related to their gambling, including activities such as embezzlement, stealing, and writing bad checks.

Comorbidity

Psychiatric comorbidity is common in individuals with pathologic gambling. Substance use disorders (especially alcohol abuse and dependence) are the most commonly seen comorbid conditions seen with pathologic gambling. There are also high estimates of co-occurring mood and anxiety disorders (mainly generalized anxiety disorder). The rates of co-occurring disorders often have wide ranges, and this may be owing to the lack of structured clinical interviews uses, the small sample sizes of gamblers assessed, and the possible heterogeneity of pathologic gambling.

Studies have shown that estimates of any personality disorder in pathologic gamblers range from 25% to 93%. Borderline, narcissistic, avoidant, and obsessive-compulsive personality disorders are most commonly reported.

Family History

High frequencies of psychiatric disorders are seen in the first-degree relatives of those with pathologic gambling (mood, anxiety, substance use, and antisocial personality disorders). Studies have also found that 20% of the first-degree relatives of pathologic gamblers also have pathologic gambling.

TREATMENT

Psychotherapy

There are no randomized controlled trials supporting the effectiveness of psychodynamic psychotherapy, Gamblers Anonymous, or self-exclusion contracts in the treatment of pathologic gambling. Psychosocial treatments such as cognitive therapy, behavioral therapy, cognitive-behavioral therapy, and brief interventions and motivational interviewing have been examined in controlled studies and some of their findings are outlined below.

Cognitive Therapy In one study, subjects involved in individual cognitive therapy combined with relapse prevention strategies appear to experience reductions in both gambling frequency and the subjects' perceived self-control over their gambling behavior at 12 months. Similar results were noted in a study employing group cognitive therapy (using a wait-list control). These studies do not include data from a significant number of subjects who completed the 12- or 24-month follow-up.

Behavioral Therapy Behavioral approaches have been examined in three controlled studies. One study reported significant reductions in gambling behaviors in a comparison of imaginal desensitization to traditional aversion therapy. At 1-year follow-up, 70% of the group assigned to imaginal desensitization was still maintaining reductions in gambling, compared to 30% of those assigned to aversion therapy. In a second study, benefits to behavioral therapy were initially observed but not maintained at a 12-month follow-up. In the third study, long-term outcomes to several behavioral approaches were assessed and there was some evidence that subjects assigned to imaginal desensitization had decreased or ceased gambling, but no difference was reported in the rates of abstinence.

Cognitive-Behavioral Therapy Studies assessing CBT demonstrate promising results for the treatment of pathologic gambling. CBT combined with interventions designed to improve treatment compliance, and CBT with mapping-enhanced treatment appear more successful than CBT alone.

Brief Interventions and Motivational Interviewing A study that looked at subjects assigned to either workbook (CBT and motivational enhancement techniques) or to workbook plus a single in-depth interview, reported significant reductions in gambling at 6 months. Another study showed a lower frequency of gambling and money lost in a workbook plus motivational intervention group, compared to a workbook alone or wait-list group.

Pharmacotherapy

No medication is currently approved by the U.S. Food and Drug Administration for treating pathologic gambling. Several placebo-controlled trials of pharmacotherapy treatment have been conducted and suggest that medications may be beneficial in treating pathologic gambling.

Opioid Antagonists Given their ability to modulate dopaminergic transmission in the mesolimbic pathway and to block μ opioid receptors, opioid receptor antagonists have been investigated in the treatment of pathologic gambling. In an 11-week, double-blind, placebo-controlled study, significant improvement was seen in 75% of naltrexone subjects, compared to 24% of placebo subjects. A second, larger study replicated these findings with significantly greater reductions in gambling urges and gambling behavior in the naltrexone group, as well as greater improvement in psychosocial functioning.

Another opioid antagonist, nalmefene, has also shown promise in the treatment of pathologic gambling.

"Antidepressants": Serotonin Reuptake Inhibitors and Buproprion Based on the proposed neurobiology of pathologic gambling, antidepressant medications have been examined as treatment. Low levels of the serotonin metabolite, 5-hydroxyindole acetic acid (5-HIAA), and blunted serotonergic response within the ventromedial prefrontal cortex (vmPFC) have been associated with impulsive behaviors. Compared to controls, individuals with pathologic gambling demonstrate diminished activation of the vmPFC during gambling-related activities.

Mixed results have been found with the drugs paroxetine (Paxil) and fluvoxamine (Luvox). A double-blind, 6-month, placebo-controlled trial using sertaline (Zoloft) demonstrated no statistical advantage over placebo.

In the only controlled study of a non-SSRI antidepressant, buproprion (Wellbutrin) was not significantly more efficacious than placebo for pathologic gambling.

The mixed results of antidepressant trials for pathologic gambling may be owing to the fact that serotonergic dysfunction is merely a peripheral aspect of pathologic gambling, the small sample sizes of the studies, or the heterogeneity of pathologic gambling.

Mood Stabilizers Mood stabilizers have been examined in pathologic gambling with the hypothesis that they are beneficial in reducing impulsivity and hypermotoric activation. Lithium reduced the thoughts and urges associated with pathologic gambling; however, no significant difference was found in the episodes of gambling per week, time spent per gambling episode, or the amount of money lost.

Glutamatergic Agents There is some suggestion that *N*-acetylcysteine (NAC), a glutamate-modulating agent that is available through health food stores without a prescription, may be beneficial in reducing pathologic gambling symptoms. This is based on the fact that improving gluamatergic tone in the nucleus accumbens has been implicated in reducing the reward-seeking behavior of animals.

Assessment of Pharmacotherapies

- Naltrexone should be considered a first-line treatment for pathologic gambling.
- No study has examined pharmacologic treatment effects for longer than 6 months.
- Preliminary data suggest that individuals with pathologic gambling and bipolar symptoms may respond to lithium.
- Pathologic gamblers and anxiety respond to escitalopram.

Treatment Recommendations

Pathologic gambling is a common, disabling psychiatric disorder that is associated with high rates of co-occurring disorders, particularly substance use disorders, and high rates of illegal activities. Psychotherapy and pharmacotherapy have shown promise in the treatment of pathologic gambling. Based on treatment literature, the off-label use of naltrexone would appear the most promising pharmacologic option. An SSRI antidepressant used off-label may also be beneficial particularly when the individual has comorbid depression or anxiety. In terms of psychosocial treatments, CBT appears promising.

Other factors may influence which treatment option is chosen for a particular patient. First, many clinicians are simply unaware of pathologic gambling. Having a list of providers who know about pathologic gambling and can provide treatment can minimize this problem. Second, there are no clear recommendations of treatment for the clinician to follow. It is unclear exactly how many sessions of CBT are most helpful for pathologic gambling. The exact dose of medication or duration of medication trial for optimal treatment is also unknown. Third, individuals with pathologic gambling exhibit high rates of placebo response in treatment studies (clinicians should monitor for several months and not assume they will continue to do well). Fourth, impulsive patients do not often follow recommendations or follow-up with treatment. (Treatment data show that dropout rates are high for pathologic gambling). This can be minimized by providing psychoeducation about the illness, detailing the expectations of treatment, and the expressing the need to stay in treatment.

CHAPTER 39

Summary Author: Christopher A. Cavacuiti
Steven J. Shoptaw

Sexual Addiction

The suggestion that some individuals can become addicted to a behavior as fundamental as sex carries controversy, in both the professional and the lay communities. Yet there are striking similarities between "sexual addiction" and substance dependence including the following:

- Repetitive, compulsive behaviors that impact on neurobiology
- The behavior continues despite knowledge of adverse medical, legal, and/or interpersonal consequences.
- Loss of control over this behavior
- Inordinate amounts of time spent engaging in, or thinking about sexual behavior
- Neglect of social-recreational activities and role responsibilities
- Consistent with the concept of tolerance: there is often a need for increased sexual activity and/or more aberrant activity to achieve the same level of pleasure.
- Extreme mood changes that are related to sexual activity (euphoria) or its abstinence (depression)

DEFINITIONS

There is a wide range of opinions on what defines abnormal or pathologic sexual behaviors. Two current boundaries that define pathologic (and illegal) sexual behavior involve inclusion of sexual partners who are children and sexual partners who are subjected to aggression, physically or emotionally. Outside of legal sanctions against behaviors that involve pedophilia, violence, or abuse, there are no agreed upon cut points that distinguish "normal" from "out-of-control" sexual behaviors. One definition of "hypersexual desire" in men is the persistence of seven or more orgasms per week for a minimum duration of 6 months or more after age 15. The definition, however, may not extend as well to females, as fewer women in the population engage in high rates of sexual behavior.

Formal definitions of human sexual urges as abnormal or excessive remain as culturally defined and historically influenced. As currently referenced in the *DSM-IV-Text Revision*, disorders consistent with sexual addiction are defined as paraphilias and paraphilia-related disorders that involve "recurrent, intense sexually arousing fantasies, urges or behaviors involving (1) nonhuman objects, (2) the suffering or humiliation of oneself or one's partner, or (3) children or other non-consenting persons." The *DSM-IV-TR* does not formally classify sexual addiction as an addictive behavior. Instead, the behavior is coded under along with other diagnoses that feature impaired impulse control or paraphilia.

While many professionals and affected individuals agree that sexual addiction is defined by repetitive, frequent, and compulsive sexual behaviors, there are few evidence-based, quantitative definitions of sexual addiction that are based on amount of sexual behaviors. Attempts to define sexual addiction are further complicated by the fact that it often co-occurs with other psychiatric disorders, particularly illnesses that involve social disinhibition (e.g., bipolar disorder, schizophrenia, stimulant dependence, and antisocial personality disorder).

DIAGNOSIS

The group of individuals easiest to diagnose with a form of sexual addiction are those (primarily men) who meet criteria for paraphilia disorders. The societal and legal sanctions on many of these sexual behaviors frequently require individuals with paraphilias to submit to the justice system for remedy and to the medical establishment for treatment (including chemical castration). Outside the paraphilias, however, sexual addiction typically presents with specific behaviors that are not necessarily illegal, but can nonetheless cause significant clinical distress and that may be concomitant with other problems, such as substance abuse or mental disorders.

Common behavioral complaints with sexual addiction include

Large amounts of time planning and/or engaging in sexual behaviors
Sexual behavior that is repetitive, persistent, compulsive, and out of control
Intrusive and obsessive thoughts about sex
Negative self-evaluation in terms of sexual behavior (i.e., feeling abnormal, sick; degraded, guilty, ashamed; regretful, depressed, numb, hollow, or empty)

There are no large-scale studies on the incidence and/or prevalence of sexual addiction. Retrospective self-reports of individuals seeking treatment for sexual addiction suggest that the condition typically begins in the late teens or early twenties and can be chronic or intermittent.

ETIOLOGY

The quality of evidence supporting the etiology of a sexual addiction is poor, with much of the literature describing etiology being based on theory rather than data.

Developmental/Adolescent Theories

Human sexual behavior typically develops in early to mid-adolescence, with most people establishing a fairly set selection of sexual preferences and sexual behaviors by early adulthood. It has been hypothesized that sexual addiction may involve abnormal "imprinting." According to this model, particular sentinel experiences during adolescence become the model of compulsive sexual behaviors in adulthood. Others have suggested that sexual addiction represents "courtship disorder" in which an adolescent fails to successfully negotiate one of the stages to establish an intimate relationship, associating with development of a specific type of compulsive sexual behavior in adulthood. One of the main criticisms of these theories is that there are currently no studies to indicate that particular adolescent sexual behaviors reliably predict those individuals who will go on to develop sexual addiction in adulthood.

Trauma Theories

There is a growing body of data documenting emotional and physical trauma in the developmental histories of individuals who develop sexual addiction. Developmental traumatic experiences commonly recognized among individuals with sexual addiction include childhood sexual abuse, early substance use, impulse inhibition problems, and traumatic peer and/or family experiences. Multiple (three or more) episodes of head trauma before the age of 13 are associated with an increased risk of pedophilia.

Genetic/Biologic Theories

When compared to the general population, individuals with sexual addiction are more likely to have family members with sexual or other types of addiction. It has also been hypothesized that sexual addiction may be related to some form of endocrine dysfunction.

Sexual Addiction and Gay Men

The presentation of sexual addiction among gay and bisexual men may differ from that of heterosexual men for several reasons: (a) easier access to sexual partners willing to sexually liaise and (b) internalized and societal homophobia may contribute to obsessive thinking and sexual compulsivity. Although sexual addiction may be expressed differently in gay and bisexual men than in heterosexual men, studies provide strong evidence that the concept of sexual addiction appears to differentiate a group of gay and bisexual men whose sexual behaviors are more compulsive, more repetitive, and more distressing than for gay and bisexual men in general.

Several studies of sexually compulsive behaviors in gay men (using the validated *Sexual Compulsivity Scale [SCS]*) have shown that high scores on this scale correspond remarkably well with a number of factors including

- Older age
- Using methamphetamine and/or cocaine before or during sex
- Going to sex venues or street corners for sex partners
- Less frequent condom use

- Low levels of self-esteem
- Higher disinhibition
- Higher number of HIV status–unknown sexual partners
- More frequent unprotected sexual acts with more partners
- Greater enjoyment of high-risk sex
- Internalized homophobia
- Greater number of male sexual partners met online

Of particular note is that across a variety of studies using different methodologies, there is a remarkably strong association in gay men between reported substance use, particularly stimulant use, and sexual behaviors consistent with sexual addiction.

There are no published reports of behaviors consistent with sexual addiction in lesbians. Indeed, it appears that lesbian women report lower numbers of sexual episodes compared to heterosexual women.

Neurobiology of Sexual Addiction

There are a variety of studies suggesting that sexual addiction has a significant neurobiological component. It has been noted that patients with brain injury in the right temporal areas are more likely to develop sexual compulsivity. This is consistent with positron emission tomography studies indicating that the right temporal lobe is also associated with male heterosexual response. Studies comparing pedophiles with nonsexual offenders as the control group showed significant reductions in white matter volume in the fiber bundles of the superior fronto-occipital fasciculus and the right arcuate in the pedophilia group. Patients with stroke and with multiple sclerosis also experience high rates of aberrant sexual behaviors. Abnormal dopamine neurotransmission has been associated a variety of behavioral compulsions. Multiple case reports have noted the development of compulsive behaviors (including gambling and aberrant sexual behavior) when patients with Parkinson disease are treated with dopamine agonists such as selegiline and pergolide.

PSYCHIATRIC COMORBIDITY

Sexual addiction has been associated with a variety of psychiatric comorbidities including Attention-Deficit Hyperactivity Disorder (ADHD), mood disorders, anxiety disorders, and substance abuse. This is not surprising, given that studies consistently implicate emotional distress and impulsivity as central issues in the expression of sexual addiction. Several of the psychiatric conditions listed above share one or more of these features. Emotional distress is a core feature of mood and anxiety disorders, while impulsivity is a core feature of ADHD, and substance abuse and dependence.

Axis II diagnoses (particularly cluster C traits) also seem to be more common in individuals with sexual addiction though this association appears to be stronger in females than in males.

ASSESSMENT

This starts with thorough review of medical history (especially regarding treatments for sexually transmitted infections), employment background and pattern, involvement with alcohol and drugs (including nicotine and marijuana) that may be used before, during, and after sexually compulsive behaviors, detailed history of legal problems (whether formal charges were or were not recorded), quality of relationships with family, friends, and intimates (if any), and mental health functioning, including both diagnosable psychiatric conditions and sub-threshold mood, affect, and cognitive disturbances. This ancillary information provides strong indications as to whether the behaviors indicating sexual addiction are localized or are more generalized across most domains of functioning for the individual and as to the extent of clinical distress caused by the behaviors.

A variety of screening tools for sexual addiction have been developed over the past 15 years or so. These include the following.

The Sexual Addiction Screening Test

A 25-item test in which respondents answer questions with yes or no regarding various aspects of their sexual behaviors.

The Sexual Outlet Inventory

A clinician-administered rating scale that quantifies sexual fantasies, urges, and behaviors to distinguish unconventional (paraphilic) from conventional (nonparaphilic) sexual behavior.

The Sexual Compulsivity Scale

This is the scale most frequently used in reports of sexual addiction. The SCS is composed of 32 items that are answered on a Likert scale ranging from 1 (not at all like me) to 4 (very much like me). There is published information indicating the SCS performs well in ethnic groups.

Compulsive Sexual Behavior Inventory

Measures factors of control (over sexual behaviors), abuse (sexual and physical), and violence (current and historical)

TREATMENT APPROACHES

Treatment approaches for sexual addictions involve behavioral and/or pharmacologic approaches. There are few randomized controlled trials to guide either behavioral or pharmacologic treatment approaches to sexual addiction.

Behavior Therapies

Behavioral models for treating sexual addiction largely draw upon existing models for treating other forms of addiction (e.g., cognitive-behavioral therapy [CBT], Twelve-Step, motivational interviewing). None of these models has undergone large-scale evaluation of efficacy in terms of sexual addiction. Literature documenting outcomes for residential treatment is also poorly developed.

Cognitive-Behavioral Therapy

CBT is a general approach to treating addictive behavioral disorders that teach patients skills to instill abstinence and to return to abstinence upon relapse. One generic CBT strategy involves identification of "triggers" (i.e., persons, places, things, or internal experiences) that are specific to sexually compulsive behavior.

Twelve-Step and Self-Help Groups

One of the primary advantages to Twelve-Step group attendance for those with sexual addiction is that the groups are convenient and are generally available both in urban and rural contexts. The Twelve-Step process of recovery involves attendance at Twelve-Step meetings and the selection of a "sponsor" to provide around-the-clock assistance in managing sexual obsessions and compulsive urges. There are currently four groups using a Twelve-Step approach to assist individuals in recovering from sexual addiction:

- Sexaholics Anonymous (*www.sa.org*)
- Sex Addicts Anonymous (*www.saa-recovery.org*)
- Sex and Love Addicts Anonymous (*www.slaafws.org*)
- Sexual Compulsives Anonymous (*www.sca-recovery.org*)

PHARMACOTHERAPY STRATEGIES

Antidepressants

One strategy to pharmacotherapy of sexual addiction involves treatment of dysphoric mood symptoms commonly experienced during initial (and perhaps sustained) abstinence.

Selective Serotonin Reuptake Inhibitors (SSRIs)

The use of SSRI as treatment for sexual addiction is based largely on the theorized mechanism of serotonergic dysfunction that may underlie the condition. Low serotonin greatly potentiates sexual behavior in laboratory animals. Conversely, use of SSRIs frequently leads to reduction in sexual libido, particularly for males but also for females. There is some initial randomized controlled trial evidence supporting use of SSRIs for sexual addiction, particularly with gay and bisexual men.

Naltrexone

Naltrexone is an opioid antagonist approved for use in treating alcoholism and opioid dependence. The mechanism of action for considering naltrexone treatment for sexual abuse involves opioid antagonist effects in dampening dopamine release, thereby reducing the euphoria associated with aberrant sexual behavior. Unfortunately, there are no randomized, placebo-controlled trials of opioid antagonists for sexual addiction.

Hormone Therapies

The strategy involves using antiandrogen medications that chemically stop production of testosterone. This approach is often referred to as *chemical castration* and is usually reserved for treating men with paraphilias that involve sexual offenses involving children or violence against adults. While there are case reports describing remission of paraphilia behaviors when patients take antiandrogen medications, there are no placebo-controlled clinical trials using hormone therapies for treatment paraphilia or any other forms of sexual addiction. There are no reports or studies on the utility of these drugs in women with sexual addiction.

Summary Author: Christopher A. Cavacuiti
Paul H. Earley

Physician Health Programs and Addiction Among Physicians

Physicians are a convenient population to study; they are accessible both prior to and after treatment and are articulate about their disease. Research on physician addiction elucidates the natural course of addiction in a highly regulated and monitored population. At the same time, physicians differ from the general population in terms of education, income, and regulatory oversight. Thus, though informative, conclusions made from physician studies cannot necessarily be extrapolated to the population at large.

PREVALENCE

There is longstanding debate about the actual and changing prevalence of addiction in physicians. Anonymous questionnaires studies have found a lifetime prevalence of alcohol abuse or dependence and drug abuse or dependence in physicians at 7.9%, somewhat less than the percentage (8%–13%) reported in the general population

Compared with the general population, physicians were *less* likely to smoke cigarettes and more likely to consume alcohol, benzodiazepines, and opiates.

Studies of complaints heard by medical boards have shown that about 15% to 20% of board disciplinary actions were alcohol or drug related, and another 10% were due to inappropriate prescribing practices—many of which are also addiction related. Alcohol- and drug-related work impairment was the primary impetus for the formation of state physician health programs (PHPs).

CHARACTERISTICS OF ADDICTED PHYSICIANS

Ethnicity

No published data about physician addiction have been reported to date using ethnicity as an independent variable.

Age

A study of doctors attending a large US physician treatment program found an age range of 25 to 83 years, with a median age of 46. Some studies suggest that physician addiction follows a standard bell curve, others have found a bimodal distribution of age at first presentation for treatment; physicians in training and early practice comprise the first wave, mid-to-late career comprise the second. These differences in findings may be due to different methodologies (i.e., age analysis of all treated physicians vs. age of first treatment). Also of interest, heavy drinking decreases with age in the general population and appears to increase with age in physicians.

Gender

Males account for the majority of physician addiction cases, with reported ratios varying between 7 to 1 and 10 to 1, male to female. This contrasts with the 3 to 1 male-to-female ratio in the physician population at large. When compared with their nonmedical counterparts, a disproportionate number of both male and female physicians have been shown to have alcohol problem late in life. Compared with addicted male doctors, addicted female physicians are more likely to be younger, to have medical and psychiatric comorbidity, to have past or current suicidal ideation, and to have attempted suicide. Interestingly, women physicians are the subject of more severe sanctions by medical boards than their male counterparts.

Specialty

A number of studies have looked at rates of addiction by specialty. To date, there is insufficient information to allow meta-analysis. However, the existing studies in this area fairly consistently suggest that psychiatry and emergency medicine physicians have higher substance problems than the physician population at large. Existing studies also suggest that family practice physicians might also be overrepresented, and pediatricians and pathologists appear to be at lower risk for addiction. Most studies suggest that anesthesiologists appear to be more frequent users of highly potent opioids.

DRUGS ABUSED

Two types of studies are generally used to assess the types of drugs abused by physicians: (a) anonymous questionnaires and (b) self-reports of drugs of choice of physicians as they appear in treatment or monitoring programs. Interestingly, physicians are more likely to become addicted to drugs that they commonly prescribe to patients. Thus, psychiatrists tend to abuse benzodiazepines more frequently than other doctors; doctors who prescribe cocaine during procedures (ENT, ophthalmology, plastics) appear more likely to abuse cocaine; family doctors tend to abuse "minor" (lower potency, oral) opioids, whereas anesthetists tend to abuse major (higher potency, injectable) opioids.

Alcohol

Alcohol is, as expected, the most frequent primary drug of abuse by physicians, just as in the general population.

Nicotine

Tobacco dependence has been suggested as a risk factor for alcohol and other drug dependence in physicians as in the general population. Tobacco use in physicians has decreased over time. Emergency medicine and surgery physicians are twice as likely to smoke as are other physicians.

Opioids

Opioids are the second most frequently abused substance by physicians arriving in treatment. This finding has been remarkably stable over several decades of studies, but the type of opioids used continues to change.

Cocaine

In one study, professions that use cocaine medicinally (ophthalmology, head and neck surgery, plastic surgery, and otolaryngology) had a (nonstatistically significant) trend to higher cocaine use.

Benzodiazepines

Psychiatrists have a greater misuse of benzodiazepines; 26.3% report using unsupervised benzodiazepines in the past year, in comparison with 11.4% in other physician groups.

Illicit Drugs

The most common street drug of abuse among medical residents is marijuana. Many kinds of specialists abuse marijuana, with emergency medicine, anesthesiology, family practice, and psychiatry physicians displaying elevated odds of marijuana abuse over physicians as a whole.

RISK FACTORS

Genetics

The strongest predictor of alcohol or drug problems in physicians is the same as in the general population: a family history of alcoholism or drug dependence.

Tobacco Use

Cigarette use of one pack or more per day was highly correlated with alcohol abuse in physicians.

Personality

All physician specialties are burdened with common stereotypes, and a number of researchers have speculated about causal personality factors in the development of physician addiction. At the outset, it must be noted that in the general population, decades of research have failed to discern an "addictive personality." Keeping that in mind, researchers have speculated that "sensation seeking" as a personality factor is correlated with recreational drug use in physicians in training. This "sensation-seeking" personality might also cause such individuals to gravitate to certain specialties such as emergency medicine.

Drug Access

It has been noted that as overall prescribing patterns and the drug availability shift, these shifts tend to be mirrored in terms of the "drugs of choice" among addicted physicians.

Biologic Effect of the Drug of Choice

The pharmacodynamic properties of particular drugs may result in a skew in the physician-patients seen in treatment programs. For example, major anesthetic opioids (such as fentanyl) when consumed parenterally produce a rapid downhill course owing to the development of a remarkable levels of tolerance. This may in part explain the high percentage of anesthesiologists seen in physician treatment programs. Moreover, major opioids tend to have a relatively narrow therapeutic window (the dose needed to achieve the desired effect is quite close to the dose that can lead to respiratory depression), which may account for the high mortality rate among opioids-abusing anesthesiologists.

ADDICTION COMORBIDITY

Thought and Mood Disorders

Although it is unclear whether physicians have higher or lower rates of unipolar depression, physicians who successfully complete suicide are more likely to have a drug abuse problem in their lives, self-prescribed psychoactive substances, a recent alcohol-related problem, a history of emotional problems prior to 18 years of age, and/or a family history of alcohol abuse and/or mental illness.

Addicted physicians rarely have comorbid primary schizophrenia and related thought disorders.

Pain

PHPs are working with an increasing number of physicians with pain and chronic opioid use, many of whom have become physiologically dependent; in turn, a percentage of those go on to become addicted. Eventual addiction is thought to be more common in patients with pain disorders and, when combined with the 25% of physicians who self-prescribe, a perfect storm of high-risk factors emerges.

Scientific data on the safety of allowing physicians to practice on opioids, whether for addiction treatment (i.e., methadone or buprenorphine) or not, are absent.

Posttraumatic Stress Disorder

Posttraumatic stress disorder (PTSD) and alcoholism are closely intertwined and PTSD increases the probability of addiction relapse. However, no studies about the prevalence of PTSD in physicians have been published.

THEORIES OF ADDICTION IN PHYSICIANS

Addiction in physicians has been correlated with a number of familial factors. Several studies have noted that a high proportion of addicted physicians experienced parental deprivation in their childhood. Additionally, approximately 25% of alcohol-dependent medical students and physicians have family histories of alcohol dependence. This is not surprising, given that genetic research literature now supports inherited genetic vulnerabilities for all major classes of addictive drugs.

Excessive alcohol consumption in medical students was positively associated with better grades in the 1st year and a strong tendency toward better scores on Part One of the National Board of Medical Examiners test. Thus, for many students, their personal experience with alcohol does not match cautionary information provided to them during their medical education. This has led to speculation that hard drinking students may be prone to discount warnings. As students progress into full-fledged physicians, the act of saving lives can lead to a feeling of "omnipotence." At the same time, these physicians develop a detailed knowledge of the drugs they prescribe and are being given increased access to a variety of pharmaceuticals. All of these factors can lead physicians to believe that a different set of rules apply to "us" (doctors) versus "them" (patients).

Stress is often cited by physicians in recovery as the primary agent that drove their self-medication. However, the correlation between physician substance use and stress is unclear. Physicians report similar levels of stress to other health professionals, and levels of physician stress do not correlate particularly well with levels of substance use. This has led to speculation that the physician's unhealthy *response* to stress is a more important determinant of addiction than the ubiquitous *presence* of stress itself.

Physicians are taught in medical school and residency (and often in their childhood) to appear self-sufficient and in control. It is therefore often particularly difficult for doctors to admit that they have lost control over their use of drugs. It is very common for actively addicted physicians (and those in early recovery) to exhibit a demeanor of superiority and knowledge, deny any loss of control, and have a need to appear competent, in stark contrast to their crumbling lives.

IDENTIFICATION, INTERVENTION, AND ASSESSMENT

Identification

In the past, denial, shame, and fear of reprisal tended to keep the physician from seeking proper help until significant external consequences coalesced. In more recent years, the emergence of clinically oriented, supportive, and confidential PHPs has stimulated earlier reporting, either by self or colleagues.

The physician's behavior tends to deteriorate first at home, then with friends, and finally surfaces at the workplace. Therefore, disturbances of social or familial functioning can be sensitive early indicators of physician substance dependence. Unfortunately, the family often protects the alcoholic or drug-addicted "bread winner" physician.

Warning signs that can help detect addiction include

- Genetic history
- Drug access
- Domestic problems
- Appearance of being drunk at social functions
- Intoxication or the odor of alcohol on the breath at work
- Highly irregular hours for rounds
- Self-prescribing, neglect of responsibilities
- Angry outbursts
- Frequent medical complaints without a reasonable diagnosis
- Staff concerns about physician behavior
- Depression or weight change
- Citations for driving while under the influence (DUI or DWI)

It is worth noting that if a physician obtains drugs at work (e.g., samples from a drug closet or drugs diverted from the OR or ICU), he or she may display a different set of behaviors—volunteering for additional shifts, arriving early for work, and signing up for more complex (i.e., easier drug access) cases.

Modes of Intervention

Tension involved in the intervention process can be reduced by directing the physician suspected of addictive disease to undergo an evaluation rather than insisting that addiction exists and treatment is indicated. The physician in question is told about the concerns (often without divulging the source of information) and the importance of resolving said concerns by undergoing a thorough and authoritative evaluation. If handled with tact, as is common with experienced PHPs, physicians can usually be "gently coerced" into an evaluation, given the alternative of possible Medical Board referral, evaluation, and possible legal action.

Most states have reporting laws that require hospitals and colleagues to report to the state PHP or their state medical board a physician who is suspected of being impaired by alcohol or drugs.

Assessment

Physicians vary on their need for assessment. Some are quickly identified and agree to cooperate with their treatment needs or at least with an outpatient evaluation. Physicians who are more entrenched in their addiction, have more complex presentations, or are frankly resistant need formal assessment. The examination process must prevent the assessed physician from hiding continued drug use, withdrawal, and addiction-related interpersonal behaviors. Because of the complexity and comprehensive nature of these evaluations, most evaluators conduct them in a residential or partial hospitalization setting where the physician can be observed continuously. Such evaluations have come to be called a "Ninety-six Hour Evaluation," a moniker derived from the time usually taken to complete this process.

Among the criteria listed by PHPs for competent evaluation are that the evaluation be performed by a multidisciplinary team composed of an addiction medicine physician and an addiction psychiatrist; include psychologic and neuropsychologic testing, family assessment, review of previous medical records, and the collection of collateral information from coworkers, hospital employees, friends, and PHPs themselves; and/or any other important source of information needed to thoroughly assess the physician. The patient then meets with one of or all members of the evaluation team to review the diagnosis and recommendations.

TREATMENT

Approximately a dozen drug treatment in the United States have special expertise in the treatment of addicted physicians and other health professionals; some programs have been used for >30 years and have treated thousands of addicted physicians. However, some states are trending toward increased law enforcement actions against addicted physicians, as opposed to treatment.

Clinical Considerations with Addicted Physicians as Patients

Working with addicted physicians requires understanding of the dynamics of addiction and the distinct but highly interactive elements between the addiction, the profession, and the personality. It has been alleged that physicians "make the worst patients." Regardless of the disease, physicians often deny symptoms of any disease, seek substandard care, and put off appropriate care for serious symptoms. As in any other medical situation, the physician-patient in addiction treatment has difficulty giving up the physician role and assuming the patient role. In treatment settings with a mixture of physician and nonphysician patients, the treatment program must set firm limits prohibiting the recovering physician from providing medical advice to other patients.

Physicians will often attempt to fit the treatment into what they know: school and testing. Physician-patients have little trouble learning the didactic parts of treatment and they often become stuck trying to obtain an "A" in treatment. This can lead to the "intellectualization" of the problem at the expense of the emotional, interpersonal, and spiritual dimensions of the addiction experience. This approach can make it difficult for physicians to make the changes that are necessary for sustained recovery. When staff attempt to correct the physician's approach to treatment, it can result in negative transference and poorly veiled contempt for "less educated" treaters.

Treatment will necessarily reacquaint the physician with their feelings. One particularly difficult emotional state is shame. A key task in recovery is an honest appraisal of how the physician's addiction has interfered with his ability to function as a physician. Often, a great deal of self-identity for physician's derives from childhood and training-induced drives for accomplishment and perfection. Thus, therapists must be aware of the risk that physicians may quickly veer from self-examination into shame and self-loathing.

Medical boards, the general public, PHPs, and the physician himself or herself have low tolerance for the potential public harm that can occur when a physician relapses. This flies in the face of the nature of addiction as a disease characterized by relapse and remission. The societal pressure to "have a perfect recovery" creates a maladaptive alliance with the physician patient's own perfectionism.

Characteristics of the Treatment Setting

The confluence of known difficulties engaging physicians in treatment, the public demand for safety, and liability issues have promoted physician-specific, long-term residential addiction treatment programs. While there is little research comparing long-term intensive treatment with less intensive treatment, the few studies that have been done suggest the outcomes are better with longer-term residential care. Because of the significant public and professional consequences that can occur from even just a single relapse, most physician patients are encouraged to attend longer treatment programs than their nonphysician brethren.

The treatment of physicians involves a prolonged continuum of care. When a physician leaves his or her initial treatment setting and returns to work, this is described by the unfortunate and inaccurate vernacular of having "completed treatment." In fact, what physicians are asked to do in the second phase of treatment is in many ways more challenging and more comprehensive care than their primary treatment. This "posttreatment" monitoring commonly involves weekly group therapy sessions, peer support groups, after-care groups, individual counseling, self-help group attendance, drug testing, and worksite monitor reports for 5 years or more.

Available evidence suggests that physician treatment programs with the best outcomes employ abstinence-based Twelve-Step model as well as family participation (i.e., family therapy). Most US physician treatment programs contain both of these elements.

Physician-specific treatment groups can be helpful in developing relapse prevention plans that address the unique triggers faced by doctors (e.g., drug access at work, prescription pads, and locations in the office or hospital where use occurred).

Physician-specific groups can also help doctors to navigate the complex and challenging issues physicians face when returning to practice, such as the difficulties of seeing their patients in A.A., Drug Enforcement Agency prescribing restrictions, and continued management of drugs and prescriptions in the office or hospital.

There is an increasing body of evidence for the safe and effective use of pharmacologic adjuncts in the treatment of alcoholism and opioid dependence. Most physician treatment programs use one or more medications including disulfiram, naltrexone, acamprosate, and/or topiramate as adjuncts for alcohol treatment and the opioid blocker naltrexone in opioid-addicted physicians.

Ultimately, long-term monitoring of physicians may be the most essential component of treatment and critical for sustained recovery. Monitoring and support groups are commonly provided by PHPs or occasionally by the treatment center itself.

Physician Health Programs

History   The beginning of the physician's health movement can be traced back to the founding of International Doctors in Alcoholics Anonymous (IDAA) by Clarence Pearson in 1949. The American and Canadian Medical Associations have jointly sponsored conferences on physician impairment every other year since 1975. By 2007, almost every state in the United States has some type of PHP. In 2007, >9,000 physicians were in monitoring by PHPs programs across the United States.

Structure   PHPs have widely different organizational structures and lines of authority. More than half (54%) of PHPs are nonprofit foundations. Others are part of their respective state medical association (35%) or the licensing board itself (13%). Most (59%) of PHPs evaluated have specific state laws that sanction their actions and guide their operation. The independent evolution of state PHPs coalesced into a federation in 1990.

Activities

Education And Referral   The core concept of PHPs has become clear: "to detect problems that lead to impairment and to intervene and encourage physicians to obtain assistance prior to damaging their careers or harming patients." Addiction continues to be the most commonly identified problem addressed by many PHPs, but most PHPs also address other psychiatric disorders, behaviorally disruptive physicians, and physicians who suffer from other compulsive, addiction-related disorders such as gambling and sexual misbehaviors. Most PHPs provide education and train local hospitals and physician organizations on techniques to help identify and report suspected impairment. PHPs offer consultation about a potential impairment, coordinate intake into treatment, and monitor physicians after treatment through statewide systems. Some PHPs also offer initial assessment and triage and ongoing therapy groups for the physicians in their state.

Abstinence Monitoring   All PHPs track the abstinence status of their recovering physicians. All programs use random witnessed body fluid analysis (most frequently through urine drug screens but often including hair and blood analysis) through an organized monitoring program. Screens commonly taper in frequency over the course of monitoring, for a period of 5 or more years. Drug screening in physician populations requires considerable expertise and accuracy, as addicted physicians can use their knowledge to evade detection.

Recovery Support   In addition to urine monitoring, most state PHPs provide support or therapy groups. Some PHPs provide group-facilitated psychotherapy, while others provide Caduceus groups that are peer-led groups similar to Twelve-Step meetings but often discussing an issue or concern of a given group member. A survey of recovering physicians noted that "A.A. was apparently perceived by respondents as the most potent element of their recovery."

Relapse Significant consequences to the physician and the public result from relapse. PHPs have developed models of assessing relapse severity. One such model divides severity of relapse in three levels:

- **Level I relapse:** missing therapy meetings, support groups, dishonesty, or other behavioral infraction
- **Level II relapse:** the reuse of drugs or alcohol but outside the context of medical practice
- **Level III relapse:** drug or alcohol use within the context of practice

Slips are not uncommon (particularly early in treatment) and they often deepen the physicians' acceptance of their disease and solidify recovery. If managed properly, singular slips are most often helpful in the long run and are not indicators of failed treatment.

Should a physician have a more extensive relapse, he or she should engage in the following:

- A reevaluation of the physician's ability to practice until he or she is more stable in recovery
- A longer and tighter monitoring contract
- A reexamination of the patient's psychiatric status, to determine whether an occult mood disorder or other addictive process or past unaddressed trauma is present.
- A reassessment of the patient's family dynamics and support system
- A reevaluation of the physician's safety to practice
- A determination of the need to repeat primary residential treatment (or to treat other elements of the addiction or other psychiatric disorder)
- Consideration to add relapse prevention medications

Relapse is part of the disease of addiction. Physicians who have difficulty maintaining abstinence should be removed from the workforce until treatment providers with experience in physician recovery feel that the physician is safe to return.

Treatment Outcome Data

Physicians appear to have much higher recovery rates (approximately 75%) than the general population. A number of studies have sought to define why physician treatment is so successful and to identify which components of the physician treatment process might also be beneficial to the public at large.

Studies suggest that approximately 25% of physicians in recovery have at least one relapse. Among those physicians who do relapse, approximately 75% have only one episode of alcohol or drug use.

Controversies

Privacy and Safety Conflict Physician treatment and abstinence monitoring is troubled by the conflict between the physician-patient's need for privacy and the public's need for safety. It has been noted that confidentiality for treatment of physician mental illness, including substance use disorders, can actually increase patient safety by encouraging early referral and safe passage into treatment.

If the perceived consequences of referral are sufficiently prejudicial (e.g., states that require that all PHP referrals be reported to the medical board, regardless of whether impairment has been proven), referral will often not occur until a major incident occurs.

The structure of PHPs facilitates a proper balance in the privacy/safety conflict. They hold the awkward middle ground between their medical board and the treatment providers. PHPs provide limited confidentiality if the physician does not pose a threat to public safety but report to the medical board should a patient become uncooperative or a risk.

Is Monitored Recovery the Same as Self-Guided Recovery? Physicians frequently enter treatment to retain their medical license. One intent of treatment is to shift the physician from this external driver to an internalized state of recovery as a lifetime's work. Some physicians remain drug and alcohol free because of the threat of drug screens and behavioral monitoring, rather than because they are truly interested in recovery.

Treatment providers should avoid pressuring patients to conform, should encourage patients to verbalize their resistance and dissatisfaction with treatment, and welcome honest self-disclosure, especially if the patient is describing how he or she is stuck in the process of change. It should not be a cardinal sin in treatment for a patient to admit to the wish that never quite goes away—that is, to drink or use drugs in a controlled and sociable manner.

Can Physicians Return to Practice on Opioid Maintenance? Unlike the general population, opioids-addicted physicians have very high sustained success rates using an abstinence-based opioids treatment model. Proponents of opioid agonist treatment therefore argue that in selected cases, when abstinence-based treatment has failed (often repeatedly), opioid agonist maintenance therapy is not only justified but also safe. A survey of 36 PHPs found that 14 of the PHP respondents were following up at least one physician on maintenance opioid-agonist medication. Usually, these cases involved complex pain issues.

Medical-legal issues come into the picture when addicted physicians are maintained on opioid medications. As one study has noted, "At least one major statewide malpractice carrier has indicated that they will not insure an addicted physician if he is on opioid maintenance therapy, due to the difficulties in defending such a physician in a malpractice case."

Currently, research on the efficacy of opioid agonist treatment for physicians does not exist.

Are Opioid-Addicted Anesthesiologists Safe to Return to Their Profession? This remains an area of considerable controversy. Studies that are based upon a survey of the memories of anesthesiology program directors (where patients had uncertain treatment and monitoring) describe poor, and often fatal, outcomes. In contrast, studies that followed anesthesiologists under close monitoring in PHPs or regulatory boards describe outcomes of anesthesiologists that are similar to other physicians. As a result of this conflicting research, some residencies lean toward retraining a resident in an alternative field once addiction to major opioids occurs.

No study has cross-correlated relapse rate with type or length of treatment or the use of opioid-blocking agents such as maintenance naltrexone.

CHAPTER

41

Summary Author: Ashok Krishnamurthy
Tara M. Wright • Jeffrey S. Cluver • Hugh Myrick

Management of Intoxication and Withdrawal: General Principles

INTOXICATION STATES

Intoxication is the result of being under the influence of, and responding to, the acute effects of alcohol or another drug of abuse.

Intoxication states can range from euphoria or sedation to life-threatening emergencies when overdose occurs.

Identification and Management of Intoxication

The identification of intoxication begins with the collection of patient data through a patient history, physical examination, and laboratory screening. It is important to determine not only the severity of the substance ingestion, but also the patient's level of consciousness, the substances involved, and any complicating medical disorders. Life-threatening intoxication or overdose is of immediate concern, and thus, the first priority is general supportive care and resuscitative actions.

Historical information regarding substance use usually can be obtained from the patient. Questions regarding the quantity and frequency of substance use provide valuable information to the clinician. Acute intoxication may impede an individual's ability to provide such information: companions or family may be able to provide important information. Toxicology screens provide valuable information regarding the type(s) of substances used.

WITHDRAWAL STATES

The signs and symptoms of withdrawal usually are the opposite of a substance's direct pharmacologic effects. Substances in a given pharmacologic class produce similar withdrawal syndromes; however, the onset, duration, and intensity are variable, depending on the particular agent used, the duration of use, and the degree of neuroadaptation.

Evidence for the cessation of or reduction in use of a substance may be obtained by history or toxicology. Additionally, the clinical picture should not correspond to any of the organic mental syndromes, such as organic hallucinosis. Withdrawal may, however, be superimposed on any organic mental syndrome.

Goals of Detoxification

Detoxification includes a set of interventions by which substances that cause physical dependence are eliminated from the body. The American Society of Addiction Medicine lists three immediate goals for detoxification of alcohol and other substances: (a) to provide a safe withdrawal from the drug(s) of dependence and enable the patient to become drug-free, (b) to provide a withdrawal that is humane and thus protects the patient's dignity, and (c) to prepare the patient for ongoing treatment of his or her dependence on alcohol or other drugs.

It also comprises three essential and sequential steps: evaluation, stabilization, and fostering patient readiness for and entry into treatment. It is important to distinguish detoxification from substance abuse treatment. *Substance abuse treatment/rehabilitation* involves a constellation of ongoing therapeutic services ultimately intended to promote recovery for substance abuse patients. Detoxification may be the first step in this process.

Important components of a humane withdrawal:

1. Caring staff
2. A supportive environment
3. Sensitivity to cultural issues
4. Confidentiality
5. Selection of appropriate detoxification medications (as needed)

Staff must be

1. Clear in their treatment goals
2. Set firm boundaries
3. Be sympathetic
4. Have experience in dealing with difficult behavior

Supportive others (family members, friends, or employers) should be enlisted whenever possible to assist in the care of the patient during outpatient detoxification.

General Principles of Management

Initial medical assessment is important to determine the need for medication and medical management. Such an assessment should include evaluation of predicted withdrawal severity and medical or psychiatric comorbidity. A history of complicated withdrawal should alert the practitioner to the likely possibility of future complicated withdrawals. For example, the CIWA-Ar, or The Clinical Institute Withdrawal Assessment of Alcohol–revised scale, rates the severity of withdrawal, as observed by the clinician. In general, low scores (<9) suggest that pharmacotherapy may not be required, whereas high scores (≥10) indicate a greater risk of seizures and delirium tremens.

The duration of detoxification is not a clearly defined, discrete period. The detoxification period usually is defined as the time during which the patient receives detoxification medications, even though some signs and symptoms may persist for a much longer period.

Many patients may have prolonged withdrawal signs or symptoms, or "protracted abstinence syndrome." Symptoms of the syndrome include disturbances of sleep, anxiety, irritability, and mood instability. The very existence of the protracted abstinence syndrome has been the subject of considerable controversy; however, there is increasing evidence in the literature supporting its existence.

The plan of care for detoxification should be individualized to account for the considerable variation among patients in terms of signs and symptoms of withdrawal.

Pharmacologic Management

Two general strategies for pharmacologic management of withdrawal are

1. Suppressing withdrawal through use of a cross-tolerant medication
2. Reducing signs and symptoms of withdrawal through alteration of another neuropharmacologic process

To suppress withdrawal with cross-tolerant medication, a longer-acting medication typically is used to provide a milder, controlled withdrawal.

Detoxification alone rarely constitutes adequate treatment!

The maintenance of abstinence can be a very difficult goal to achieve: it has been estimated that approximately *50% of alcohol-dependent patients relapse within 3 months of detoxification.*

Detoxification Settings

In determining the most appropriate setting, the practitioner should match the patients' clinical needs with the least restrictive and most cost-effective setting.

Detoxification is conducted in both inpatient and outpatient settings: both types of settings initiate recovery programs that may include referrals for problems such as medical, legal, psychiatric, and family issues.

Inpatient Detoxification

Inpatient detoxification is offered in medical hospitals, psychiatric hospitals, and medically managed residential treatment programs. It allows 24-hour supervision, observation, and support for patients who are intoxicated or experiencing withdrawal.

Inpatient detoxification may have several advantages to outpatient detoxification:

1. The inpatient detoxification restricts the patient's access to substances of abuse.
2. Inpatient detoxification allows the clinician to closely monitor the patient for serious withdrawal symptoms and adjust medications as indicated.
3. Detoxification in an inpatient facility can be accomplished more rapidly than in an outpatient setting.

Relative indications for inpatient treatment re: ALCOHOL: (NB: 20% of those undergoing treatment for alcohol withdrawal must be treated as inpatients)

1. History of alcohol withdrawal seizures or delirium
2. Pregnancy
3. Medical or psychiatric illness
4. Lack of a reliable support system

Inpatient care of alcohol withdrawal can be *10 to 20 times as expensive* as outpatient care. Generally, therefore, it is *reserved for those expected to have severe withdrawal symptoms* and to *require a more intensive level of care* (such as patients with a history of severe withdrawal symptoms).

Outpatient Detoxification

Essential components to a successful outpatient detoxification include a positive and helpful social support network and regular accessibility to the treatment provider.

Advantages of outpatient detoxification:

1. Much less expensive than inpatient treatment
2. Less life disruption as compared with inpatient setting
3. Avoids abrupt transition from a protected inpatient setting to the everyday home and work settings

For the substance-abusing individual who has overdosed or who is experiencing a medical complication of abuse, the emergency department may be the initial point of contact with the health care system and serve as a source of case identification and referral to detoxification.

Considerations in Selecting a Setting

The patient's needs should drive the selection of the most appropriate detox setting as follows:

1. Severity of the patient's withdrawal symptoms
2. The intensity of care required to ensure appropriate management of these symptoms

The use of the ASAM Patient Placement Criteria

ASAM PPC-2R is intended for use as a clinical tool for matching patients to appropriate levels of care.

The ASAM criteria describe levels of treatment that are differentiated by the following characteristics: (a) degree of direct medical management provided; (b) degree of structure, safety, and security provided; and (c) degree of treatment intensity provided.

Relapse

Many individuals undergo detoxification more than once, and some do so many times. When recently dependent persons return for repeat detoxification, it generally is with a more realistic expectation of what is needed to remain free from alcohol and other drugs.

SPECIAL POPULATIONS

Pregnant and Nursing Women

Withdrawal from opioids can result in fetal distress, which can lead to premature labor or miscarriage. Federal panels recommend that all pregnant and nursing women be advised of the potential risks of drugs that are excreted in breast milk. Nevertheless, they advise that detoxification protocols should not be modified for nursing women unless there is specific evidence that the detoxification medication enters the breast milk in amounts that could be harmful to the nursing infant.

Persons who are HIV Positive

A diagnosis of HIV infection does not change the indications for detoxification medications, which can be used in HIV-positive persons in the same way they are used in uninfected patients. However, the treatment provider does need to be aware of the possible drug interactions between antiretroviral agents used to treat HIV and medications used in detoxification and adjust dosages accordingly.

Patients with Other Medical Conditions

Neurologic Disorders

- Brain-injured patients are at risk for seizures; therefore, *slower medication tapers should be used in these patients.*
- Doses of anticonvulsant medications should be stabilized before sedative-hypnotic withdrawal begins.

Cardiovascular Disorders

- Require continued clinical assessment
- Underlying cardiac disease may be worsened by the symptoms of autonomic arousal (elevated blood pressure, increased pulse and sweating) as seen in alcohol, sedative, and opioid withdrawal.
- May be necessary to withdraw the medication at a slower than normal rate

Hepatic or Renal Disorders

- The use of shorter-acting detoxification drugs and a slower taper are appropriate for such patients but require precautions against drug accumulation and oversedation.

Chronic Pain

- Treatment providers should exercise caution when prescribing medications for chronic pain in patients who have a history of addictive disorders.
- In a large secondary data analysis of chronic users of opioids for chronic noncancer pain, a diagnosis of nonopioid substance abuse was the strongest predictor of opioid abuse/dependence. Mental health disorders were also moderately strong predictors of opioid abuse/dependence in this group.

Patients with Psychiatric Comorbidities

It is difficult to accurately assess underlying psychopathology in a patient who is undergoing detoxification. *Thorough psychiatric evaluation should be conducted after 2 to 3 weeks of abstinence.*

Abrupt cessation of psychotherapeutic medications may cause withdrawal symptoms or reemergence of symptoms of the underlying psychopathology.

During detoxification, some patients decompensate into psychosis, depression, or severe anxiety. In such cases, careful evaluation of the withdrawal medication regimen is of paramount importance.

If withdrawal medications are adequate and appropriate but the patient continues to decompensate, nonaddicting psychotropic medications (such as antipsychotics, anticonvulsants, or antidepressants) may be indicated for the treatment of psychoses, depression, or anxiety emerging during withdrawal.

Adolescents Physical dependence is often not as severe in the adolescent compared with the adult, and *the adolescent patient's response to detoxification usually is more rapid than that of the adult.*

Inquiring about academic performance, school attendance, and disciplinary problems can be particularly important to help the practitioner ascertain the adolescent's risk of a substance use disorder. Behavioral problems may be more indirect, and the potential for suicide needs to be evaluated carefully.

Substance abuse, particularly when comorbid with depression, contributes to an increased rate of suicide in this age group.

Adolescents should be housed separately from adults.

Older Adults

(1) Increased likelihood of medical comorbidities with multiple prescribed medications and prescribing physicians.
(2) Greater access to prescription medications (which may be abused).
(3) Possible impaired mobility from either social isolation or general medical conditions resulting in difficulty accessing clinic or office-based treatment.
(4) The possibility of drug interactions cannot be ignored.
(5) *Detoxification in a medically monitored or medically managed setting often is required.*
(6) The cumulative effects of years of drinking may lead to more severe withdrawal symptoms in elderly persons.
(7) May be necessary to reduce the doses of detoxification medications because of older patients' slowed metabolism or coexisting medical disorders.

Persons in Criminal Justice Settings Prevalence of dependence in these settings is higher than in the general population. In fact, an estimated 70% of people arrested for violent offenses test positive for substances. According to data from the Arrestee Drug Abuse Monitoring program in 2000, 64% of male arrestees tested positive for at least one of five illicit drugs (cocaine, opioids, marijuana, methamphetamines, and PCP) and 36% reported heavy drinking in the 30 days before arrest. Detoxification protocols need not be modified for incarcerated persons, except to the extent that state laws restrict the use of methadone or buprenorphine in criminal justice settings. In such cases, linkages with local methadone detoxification programs are advised.

CONCLUSIONS

The recognition and treatment of intoxication and withdrawal states represent important initial steps in the treatment of alcohol or other drug addiction. The primary goal of managing intoxication and withdrawal states is the prevention of morbidity and mortality.

The ASAM PPC-2R can aid the clinician in matching patients to the appropriate levels of care for ongoing treatment of their addictive disorders.

Summary Author: Ashok Krishnamurthy
Michael F. Mayo-Smith

Management of Alcohol Intoxication and Withdrawal

ALCOHOL INTOXICATION

Clinical Picture

As blood alcohol concentration rises, so too does the clinical effect on the individual (Table 42.1).

Management

The medical management of alcohol intoxication and overdose is supportive. The most important goal of management of alcohol intoxication is to prevent harm to the patient from severe respiratory depression, and to protect the airway against aspiration.

Intravenous glucose should be given if rapid testing of blood glucose is not immediately available, as well as intravenous thiamine. Ethanol can impair gluconeogenesis, with an increased risk of hypoglycemia, and chronic alcoholism places the individual at increased risk of thiamine deficiency.

TABLE 42.1	Clinical Effects of Alcohol
Blood alcohol level mg%	**Clinical manifestations**
20–99	Loss of muscular coordination
	Changes in mood, personality, and behavior
100–199	Neurologic impairment with prolonged reaction time, ataxia, incoordination, and mental impairment
200–299	Very obvious intoxication, except in those with marked tolerance
	Nausea, vomiting, marked ataxia
300–399	Hypothermia, severe dysarthria, amnesia, Stage 1 anesthesia
400–799	Onset of alcoholic coma, with precise level depending on degree of tolerance
	Progressive obtundation, decreases in respiration, blood pressure, and body temperature
	Urinary incontinence or retention, reflexes markedly decreased or absent
600–800	Often fatal because of loss of airway protective reflexes from airway obstruction by flaccid tongue, from pulmonary aspiration of gastric contents, or from respiratory arrest from profound central nervous system depression

Alcohol is rapidly absorbed into the bloodstream, so induction of emesis or gastric lavage usually is not indicated unless a substantial ingestion has occurred within the preceding 30 to 60 minutes, or unless other drug ingestion is suspected.

In extreme cases of alcohol intoxication, hemodialysis can be used, because it efficiently removes alcohol, but it is needed only rarely because supportive care usually is sufficient.

Hemoperfusion and forced diuresis are not effective.

There is no known agent that is effective as an alcohol antagonist. Benzodiazepine antagonists such as **flumazenil** do not block or reverse alcohol intoxication.

The acutely intoxicated patient may exhibit some agitation as part of the intoxication syndrome. This is best managed nonpharmacologically. Support and reassurance can go a long way in dealing with agitation in an acutely intoxicated patient.

On rare occasions, if pharmacologic intervention is needed to manage a mildly or moderately intoxicated individual's behavior in a medical setting, intramuscular administration of a rapid-onset, short-acting benzodiazepine (such as **lorazepam**), alone or in combination with a neuroleptic agent such as **haloperidol**, can be useful.

HANGOVER

Hangover is a constellation of unpleasant physical and mental symptoms that occur after a bout of heavy alcohol intake.

Headache, malaise, diarrhea, nausea, and difficulty concentrating are the most common symptoms, often accompanied by sensitivity to light or sound, sweating, and anxiety.

The primary alcohol-related morbidity in light-to-moderate drinkers is hangover.

The pathophysiology of hangover is not completely understood. In part, it is believed to be the effect of the intermediate product of ethanol metabolism, acetaldehyde. In addition congeners, by-products of individual alcohol preparations found primarily in dark liquors such as brandy, whiskey, wine, and tequila, appear to play a role because they increase the frequency and severity of hangover. Clear liquors, such as rum, vodka, and gin, cause hangover less frequently.

Dehydration, electrolyte imbalance, disruption of sleep and other biologic rhythms, increased physical activity while intoxicated, hypoglycemia, and the many hormonal disruptions caused by alcohol may also play contributing roles.

Attentiveness to the quantity and quality of alcohol consumed can have a significant effect on preventing hangover.

ALCOHOL WITHDRAWAL

Clinical Presentation

Alcohol Withdrawal Syndrome In those with physiologic dependence on alcohol, the clinical manifestations of alcohol withdrawal begin 6 to 24 hours after the last drink (Table 42.2).
Early withdrawal signs and symptoms include

- Anxiety
- Sleep disturbances
- Vivid dreams
- Anorexia
- Nausea
- Headache

Physical signs include

- Tachycardia
- Elevation of blood pressure
- Hyperactive reflexes
- Sweating
- Hyperthermia
- Tremors (best brought out by extension of the hands or tongue)

TABLE 42.2 *DSM-IV-TR* Diagnostic Criteria for 291.81 Alcohol Withdrawal

A. Cessation of (or reduction in) alcohol use that has been heavy and prolonged
B. Two (or more) of the following, developing within several hours to a few days after Criterion A:
   (1) Autonomic hyperactivity (e.g., sweating or pulse rate >100)
   (2) Increased hand tremor
   (3) Insomnia
   (4) Nausea or vomiting
   (5) Transient visual, tactile, or auditory hallucinations or illusions
   (6) Psychomotor agitation
   (7) Anxiety
   (8) Grand mal seizures
C. The symptoms in Criterion B cause clinically significant distress or impairment in social, occupational, or other important areas of functioning.
D. The symptoms are not due to a general medical condition and are not better accounted for by another mental disorder.

The following specifier may be applied to a diagnosis of alcohol withdrawal.

With Perceptual Disturbances. This specifier may be noted in the rare instance when hallucinations with intact reality testing or auditory, visual, or tactile illusions occur in the absence of a delirium. *Intact reality testing* means that the person knows that the hallucinations are induced by the substance and do not represent external reality. When hallucinations occur in the absence of intact reality testing, a diagnosis of substance-induced psychotic disorder, with hallucinations, should be considered.

DSM-IV-TR Diagnostic Criteria for Alcohol Withdrawal Delirium

A. Disturbance of consciousness (i.e., reduced clarity of awareness of the environment) with reduced ability to focus, sustain, or shift attention.
B. A change in cognition (such as memory deficit, disorientation, language disturbance) or the development of a perceptual disturbance that is not better accounted for by a preexisting, established, or evolving dementia.
C. The disturbance develops over a short period (usually hours to days) and tends to fluctuate during the course of the day.
D. There is evidence from the history, physical examination, or laboratory findings that the symptoms in Criteria A and B developed during, or shortly after, an alcohol withdrawal syndrome.

Note: This diagnosis should be made instead of a diagnosis of substance withdrawal only when the cognitive symptoms are in excess of those usually associated with the withdrawal syndrome and when the symptoms are sufficiently severe to warrant independent clinical attention.

From American Psychiatric Association. *Diagnostic and statistical manual of mental disorders*, 4th ed. (Text revision). Washington, DC: American Psychiatric Association, copyright © 2000.

Hallucinations

In mild alcohol withdrawal, patients may experience perceptual distortions of a visual, auditory, and tactile nature.

Visual hallucinations are most common and frequently involve some type of animal life, such as seeing a dog or rodent in the room.

Auditory hallucinations may begin as unformed sounds (such as clicks or buzzing) and progress to formed voices. In contrast to the auditory hallucinations of schizophrenia, which may be of religious or political significance, these voices often are of friends or relatives and frequently are accusatory in nature.

Tactile hallucinations may involve a sensation of bugs or insects crawling on the skin.

Alcohol Withdrawal Seizures These most often present as Grand mal seizures. Withdrawal seizures usually begin within 8 to 24 hours after the patient's last drink and may occur before the blood alcohol level has returned to zero. Although 3% of withdrawal seizures evolve into status epilepticus, alcohol withdrawal has been found to be a contributing cause in up to 15% of status epilepticus patients. *Seizures peak 24 hours after the last drink.* The risk of withdrawal seizures appears to be in part genetically determined and is increased in patients with a history of prior withdrawal seizures, or in those who are undergoing concurrent withdrawal from benzodiazepines or other sedative-hypnotic drugs.

Also, evidence exists that the risk of seizures increases as an individual undergoes repeated withdrawals. This association has been described as a "kindling effect."

Alcohol Withdrawal Delirium

For up to 90% of patients, withdrawal does not progress beyond the mild to moderate symptoms described previously, peaking between 24 and 36 hours and gradually subsiding. In other patients, however, manifestations can include delirium.

In the classic cases of withdrawal delirium, the manifestations of withdrawal steadily worsen and progress into a severe life-threatening delirium accompanied by an autonomic storm, hence the term *delirium tremens* (DTs).

DTs generally appear 72 to 96 hours after the last drink. In their classic presentation, *DTs are marked by all the signs and symptoms of mild withdrawal but in a much more pronounced form,* with the development of marked tachycardia, tremor, diaphoresis, and fever. The patient develops global confusion and disorientation to place and time.

Hallucinations are frequent, and the patient may have no insight into them. Marked psychomotor activity may develop, with severe agitation in some cases. Severe disruption of the normal sleep-wake cycle also is common.

The duration of the delirium is variable, but averages 2 to 3 days in most studies.

Alcohol Withdrawal Severity Scales

The most extensively studied of the scales and best known is the Clinical Institute Withdrawal Assessment-Alcohol, or CIWA, and a shortened version known as the CIWA-A Revised, or CIWA-Ar.

CIWA-Ar has well-documented reliability, reproducibility, and validity based on comparisons to ratings of withdrawal severity by experienced clinicians.

In the case of the CIWA-Ar, a score of 9 indicates mild withdrawal; a score of 10 to 18 moderate withdrawal; and a score of greater than 18 severe withdrawal.

Predictors of Severe Withdrawal

Withdrawal scales can also contribute to appropriate triage of patients as it has been shown that *high scores early in the course are predictive of the development of seizures and delirium.*

Those with low scores on withdrawal scales over the first 24 hours have consistently been found to be at little or no risk for severe withdrawal.

Other risk factors for severe withdrawal include

- A history of prior DTs or withdrawal seizures
- Marked autonomic hyperactivity
- Elevated blood alcohol level of 100 mg/dL or higher at the time of admission
- Serum electrolyte abnormalities
- Medical comorbidity, particularly infection

Pathophysiology

Alcohol exerts its effects in part by directly or indirectly enhancing the effect of GABA, a major inhibitory neurotransmitter.

GABA mediates typical sedative-hypnotic effects such as sedation, muscle relaxation, and a raised seizure threshold.

Chronic alcohol intake leads to an adaptive suppression of GABA activity.

A sudden relative deficiency in GABA neurotransmitter activity is produced with alcohol abstinence and is believed to contribute to the anxiety, increased psychomotor activity, and predisposition to seizures seen in withdrawal.

Although alcohol enhances the effect of GABA, it inhibits the sensitivity of autonomic adrenergic systems, with a resulting upregulation with chronic alcohol intake. The discontinuation of alcohol leads to rebound overactivity of the brain and peripheral noradrenergic systems. Increased sympathetic autonomic activity contributes to such acute manifestations as tachycardia, hypertension, tremor, diaphoresis, and anxiety.

TABLE 42.3   **Examples of Specific Pharmacologic Treatment Regimens**

Monitoring

Monitor the patient every 4–8 h using the CIWA-Ar until the score has been below 8–10 for 24 h; use additional assessments as needed.

Symptom-Triggered Medication Regimens

Administer one of the following medications every hour when the CIWA-Ar is >8–10:

- Chlordiazepoxide, 50–100 mg
- Diazepam, 10–20 mg
- Oxazepam, 30–60 mg
- Lorazepam, 2–4 mg

(Other benzodiazepines may be used at equivalent substitutions.)

Repeat the CIWA-Ar 1 hour after every dose to assess need for further medication.

Structured Medication Regimens

The physician may feel that the development of even mild-to-moderate withdrawal should be prevented in certain patients (e.g., in a patient experiencing a myocardial infarction) and thus may order medications to be given on a predetermined schedule. One of the following regimens could be used in such a situation:

- Chlordiazepoxide, 50 mg, every 6 h for four doses, then 25 mg every 6 h for eight doses.
- Diazepam, 10 mg, every 6 h for four doses, then 5 mg every 6 h for eight doses.
- Lorazepam, 2 mg, every 6 h for four doses, then 1 mg every 6 h for eight doses.

(Other benzodiazepines may be substituted at equivalent doses.)

- Carbamazepine, 300–400 mg, twice daily on day 1, tapering to 200 mg as single dose on day 5.

It is very important that patients receiving medication on a predetermined schedule be monitored closely and that additional benzodiazepine be provided should the doses given prove inadequate.

Agitation and Delirium

For the patient who displays increasing agitation or hallucinations that have not responded to oral benzodiazepines alone, one of the following medications may be used:

- Haloperidol, 2–5 mg, intramuscularly alone or in combination with 2–4 mg of lorazepam.
- Intravenous diazepam given slowly every 5 min until the patient is lightly sedated. Begin with 5 mg for two doses. If needed, increase to 10 mg for two doses, then 20 mg every 5 min. Given the risk of respiratory depression, the patient on this regimen should be closely monitored, with equipment for respiratory support immediately available.

(Other phenothiazines and benzodiazepines may be substituted at equivalent doses.)

Genetics

The role of genetics in alcohol withdrawal is a topic of active investigation. To date, no relationship with genes involved in the serotonin, GABAergic or opioidergic systems have been found. Although these findings are not of immediate clinical use, genetic studies may shed light on basic pathophysiology and at some point assist in identifying high-risk individuals who may benefit from tailored therapy.

MANAGEMENT OF ALCOHOL WITHDRAWAL SYNDROMES (SEE TABLE 42.3)

Pharmacologic Management of Uncomplicated Withdrawal Syndrome

Benzodiazepines are pharmacologically cross-tolerant with alcohol and have the similar effect of enhancing the effect of GABA-induced sedation.

Benzodiazepines alleviate the acute deficiency of GABA neurotransmitter activity that occurs with sudden cessation of alcohol intake.

Trials comparing different benzodiazepines indicate that all are similarly efficacious in reducing signs and symptoms of withdrawal.

Longer-acting agents such as **diazepam** and **chlordiazepoxide** may be more effective in preventing seizures. Longer-acting agents also may contribute to an overall smoother withdrawal course, with a reduction in breakthrough or rebound symptoms. Longer-acting agents can pose a risk of excess sedation in some patients, including elderly persons and patients with significant liver disease. In such patients, shorter-acting agents such as **lorazepam** or **oxazepam** may be preferable.

Certain agents with rapid onset of action (such as **diazepam**, **alprazolam**, and **lorazepam**) demonstrate greater abuse potential than do agents with a slower onset of action (such as **chlordiazepoxide** and **oxazepam**).

Benzodiazepines have a greater margin of safety, with a lower risk of respiratory depression, as well as overall lower abuse potential than do the nonbenzodiazepine agents. Phenobarbital, a long-acting barbiturate, still is used by some programs, as it is long acting, has well-documented anticonvulsant activity, is inexpensive, and has low abuse liability.

Determining the Dosing Schedule
Symptom-triggered therapy is preferred.

Symptom-triggered therapy also facilitates the delivery of large amounts of medication quickly to patients who evidence rapidly escalating withdrawal and thus reduces the risk of undertreatment that may arise with the use of fixed doses.

However, there may be situations in which the provision of fixed doses remains appropriate. For example, with patients admitted to general medical or surgical wards, the nursing staff may not have the training or experience to implement the regular use of scales to monitor patients. Other patients warranting fixed-dose regimens include those with a history of withdrawal seizures or those with serious medical conditions that could be exacerbated by withdrawal syndrome, such as severe coronary disease.

Whenever fixed doses are given, it is very important that allowances be made to provide additional medication if the fixed dose should prove inadequate to control symptoms.

Treatment should allow for a degree of individualization so that patients can receive large amounts of medication rapidly if needed. In all cases, *medications should be administered by a route that has been shown to have reliable absorption.* Therefore, the benzodiazepines should be administered orally or, when necessary, intravenously. An exception is **lorazepam**, which has good intramuscular and sublingual absorption.

Anticonvulsants
Carbamazepine has been widely used in Europe for alcohol withdrawal and has been shown to be equal in efficacy to benzodiazepines for patients with mild to moderate withdrawal.

Carbamazepine does not potentiate the central nervous system and respiratory depression caused by alcohol, does not inhibit learning (an important side effect of larger doses of benzodiazepines), and has no abuse potential.

Although the evidence base is smaller, tapering doses of sodium valproate could be used in similar fashion.

Patients treated with **carbamazepine** or **sodium valproate** should be monitored using withdrawal scales and receive benzodiazepines should more severe withdrawal symptoms emerge. Both these agents have interactions with other drugs and have hepatic and hematologic toxicities, and thus must be used carefully, if at all, in patients with certain comorbid medical and psychiatric disorders.

Other Agents
Beta-blocking (BB) agents (**atenolol** and **propanolol**) and centrally acting alpha-adrenergic agonists (**clonidine**) limit automonic nervous system activation and are effective in helping with withdrawal symptoms in mild to moderate withdrawal. These agents do not have anticonvulsant activity. BB agents can rarely cause delirium.

Neuroleptic agents slightly reduce withdrawal symptoms, but do not prevent delirium, and may actually increase rate of seizures. They are primarily used to calm agitated patients in withdrawal. They should be used with a benzodiazepine; and preferably one with low risk of seizure activation (**haloperidol**) should be used.

Thiamine
Alcohol-dependent patients are at risk for thiamine deficiency (leading to Wernicke disease and/or Korsakoff syndrome). Wernicke disease is an illness of acute onset characterized by the triad of *mental disturbance, paralysis of eye movements, and ataxia.* The ocular abnormality usually is weakness or paralysis of abduction (sixth nerve palsy), which invariably is bilateral, although rarely symmetric. It is accompanied by diplopia, strabismus, and nystagmus. Mental status changes typically involve a global confusional-apathetic state, but in some patients, a disproportionate disorder of retentive memory (known as Korsakoff psychosis) is apparent. Wernicke disease is a neurologic emergency that should be treated by the immediate parenteral administration of thiamine, with a dose of 50 mg intravenously and 50 mg intramuscularly. The provision of intravenous glucose solutions may exhaust a patient's reserve of B vitamins, acutely precipitating Wernicke disease. *Therefore, intravenous glucose always should be accompanied by the administration of thiamine in the alcohol-dependent patient.*

All patients presenting with alcohol withdrawal should receive 50 to 100 mg of thiamine at the time of presentation, followed by oral supplementation for several weeks. Patients with symptoms of Wernicke disease, those who are to receive glucose containing intravenous solutions, and those at high risk of malnutrition should receive their initial dose parenterally.

Management of the Patient after a Withdrawal Seizure

A careful history of the temporal relationship of alcohol intake to the seizure should be obtained, and the diagnosis of withdrawal seizure should be made *only if there is a clear history of a marked decrease or cessation of drinking in the 24 to 48 hours preceding the seizure.* If a seizure was generalized and without focal elements and if a careful neurologic examination reveals no evidence of focal deficits, there is no suspicion of meningitis and there is no history of recent major head trauma; additional testing has an extremely low yield and may be safely omitted in a pt with alc-related w/d seizure. *Withdrawal seizures often are multiple,* with a second seizure occurring in one case out of four. For the patient who presents with a withdrawal seizure, rapid treatment is indicated to prevent further episodes. The parenteral administration of a rapid-acting benzodiazepine such as **diazepam** or **lorazepam** is effective.

Initial treatment should be followed by oral doses of long-acting benzodiazepines over the ensuing 24 to 48 hours. Early studies indicated that a withdrawal seizure placed the patient at increased risk for progression to DTs, so close monitoring is warranted.

Management of the Patient with Delirium

Though initially tagged with higher mortality rates, mortality has been reduced to <1%.

The principles of successful treatment involve adequate sedation and meticulous supportive medical care.

Such patients require close nursing observation and supportive care, which frequently necessitates admission to an ICU. Careful management of fluids and electrolytes is important, given the patient's inability to manage his own intake and the presence of marked autonomic hyperactivity.

Delirium often is encountered in patients admitted for acute medical problems whose alcohol dependence was not recognized and whose withdrawal was not adequately treated.

The use of cross-tolerant sedative-hypnotics has been shown to reduce mortality in DTs and is recommended.

The use of intravenous benzodiazepines with rapid onset, such as **diazepam**, has been shown to provide more rapid control of the patient's symptoms.

The main complication of therapy with **diazepam** is respiratory depression. Whenever this approach is used, providers should have equipment and personnel immediately available to provide respiratory support if needed. One advantage of **diazepam** is that its peak onset occurs within 5 minutes of intravenous administration. This allows the provider to deliver repeat boluses and titrate sedation quickly without fear of a delayed appearance of oversedation.

Once established, delirium can be expected to last for a number of hours, so **diazepam** offers another advantage in that its longer half-life helps maintain sedation with less chance of breakthrough agitation.

In the agitated patient, benzodiazepines can be supplemented with the addition of neuroleptic agents such as **haloperidol**.

COMMON TREATMENT ISSUES

Location of Treatment Services

All patients presenting for management of withdrawal should undergo a comprehensive history and medical evaluation. For patients with only mild withdrawal symptoms, no history of seizures or DTs, and no concurrent significant medical or psychiatric problems, management on an outpatient basis is reasonable. Such patients should have a responsible individual to monitor them, they should be seen daily until they have stabilized, and ready access, including transportation, to emergency medical services should be available.

In addition, many programs concentrate on sharply reducing the length of stay for patients undergoing withdrawal. Patients may be treated in an observation unit or admitted for a 1-day stay. If significant withdrawal symptoms do not develop and the withdrawal is easily controlled with little or no medication, patients can be discharged or transferred to an intensive outpatient rehabilitation program.

Patients Admitted for Medical/Surgical Treatment

Studies have shown that about 20% of patients admitted to the hospital have alcohol use disorders. As a result, hospital admission is a frequent precipitating event for alcohol withdrawal.

Screening for alcohol problems should be universal at the time of hospital admission but is not yet a common practice.

Patients thus may develop withdrawal that goes unrecognized or becomes far advanced before being recognized and treated. Withdrawal has been shown to contribute to higher postoperative complications, mortality, and length of stay.

The use of alcohol withdrawal scales in general medical/surgical patients have been studied and found to be valuable in selected patients.

Given the frequency of alcohol problems in hospitalized patients, instituting standard screening, assessment, and management protocols is appropriate and has been found to be helpful.

Alcohol Withdrawal in US Jails

Another event that frequently precipitates alcohol withdrawal is arrest and incarceration.

In 1997, surveys showed that of the 11 million individuals arrested, approximately 1.2 million were alcohol-dependent.

In 1997, only 28% of jail administrators reported that their institutions ever provided medically managed withdrawal for arrestees.

Overall in 1997, 750,000 arrestees were at risk for untreated alcohol withdrawal. Because this situation has not changed significantly in the intervening years, it is not surprising that inadequately treated alcohol withdrawal has been shown to contribute to deaths among newly arrested individuals.

That this population is at high risk should be kept in mind as health care professionals encounter patients referred from jails with possible withdrawal symptoms.

CHAPTER 43

Summary Author: Ashok Krishnamurthy
William E. Dickinson • Steven J. Eickelberg

Management of Sedative-Hypnotic Intoxication and Withdrawal

INTRODUCTION

Sedative hypnotics stimulate the inhibitory neurotransmitters in the GABA receptors.

Although all sedatives and hypnotics have mild stimulant properties at low doses, their primary effect is to inhibit central nervous system function.

SEDATIVE-HYPNOTIC INTOXICATION AND OVERDOSE

Clinical Picture

The signs and symptoms of sedative-hypnotic intoxication and overdose are similar for the various drugs in the class (Table 43.1).

Mild to moderate toxicity

- Slurred speech
- Ataxia
- Uncoordination(similar to that seen with alcohol intoxication)

On occasion, particularly in the older adults

- Paradoxical agitation
- Confusion
- Delirium

More severe intoxication

- Stupor
- Coma develop

TABLE 43.1 Diagnosis of Sedative-Hypnotic Overdose
History
• Sedative-hypnotic use (ask about drug, amount, time of last use)
• Polydrug abuse
• Use multiple sources of information (family, hospital records, etc.)
Physical Examination
• Central nervous system depression
• Respiratory depression
Laboratory Tests
• Rule out hypoglycemia, acidemia, and fluid and electrolyte abnormalities
• Toxicology screens for sedative hypnotics and other drugs

With the older nonbenzodiazepine agents, toxicity may progress, ultimately leading to fatal respiratory arrest or cardiovascular collapse.

An additional problem with several of the older sedative hypnotics is that with regular use, tolerance may develop to the drugs' therapeutic effects, but not to their lethal effects. The maintenance dose then may approach the lethal dose and the therapeutic index decreases. Toxicity and overdose thus can occur with only small increases over the individual's regular intake.

On the other hand, benzodiazepines rarely lead to death when ingested by themselves.

A lethal dose has not been established for any of the benzodiazepines and there are very few well-documented cases of death from ingestion of benzodiazepines alone.

The few deaths that have occurred all involved short-acting, high-potency benzodiazepines such as **alprazolam** and **triazolam** or administration of benzodiazepines by an intravenous route.

Mixed overdoses—such as those involving benzodiazepines in combination with alcohol, major tranquilizers, antidepressants, or opiates—can be fatal. This result is true for the nonbenzodiazepine agents as well.

Management

Sedative-Hypnotic Overdose Most important: assessment and maintenance of the airway and, ± ventilatory support

Phenobarbital, **meprobamate**, **glutethimide**, and **ethchlorvynol** can form concretions in the stomach. Evacuation of the gastrointestinal tract with a large-bore orogastric tube is the next step, provided an active gag reflex is elicited or the airway is protected by intubation.

Flumazenil is a competitive benzodiazepine receptor antagonist with very weak agonist properties at the benzodiazepine receptor. It can reverse the sedative effects of benzodiazepines, but not of the other agents or alcohol.

- It has found a role in reversing the effects of short-acting benzodiazepines, such as **midazolam**, after medical procedures. It also may be used when benzodiazepines have been ingested alone as an overdose.
- The effects of **flumazenil** are short-lived, and symptoms may return in 30 to 60 minutes. Moreover, its use has been associated with seizures and cardiac arrhythmias.
- Persons who are physiologically dependent on benzodiazepines are at higher risk of seizures.

SEDATIVE-HYPNOTIC WITHDRAWAL

Overview

The use of most sedative, hypnotic, or anxiolytic agents can result in the development of psychological dependence, physical dependence, or addiction.

The development of dependence to sedative-hypnotic compounds is similar across the classes of the benzodiazepines, the barbiturates, and the nonbarbiturate/nonbenzodiazepine agents.

Differences in withdrawal syndrome characteristics among sedative-hypnotic compounds primarily reflect differences in the rate at which dependence is induced, the rapidity with which symptoms occur on discontinuation of the drug, and the severity of those symptoms.

A clinically significant withdrawal syndrome is most apt to occur after discontinuation of daily therapeutic dose (low dose) use of a sedative hypnotic for at least 4 to 6 months or, at doses that exceed two to three times the upper limit of recommended therapeutic use (high dose), for >2 to 3 months.

The time course and severity of the sedative-hypnotic withdrawal syndrome reflect the influences of three pharmacologic factors:

- Dose
- Duration of use
- Duration of drug action

Latency to onset of withdrawal is related to the elimination half-life.

Signs and Symptoms of Discontinuation

Most patients experience significant moment-to-moment quantitative and qualitative variations in their signs and symptoms (see Table 43.2).

Very Frequent: Anxiety, insomnia, restlessness, agitation, irritability, and muscle tension.

Less Frequent: Nausea, diaphoresis, lethargy, aches and pains, coryza, hyperacusis, blurred vision, nightmares, depression, hyperreflexia, and ataxia.

TABLE 43.2	**Clinical Manifestations of Sedative-Hypnotic Withdrawal**

Vital Signs
- Tachycardia
- Hypertension
- Fever

Central Nervous System
- Agitation
- Anxiety
- Delirium
- Hallucinations
- Insomnia
- Irritability
- Nightmares

- Sensory disturbances
- Tremor

Ears
- Tinnitus

Gastrointestinal
- Anorexia
- Diarrhea
- Nausea

High-Dose (Severe) Withdrawal
- Seizures
- Delirium
- Death

Benzodiazepine Discontinuation

The signs and symptoms experienced after the discontinuation of benzodiazepines have been described as falling into four categories:

1. *Symptom recurrence or relapse*
2. *Rebound*
3. *Pseudowithdrawal*
4. *True withdrawal*

Symptom recurrence or relapse is characterized by the recurrence of symptoms (such as insomnia or anxiety) for which the benzodiazepine initially was taken. Symptom recurrence can present rapidly or slowly over days to months after drug discontinuation.

Rebound is marked by the development of symptoms, within hours to days of drug discontinuation, which are qualitatively similar to the disorder for which the benzodiazepine initially was prescribed. However, the symptoms are transiently more intense than they were before drug treatment. Rebound symptoms are of short duration and are self-limited, which distinguishes this syndrome from recurrence.

Pseudowithdrawal and overinterpretation of symptoms may occur when expectations of withdrawal lead to the experiencing of abstinence symptoms.

True withdrawal: Psychological and somatic signs and symptoms after the discontinuation of benzodiazepines in an individual who is physically dependent on the drug. The withdrawal syndrome can be suppressed by the reinstitution of the discontinued benzodiazepine or another cross-tolerant sedative hypnotic. Withdrawal reflects a relative temporal and temporary diminution of central nervous system GABAergic neuronal inhibition coupled with an increased glutamate response to balance the benzodiazepine-induced GABA release.

Any combination of signs and symptoms (Table 43.2) may be experienced with varying severity throughout the initial 1 to 4 weeks of abstinence.

None of the signs or symptoms of the abstinence syndrome are pathognomonic of benzodiazepine withdrawal.

The clinical withdrawal picture can consist primarily of subjective symptoms, accompanied by few or no concurrently observable hyperadrenergic signs or vital sign fluctuations (as seen with acute alcohol withdrawal).

Considerable overlap exists between the symptoms of recurrence in anxiety and insomnia disorders and the signs and symptoms of rebound and withdrawal.

Clinical techniques that treat, minimize, and attenuate benzodiazepine abstinence symptoms also effectively alleviate rebound.

As a result, attention to sorting out rebound from withdrawal is unnecessary (if not impossible). However, symptom recurrence or relapse is common. Clinicians must be attuned to the emergence or persistence of clinically important symptoms of relapse during and after the period of acute withdrawal.

Prolonged Withdrawal The signs and symptoms may persist for weeks to months after discontinuation.

The syndrome is notable for its irregular and unpredictable day-to-day course and qualitative and quantitative differences in symptoms from both the prebenzodiazepine use state and the acute withdrawal period.

Patients with prolonged withdrawal often experience slowly abating—albeit characteristic waxing and waning—symptoms of insomnia, perceptual disturbances, tremor, sensory hypersensitivities, and anxiety.

Role of the GABA-Benzodiazepine Receptor Complex

Benzodiazepine action in the central nervous system is mediated by the γ-aminobutyric acid–benzodiazepine receptor-complex (GABA-BDZ-R-complex) primarily the $GABA_A$ receptor.

GABA is the primary central nervous system inhibitory neurotransmitter.

The amino acid L-glutamate is the major excitatory neurotransmitter in the central nervous system.

Benzodiazepine administration increases the inhibition effect of the GABA system while also beginning a compensatory excitation effect of the glutamate system as a counterbalancing response.

The continued or increased use of benzodiazepines results in a new balance of these neuronal systems.

When the benzodiazepine is lessened or stopped, the increased activity of the glutamate system is seen.

Thus rebound anxiety, increased muscle tone, sensory disturbances, tremors, and seizures can be related to the increased glutamate.

Pharmacologic Characteristics Affecting Withdrawal

Pharmacokinetics Benzodiazepine pharmacokinetics determines the onset of discontinuation symptoms following chronic use.

The onset, duration, and severity of the withdrawal syndrome correlate with declining serum levels of drug.

Onset of withdrawal from short-acting benzodiazepines (such as **lorazepam**, **oxazepam**, **triazolam**, **alprazolam**, and **temazepam**) *occurs within 24 hours of cessation,* with *peak severity of withdrawal occurring within 1 to 5 days* after cessation.

Long-acting benzodiazepines (such as **diazepam**, **chlordiazepoxide**, and **clonazepam**): onset of withdrawal *occurs within 5 days* of cessation and *withdrawal severity peaks at 1 to 9 days.*

Duration of acute withdrawal, from the temporal onset to the resolution of symptoms, can *be as long as 7 to 21 days for short-acting* and *10 to 28 days for long-acting benzodiazepines.*

Dose and Duration of Use Higher doses and longer use place patients at greater risk for increased withdrawal severity.

Daily benzodiazepine use for 10 days or less can lead to transient insomnia when the medications are stopped.

Subjects with lower benzodiazepine doses and no previous withdrawal attempts were more successful with discontinuation.

On discontinuation of long-term (>1 year) therapeutic (low-dose) use, withdrawal is common and is accompanied by moderate to severe symptoms in 20% to 100% of patients.

Discontinuation of high-dose (more than four or five times the high end of the therapeutic range for longer than 6–12 weeks) benzodiazepine use leads to moderate withdrawal in all patients, and severe withdrawal signs and symptoms in most patients.

Beyond 1 year of continuous benzodiazepine therapy, the duration of use becomes a less important factor in the severity of withdrawal.

Potency Tolerance to the sedative and hypnotic effects develops most rapidly to shorter-acting, higher-potency benzodiazepines (such as **triazolam** and **alprazolam**). *Withdrawal from these agents may be more intense* and require more aggressive attention and longer periods of medical monitoring than is the case with other benzodiazepines.

Host Factors Affecting Withdrawal

Psychiatric Comorbidity Numerous benzodiazepine discontinuation studies highlight the high (40%–100%) prevalence of active concurrent psychiatric disorders seen at intake of study participants. Most of these studies demonstrate a correlation between the patients' degree of psychopathology and their withdrawal symptom severity and difficulty in discontinuing use.

The intensity of the withdrawal syndrome is often partially a function of the degree of psychopathology and other premorbid personality variables.

Increased withdrawal symptoms also have been associated with high initial anxiety or depression and decreased educational level.

Clinicians conducting benzodiazepine discontinuation thus must obtain psychiatric histories while remaining vigilantly watchful for, and prepared to manage, the emergence or reemergence of psychiatric disorders.

The reduction of fear and anxiety symptoms during withdrawal was the best predictor of a patient's success for achieving and maintaining abstinence.

Concurrent Use of Other Substances Concurrent regular use of other dependence-producing substances increases the complexity of the benzodiazepine abstinence syndrome and the clinical situation as a whole.

Additional sedative-hypnotic substance use contributes to a withdrawal syndrome of increased severity and less predictable course.

For example, anxiety, agitation, irritation, hyperarousal, and the adrenergic components of opioid and benzodiazepine withdrawal are additive, often overlap, and lead to an exacerbation of symptoms.

Psychomotor stimulant withdrawal symptoms contribute factors from the opposite end of the withdrawal spectrum (e.g., apathy, hypersomnia, and lethargy). When stimulant withdrawal is combined with sedative-hypnotic withdrawal, the clinical picture is variable, with hypersomnolence and lethargy mixed with symptoms of severe agitation, depression, irritability, and somatosensory hypersensitivity.

Moderate alcohol use (exceeding one beer or drink per day) is a more significant predictor of benzodiazepine withdrawal severity than dose or half-life of the drug.

- A high percentage of alcohol-dependent patients use benzodiazepines regularly, ranging from 29% to 76%.
- Alcohol-dependent patients have a high propensity for dependence on benzodiazepines.

It is uncommon for patients with drug addictions to use a benzodiazepine as an initial or primary drug of use.

Consequently, clinicians must be aware of, and suspect, benzodiazepine use in patients with any substance use disorders.

Conversely, in high-dose benzodiazepine users, other substance use must be assumed until ruled out.

Family History of Alcohol Dependence Studies show a predisposition to abuse benzodiazepines in those with family history of alcoholism.

There has been a linkage of paternal history of alcoholism with increased withdrawal severity in patients discontinuing alprazolam use.

Concurrent Medical Conditions Benzodiazepine withdrawal should be avoided during acute medical or surgical conditions because the physiologic stress of withdrawal can adversely and unnecessarily affect the course of the medical condition.

Continued benzodiazepine use rarely has a negative effect on acute medical conditions.

In an acute medical situation, the goal of therapy for a patient dependent on benzodiazepines is to provide adequate stabilization of the benzodiazepine dose so as to prevent withdrawal.

In general, patients with chronic medical conditions experience benzodiazepine withdrawal more severely than others.

The rate of discontinuation is an important factor. Slower rates can improve the success of detoxification. Achieving lower doses of benzodiazepine use is an acceptable intermediate (and, in some patients, final) goal.

Age Elderly patients may have elimination half-lives that are two to five times slower than the rate in younger adults for benzodiazepines eliminated through the microsomal enzyme oxidase system (all benzodiazepines except for **lorazepam**, **temazepam**, and **oxazepam**.)

The withdrawal course can become especially pernicious after discontinuation of long-acting benzodiazepines that are metabolized to sedative-hypnotic compounds with longer elimination half-lives (such as **diazepam**, **chlordiazepoxide**, and **flurazepam**).

In general, younger age is associated with favorable withdrawal outcomes.

Gender Worldwide, *women are prescribed benzodiazepines twice as often as men*; hence, *twice as many women as men are likely to become dependent.*

Female gender is a significant predictor of increased withdrawal severity in patients undergoing tapered cessation of long-term, therapeutic benzodiazepine use. (However, gender has not been implicated as an influential factor in abrupt cessation of long-term, therapeutic dose use.)

PATIENT EVALUATION AND MANAGEMENT

Evaluation and Assessment

To be effective, the clinician must be flexible and able to tolerate ambiguities and variations in the course of withdrawal, while supporting the patient (who generally experiences significant apprehension and anxiety).

Step 1

1. Determine the reasons the patient or referral source is seeking evaluation of sedative-hypnotic use.
2. Determine the indications for the patient's drug use.
3. A discussion with the referring physician should be standard practice.
4. Discuss the patient's expectations.

Step 2

1. Take a sedative-hypnotic use history, including, at a minimum, the dose, duration of use, substances used, and the patient's clinical response to sedative-hypnotic use at present and over time.
2. History highlights

- Attempts at abstinence (including previous detoxifications)
- Symptoms experienced with changing the dose
- Reasons for increasing or decreasing the dose
- Behavioral responses to sedative-hypnotic use
- Adverse or toxic side effects

Step 3

1. Elicit a detailed accounting of other alcohol or psychoactive drug use.
2. Include prior periods of abstinence and abstinence attempts.

Step 4

1. Take a psychiatric history.
2. Ask if alcohol or other drugs were used during or near the time any psychiatric diagnoses were made.
3. Personality assessments may help identify patients who may be more suitable to attempt withdrawal. High levels of dependency, passivity, neuroticism, and harm avoidance on the Minnesota Multiphasic Personality Inventory contributed to increased withdrawal severity.

Step 5 Take a family history of substance use, psychiatric disorders, and medical disorders.

Step 6 Take a medical history of the patient, including illnesses, trauma, surgery, medications, allergies, and history of loss of consciousness, seizures, or seizure disorder.

Step 7 Take a psychosocial history, including current social status and support system.

Step 8 Perform a physical and mental status examination.

Step 9 Conduct a laboratory urine drug screen for substances of abuse. Depending on the patient's profile, a complete blood count, blood chemistry panel, liver enzymes, viral hepatitis panel, HIV test, tuberculosis test, pregnancy test, or electrocardiogram test may be indicated.

Step 10 Complete an individualized assessment.

Step 11 Arrive at a differential diagnosis.

Step 12 Determine the most efficacious detoxification method. In addition to proven clinical and pharmacologic efficacy, the method selected should be one that the physician and clinical staff in the detoxification setting are comfortable with and experienced in administering.

Step 13 Obtain the patient's informed consent.

Step 14 Initiate detoxification. An individualized discontinuation program should be initiated. To achieve optimal results, the physician and patient will need to establish a close working relationship. A withdrawal contract is a useful tool.

Management
Strategies for discontinuation fall into two categories: *minimal intervention* and *systematic discontinuation*.

- Minimal intervention delivers simple advice to discontinue the benzodiazepine.
- *Minimal interventions are more effective in low dose users.*

Systematic Discontinuation
For patients who are dependent on sedative hypnotics, there are two primary options for the detoxification process: *tapering* or *substitution and tapering*.

Gradual dose reduction (tapering) is the most widely used and most logical method of benzodiazepine discontinuation—indicated for use in

- Ambulatory setting
- Patients on a therapeutic dose
- Benzodiazepine-only patients
- Patients with proper follow-up

Tapering
- Fixed-dose taper schedule used.
- The dose is decreased on a weekly to every-other-week basis.
- The rate of discontinuation for long-term users (>1 year) should not exceed 5 mg **diazepam** equivalents per week (12.5 mg **chlordiazepoxide** or 15 mg **phenobarbital** equivalents) or 10% of the current (starting) dose per week, whichever is smaller.
- *The first 50% of the taper is usually smoother, quicker, and less symptomatic than the last 50%.*
- For the final 25% to 35% of the taper, the rate or dose reduction schedule should be slowed to half the previous dose reduction per week and the reduction accomplished at twice the original tapering interval.
- If symptoms of withdrawal occur, the dose should be increased slightly until the symptoms resolve and the subsequent taper schedule commenced at a slower rate.
- As a general rule, patients tolerate more dose reduction and with shorter intervals early in the tapering process and then require decreased dose reduction over longer intervals as the taper progresses and the dose is reduced.
- A common error is trying to push the taper process too quickly.
- Brief office visits should be conducted at least weekly.
- Prescriber should give a clear message to the patient that lost or stolen medication will not be replaced.

Substitution and Taper
Substitution and taper methods employ cross-tolerant long-acting benzodiazepines (such as **chlordiazepoxide** or **clonazepam**) or **phenobarbital** to substitute, at equipotent doses, for the sedative hypnotics on which the patient is dependent (Table 43.3).
Chlordiazepoxide, clonazepam, and **phenobarbital** are the most widely used substitution agents for a number of important reasons.

- At steady state, there is negligible interdose serum level variation with these drugs; with tapering, a more gradual reduction in serum levels, reducing the risk of that withdrawal symptoms will emerge.
- Each of the drugs has a low abuse potential (**phenobarbital** is lowest, followed by **clonazepam** and then **chlordiazepoxide**).

Clinical experience shows that **phenobarbital** is most useful and effective in patients with polysubstance dependence, high-dose dependence, and in patients with unknown dose or erratic "polypharmacy" drug use.

TABLE 43.3 Sedative-Hypnotic Withdrawal Substitute Dose Conversions	
Drug	**Dose equal to 30 mg of Phenobarbital (mg)**
Benzodiazepines	
Alprazolam (Xanax)	0.5–1
Chlordiazepoxide (Librium)	25
Clonazepam (Klonopin)	1–2
Clorazepate (Tranxene)	7.5
Diazepam (Valium)	10
Estazolam (ProSom)	1
Flurazepam (Dalmane)	15
Lorazepam (Ativan)	2
Oxazepam (Serax)	10–15
Quazepam (Doral)	15
Temazepam (Restoril)	15
Triazolam (Halcion)	0.25
Barbiturates	
Pentobarbital (Nembutal)	100
Secobarbital (Seconal)	100
Butalbital (Fiorinal)	100
Amobarbital (Amytal)	100
Phenobarbital	30
Nonbarbiturates-nonbenzodiazepines	
Ethchlorvynol (Placidyl)	500
Glutethimide (Doriden)	250
Methyprylon (Noludar)	200
Methaqualone (Quaalude)	300
Meprobamate (Miltown)	1,200
Carisoprodol (Soma)	700
Chloral hydrate (Noctec)	500

Uncomplicated Substitution and Taper Used in *outpatient settings* for patients who are discontinuing use of *short half-life benzodiazepines* or for those who are *unable to tolerate gradual tapering*

1. Calculate the equivalent dose of **chlordiazepoxide, clonazepam,** or **phenobarbital** using the Substitution Dose Conversion Table (Table 43.3). Individual variation in clinical responses to "equivalent" doses can vary, so close clinical monitoring of patient response to substitution is necessary. Adjustments to the initially calculated dose schedule are to be expected.

2. Provide the substituted drug in a divided dose. For **chlordiazepoxide, oxazepam,** or **phenobarbital,** give three to four doses per day. For **clonazepam,** two to three doses per day usually are sufficient.

3. While the substituted agent is achieving steady-state levels on a fixed dose schedule, provide the patient with as-needed (PRN) doses of the benzodiazepine he or she has been using. This will help to suppress breakthrough symptoms of withdrawal. *Do this for the 1st week only* and then discontinue PRN drug dosing.

4. Stabilize the patient on an adequate substitution dose (same dose on consecutive days without the need for regular PRN doses). This usually is accomplished within 1 week.

5. Gradually reduce the dose. The dose is decreased on a weekly to every-other-week basis, as in the simple taper model. The *rate of discontinuation is 5 mg* **diazepam** *equivalents per week* (or 12.5 mg **chlordiazepoxide** equivalents or 15 mg **phenobarbital** equivalents, as shown in Table 43.3, *or 10% of the current* (starting) dose per week. NOTE: The first half of the taper usually is smoother, quicker, and less symptomatic than the latter half.

6. For the final 25% to 35% of the taper, the rate, or dose reduction should be slowed. If symptoms of withdrawal occur, hold the taper for 3 to 4 days to stabilize the patient and then resume the process. Some

patients may wish to accelerate the reduction. This is better tolerated early in the taper. Care should be taken not to push the taper too quickly.

7. Support the patient with short but frequent visits, as described above. *Taper medication should be closely controlled by prescribing only enough medication for the time period until the next visit.*

Sedative-Hypnotic Tolerance Testing   Employed when the degree of dependence is difficult to determine

Useful in high-dose, erratic-dose, illicit source, polysubstance, or alcohol plus sedative-hypnotic use

Testing is best done in a setting that offers 24-hour medical monitoring.

Pentobarbital is used because of

- Rapid onset of action
- Short half-life
- Ease with which signs of toxicity can be monitored
- Ease with which it can be replaced by **phenobarbital** after the patient has been stabilized

1. A 200-mg **pentobarbital** dose is given orally every 2 hours for up to 24 to 48 hours.
2. Doses are held for signs of toxicity (intoxication), which develop in the following progression at increasing serum levels: fine lateral sustained nystagmus, coarse nystagmus, slurred speech, ataxia, and somnolence. Doses are held with the development of coarse nystagmus and slurred speech and subsequently resumed with the resolution of the signs of toxicity.
3. After 24 to 48 hours, the total amount of administered pentobarbital is divided by the number of days it was administered. This amount is the 24-hour stabilizing dose.
4. The stabilizing dose is administered in divided doses over the next 24 hours to ensure adequate substitution. The patient's response determines the indications for upward or downward adjustments in the dose.
5. After the patient is stable on a consistent dose for 24 hours, **phenobarbital** is substituted for **pentobarbital** with 30 mg of **phenobarbital** substituting for 100 mg of **pentobarbital** (Table 43.3).
6. A gradual dose reduction of **phenobarbital** is conducted, as described under Substitution and Tapering above.

Withdrawal Emergence PRN Phenobarbital Substitution   Used in a 24-hour medically monitored setting

It provides the smoothest and most effective treatment for sedative-hypnotic withdrawal for patients who

- are unable to complete outpatient tapering regimens
- are high-dose users
- are polysubstance-dependent
- are experiencing considerable comorbid psychopathology

1. Signs and symptoms of withdrawal are treated PRN with 30 to 60 mg of **phenobarbital** every 1 to 4 hours. (The period of PRN dosing is determined by the elimination of most withdrawal signs and symptoms and is influenced by the duration of action of the substances the patient is discontinuing.)
2. The patient is monitored hourly to ensure adequate dosing and to prevent oversedation. Ideally, a balance is achieved between the signs and symptoms of withdrawal and those of **phenobarbital** intoxication.
3. When the patient has received similar 24-hour **phenobarbital** dose totals for 2 consecutive days, the total dose for those 2 days is divided by 2 to arrive at the stabilizing dose.
4. The stabilizing dose is given in divided-dose increments over the next 24 hours, which may require medication administration every 3 to 4 hours for patients with high tolerance. After the patient is stabilized, a gradual taper is initiated, as described previously.

Appropriate Clinical Setting

Inpatient facility that offers 24-hour medical monitoring is most required in the following cases:

- Polysubstance dependence (including sedatives and hypnotics)
- Mixed alcohol with other sedative-hypnotic use
- High-dose hypnotic sedative use
- Erratic behavior
- Incompatible use histories
- Involvement with illicit sources
- Extensive mental health issues

Adjunctive Withdrawal Management Measures

Anticonvulsants Some anticonvulsants are also beneficial in treating alcohol withdrawal and cocaine intoxication.

There appears to be *no addiction potential with anticonvulsants* and this is a great advantage.

Carbamazepine Initial reports on small clinical trials using *carbamazepine* showed encouraging but mixed effectiveness and utility.

Ries et al. reported protocols for the use of **carbamazepine**: 600 mg per day (usually 200 mg three times per day) is used alone or in combination with a 3-day benzodiazepine taper.

Chlordiazepoxide is useful because of its longer half-life and low abuse potential.

Phenobarbital can be added PRN to this protocol for breakthrough withdrawal symptoms.

Carbamazepine is continued for a minimum of 2 to 3 weeks after the 3-day benzodiazepine taper is completed and can be tapered to monitor for return of withdrawal symptoms.

Elderly patients who are discontinuing benzodiazepines have been treated successfully with **carbamazepine** at doses of 400 to 500 mg per day.

Adverse consequences of **carbamazepine** use can include

• Gastrointestinal upset
• Neutropenia
• Thrombocytopenia
• Hyponatremia

Therefore, initial and ongoing laboratory evaluation and monitoring is necessary.

Sodium Valproate **Sodium valproate** is effective in attenuating the benzodiazepine withdrawal syndrome.

Valproate possesses GABAergic actions and anticonvulsant effects.

Valproate also may suppress NMDA and reduce L-glutamate responses.

Valproate-treated patients were 2.5 times more likely to be benzodiazepine-free at 5 weeks after taper, compared with a placebo group.

Valproate doses of 250 mg three times per day (250 mg two times per day if older than age 60) can be used in combination with a 3-day benzodiazepine taper.

Chlordiazepoxide is a useful choice because of its *long half-life and low abuse potential.*

Calculate the equivalent **chlordiazepoxide** dose for the amount of current benzodiazepine being discontinued. Give one half to two thirds of this dose spaced equally over the 1st day (24 hours), one third spaced equally over the 2nd day (second 24 hours), and 10% to 20% spaced equally over the 3rd day (third 24 hours).

Phenobarbital can be used for breakthrough withdrawal symptoms. **Valproate** is continued for a minimum of 2 to 3 weeks after the 3-day benzodiazepine taper is completed.

Longer treatment may improve the proportion of patients who remain benzodiazepine-free.

Valproate can be tapered to monitor for return of withdrawal symptoms.

Advantages of **Valproate**

1. Treats anxiety
2. Fewer side effects than carbamazepine
3. Both inpatient and outpatient tx possible.

Propranolol **Propranolol** can be used in doses of 60 to 120 mg per day, divided three or four times per day, as an adjunct to one of the aforementioned withdrawal methods.

Propranolol treatment may diminish the severity of adrenergic signs and symptoms of withdrawal.

Clonidine **Clonidine** has been shown to be ineffective in treating benzodiazepine withdrawal

Buspirone **Buspirone** is a nonbenzodiazepine anxiolytic drug that is not cross-tolerant with benzodiazepines or other sedative-hypnotic drugs. **Buspirone** substitution in patients undergoing abrupt or gradual benzodiazepine discontinuation *fails to protect against the symptoms of withdrawal.*

Trazodone Trazodone:

1. Decreased anxiety in benzodiazepine-tapered patients.
2. Improved patients' ability to remain benzodiazepine-free after a 4-week taper of the benzodiazepine.
3. Can be used to improve sleep during benzodiazepine tapering and when benzodiazepine-free.
4. Side effects may include dry mouth, morning hangover, drowsiness, dizziness, and priapism.

Prolonged Benzodiazepine Withdrawal

A small proportion of patients, after long-term benzodiazepine use, experience a prolonged syndrome in which withdrawal signs and symptoms persist for weeks to months after discontinuation.

Irregular and unpredictable day-to-day course and qualitative and quantitative differences in symptoms from both the prebenzodiazepine use state and the acute withdrawal period.

Patients with prolonged withdrawal often experience slowly abating, albeit characteristic, waxing and waning symptoms of insomnia, perceptual disturbances, tremor, sensory hypersensitivities, and anxiety.

Management Before entertaining the existence of a prolonged withdrawal syndrome, physicians must rule out psychiatric conditions.

Propranolol in doses of 10 to 20 mg four times per day often is helpful in attenuating anxiety or tremors.

Lower doses of sedating antidepressant medications—such as **trazodone**, **amitriptyline**, **imipramine**, or **doxepin**—are helpful in treating insomnia

Frequent clinical follow-up for education, supportive psychotherapy, and regular reassurance are strongly advised.

COMMON TREATMENT ISSUES

Among sedative-hypnotic users, treatment most often is indicated for polysubstance users, high-dose users, or patients in whom addiction is diagnosed.

Prevention

The best prevention for prescribed benzodiazepine dependence is careful prescribing.

Benzodiazepines are rarely the first-line treatment for any of the anxiety disorders. Cognitive-behavioral therapy, group therapy, relaxation therapy, stress management, structured problem solving, selective serotonin reuptake inhibitors, tricyclic antidepressants, and buspirone are all potential options that should be employed as appropriate based on the level of severity.

If used, benzodiazepines should be closely monitored for effectiveness and duration.

A plan to reassess or taper the benzodiazepine when it is first given is wise.

Reevaluate the need for the benzodiazepine when the initial indication has changed or the patient shows improvement.

Summary Author: Ashok Krishnamurthy
Jeanette M. Tetrault • Patrick G. O'Connor

Management of Opioid Intoxication and Withdrawal

OPIOID INTOXICATION AND OVERDOSE

Clinical Picture

Opioid intoxication and overdose may present in a variety of settings.

Although mild to moderate intoxication (as evidenced by euphoria or sedation) usually is not life threatening, severe intoxication or overdose is a medical emergency that causes many preventable deaths and thus requires immediate attention.

As the prevalence of opioid use has increased in the United States, the incidence of opioid overdose has increased as well.

Nonfatal opioid overdose is an additional cause of significant morbidity and the true prevalence may not be well understood.

Many nonfatal overdoses are not brought to medical attention. The factors associated with nonfatal opioid overdose include injection route of administration, sporadic heroin use, needing help with injection, prior overdose, and polydrug use.

The pharmacologic actions responsible for opioid intoxication and overdose involve a specific set of opioid receptors, particularly those in the central nervous system.

These opioid receptors include the μ, κ, and δ types, which also interact with endogenous substances, including the endorphins.

The level of tolerance to opioids can have a significant effect on an individual's risk of opioid overdose.

In addition, tolerance to respiratory depression may be slower than tolerance to euphoric effects, thus explaining why overdose occurs so often, even among "experienced" opioid users.

Detoxified-patients or those who have experienced intentional or unintentional abstinence from opioids for any reason (e.g., incarceration) may be particularly susceptible to death from heroin overdose (when reintroduced to heroin).

Diagnosis (Table 44.1)

1. Evaluation of opioid intoxication begins with the collection of patient data through a detailed history and physical examination.
2. In addition to opioid abuse, it is important to ask about use of other drugs or alcohol because of the likelihood of polydrug abuse.
3. Physical examination of the intoxicated patient may find central nervous system (CNS) and respiratory depression, as well as miosis and direct evidence of drug use, such as needle tracks or soft-tissue infection.
4. Heroin overdose syndrome = abnormal mental status, depressed respiration, and miotic pupils = sensitivity of 92%, specificity of 76% for heroin overdose.
5. Patients who present with symptoms of such intoxication also may have other important causes of depressed mental status, such as hypoglycemia, acidemia or other fluid and electrolyte disorders, or complications from end-stage liver disease.

TABLE 44.1	Diagnosis of Opioid Overdose

History

- Opioid use (ask about drug, amount, time of last use)
- Polydrug abuse
- Use multiple sources of information (family, hospital records, etc.)

Diagnosis

- Altered level of consciousness plus one of the following:
- Respiratory depression (respiratory rate <12/min)
- Miotic pupils
- Circumstantial evidence of opioid use (i.e., needle tracks)

Laboratory Tests

- Rule out hypoglycemia, acidemia, and fluid and electrolyte abnormalities
- Toxicology screens for opioids and other drugs

6. Toxicology screening should be performed immediately in emergency settings.
7. Opioid use and overdose also may be complicated by the effects of substances employed to "cut" drugs purchased on the street. Along with inert substances present to add bulk, active substances—including **dextromethorphan, lidocaine,** and **scopolamine**—may be present.

Management (Table 44.2)

1. General supportive management must be instituted simultaneously with the specific antidote, **naloxone**.
2. Adult basic life support and adult advanced cardiac life support need to be available.

TABLE 44.2	Management of Opioid Overdose

Initial Approach

- Assessment of ventilation
  - For patients with adequate ventilation
    - Monitor until normal level of arousal
  - For patients with inadequate ventilation
    - Supportive ventilation with 100% oxygenation
    - **Naloxone hydrochloride:** 0.4–0.8 mg initially, repeated as necessary
    - Consider mechanical ventilation if persistent respiratory depression despite **naloxone** or if inadequate oxygenation
- Assessment of perfusion
- Intravenous access and fluids
- Assessment for comorbid conditions

For patients with a complete naloxone response

- Observe for 2–3 h after response if no other complications
- Repeat **naloxone** if clinically significant sedation recurs
- Chest x-ray for patients with pulmonary symptoms
- Referral for substance abuse treatment

For patients with incomplete naloxone response

- *Trial of 2-mg dose of* **naloxone**
- Consider polysubstance overdose or alternative diagnosis
- Referral for substance abuse treatment if polysubstance overdose a consideration

3. Adequate airway must be established and respiratory and cardiac-function must be appropriately assessed and managed.
4. Adequate intravenous access is essential.
5. Frequent monitoring of vital signs and cardiorespiratory status is required.

Pharmacologic Therapies

Naloxone hydrochloride:

- Pure opioid antagonist
- Reverses the CNS effects of opioid intoxication and overdose
- An initial intravenous dose of 0.4 to 0.8 mg will quickly reverse neurologic and cardiorespiratory depression.
- Onset of action of IV **naloxone**, as manifested by antagonism of opioid overdose, is approximately 2 minutes.
- Overdose with opioids that are more potent (such as **fentanyl**) or longer acting (such as **methadone**) may require higher doses of **naloxone** given over longer periods of time, as by ongoing **naloxone** infusion.
- In patients who do not respond to multiple doses of **naloxone**, alternative causes of the failure to respond must be considered.

Follow-Up Care

Patients with major acute medical or psychiatric comorbidities, including suicidal ideation, should be hospitalized for further treatment.

In the absence of these issues, resolution of the symptoms of intoxication and establishment of follow-up referrals for addiction, medical , and psychiatric care are necessary before a patient can be discharged safely.

OPIOID WITHDRAWAL

Acute Withdrawal

Consists of a range of symptoms for various lengths of time, part of a syndrome known as opiate withdrawal syndrome

- Gastrointestinal distress (such as diarrhea and vomiting)
- Thermoregulation disturbances
- Insomnia
- Muscle and joint pain
- Marked anxiety
- Dysphoria

The opiate withdrawal syndrome causes marked discomfort, often prompting continuation of opioid use even in the absence of any opioid-associated euphoria.

Opiate withdrawal syndrome is not fatal.

Chronic Dependence and Protracted Abstinence

In patients with a chronic history of opiate dependence, acute withdrawal and detoxification *are only the beginning of treatment.*

Martin and Jasinski also postulated a relationship between the protracted abstinence syndrome and relapse. Based on similar observations, Dole concluded that "human addicts almost always return to use narcotics" after hospital detoxification.

Clinical Picture

The severity of opioid withdrawal *varies with the specific opioid used* and the *dose and duration of drug use.*

The time to onset of opioid withdrawal symptoms *depends on the half-life of the drug being used.* For example, withdrawal may begin 4 to 6 hours after the last use of heroin, but up to 36 hours after the last use of methadone.

Neuropharmacologic studies of opioid withdrawal have supported the clinical picture of CNS noradrenergic hyperactivity.

Therapies to alter the course of opioid withdrawal (such as **clonidine**) are designed to decrease this hyperactivity, which occurs primarily at the *locus ceruleus.*

Diagnosis

Several clinical tools are available to measure the severity of opiate withdrawal syndrome:

Clinical Opiate Withdrawal Scale (COWS)
10-item Short Opioid Withdrawal Scale
16-item Subjective Opioid Withdrawal Scale
13-item Objective Opioid Withdrawal Scale

Opiate Withdrawal Syndrome Symptoms Early abnormalities in vital signs: tachycardia and hypertension
  Bothersome CNS system symptoms: restlessness, irritability, and insomnia
  Opioid craving also occurs in proportion to the severity of physiologic withdrawal symptoms.
  Pupillary dilation
  Cutaneous and mucocutaneous symptoms (including lacrimation, rhinorrhea, and piloerection—also
known as "gooseflesh")
  Yawning and sneezing
  GI symptoms include nausea, vomiting, and diarrhea, severity increasing with opiate withdrawal syndrome
severity.

Duration of Opiate Withdrawal Syndrome The duration also varies with the *half-life of the drug* used and the
duration of drug use. For example, the **meperidine** abstinence syndrome may peak *within 8 to 12 hours* and last *only
4 to 5 days*, whereas heroin withdrawal symptoms generally peak within *36 to 72 hours* and may last for *7 to 14 days*.

Protracted Opiate Withdrawal Syndrome A protracted abstinence syndrome has been described, in
which a variety of symptoms may last beyond the typical acute withdrawal period. Findings in prolonged and
protracted abstinence may include mild abnormalities in vital signs and continued craving.

Management

- Management of opioid withdrawal involves a combination of general supportive measures and specific phar-
  macologic therapies.
- Rule out other medical problems that may be complicating the opioid withdrawal.
- Physical examination should be performed to detect specific findings consistent with withdrawal to establish
  the diagnosis.
- General supportive measures (safe environment, adequate nutrition, reassurance)
- The decision as to outpatient or inpatient detoxification depends on availability of social supports (such as
  family members to provide monitoring and transportation) and the presence of polydrug abuse.

Pharmacologic Therapies

These therapies involve

- The use of opioid agonists (such as **methadone**)
- An alpha-2 adrenergic agonist (such as **clonidine**)
- An opioid antagonist (such as **naltrexone** or **naloxone**) in combination with **clonidine**, with sedation, or
  with general anesthesia
- Or a mixed opioid agonist/antagonist (**buprenorphine**)

Slow Methadone Detoxification For short-acting opioids, the natural course of withdrawal generally is
relatively brief, but more intense and associated with a higher degree of discomfort than with equivalent doses
of long-acting opioids.

  However, there is considerable individual variation, so that strong early withdrawal symptoms from
methadone are possible, as are delayed severe **heroin** withdrawal symptoms.

  The protocol for slow **methadone** detoxification is similar to the strategy used for withdrawal from
methadone maintenance treatment. After a stabilizing dose has been reached, **methadone** is tapered by 20% a
day for inpatients, leading to a 1- to 2-week procedure.

  Alternatively, the dose is tapered by 5% per day for outpatients, in a gradual cessation phase lasting as long
as 6 months.

  The longer duration of the procedure and the greater discomfort make the outpatient detoxification with
methadone especially vulnerable to patient dropout and continuing illicit opioid use.

One study showed that even when coupled with enhanced psychosocial counseling, patients enrolled in 6-month **methadone** detoxification programs demonstrated greater illicit opioid use and greater drug-related HIV-risk behaviors than patients enrolled in **methadone** maintenance.

Clonidine Detoxification
Morphine and **clonidine** blocked activation of the locus coeruleus, a major noradrenergic nucleus that shows increased activity during opioid withdrawal.

Although opioids exert their effect through opiate receptors, **clonidine** activates alpha-2 adrenergic receptors.

Consequently, **clonidine** does not possess the potential for physical dependence and abuse seen with opioids.

Clonidine *reduces or eliminates most of the commonly reported opiate withdrawal syndrome* symptoms, including lacrimation, rhinorrhea, restlessness, muscle pain, joint pain, and GI symptoms. Symptoms such as lethargy and insomnia persist.

Sedation and dizziness from orthostatic hypotension are the most common side effects of **clonidine**.

Though **clonidine** has been shown to be useful to decrease symptoms associated with opioid withdrawal, its use for this purpose is considered off-label.

Combined Clonidine and Naltrexone Treatment
The authors found that addition of the opioid antagonist **naltrexone** to **clonidine** shortened the duration of withdrawal without increasing patient discomfort.

In the 4-day protocol, subjects underwent a **naloxone** challenge test, followed by **clonidine** therapy administered three times a day. The first **naltrexone** dose (12.5 mg) was given the afternoon of the 1st day, after preloading with **clonidine** at 0.2 to 0.3 mg. **Naltrexone** was increased to 25 mg on the 2nd day, 50 mg on the 3rd day, and 100 mg on the 4th day. **Clonidine** was given at 0.1 to 0.3 mg three times per day, as needed, for the first 3 days, and three times at 0.1 mg on the 4th day.

The authors reported that 75% of patients successfully completed detoxification and were discharged on maintenance doses of **naltrexone**.

In summary, the authors found that combined **clonidine** and **naltrexone** therapy had the advantage of "being more rapid and probably more successful in the outpatient setting."

Given the intensive approach to this rapid method of detoxification, it has been suggested that only clinicians with significant experience in treatment of opioid withdrawal should offer this intervention.

Buprenorphine Detoxification
A recent Cochrane systematic review of 18 studies (14 randomized clinical trials) of the use of **buprenorphine** for opioid withdrawal found that **buprenorphine** treatment was superior to **clonidine** and as effective as **methadone** for ameliorating withdrawal symptoms, treatment retention, and treatment completion.

The *duration of withdrawal symptoms may be significantly less* with **buprenorphine** compared with that with **methadone**.

Buprenorphine's ceiling on agonist activity *reduces the danger of overdose, may limit its abuse liability, and has low toxicity even at high intravenous doses, thereby increasing the* dose range over which it may be administered safely.

Buprenorphine also can produce sufficient tolerance to block the effects of exogenously administered opioids, suggesting that it reduces illicit opioid use.

Buprenorphine's slow dissociation from mu opioid receptors results in a long duration of action (ideal for a maintenance medication) and also diminishes withdrawal signs and symptoms on discontinuation, making it particularly useful for opioid detoxification.

In conclusion, **buprenorphine** is more effective than **clonidine** in reducing symptoms of withdrawal, retaining patients in treatment, and allowing patients to reach treatment completion.

Additionally, it is as effective as **methadone** in tapering doses for the treatment of opioid withdrawal, although withdrawal symptoms may resolve more quickly with **buprenorphine** than with **methadone**.

Gradual **buprenorphine** taper appears to be more effective than rapid taper to treat opioid withdrawal.

Finally, **buprenorphine** is an attractive alternative to **methadone** for use in special treatment populations and settings.

Rationale for Methadone-to-Buprenorphine Transfer
Reasons for this occurring:

1. Unique pharmacology of **buprenorphine**, leading to its more favorable safety profile and longer duration of action (thus permitting less frequent dosing) relative to **methadone**
2. **Buprenorphine** may engender less fear of stigma than **methadone**
3. **Buprenorphine** may also be administered in office-based settings and patients may prefer this setting, rather than **methadone** treatment settings, for their ongoing opioid agonist maintenance treatment

Buprenorphine in Agonist-to-Antagonist Treatment Buprenorphine has been used in several experimental studies as a transitional agent between agonists (such as **methadone** or **heroin**) and antagonists (such as **naloxone** or **naltrexone**).

After chronic administration, **buprenorphine** produces less physical dependence than do pure agonists, as suggested by the minimal withdrawal symptoms that occur when **buprenorphine** is stopped, and by the use of relatively higher antagonist doses that are needed to precipitate withdrawal in **buprenorphine**-maintained volunteers.

The use of **buprenorphine** stabilization of opioid addicts before switching to **naltrexone** has the advantage of psychosocial stabilization prior to detoxification. This approach thus may represent a compromise approach between acute detoxification and long-term treatment of chronic dependence.

Follow-Up Care

Detoxification alone, without plans for ongoing drug treatment, is not adequate to manage patients.

At the initiation of detoxification, arrangements for ongoing treatment need to be assured.

Role of Detoxification in the Treatment of Opioid Dependence

In general, detoxification programs focus solely on one aspect of opioid dependence (i.e., treatment of withdrawal) and often lack appropriate linkages to ongoing treatment services. The addition of psychosocial interventions to opioid substitution detoxification treatment improved treatment retention, abstinence from drugs, and adherence to clinic visits.

Summary Author: Ashok Krishnamurthy
Jeffery N. Wilkins • Itai Danovitch • David A. Gorelick*

Management of Stimulant, Hallucinogen, Marijuana, Phencyclidine, and Club Drug Intoxication and Withdrawal

STIMULANTS

Stimulant Intoxication

The acute psychologic and medical effects of cocaine, amphetamines, and other stimulants are attributable principally to increases in catecholamine neurotransmitter activity. Enhanced catecholamine activity occurs through blockade of the presynaptic neurotransmitter reuptake pumps (as by cocaine) and by presynaptic release of catecholamines (as by amphetamines).

The resulting stimulation of brain reward circuits (the corticomesolimbic dopamine circuit) is thought to mediate the desired (and addicting) psychologic effects of stimulants (see Table 45.1).

Blockade of presynaptic catecholamine reuptake sites or postsynaptic receptors should, in principle, be an effective treatment for stimulant intoxication. Several medications have shown promise in attenuating the acute subjective effects of stimulants, for example, **bupropion**, **aripiprazole**, **risperidone**, **topiramate**, and **modafinil** (Table 45.2).

Another method of attenuating the effects of stimulant intoxication might be to decrease drug availability in the central nervous system by binding it peripherally with antidrug antibodies or by increasing its catabolism.

Psychologic and Behavioral Effects of Stimulant Intoxication The initial desired effects of stimulant intoxication include increased energy, alertness, and sociability; elation; euphoria; and decreased fatigue, need for sleep, and appetite.

With high dose or repeated use, stimulant intoxication usually progresses to unwanted effects such as anxiety, irritability, interpersonal sensitivity, hypervigilance, suspiciousness, grandiosity, impaired judgment, stereotyped behavior, and psychotic symptoms such as paranoia and hallucinations.

Stimulant users typically remain alert and oriented, but the delusional state may impair judgment, cognition, and attention.

Patients with stimulant-induced psychoses may closely resemble those with acute schizophrenia and may be misdiagnosed as such.

Cocaine-induced psychosis may differ from acute schizophrenic psychosis in having less thought disorder and bizarre delusions and fewer negative symptoms such as alogia and inattention. Stimulant-induced hallucinations may be auditory, visual, or somatosensory. Tactile hallucinations are especially typical of stimulant psychosis, such as the sensation of something crawling under the skin (formication).

Panic reactions are common and may evolve into a panic disorder.

---

*Dr. Gorelick is supported by the Intramural Research Program, NIH, National Institute on Drug Abuse.

TABLE 45.1	Acute Medical Complications of Stimulant Intoxication

Organ system	Medical effects
Head, ears, eyes, nose, throat	Pupil dilation; headache; bruxism
Pulmonary[a]	Hyperventilation; dyspnea; cough; chest pain; wheezing; hemoptysis; acute exacerbation of asthma; barotrauma (pneumothorax, pneumomediastinum); pulmonary edema
Cardiovascular	Tachycardia; palpitations; increased blood pressure; arrhythmia; chest pain; myocardial ischemia or infarction; ruptured aneurysm; cardiogenic shock
Neurologic	Headache; agitation; psychosis; tremor, hyperreflexia; small muscle twitching; tics; stereotyped movements; myoclonus; seizures; cerebral hemorrhage or infarct (stroke); cerebral edema
Gastrointestinal	Nausea; vomiting; mesenteric ischemia; bowel infarction or perforation
Renal	Diuresis; myoglobinuria; acute renal failure
Body temperature	Mild fever; malignant hyperthermia
Other	Rhabdomyolysis

[a]All pulmonary complications except hyperventilation and pulmonary edema come primarily from the smoked route of administration. *Sources*: Ghuran A, Nolan J. Recreational drug misuse: issues for the cardiologist. *Heart* 2000;83:627–633; Neiman J, Haapaniemi HM, Hillblom M. Neurological complications of drug abuse: pathophysiological mechanisms. *Eur J Neurol* 2000;7:595–606; Schuckit MA. *Drug and alcohol abuse. A clinical guide to diagnosis and treatment*, 6th ed. New York: Springer, 2006; Tashkin DP. Airway effects of marijuana, cocaine, and other inhaled illicit agents. *Curr Opin Pulm Med* 2001;7:43–61.

Very severe stimulant intoxication may produce an excited delirium or organic brain syndrome that can be fatal. Patients should be evaluated promptly for an acute neurologic lesion (e.g., intracranial bleeding) or a preexisting neuropsychiatric condition and treated aggressively.

Management of Psychologic and Behavioral Effects of Stimulant Intoxication The initial treatment approach is nonpharmacologic. The patient should be observed in a quiet environment with minimal sensory stimulation to avoid exacerbating symptoms.

Treatment staff should interact in a calm and confident manner, using the "ART" approach developed at the Haight Ashbury Free Clinic in San Francisco: *A*cceptance of the patient's immediate needs (such as pain relief or use of the bathroom), *R*eassurance that the condition is due to the drug and likely will dissipate within a few hours, and *T*alk down, to provide reality orientation and avoid hostility.

Physical restraints to control agitation should be avoided unless absolutely necessary. The use of restraints can increase risk of hyperthermia and rhabdomyolysis, with resulting severe medical complications.

If medication is needed, most experts prefer benzodiazepines (such as **diazepam** [10–30 mg PO or 2–10 mg IM or IV] or **lorazepam** [2–4 mg PO, IM, or IV]) over antipsychotics to control severe agitation, anxiety, or psychotic symptoms.

The former protect against the CNS and cardiovascular toxicities of cocaine, whereas the latter may worsen the sympathomimetic and cardiovascular effects, lower the seizure threshold, and increase the risk of hyperthermia. Parenteral benzodiazepine dosing may be repeated every 5 to 10 minutes until light sedation is achieved. If an antipsychotic is needed to control psychosis, high-potency agents such as **droperidol**, **haloperidol** (5–10 mg PO, IM, or IV), or **risperidone** (2–4 mg PO) are preferred because of their minimal anticholinergic activity.

A psychotic or agitated patient who has not responded to initial treatment should be hospitalized until the episode has resolved. This usually occurs within a few days if no more stimulants are ingested.

Psychiatric symptoms that persist beyond a few days suggest an etiology other than stimulant use.

Medical Effects of Stimulant Intoxication Mild stimulant intoxication (the state desired by users) may be accompanied by one or more self-limiting physiologic effects such as restlessness, sinus tachycardia,

TABLE 45.2   Treatment of Acute Stimulant Intoxication

Clinical problem	Moderate syndrome	Severe syndrome
Anxiety; agitation	Provide reassurance; place in a quiet, nonthreatening environment	Diazepam (10–30 mg PO, 2–10 mg IM, IV) or lorazepam (2–4 mg PO, IM, IV); may repeat every 1–3 h
Paranoia; psychosis	Place in a quiet, nonthreatening environment; benzodiazepines for sedation	High-potency antipsychotic (e.g., haloperidol) or second-generation antipsychotic
Hyperthermia	Monitor body temperature; place in a cool room	If temperature >102°F (oral), use external cooling with cold water, ice packs, hypothermic blanket; if >106°F, use internal cooling; epigastric lavage with iced saline
Seizures	Diazepam (2–20 mg IV, <5 mg/min) or lorazepam (2–8 mg)	For status epilepticus, IV diazepam or phenytoin (15–20 mg/kg IV, < 150 mg/min; or phenobarbital (25–50 mg IV)
Hypertension	Monitor blood pressure closely; benzodiazepines for sedation	If diastolic >120 for 15 min, give phentolamine (2–10 mg IV over 10 min)
Cardiac arrhythmia	Monitor electrocardiogram, vital signs; benzodiazepines for sedation	As appropriate for specific rhythm, based on advanced cardiac life-support criteria
Myocardial infarction	Benzodiazepines for sedation; supplemental oxygen; sublingual nitroglycerin for vasodilation; aspirin for anticlotting; morphine for pain	Give nitrates IV for coronary artery dilation; phentolamine (2–10 mg IV) to control blood pressure; thrombolysis, angioplasty (if clot confirmed and no hemorrhage)
Rhabdomyolysis	IV hydration to maintain urine output >2 mL/kg/h	Force diuresis with aggressive intra-venous hydration
Increased urinary drug excretion	Cranberry juice (8 oz TID) or ammonium chloride (500 mg PO every 3–4 h) until urine pH < 6.6 (if renal and hepatic function are normal)	Same as for moderate intoxication
Recent (few hours) oral drug ingestion	Activated charcoal orally or gastric lavage via nasogastric tube (if the patient is awake and cooperative)	Gastric lavage via nasogastric tube after endotracheal intubation (if the patient is unconscious)

hyperventilation, mydriasis, bruxism, headache, diaphoresis, or tremor—these do not usually bring the individual to medical attention or require treatment.

Nontraumatic chest pain is a common presenting complaint among stimulant users who seek acute medical care.

The differential diagnosis includes

Acute coronary syndrome
Acute aortic dissection
Pneumothorax
Pneumomediastinum (especially among drug smokers)
Endocarditis or pneumonia (especially among injection drug users)

Pulmonary embolus
Myocarditis
Cardiomyopathy
Musculoskeletal pain after seizure
About 1% to 6% of patients with cocaine-associated chest pain and up to one fourth of those with methamphetamine-associated chest pain will have an acute myocardial infarction.

The risk for infarction is greatest during the first 1 to 3 hours after cocaine use and then declines rapidly.

The electrocardiogram is not always helpful diagnostically because of its low sensitivity and low positive predictive value and the high frequency of benign early repolarization among patients presenting with cocaine-associated chest pain. The best laboratory test for acute myocardial infarction is serial blood levels of cardiac troponin.

Patients who present with nontraumatic stimulant-associated chest pain usually should be observed for 9 to 12 hours while undergoing evaluation. Delayed complications are rare, so resolution of symptoms with a negative evaluation warrants discharge.

Rhabdomyolysis may be due to a direct effect of the drug, hyperthermia, excessive muscle activity, or trauma. The usual symptoms of myalgia and muscle tenderness and swelling often are absent in rhabdomyolysis associated with stimulants. The diagnosis is suggested by a plasma CK level greater than five times normal (with other tissue sources ruled out) and a urine dipstick positive for heme but without red blood cells (indicating free myoglobin [or hemoglobin] in the urine).

Management of Medical Effects of Stimulant Intoxication

1. *The first priority in the management of severe acute stimulant intoxication* is maintenance of basic life-support functions. Vital signs, hydration status, and neurologic status should be monitored closely.

   Severe hypertension (e.g., diastolic blood pressure >120 mm Hg) that lasts >15 minutes should be treated promptly to avoid CNS hemorrhage.

   Rhabdomyolysis should be treated vigorously with intravenous fluid to maintain a urine output of >2 mL/kg/hour to avoid myoglobinuric renal failure. Maintenance of urine pH > 5.6 with **sodium bicarbonate** (1 mmol/kg IV) helps to prevent the dissociation and precipitation of myoglobin.

   Benzodiazepines in sedative doses are the initial treatment of choice for both acute cardiovascular and CNS toxicity from stimulants.

   β-Adrenergic blockers such as **propranolol** or **esmolol** are contraindicated because of the risk of unopposed α-adrenergic stimulation by the stimulant, resulting in vasoconstriction and worsening hypertension.

   The combined α- and β-adrenergic blocker **labetalol** actually shows little α-adrenergic antagonism in clinical practice and also should be avoided.

   If α-adrenergic blockade is ineffective, direct vasodilation with **sodium nitroprusside** infusion (0.25–10 g/kg/min) or **nitroglycerin** (5–100 g IV) can be used.

2. *Treatment of cocaine-induced cardiac tachydysrhythmias* begins with correction of any exacerbating conditions such as myocardial ischemia, hypoxia, electrolyte abnormalities, or acid-base disturbance.

   Dysrhythmias occurring immediately after cocaine use are usually from the sodium channel–blocking action of cocaine. **Lidocaine** (which also blocks sodium channels) should be used cautiously in this context because of animal studies suggesting it may exacerbate cocaine-associated dysrhythmias and seizures.

   Class IA antidysrhythmic medications (such as **quinidine**, **procainamide**, or **disopyramide**) should be avoided because of their potential additive effect on QRS and QT interval prolongation.

3. *The treatment of stimulant-associated acute coronary syndrome* largely resembles that for the non–drug-associated syndrome, with the exception of avoiding use of β-adrenergic blockers and **labetalol**.

   Initial treatment includes oxygen, benzodiazepine for sedation, morphine for pain, sublingual nitroglycerin for vasodilation, and aspirin, while evaluation continues.

   Both fibrinolytic therapy and percutaneous transluminal coronary angioplasty have a role in the treatment of confirmed myocardial infarction. *Fibrinolysis should be used cautiously because of the increased risk of intracranial hemorrhage in cocaine users.*

4. Intravenous benzodiazepines (**diazepam** 5–10 mg or **lorazepam** 2–10 mg over 2 minutes, repeated as needed) are recommended to *control seizures stemming from stimulant intoxication.*

STIMULANT WITHDRAWAL

Abrupt cessation of stimulant use is associated with depression, anxiety, fatigue, difficulty concentrating, anergia, anhedonia, increased drug craving, increased appetite, hypersomnolence, and increased dreaming (because of increased REM sleep).

Most symptoms are mild and self-limited, resolving within 1 to 2 weeks without treatment.

Hospitalization for stimulant withdrawal is rarely indicated on medical grounds and has not been shown to improve the short-term outcome for stimulant addiction.

Medical Effects of Stimulant Withdrawal The 1st week of stimulant withdrawal has been associated with myocardial ischemia, possibly because of coronary vasospasm.

Management of Stimulant Withdrawal The stimulant withdrawal syndrome has been hypothesized to be the result of decreased levels of brain dopamine activity resulting from chronic stimulant exposure. This so-called "dopamine deficiency" hypothesis of withdrawal has not been consistently supported by clinical studies.

Symptoms of stimulant withdrawal are best treated supportively with rest, exercise, and a healthy diet.

Short-acting benzodiazepines such as **lorazepam** may be helpful in selected patients who develop agitation or sleep disturbance. Severe (suicidal ideation) or persistent (>2–3 weeks) depression may require antidepressant treatment and inpatient psychiatric care.

The risk of relapse is high during the early withdrawal period, in part because drug craving is easily triggered by encounters with drug-associated stimuli. This issue is better addressed by psychosocial treatment, such as supportive therapy, cognitive-behavioral therapy, relapse prevention, and contingency management, than by medication.

HALLUCINOGENS

Hallucinogen Intoxication

Hallucinogens fall into two different chemical groups:

I. serotonin or tryptamine related (including LSD, psilocybin, or N,N-dimethyltryptamine)

II. phenylethylamine or amphetamine related (including 3,4,5-trimethoxyphenylethylamine [mescaline], 2,5-dimethoxy-4-methylamphetamine [DOM, STP], or 3,4,5-trimethoxyamphetamine)

All share enough clinical similarities with LSD to be classified as LSD-like hallucinogens.

NB: 3,4-methylenedioxymethamphetamine (MDMA, "Ecstasy") has characteristics of both a hallucinogen and a stimulant and is considered below.

Psychologic and Behavioral Effects of Hallucinogen Intoxication The subjective experience is influenced greatly by set and setting, that is, the expectations and personality of the user, coupled with the environmental and social conditions of use.

Mood can vary from euphoria and feelings of spiritual insight to depression, anxiety, and terror. Perception usually is intensified and distorted, with alterations in the sense of time, space, and body boundaries. Hallucinations (especially visual and auditory) are common. Cognitive function may range from clarity to confusion and disorientation, although reality testing usually remains intact.

An experience of depersonalization may precipitate the fear of losing one's mind permanently. Panic reactions are more common in those who have limited experience with hallucinogens, but previous "positive" experiences provide no protection against an adverse reaction.

Hallucinogens may trigger a transient psychosis even in psychologically normal users; *however, a true psychotic episode is rare.* Hallucinogen-induced psychosis may resemble acute paranoid schizophrenia.

The two usually can be distinguished because patients with schizophrenia tend to have auditory (rather than visual) hallucinations and a history of prior mental illness. Hallucinogen users, unlike patients with schizophrenia, usually retain at least partial insight that their psychosis is drug related.

Hallucinogen ingestion may result in an acute toxic delirium that is characterized by delusions, hallucinations, agitation, confusion, paranoia, and inadvertent suicide attempts (e.g., attempts to fly or perform other impossible activities).

Medical Effects of Hallucinogen Intoxication Complications that require treatment are rare in the absence of overdose. See Table 45.3.

TABLE 45.3   Acute Medical Complications of Intoxication with LSD, MDMA, Marijuana, or Phencyclidine (PCP)

Organ system	LSD	MDMA	Marijuana	PCP (Stage I)	PCP (Stage II)	PCP (Stage III)
Head, eyes, ears, nose, throat	Pupil dilation	Bruxism; headache; trismus; dry mouth	Pupil constriction; conjunctival injection; headache	Horizontal nystagmus; lid reflex lost; variable pupil size; laryngeal/pharyngeal reflexes hyperactive; ↑ tearing; ↑ saliva	Corneal reflex lost; disconjugate gaze; pupils mid-position and reactive; laryngeal/pharyngeal reflexes diminished; ↑ tearing; ↑ saliva	"Eyes open" coma; pupil dilation; laryngeal/pharyngeal reflexes absent; ↑ tearing; ↑ saliva
Skin	Piloerection; diaphoresis	Diaphoresis; flushing		Diaphoresis; flushing	Diaphoresis; flushing	Diaphoresis; flushing
Pulmonary			Mild tachypnea	Moderate tachypnea	Periodic breathing; apnea; pneumonia; edema	
Cardiovascular	↑ HR; ↑ BP	↑ HR; ↑ BP (rarely, ↓ BP)	↑ HR; ↓ BP orthostatic hypotension	Mildly ↑ HR, BP	Moderately ↑ HR, BP	Greatly ↑ HR, BP; high-output cardiac failure
Neurologic	Hyperreflexia; tremors; seizures	Tremor; trismus; ↑ muscle tone	Tremor; ↓ coordination; ataxia	Conscious; muscle rigidity; repetitive movements; hyperreflexia	Stupor to mild coma; tonic-clonic seizures; deep pain response intact; muscle rigidity; muscle twitching	Deep coma; tonic-clonic seizures; stroke; deep pain response absent; generalized myoclonus, opisthotonus, or decerebrate posturing; deep tendon reflexes absent
Gastrointestinal	Nausea; vomiting	Nausea; ↓ appetite	↑ Appetite	Nausea; vomiting	Protracted vomiting	
Renal	Urinary retention	Acute renal failure	Urinary retention	Acute renal failure		
Body temperature	↑ or ↑	↑ (possible malignant hyperthermia)		Mild ↑	Moderate ↑	Possible malignant hyperthermia
Other		Rhabdomyolysis		Rhabdomyolysis		

MDMA, 3,4-methylenedioxymethamphetamine; HR, heart rate; BP, blood pressure.

Sources: Brust JCM. Acute neurologic complications of drug and alcohol abuse. *Neurol Clin N Am* 1998;16(2):503–519; Frecska E, Luna LE. The adverse effects of hallucinogens from intramural perspective. *Neuropsychopharmacol Hung* 2006;8: 189–200; Ghuran A, Nolan J. Recreational drug misuse: issues for the cardiologist. *Heart* 2000;83:627–633; Kalan H. The pharmacology and toxicology of "ecstasy" (MDMA) and related drugs. *Canad Med Assoc J* 2001;165(7):917–926; Schuckit MA. *Drug and alcohol abuse. A clinical guide to diagnosis and treatment,* 6th ed. New York: Springer, 2006; Selden BS, Clark RF, Curry SC. Marijuana. *Emerg Med Clin North Am* 1990;8(3):527–539.

Management of Hallucinogen Intoxication Initial treatment is nonpharmacologic. The patient should be placed in a quiet environment with minimal sensory stimulation but should be observed because of the risk of unintended self-injury (as the result of delusions or hallucinations) or of suicide (as the result of depression). The presence of a familiar person usually is comforting. Unless the patient presents in an acutely agitated or threatening state, physical restraints are contraindicated because they may exacerbate anxiety and increase the risk of rhabdomyolysis.

The "talk-down" or reassurance technique may be helpful.

For patients who do not respond to reassurance alone, oral benzodiazepines such as **lorazepam** or **diazepam** are the drugs of choice. IM **lorazepam** may be effective. If benzodiazepines are insufficient, a high-potency antipsychotic such as **haloperidol** may be needed. *Phenothiazines should be avoided because they have been associated with poor outcomes and may exacerbate unsuspected anticholinergic poisoning.*

If psychosis does not resolve within 1 or 2 days, ingestion of a longer-acting drug such as PCP or DOM should be suspected. Symptoms that persist beyond a few days raise the strong likelihood of a preexisting or concurrent psychiatric or neurologic condition.

Hallucinogen Withdrawal

Withdrawal symptoms, including fatigue, irritability, and anhedonia, are reported by about 10% of hallucinogen users; however, *there is no evidence to suggest a clinically significant hallucinogen withdrawal syndrome.* There is no role for medication in the treatment of hallucinogen withdrawal.

MARIJUANA

Marijuana Intoxication

Psychologic and Behavioral Effects of Marijuana Intoxication The initial—usually desired—psychologic effects of marijuana intoxication include relaxation, euphoria, slowed time perception, altered (often intensified) sensory perception, increased awareness of the environment, and increased appetite. Undesired effects may include impaired concentration, anterograde amnesia, and motor incoordination.

Psychologic set and social setting and prior experience with the drug can substantially influence the quality of the experience.

Marijuana-associated psychosis may be more likely to exhibit derealization/depersonalization experiences and visual, rather than auditory, hallucinations.

In addition, marijuana use is probably an independent risk factor for subsequent development of a psychotic disorder.

Medical Effects of Marijuana Intoxication

1. Conjunctival injection ("red eye")
2. Tachycardia
3. Orthostatic hypotension
4. Dry mouth
5. Poor motor coordination
6. Head jerks
7. Impairment of smooth pursuit eye movements

There are no well-established cases of human fatalities from exclusively marijuana overdose.

Marijuana smoking has been associated with atrial fibrillation and other tachydysrhythmias.

Intravenous use of marijuana, although rare, can be associated with cardiovascular shock and renal failure.

Management of Marijuana Intoxication Adverse effects tend to be self-limited and often can be managed without medication.

Psychosis usually responds to low doses of second-generation antipsychotics.

Marijuana Withdrawal

- Reported by up to one third of heavy marijuana users in the community
- Seen in more than half of those seeking treatment for marijuana dependence
- Not a recognized syndrome in the *DSM-IV-TR*
- Symptoms are primarily psychologic:
  - Irritability
  - Anxiety

- Depression
- Restlessness
- Anorexia
- Insomnia
- Vivid disturbing dreams

The syndrome is often relatively mild and has been compared to tobacco withdrawal.

Management of Marijuana Withdrawal

- Rarely requires treatment for intrinsic medical or psychiatric reasons
- Treatment might be warranted to reduce the risk of relapse
- In non–treatment-seeking research subjects, agonist substitution with oral synthetic THC (**dronabinol**) does *substantially suppress withdrawal symptoms*

DISSOCIATIVE ANESTHETICS

Phencyclidine, Ketamine, and Dextromethorphan Intoxication

Psychologic and Behavioral Effects of Dissociative Anesthetic Intoxication Stage I—conscious, with psychologic effects but (at most) mild physiologic effects

Stage II—stuporous or in a light coma, yet responsive to pain

Stage III—comatose and unresponsive to pain

The time course of psychologic effects is highly variable and unpredictable, so that even a recovering patient should be kept under observation until all symptoms have resolved, typically at least 12 hours.

The psychiatric manifestations of Stage I intoxication can resemble a variety of psychiatric syndromes, making differential diagnosis difficult in the absence of toxicology results or a history of recent PCP, *ketamine*, or DXM intake.

Common syndromes are delirium, psychosis without delirium, catatonia, hypomania with euphoria, and depression with lethargy. Because of the analgesic effect of PCP, patients may not report the existence of even serious injuries (which may be self-inflicted).

Medical Effects of Dissociative Anesthetic Intoxication Intoxication at the mild Stage I desired by users is associated with few serious medical complications.

Higher stages are associated with severe medical effects, including hypertension, stroke, cardiac failure, seizures, rhabdomyolysis, acute renal failure, coma, and death.

The acute effects of **ketamine** tend to be less severe and of shorter duration than those of PCP, possibly due to its shorter half-life.

Management of Psychologic and Behavioral Effects of Dissociative Anesthetic Intoxication
Treatment of intoxication with dissociative anesthetics is largely supportive and aimed at controlling or reversing specific signs and symptoms.

No clinically useful antagonist is yet available.

Mild Stage I intoxication is best treated without medication.

The patient should be isolated in a quiet room with unobtrusive observation and minimal external stimuli. Reassuring, reality-oriented communication ("talking down") rarely works with such patients.

Benzodiazepines should be used if medication is needed to control severe anxiety, agitation, or psychotic behavior, although they may delay renal clearance of PCP at high doses.

If benzodiazepines are insufficient to control psychosis, high-potency first-generation antipsychotics, such as **haloperidol** or **droperidol**, or second-generation antipsychotics, such as **risperidone** or **olanzapine**, may be used.

Management of Medical Effects of Dissociative Anesthetic Intoxication Stage I intoxication usually does not need specific medical treatment.

Stage II and III intoxication are medical emergencies that require treatment in a comprehensive medical setting to maintain life-support functions until the drug has been eliminated from the body.

Dissociative Anesthetic Withdrawal

- A dissociative anesthetic withdrawal syndrome is not recognized in the *DSM-IV-TR.*
- Despite this, about one fourth of heavy PCP users report withdrawal symptoms (depression, anxiety, irritability, hypersomnolence, diaphoresis, and tremor).
- DXM withdrawal has been associated with craving, dysphoria, and insomnia.
- Tricyclic antidepressants such as **desipramine** may reduce the psychologic symptoms associated with discontinuation of PCP use, but there is no evidence that such treatment improves the outcome of PCP addiction.

Prolonged Psychiatric Sequelae

Hallucinogens and dissociative anesthetics (e.g., PCP) have the potential to trigger psychiatric sequelae that last beyond the period of acute intoxication, including prolonged states of anxiety, depression, or psychosis.

The risk of a prolonged psychiatric reaction appears to depend on several factors: the patient's premorbid psychopathology, the number of prior exposures to the drug, and a history of polydrug use.

Treatment of prolonged anxiety or depression usually is psychosocial, but may involve medication if symptoms become sufficiently severe.

Treatment of prolonged psychosis essentially follows guidelines for treatment of chronic functional psychosis.

"Flashbacks" are brief episodes (often lasting a few seconds) in which perceptual aspects of a previous hallucinogenic drug experiences are unexpectedly reexperienced after acute intoxication has resolved.

Flashbacks are associated principally with LSD. They can occur after use of other hallucinogens, MDMA, PCP, and, occasionally, marijuana.

Flashbacks usually are brief and self-limiting.

Over time, flashbacks tend to decrease in frequency, duration, and intensity, as long as no further hallucinogens are taken.

INHALANTS

Inhalant Intoxication

Inhalant intoxication produces initial euphoria or "rush," followed by light-headedness, excitability, and perceptual changes.

Higher doses may cause dizziness, slurred speech, and motor incoordination, followed by drowsiness and headache.

Intoxicated users rarely seek medical attention, in part because exposure tends to be self-limited and the duration of effect from a single exposure is usually only a few minutes.

There is no specific treatment for inhalant intoxication.

Inhalants may sensitize the myocardium, so pressor medications and bronchodilators are relatively contraindicated.

Inhalant Withdrawal

Inhalant withdrawal is primarily associated with drug craving and occasional tachycardia and diaphoresis.

Prominent psychologic or physical symptoms are rare. There is no specific treatment for inhalant withdrawal.

CLUB DRUGS

"Club drugs" are a pharmacologically heterogeneous group of drugs associated with a youth subculture that revolves around late-night dance parties known as "raves" or "trances."

Common club drugs are MDMA ("Ecstasy"), an amphetamine analogue with stimulant and hallucinogenic properties, as well as GHB and **flunitrazepam** (Rohypnol), both of which are CNS depressants.

MDMA ("ECSTASY")

Ecstasy is the common street name for 3,4-methylenedioxymethamphetamine (MDMA).

The effects of MDMA are *those of a stimulant combined with a mild hallucinogen.*

"Herbal Ecstasy" often refers to preparations containing the stimulant ephedrine. "Liquid Ecstasy" is a street name for GHB.

MDMA often is taken concurrently with other drugs, such as LSD (in a combination called "candyflipping"), for enhanced effect.

Dextromethorphan (available in over-the-counter cough medicines) is a frequent concomitant drug and may be substituted for MDMA in street preparations.

"Stacking" refers to the practice of taking multiple MDMA doses over a short period, often alternating with other drugs to enhance the experience. For example, amphetamine or cocaine may be used initially to augment the experience, followed later by a CNS depressant, such as alcohol, marijuana, or GHB, to temper the "coming down".

MDMA has good oral bioavailability and readily crosses the blood–brain barrier.

The onset of action is within 30 minutes and peak plasma concentrations are achieved in 1 to 3 hours. The elimination half-life is 7 to 8 hours.

Individuals who are genetically deficient in CYP2D6 (up to 10% of whites) are theoretically at increased risk of developing MDMA toxicity because MDMA is metabolized by CYP2D6.

A major MDMA metabolite is methylenedioxyamphetamine (MDA), which also is pharmacologically active and has a longer elimination half-life of 16 to 38 hours.

MDMA Intoxication

The diagnosis of MDMA intoxication is made by history of drug intake and/or analysis of unused drug. *MDMA is not detected by routine urine or blood drug screens*, which may be positive for amphetamines (products of MDMA metabolism).

Gastric lavage with activated charcoal may be helpful within the 1st hour after ingestion, especially if other drugs also have been taken. Induced emesis is not recommended because of the risk of CNS depression.

Psychologic and Behavioral Effects of MDMA Intoxication
Low to moderate oral doses of MDMA (50–150 mg) typically produce an intense initial effect (known as "coming on" or "rush"), especially if taken on an empty stomach, that may last 30 to 45 minutes.

These desired effects include increased wakefulness and energy, euphoria, increased sexual desire and satisfaction, heightened sensory perception, sociability, and increased empathy and sense of closeness to others.

The initial phase is followed by several hours of less intense experience ("plateau"), during which repetitive dancing is common. Users start to "come down" 3 to 6 hours after ingestion.

Undesired effects may occur with repeated use or at higher doses.

These include hyperactivity, fatigue, insomnia, anxiety, agitation, impaired decision making, flight of ideas, hallucinations, depersonalization, derealization, and bizarre or reckless behavior.

Initial treatment should be the same as for hallucinogen intoxication: placement in a quiet, reassuring environment, with observation to reduce the risk of unintended self-injury.

Physical restraints are contraindicated because they may exacerbate anxiety and increase the risk of rhabdomyolysis. If severe or persisting symptoms require medication, benzodiazepines are preferred. Antipsychotics should be avoided as much as possible because they may increase the risk of hyperthermia and seizures. A high-potency antipsychotic such as **haloperidol** should be used if necessary.

Medical Effects of MDMA Intoxication
The acute physical effects of MDMA at low to moderate doses resemble those of a stimulant: increased muscle tension, jaw clenching, bruxism, restlessness, insomnia, ataxia, headache, nausea, decreased appetite, dry mouth, dilated pupils, increased heart rate, and blood pressure.

Doses >200 mg are associated with life-threatening toxicities that can be grouped into four major syndromes.

Most dangerous are hyperthermia, rhabdomyolysis, liver damage, and disseminated intravascular coagulation.

Treatment is based on early recognition, close monitoring of serum creatinine kinase levels (to detect rhabdomyolysis), and reversal of the hyperthermia and may involve the use of benzodiazepines and antipsychotics. **Dantrolene** (1 mg/kg IV) may be helpful. Because of similarities between MDMA toxicity and the serotonin syndrome, serotonin antagonists such as **methysergide** and **cyproheptadine** have been used successfully.

Acute cardiovascular toxicity from MDMA is the result of increased catecholamine activity.

The preferred treatment is an adrenergic antagonist with both α- and β-blocking activity, combined with a vasodilator such as nitroglycerin or nitroprusside if needed to control blood pressure.

A pure β-adrenergic blocker should be avoided because of the remaining unopposed α-adrenergic stimulation, resulting in vasoconstriction and worsening hypertension.

In addition to direct MDMA-mediated neurotoxicity, acute toxicity can result from hyponatremia.

The conservative initial treatment is fluid restriction. Profound hyponatremia has been treated with hypertonic saline solution.

MDMA Withdrawal

Medical Effects of MDMA Withdrawal There is no withdrawal syndrome associated with MDMA that would require specific pharmacologic treatment.

Users may complain of muscle pain and stiffness in the jaw, neck, lower back, and limbs for the first 2 to 3 days after use. There is some evidence of increased variability of heart rate and blood pressure for several days after MDMA use.

γ-HYDROXYBUTYRATE (GHB)

GHB (or "liquid Ecstasy") is a naturally occurring metabolite of the neurotransmitter γ-aminobutyric acid (GABA). It is approved for the treatment of narcolepsy.

GHB became popular in the late 1980s in part because of its reputed aphrodisiac, disinhibitory, and amnestic effects; short duration of action; absence of "hangover;" and nondetectability by standard drug screens.

GHB is taken orally as a liquid or in a powder mixed into drinks. A typical dose is one to three teaspoons or capfuls. GHB is rapidly absorbed from the gastrointestinal tract and readily crosses the blood–brain barrier. Effects begin within 15 minutes of ingestion and last 2 to 4 hours.

The blood elimination half-life is about 30 minutes, largely because of rapid redistribution into other tissues.

GHB Intoxication

The diagnosis of GHB intoxication is based on clinical suspicion, a history of drug intake, or analysis of unused drug. The signs and symptoms are not specific for GHB, but resemble those of any CNS depressant. *GHB is not detected by routine drug toxicology assays.*

There is no proven antidote for GHB intoxication.

Psychologic and Behavioral Effects of GHB Intoxication The desired acute effects of GHB at low oral doses include relaxation, euphoria, sedation, disinhibition, sociability, and anterograde amnesia.

Higher doses produce somnolence, confusion, and hallucinations.

Unintended overdose may occur because of GHB's very steep dose-response curve and the great variability in potency of street preparations.

First-time users often underestimate the potency of GHB.

The effects are prolonged and intensified when taken with other CNS depressants, such as alcohol.

Medical Effects of GHB Intoxication Low to moderate oral doses of GHB may cause headache, dizziness, ataxia, hypotonia, and vomiting.

Higher doses may cause incontinence, myoclonic movements, bradycardia, hypotension, hypothermia, generalized tonic-clonic seizures, and coma.

Most patients recover completely within several hours with supportive care and do not require intubation.

However, death may result from respiratory depression, so that intubation and mechanical ventilation may be indicated in severe cases.

GHB Withdrawal

Cessation of chronic GHB use leads to a discrete withdrawal syndrome resembling that of sedative-hypnotic withdrawal.

Anxiety, restlessness, insomnia, tremor, nystagmus, tachycardia, and hypertension usually appear 2 to 12 hours after the last dose. Mild symptoms usually resolve gradually over 1 to 2 weeks.

More severe withdrawal may cause delirium with hallucinations, psychosis, agitation, and autonomic instability. GHB withdrawal seizures have not been reported.

Most cases of GHB withdrawal can be effectively managed through use of a long-acting benzodiazepine, on a tapering protocol.

Severe cases may require high doses (several hundred milligrams) or parenteral administration.

Patients unresponsive to benzodiazepines may benefit from barbiturates, a mood stabilizer such as **gabapentin**, or low-dose antipsychotics.

HERBS OF ABUSE

Many herbs contain psychoactive compounds with stimulant, anxiogenic, anxiolytic, hallucinogenic, euphoric, or dissociative effects.

The perception that herbs are safer than illicit drugs, coupled with the absence of clearly established dosing parameters, may contribute to their misuse.

Routine toxicology screens do not detect many of these substances. Accurate diagnosis may rest on collateral information from family, friends, and first responders, in addition to a thorough clinical examination.

Herbs of Abuse Intoxication

Herbs of abuse may be categorized as predominantly hallucinogenic or stimulating (see Table 45.4).

Management of Psychologic, Behavioral, and Medical Effects   Management of intoxication with hallucinogenic herbs is largely supportive. Symptoms, including psychosis, are usually self-limited.

A quiet environment often avoids the need for pharmacologic interventions.

Medications with anticholinergic properties are usually avoided to minimize the possibility of exacerbating substance-induced delirium.

Patients who are agitated, in severe panic, or having distressing psychotic symptoms may be relieved by benzodiazepines.

Management of intoxication with stimulant herbs is similar to that with hallucinogenic herbs, except that the former are more likely to generate hyperexcitable, agitated, and psychotic states.

With one exception, there are no specific antidotes to intoxication with psychoactive herbs.

Intoxication with herbs having anticholinergic activity (e.g., jimsonweed) has been successfully treated with **physostigmine**, a short-acting acetylcholinesterase inhibitor.

Severe intoxication with betel nut, which has cholinergic activity, can be treated with **atropine**, a cholinergic antagonist.

Herbs of Abuse Withdrawal

Most users of psychoactive herbs do not experience withdrawal symptoms.

Some users of khat and betel nuts do experience a withdrawal syndrome, often including irritability, fatigue, and rhinorrhea.

Protracted withdrawal symptoms (e.g., psychosis, depression, anxiety) should be treated symptomatically while the patient is evaluated for an underlying psychiatric disorder.

FLUNITRAZEPAM

Flunitrazepam (**Rohypnol**, also known as "roofies" or the "date rape pill")

- Potent, fast-acting benzodiazepine that frequently causes anterograde amnesia
- Legally manufactured and marketed in Europe and Latin America
- Illegal in the United States because of its association with date rape
- Difficult to detect with routine toxicology screens because of its low concentration

Flunitrazepam Intoxication

- Features sedation, disinhibition, anterograde amnesia, confusion, ataxia, bradycardia, hypotension, and respiratory depression
- Overdose rarely is life threatening unless the drug is combined with another CNS depressant, such as alcohol.
- Treatment is supportive; activated charcoal and gastric lavage may be helpful.
- When respiratory depression or circulatory compromise is severe, the benzodiazepine antagonist **flumazenil** may be used, albeit cautiously.

TABLE 45.4   Common Herbal Drugs of Abuse

Herb	Street names	Predominant psychoactive compound	Predominant mechanism of action	Typical duration of action	Dosage at which toxicity becomes more prominent	Urine toxicology screen
Salvia divinorum	Magic mint; Sally-D; Ska	Salvinorin A	Kappa opioid agonist	15 min	>500 µg	Negative
Myristica fragrans	Nutmeg	Myristicin, elemicin, safrole	MAO inhibition, serotonergic	24–72 h	>20 g (5 teaspoons)	Negative
Lophophora williamsii	Peyote; buttons; mescal	Mescaline	Serotonergic; dopaminergic	1–12 h	400–500 mg (6–12 buttons)	Negative
Psilocybe mushrooms	Magic mushrooms, shrooms	Psilocybin, psilocin	Serotonergic	2–6 h	>50 mg (>5 g mushrooms)	Negative
Amanita muscaria	Fly agaric	Ibotenic acid, muscimol	Glutamatergic GABAergic	0.5–3 h	(100 g dried mushrooms)	Negative
Ayahuasca (mixture of various plants)	Huasca, yage, brew, daime	DMT + MAO inhibitor	Serotonergic; anticholinergic	20–60 min	Varies	Negative
Ipomea violacea	Morning glory	LSA	Serotonergic	6–10 h	3–6 g (25–200 seeds)	Negative
Argyreia nervosa	Hawaiian baby	LSA	Serotonergic	6–10 h	3–6 g (5–10 seeds)	Negative
Datura stramonium	Jimsonweed, locoweed, stinkweed	Atropine, scopolamine, hyoscyamine	Anticholinergic	1 h–several days	Varies	Negative
Ephedra species	Ma-huang, herbal ecstasy	Ephedrine, pseudoephedrine	Sympathomimetic	6 h	>8 mg at one time, or >100 mg	MA+
Pausinystalia yohimbe	Yohimbine	Yohimbine	Adrenergic, serotonergic	3–4 h	>35 mg	Negative
Catha edulis	Khat; qat	Cathinone, cathine	Sympathomimetic	1–4 h	>100 mg	Negative
Areca catechu	Betel nut	Arecoline	Cholinergic	2–17 min	Varies	Negative

DMT, *N*,*N*-dimethyltryptamine; GABA, *γ*-aminobutyric acid; LSA, lysergic acid hydroxyethylamide; MA, methamphetamine; MAO, monoamine oxidase.
Sources: Halpern JH. Hallucinogens and dissociative agents naturally growing in the United States. *Pharmacol Ther* 2004;102:131–138; Richardson WH, Slone CM, Michels JE. Herbal drugs of abuse: an emerging problem. *Emerg Med Clin N Am* 2007;254:35–57.

- **Flumazenil** precipitates acute withdrawal in patients who are physically dependent on benzodiazepines and lowers the seizure threshold, thus increasing the risk of withdrawal seizures.
- **Flumazenil** is effective for about 20 minutes, so that repeated dosing is necessary to avoid re-sedation by **flunitrazepam**.

Flunitrazepam Withdrawal

Withdrawal symptoms can develop up to 36 hours after the last dose and include anxiety, restlessness, tremors, headache, insomnia, and paraesthesias.

Treatment of this withdrawal is as with other benzodiazepines.

SEROTONIN SYNDROME

The serotonin syndrome may account for some of the severe complications associated with intoxication and overdose on amphetamines or MDMA.

The serotonin syndrome is a triad of signs and symptoms, consisting of

1. Mental status changes (e.g., anxiety, confusion, agitation, lethargy, delirium, coma)
2. Autonomic hyperactivity (e.g., low-grade fever, tachycardia, diaphoresis, nausea, vomiting, diarrhea, dilated pupils, abdominal pain, hypertension, tachypnea)
3. Neuromuscular abnormalities (e.g., myoclonus, nystagmus, hyperreflexia, rigidity, trismus, tremor)

The clinical presentation is highly variable; neuromuscular signs are usually prominent.

The differential diagnosis includes

- Neuroleptic malignant syndrome (with which it is most commonly confused)
- Sepsis
- Heat stroke
- Delirium tremens
- Sympathomimetic or anticholinergic poisoning

Patients with neuroleptic malignant syndrome differ from those with serotonin syndrome in that they are more likely to present with extrapyramidal signs and autonomic instability and rarely present with the neuromuscular changes common in serotonin syndrome.

The serotonin syndrome is the result of excessive stimulation of 5-HT_{2A}, possibly with some contribution also from 5-HT_{1A}, receptors.

Mechanisms for excess serotonin/stimulation by serotonin include

- Activation of serotonin receptors by agonists
- Enhanced release of serotonin (by MDMA or amphetamines)
- Decreased presynaptic serotonin reuptake (by cocaine or SSRIs)
- Decreased serotonin metabolism (by amphetamines or monoamine oxidase inhibitors)
- Increased serotonin synthesis

The serotonin syndrome is most commonly seen after ingestion of two or more drugs with such actions but also may occur with a single drug.

Laboratory abnormalities are nonspecific, but elevated CPK, liver transaminases, white blood cell count, serum bicarbonate, and evidence of disseminated intravascular coagulation may occur in severe cases.

In the absence of appropriate diagnosis and treatment, there may be progression to rhabdomyolysis, hyperthermia, renal failure, disseminated intravascular coagulation, and death.

Effective treatment requires

1. Early identification
2. Immediate discontinuation of all serotonergic medications
3. Close monitoring
4. Supportive care (usually including intravenous hydration)

WITHDRAWAL FROM MULTIPLE DRUGS

Multiple Sedative Hypnotics

Withdrawal from dependence on multiple sedative-hypnotic agents, including alcohol, is best managed in the same way as withdrawal from a single such drug: by using tapering dosages of a single, longer-acting sedative hypnotic.

Focus on managing withdrawal of the longer-acting drug.

The rate at which the dose is tapered usually should not exceed 10% per day.

Sedative Hypnotics with Other Drugs

In the management of patients withdrawing from both sedative hypnotics and CNS stimulants, treat the sedative-hypnotic withdrawal first, because this poses the greatest difficulty and medical risk.

For concurrent addiction to sedative hypnotics and opiates, concurrent pharmacologic treatment is recommended. The patient may be stabilized on an opiate (preferably oral **methadone**, although **codeine** can be used if **methadone** is not available) at the same time that the sedative-hypnotic dose is tapered by 10% per day. After the sedative-hypnotic withdrawal is completed, opiate withdrawal can begin.

POPULATION-SPECIFIC CONSIDERATIONS

Neonates

Perinatal drug use by the mother raises the possibility of drug intoxication or withdrawal in the newborn.

Obtaining an accurate maternal drug use history for the period preceding delivery is essential.

Meconium is the most accurate substrate for neonatal toxicology through the 3rd to 4th day of life, but such testing is not widely available.

Neonatal intoxication signs and symptoms are nonspecific:

- Sedation
- Irritability
- Restlessness
- Hypertonia
- Hyperreflexia
- Tremors
- Poor feeding
- Abnormal sleep patterns
- Respiratory difficulty
- Seizures

Stimulants (such as cocaine), marijuana, LSD, and PCP all have been associated with a neonatal withdrawal syndrome, although one that usually is less intense than the opiate withdrawal syndrome.

Perinatal use of stimulants is associated with either bradycardia or tachycardia in the newborn.

The additive cardiovascular effects of the stimulant and the normal catecholamine surge during labor may cause fetal distress and retard delivery.

These cardiac effects usually resolve as the drug is eliminated from the body.

Neonatal stimulant intoxication may be associated with irritability, tremors, hyperactivity, abnormal movements, excessive sucking, and high-pitched and excessive crying for 1 to 2 days, followed by a period of lethargy and hyporeactivity.

Treatment of drug-exposed newborns is largely supportive, with avoidance of overstimulation.

Phenobarbital is the preferred medication for newborns with nonopiate drug withdrawal, especially when seizures are a factor.

A loading dose of 5 mg/kg/day is given until withdrawal is controlled, with adjustments of 10% to 20% every 2 to 3 days based on the response. **Phenobarbital** has a long half-life, so plasma concentrations should be checked periodically to avoid drug accumulation and over treatment.

Older Adults

There is little published data on the treatment of drug intoxication or withdrawal in this age group.

The recommended dosing approach is "start low and go slow"; that is, start medication at a lower dose and increase the dose in smaller increments than would be used in younger individuals.

Adolescents

Adolescence is the common age of onset for illegal drug use and abuse. Adolescents experience symptoms of drug withdrawal similar to those in adults, including physical symptoms. There are few published data on the treatment of drug intoxication or withdrawal in adolescents.

Women

Limited anecdotal evidence suggests that pharmacologic treatment for women is similar to that for men, taking into account possible gender differences in medication pharmacokinetics.

CHAPTER

46

Summary Author: Ashok Krishnamurthy
Henry R. Kranzler • Domenic A. Ciraulo • Jerome H. Jaffe

Medications for Use in Alcohol Rehabilitation

One pharmacological approach for alcohol treatment involves direct efforts to reduce or stop drinking behavior by producing adverse effects when alcohol is consumed or by modifying the neurotransmitter systems that mediate alcohol reinforcement.

A second pharmacological approach to the treatment of alcohol dependence involves the treatment of persistent psychiatric symptoms, which aims to stop or reduce drinking by modifying the motivation to use alcohol to "self-medicate" such symptom.

MEDICATIONS USED TO REDUCE OR STOP DRINKING

Alcohol-Sensitizing Agents

Alcohol-sensitizing agents alter the body's response to alcohol, thereby making its ingestion unpleasant or toxic.

Disulfiram (**Antabuse**) is the only alcohol-sensitizing medication approved in the United States for the treatment of alcohol dependence and is widely used clinically.

Mechanism: inhibits the enzyme *aldehyde dehydrogenase* (sometimes also referred to as *acetaldehyde dehydrogenase* or *alcohol dehydrogenase*), which catalyzes the oxidation of acetaldehyde to acetic acid

Effect: raises blood acetaldehyde concentration, resulting in the **disulfiram**-ethanol reaction (DER)

The intensity of the DER varies both with the dose of **disulfiram** and the volume of alcohol ingested.

Most DERs are self-limited, lasting about 30 minutes.

Symptoms and signs of the DER:

Warmness and flushing of the skin, especially that of the upper chest and face
Increased heart rate
Palpitations
Decreased blood pressure
Nausea
Vomiting
Shortness of breath
Sweating
Dizziness
Blurred vision
Confusion

Occasionally, the DER may be severe, with marked tachycardia, hypotension, or bradycardia; rarely, it may result in cardiovascular collapse, congestive failure, and convulsions.

Severe reactions are usually associated with high doses of **disulfiram** (over 500 mg per day), combined with >2 oz of alcohol; deaths have occurred with lower dosage and after a single drink.

The efficacy of alcohol-sensitizing agents in the prevention of relapse in alcohol-dependent individuals remains to be demonstrated in placebo-controlled, double-blind studies.

However, in selected samples of such individuals with whom special efforts, such as supervised administration, are made to ensure compliance, these medications may be useful.

Pharmacology of Disulfiram

- Almost completely absorbed orally
- Binds irreversibly to *aldehyde dehydrogenase;* renewed enzyme activity requires the synthesis of new enzyme, so that the potential exists for a DER to occur at least 2 weeks from the last ingestion of **disulfiram**. Alcohol should be avoided during this period.
- Patients treated with **disulfiram** should be monitored regularly for visual changes and symptoms of peripheral neuropathy and the medication discontinued if they appear.
- Liver enzymes should be monitored at quarterly intervals to identify hepatotoxic effects, which may also warrant discontinuation of the medication. The risk of hepatic injury does not appear to be related to dose.
- Inhibits dopamine β-hydroxylase, which *increases* dopamine concentrations, which in turn can exacerbate psychotic symptoms in patients with schizophrenia and rarely result in psychotic or depressive symptoms among individuals without a psychotic disorder. Such symptoms should also lead to discontinuation of the medication
- The daily dosage prescribed in the United States limited to 250 to 500 mg per day out of concerns about dose-related effects; however, titrated to DER effect in some individuals, doses >1 g per day are required.

Clinical Use of Disulfiram In the controlled studies conducted, the difference in outcome between subjects receiving **disulfiram** and those given placebo has generally been modest.

Disulfiram may be of clinical value in selected samples of alcohol-dependent patients with whom special efforts are made to ensure compliance.

Specific behavioral efforts to enhance compliance with **disulfiram** include

Contacting with the patient and a significant other to work together to ensure compliance
Provision to the patient of incentives
Regular reminders and other information
Behavioral training and social support

Decision to use **disulfiram** in alcohol treatment must be made only if
    Patients are made aware of the hazards of the medication.
    They are aware that they must avoid over-the-counter preparations with alcohol and drugs.
    The administration of **disulfiram** to anyone who does not agree to use it, who does not seek to be abstinent from alcohol, or who has any psychological or medical contraindications is not recommended.

Opioidergic Agents

Naltrexone and, to a lesser extent, **nalmefene**, both of which are opioid antagonists with no intrinsic agonist properties, have been studied for the treatment of alcohol dependence.

Naltrexone

- Approval based on two single-site studies that showed it to be efficacious in the prevention of relapse to heavy drinking
- Studies found **naltrexone** to be well tolerated and to result in significantly less craving for alcohol and fewer drinking days than placebo.
- Presumed mechanism: less euphoric effects of alcohol while using **naltrexone**, suggesting that it blocked the endogenous opioid system's contribution to alcohol's "priming effect"
- Reduced craving for alcohol, alcohol's reinforcing properties, the experience of intoxication, and the chances of continued drinking following a slip
- During a 6-month, posttreatment follow-up period, the effects of **naltrexone** treatment for 12 weeks diminished gradually over time, suggesting that patients may benefit from treatment with **naltrexone** for longer than 12 weeks.
- Literature on **naltrexone** treatment of alcohol dependence has been reviewed in detail in a number of meta-analyses.
- It appears that targeted medication administration (medication given during periods of high risk craving) may be useful both for the initial treatment of problem drinking and for maintenance of the beneficial effects of an initial period of daily naltrexone.

- A series of RCTs have shown that the beneficial effects of treatment with **naltrexone** can be maintained during an extended period through the use of either a more intensive, skills-oriented treatment (i.e., CBT) or a less intensive, supportive treatment combined with continued **naltrexone** administration.
- Poor compliance with oral **naltrexone** has been shown to reduce the potential benefits of the medication.
- As a result of poor compliance, interest in the development and evaluation of long-acting injectable formulations of the medication has increased; monthly, compared with daily, administration would improve medication adherence and parenteral administration would increase bioavailability by avoiding first-pass metabolism.
- FDA approved long-acting **naltrexone** for monthly administration at a dosage of 380 mg: the package insert states that the medication should be used only in alcohol-dependent patients who are abstinent at treatment initiation (for at least 7 days) since studies showed the most effect with this entry condition.

Clinical Considerations in the Use of Naltrexone The medication should be prescribed at the time that psychosocial treatment is initiated.

Because of adverse effects of the medication that could compound the adverse effects of alcohol withdrawal, the initiation of **naltrexone** therapy is probably best delayed until after the acute withdrawal period.

Initial testing for liver enzyme abnormalities is warranted to avoid prescribing the medication in the context of extreme elevations.

Ongoing monitoring is required only if symptoms warrant it, because the consistent effect of **naltrexone** in studies of alcohol dependence has been to decrease liver enzyme concentrations.

Oral **naltrexone** should be administered initially at a dosage of 25 mg per day to minimize adverse effects. The dosage can then be increased in 25-mg increments every 3 to 7 days.

Increase to maximum dosage of 150 mg per day using desire to drink or another symptom that the patient identifies as reflective of risk of relapse to heavy drinking.

No clear evidence that a higher dosage is more efficacious than the FDA-approved dosage of 50 mg per day.

Initial side effects Nausea, gastrointestinal symptoms, and neuropsychiatric symptoms (e.g., headache, dizziness, light-headedness, weakness) are most common in early treatment and are usually transient.

Delaying or avoiding a dosage increase can be used to address more persistent adverse events.

Long-acting **naltrexone** is only available as a 380-mg dose, which should be administered intramuscularly in the buttock every 4 weeks. The medication is approved for use in patients who are abstinent from alcohol and who are also receiving psychosocial treatment. Local interventions, such as warm compresses, and nonsteroidal anti-inflammatory medications can be used to treat such injection site reactions.

Nalmefene As with **naltrexone**, **nalmefene** is an opioid antagonist without agonist properties.

Nalmefene's affinity for the delta opioid receptor is greater than that of **naltrexone**.

A pilot study of **nalmefene** 40 mg per day showed it to be superior to both 10 mg per day of the medication and placebo in the prevention of relapse to heavy drinking in alcohol-dependent patients.

Recently, targeted **nalmefene** (where subjects were encouraged to use 10–40 mg of the medication when they believed drinking to be imminent) was combined with a minimal psychosocial intervention in a multi-center, placebo-controlled, randomized trial; effects were similar to that of **naltrexone**.

For both **naltrexone** and **nalmefene**, the optimal dosage and duration of treatment and the relative benefit accruing to combining the medication with different types and intensities of psychosocial treatment are important clinical questions that have not yet been adequately addressed.

Acamprosate

Acamprosate (calcium acetylhomotaurinate) is an amino acid derivative that increases γ-aminobutyric acid (GABA) neurotransmission and also has complex effects on excitatory amino acid (i.e., glutamate) neurotransmission.

Acamprosate was first shown in a single-site study to be twice as effective as placebo in reducing the rate at which alcohol-dependent patients returned to drinking.

Studies in >4,000 patients in Europe provided evidence of a beneficial effect of **acamprosate** in the prevention of relapse to drinking and in the reduction of drinking among patients who relapse.

A meta-analysis of continuous abstinence showed a significant advantage for **acamprosate** over placebo, and although the effects were modest, they increased progressively as treatment duration increased from 3 to 6 and then to 12 months.

Two multicenter trials conducted in the United States, the first being a multicenter trial of two active dosages of **acamprosate** and the second being the COMBINE (Combining Medications and Behavioral Interventions for Alcoholism) Study, the largest alcohol treatment trial to date (described in the following section), failed to show an advantage of **acamprosate** over placebo on an intent-to-treat basis.

Clinical Considerations in the Use of Acamprosate
Acamprosate is FDA approved at a dosage of 1,998 mg per day (i.e., two 333-mg capsules three times per day) in patients who are abstinent from alcohol and are receiving psychosocial treatment.

Most common adverse effects of the drug are generally mild and transient and include gastrointestinal (e.g., diarrhea, bloating) and dermatologic (e.g., pruritus) complaints.

In contrast to **disulfiram** and **naltrexone**, which are metabolized in the liver, **acamprosate** is excreted unmetabolized, so that renal function is the rate-limiting factor in the drug's elimination.

Evaluation of renal function prior to initiation of the drug is warranted, particularly in individuals who have a history or are otherwise at risk of renal disease and in the elderly.

Studies Comparing Acamprosate with Naltrexone and the Two Medications Combined
The COMBINE Study, a 4-month, multicenter, placebo-controlled study conducted at 11 sites in the United States, compared naltrexone, **acamprosate**, and their combination in a sample of nearly 1,400 abstinent alcohol dependent.

Overall, when on study treatment, subjects significantly increased the percentage of abstinent days. The study found an advantage for naltrexone but not for acamprosate compared to placebo or when combined with naltrexone.

Anticonvulsants
Medications studied in this class include **carbamazepine**, **divalproex**, and **topiramate**.

Although these medications have different mechanisms of action, it is likely that they exert beneficial effects in alcohol dependence through their actions as glutamate antagonists and GABA agonists, helping to normalize the abnormal activity in these neurotransmitter systems seen following chronic heavy drinking.

- Twelve-month pilot study found **carbamazepine** to be superior to placebo in increasing the time to the first heavy drinking day and in reducing drinks/drinking day and the number of consecutive days of heavy drinking.
- Twelve-week, double-blind pilot study found that a significantly lower percentage of patients receiving **divalproex** than placebo relapsed to heavy drinking.
- Twelve-week, placebo-controlled study of **topiramate**, with the dosage gradually increased over 8 weeks to a maximum of 300 mg. **Topiramate**-treated patients showed significantly greater reductions than placebo-treated patients in drinks per day, drinks/drinking day, drinking days, heavy drinking days, and GGT levels.

The most common adverse effect of **topiramate** is numbness and tingling (which is secondary to the commonly observed metabolic acidosis produced by the antagonism by **topiramate** of carbonic anhydrase).

Other common side effects include a change in the sense of taste, tiredness/sleepiness, fatigue, dizziness, loss of appetite, nausea, diarrhea, weight decrease, and difficulty concentrating, with memory, and in word finding.

Of clinical concern also are suicidal thoughts or actions, which have been reported uncommonly.

Baclofen
In a small trial, randomly assigned recently abstinent alcohol-dependent individuals received up to 30 mg per day of the medication or placebo divided into three daily doses. The medication was well tolerated and the **baclofen**-treated group was more likely to remain abstinent over the 1-month treatment period (also showing a greater number of cumulative abstinence days) than the placebo group.

There is, however, evidence of misuse, overdose, and other complications (e.g., withdrawal reactions, including delirium) associated with **baclofen**, which underscores the need for more research on this medication before it can be recommended as a safe and efficacious treatment for alcohol dependence.

Serotonergic Agents
A recent meta-analysis concluded that there was no benefit to the use of any antidepressant in alcohol-dependent patients without comorbid depression. However, some studies suggest that antidepressants may have benefits in selective subtypes of alcoholics.

Alcohol Dependence Subtypes

Low-risk/severity alcohol-dependent patients (i.e., those with later age of onset) drank on fewer days and were more likely to be completely abstinent in the 12-week treatment trial when treated with **sertraline** compared with placebo.

In a 6-month posttreatment follow-up of these patients, the beneficial effects of **sertraline** treatment persisted in this subgroup.

Using a subtyping approach, it was found that **ondansetron** (a 5-HT3 receptor antagonist) selectively reduced drinking among patients with early onset of problem drinking (i.e., before age 25; early-onset alcohol-dependent patients). Specifically, **ondansetron** was superior to placebo on the proportion of days abstinent and on the intensity of alcohol intake.

In contrast, late-onset alcohol-dependent patients showed effects of ondansetron on drinking behavior that were comparable to those of placebo.

Prospective studies are needed to evaluate whether there is a clearer role for the serotonergic medications in the treatment of heavy drinking or alcohol dependence in individuals differentiated by alcohol dependence subtype.

MEDICATIONS TO TREAT CO-OCCURRING PSYCHIATRIC SYMPTOMS OR DISORDERS IN ALCOHOL-DEPENDENT PATIENTS

Some patients report persistence in mood and anxiety symptoms well after acute withdrawal period is over.

These low-level mood or anxiety symptoms may develop into a condition that has been called "subacute withdrawal."

Although medications (e.g., SSRIs) are often prescribed during the postwithdrawal period in hopes of relieving these symptoms, there is no good evidence that the treatment of persistent or subacute withdrawal symptoms that do not meet diagnostic criteria for a co-occurring psychiatric disorder results in better outcome in alcohol-dependent patients.

Community studies have shown high rates of co-occurrence of psychiatric disorders in alcohol-dependent individuals in the community.

Further, the majority of such individuals who seek treatment meet lifetime criteria for one or more psychiatric disorders in addition to alcohol dependence, most commonly mood disorders, drug dependence, antisocial personality disorder, and anxiety disorders.

Antidepressants, benzodiazepines (BZs) and other anxiolytics, antipsychotics, and lithium have been used to treat anxiety and depression in the postwithdrawal state.

The choice of medications should take into account the increased potential for adverse effects when prescribed to individuals who are actively drinking heavily.

Adverse effects can result from pharmacodynamic interactions with medical disorders that commonly occur in the course of alcohol dependence, as well as from pharmacokinetic interactions with medications prescribed to treat these disorders.

Antidepressant Treatment of Unipolar Depression and Alcohol Dependence

There is evidence that most episodes of postwithdrawal depression will remit without specific treatment if abstinence from alcohol is maintained for a period of days or weeks.

Persistent depression requires treatment.

SSRIs and newer generation antidepressants have become the first-line treatment of depression because they have a favorable adverse event profile, but their efficacy compared to placebo is not well supported.

These medications do not have the anticholinergic, hypotensive, or sedative effects of the tricyclic antidepressants, nor do they have the adverse cardiovascular effects, which in overdose can be lethal.

However, SSRIs can exacerbate the tremor, anxiety, and insomnia often experienced by recently detoxified alcohol-dependent patients and may slightly increase the risk of gastrointestinal bleeding (particularly in combination with nonsteroidal anti-inflammatory drugs or aspirin.)

Mood-Stabilizer Treatment of Bipolar Disorder and Alcohol Dependence

Bipolar disorder co-occurs commonly with alcohol dependence.

Presence of alcohol dependence is associated with an increased rate of mixed or dysphoric mania and rapid cycling, as well as greater bipolar symptom severity, suicidality, and aggressivity.

Controlled trials of medication to treat these comorbid disorders are difficult to conduct.

Treatment of Co-Occurring Anxiety Disorders and Alcohol Dependence

Benzodiazepines and Other Anxiolytics

The relative merits of the use of BZs in alcohol-dependent and other substance abuse patients during the postwithdrawal period for the management of anxiety or insomnia have been debated in the medical literature.

Although generally opposed by non-medical personnel, judicious use of the drugs in this setting may be justified.

Early relapse, which commonly disrupts alcohol rehabilitation, can result from protracted withdrawal-related symptoms (e.g., anxiety, depression, insomnia). To the extent that these symptoms can be suppressed by low doses of BZs, retention in treatment could be increased.

Although there is little doubt that alcohol-dependent individuals are more vulnerable to develop dependence on the BZs than the average person, the potential for abuse and dependence may be lower than is generally believed.

However, dependence on both alcohol and BZs may increase depressive symptoms, and co-occurring alcohol and BZ dependence may be more difficult to treat than alcoholism alone.

Diazepam, **lorazepam**, and **alprazolam** may have greater abuse potential than **chlordiazepoxide** or **clorazepate**. **Oxazepam** was reported to produce low levels of abuse.

Buspirone, a non-BZ anxiolytic, exerts its effects largely via its partial agonist activity at serotonergic autoreceptors. Although comparable in efficacy to **diazepam** in the relief of anxiety and associated depression in outpatients with moderate-to-severe anxiety, **buspirone** is less sedating than **diazepam** or **clorazepate**, does not interact with alcohol to impair psychomotor skills, and does not have abuse liability.

This pharmacologic profile makes **buspirone** more suitable than BZs to treat anxiety symptoms among alcohol-dependent patients.

In contrast to BZs, however, **buspirone** does not have acute anxiolytic effects, is not useful in the treatment of alcohol withdrawal, and is not useful for treating the insomnia that is commonly reported by alcohol-dependent patients during acute and protracted withdrawal.

Although **buspirone** appears to be useful in the treatment of anxiety symptoms in alcohol-dependent patients, it has not been possible to identify clinical features that differentiate individuals for whom **buspirone** may be most efficacious from those who are not responsive to the medication.

CHAPTER 47

Summary Author: Ashok Krishnamurthy
Jeffrey S. Cluver • Tara M. Wright • Hugh Myrick

Pharmacologic Interventions for Sedative-Hypnotic Addiction

PHARMACOLOGY

The effects of benzodiazepines and other sedative-hypnotics are mediated by their binding to the GABA receptor.

When an agonist such as a benzodiazepine or a barbiturate binds to the GABA receptor, the receptor opens its chloride channel, which then decreases neuronal excitability. Clinically this leads to the effects of

1. Decreased anxiety
2. Increased sedation
3. Muscle relaxation
4. Increased seizure threshold

The toxic effects of these compounds are caused by excessive opening of chloride channels and can lead to respiratory depression, coma, and death.

One essential difference between benzodiazepines and barbiturates is that high doses of barbiturates *lead to excessive activity of GABA at the GABA-A receptor, which directly leads to respiratory depression, whereas high doses of benzodiazepines do not.*

A compound with a high affinity for the GABA receptor that does not exert an agonist or inverse agonist effects is **flumazenil**: it is marketed to reverse the effects of benzodiazepines, including sedation and respiratory depression.

Both *physical dependence* and *tolerance* are inevitable with prolonged and regular use of medications in the class of benzodiazepines and other sedative-hypnotics.

ISSUES OF ABUSE AND DEPENDENCE

Overall, there has been a trend toward decreased use of benzodiazepines and other sedative-hypnotics, but their use is still widespread.

Lorazepam, **alprazolam**, and **diazepam** all appear to have a greater potential for abuse, based on their inherent properties (i.e., their lipophilic properties and therefore more rapid onset of action).

Misuse and abuse of benzodiazepines and sedative-hypnotics is commonly seen in individuals with other substance use disorders.

In this context, sedative-hypnotics are often used to enhance the effects of other drugs and alleviate unpleasant side effects from use of or withdrawal from other substances.

The majority of patients who develop benzodiazepine and sedative-hypnotic dependence were initially being treated for problems with sleep and anxiety disorders.

Individuals seeking treatment for anxiety disorders, sleep disorders, and depression are at higher risk for developing sedative-hypnotic dependence if they have a history of substance use disorders. A family history of substance use disorders also places an individual at higher risk for developing dependence.

INTERVENTIONS

In a state of intoxication, a patient may require monitoring and even intervention to ensure a safe recovery.

In patients experiencing acute withdrawal, pharmacologic management is often recommended because of the risk of serious consequences, including seizures and delirium tremens.

Sedative-hypnotics are commonly *recommended for the shortest period of time possible*, and these medications are often seen as *short-term therapies that should be discontinued as soon as the clinical situation permits.*

MANAGEMENT OF INTOXICATION

The signs and symptoms of benzodiazepine and sedative-hypnotic intoxication are very similar to those of alcohol intoxication.

Severe intoxication can lead to respiratory depression, coma, and death, especially with the barbiturates and other older, nonbenzodiazepine agents.

Benzodiazepine intoxication, even in the situation of an overdose, rarely leads to death, unless the benzodiazepines are combined with other CNS depressants.

The management of acute intoxication is mostly supportive.

In overdose, it is also critical to know what other psychoactive agents (especially CNS depressants) may have been acutely or chronically ingested. **Flumazenil** can be used in the case of benzodiazepine intoxication, but *its use is limited by the risk of precipitating withdrawal symptoms, including seizures.*

WITHDRAWAL

Withdrawal symptoms are most often seen in patients who abruptly discontinue taking benzodiazepines and other sedative-hypnotics.

Individuals are likely to develop withdrawal symptoms when they have been taking high doses of sedative-hypnotics or if they have been taking low or moderate doses for a prolonged period of time.

The signs and symptoms of withdrawal manifest differently in each patient: characteristics like age and overall state of health and the properties of the unique pharmacologic properties of each medication affect this.

The half-life of the medication is of particular importance, especially when discussing the *onset* of withdrawal symptoms.

1. The withdrawal from agents with short half-lives usually begins within 12 to 24 hours and reaches peak intensity within 1 to 3 days.
2. With longer-acting agents, withdrawal symptoms may begin later and not peak until 4 to 7 days after discontinuation.
3. Symptoms may then continue for several more days or even weeks, depending on the half-life of drug.

Prolonged or protracted withdrawal symptoms may include anxiety, sensitivity to light, sound, touch, and tinnitus. In contrast to *symptom reemergence*, protracted withdrawal symptoms often wax and wane and slowly resolve with continued abstinence.

It has been estimated that up to 50% of regular benzodiazepine users will experience clinically significant signs of withdrawal with sudden discontinuation.

MANAGEMENT OF WITHDRAWAL

A. The most straightforward approach is to initiate a taper that uses decreasing doses of the therapeutic agent over the course of 6 to 12 weeks. This is most often used in settings of long-term use and physical dependence, where there is not an urgent need to discontinue the current medication.

For this strategy to be effective, the patient must be able to follow complex dosing regimens, adhere to regular follow-up appointments, and be free of other active substance use disorders.

As lower doses are achieved, the dose reduction at each stage should be more modest, especially if short-half-life drugs are being prescribed.

More frequent dosing intervals can also be used in the later stages to help prevent the emergence of any withdrawal symptoms.

B. Another withdrawal strategy is to convert the therapeutic agent to an equivalent dose of a longer-acting agent and then gradually reduce the dose of the latter, using the principles described earlier. Agents such as **clonazepam** and **chlordiazepoxide** are especially good choices given their slower onset of action and therefore relatively limited abuse potential.

C. Another option for withdrawal treatment is the use of **phenobarbital**.

The starting daily dose of **phenobarbital** should be based on the patient's drug use during the previous month.

In cases when this is not known, a **pentobarbital** challenge test can be used to determine the starting dose. The maximum starting dose is 500 mg daily. The daily dose should be administered in divided doses, three times a day, and then tapered by 30 mg a day.

Signs of **phenobarbital** intoxication are similar to those seen with other sedative hypnotics and include *slurred speech, ataxia, and nystagmus.* If signs and symptoms of intoxication are present, then the total daily dose should be decreased by 50% (or more) and the patient reassessed at frequent intervals until the intoxication resolves.

D. Another strategy for the treatment of withdrawal is the use of **carbamazepine**.

This anticonvulsant has been shown to be as effective as **oxazepam** in the treatment of alcohol withdrawal, and two open-label studies also demonstrated the effectiveness of this agent in the management of complicated benzodiazepine withdrawal.

On the basis of initial studies, the suggested dosing of **carbamazepine** is in the range of 200 mg three times a day for 7 to 10 days. Because of the potential for serious adverse events during sedative-hypnotic withdrawal, patients should be monitored closely, and benzodiazepines should be used as needed.

Carbamazepine has *low abuse potential and limited cognitive side effects,* especially during short-term use. These properties make **carbamazepine** an attractive option in patients who are beginning a treatment program while also undergoing medically supervised withdrawal.

E. Both **gabapentin** and **divalproex** compare favorably to **carbamazepine** in terms of research supporting their use in the treatment of alcohol withdrawal. This suggests that these agents would also be efficacious in the treatment of the symptoms of sedative-hypnotic withdrawal.

TREATMENT SETTING

Inpatient treatment of withdrawal should be limited to cases in which the patient is medically compromised or a high risk of the patient's developing severe symptoms, such as seizures, exists.

Other conditions:

1. Patients taking high doses of sedative-hypnotics for a long period and who require rapid medically supervised withdrawal.
2. Patients have been taking multiple sedative-hypnotics or are alcohol dependent.
3. Patients who have a history of experiencing severe withdrawal when they have previously stopped using sedative-hypnotics

Medically supervised outpatient withdrawal is reasonable if

1. The patient does not appear to be at risk for severe withdrawal
2. The method of slowly reducing the sedative-hypnotic dose can be utilized
3. The patient should be given clear instruction and close follow-up appointments

POSTWITHDRAWAL TREATMENT

Medically supervised withdrawal should not be seen as definitive treatment in the case of sedative-hypnotic dependence.

This is the first step in the management of patients who often have other substance use disorders, anxiety and sleep disorders, and other co-occurring medical and psychiatric disorders.

In the case of other substance use disorders, a treatment plan should include co-occurring medically supervised withdrawal from other substances and substance abuse treatment in an appropriate setting.

When treating patients with underlying anxiety and sleep disorders, other pharmacologic and psychotherapeutic treatments, particularly cognitive-behavioral therapy, should be initiated.

Co-occurring psychiatric disorders should also be addressed during or soon after withdrawal.

CHAPTER

48

Summary Author: Ashok Krishnamurthy
Susan M. Stine • Thomas R. Kosten

Pharmacologic Interventions for Opioid Dependence

ABSTINENCE SYNDROMES AND MEDICALLY SUPERVISED WITHDRAWAL

The opioid abstinence syndrome is characterized by two phases: (a) a relatively brief initial phase in which opioid-dependent patients experience acute withdrawal, followed by (b) a protracted abstinence (PA) syndrome. The acute withdrawal syndrome lasts from 5 to 14 days and consists of

1. Gastrointestinal distress (such as diarrhea and vomiting)
2. Disturbances in thermal regulation
3. Insomnia
4. Myalgia
5. Arthralgia
6. Marked anxiety
7. Dysphoria

Though not life threatening, the acute withdrawal syndrome causes marked discomfort, often prompting continuation of opioid use, even in the absence of any opioid-associated euphoria.

Opioid Agonists and Partial Agonists

Opioid-based medically supervised withdrawal is based on the principle of cross-tolerance, in which one opioid is replaced with another that is slowly tapered.

Methadone is usually used because it has a long half-life and can be administered once daily.

Withdrawal from heroin is usually managed with initial dosages of **methadone** in the range of 15 to 30 mg per day. This starting dose does not usually excess 40 mg per day. A simple conversion of short-acting prescription medications into an equivalent dosage of **methadone** can lead to overdose as the **methadone** accumulates over the first several days of dosing. Peak dosing usually takes at least 2 to 3 days to achieve, with steady state achieved at about 5 days.

In acute medical settings, this starting dosage should be maintained through the 2nd or 3rd day after the peak dose is attained and then the **methadone** can be slowly tapered by approximately 10% to 15% per day.

Outpatient withdrawal using **methadone** must be performed in a federally licensed opioid treatment program.

Buprenorphine's slow dissociation from μ opioid receptors results in a long duration of action and also has milder withdrawal signs and symptoms on discontinuation than full agonists. Such qualities may make **buprenorphine** an advance in medically supervised withdrawal treatment by permitting accelerated withdrawal without significant distress.

Several studies have supported the benefits of **buprenorphine** and **buprenorphine/naloxone** for medically supervised opioid withdrawal.

The optimum dose of **buprenorphine** for acute inpatient heroin withdrawal has not been determined.

Nonopioid Medication Treatments

Nonopioid methods of medically supervised opioid withdrawal have focused primarily on **clonidine**, an α_2-adrenergic agonist.

Therefore, α_2-adrenergic agonists act centrally at the locus coeruleus via presynaptic receptors to moderate the symptoms of noradrenergic hyperactivity during medically supervised opioid withdrawal.

Clonidine Early clinical studies demonstrated that **clonidine** diminished withdrawal symptoms in patients who were withdrawn from methadone.

Clonidine seems to be most effective in suppressing autonomic signs and symptoms of opioid withdrawal but is less effective for subjective withdrawal symptoms.

Initial daily doses of up to 1.2 mg per 24 hours in divided doses are commonly suggested. For example, a regimen of 0.1 to 0.2 mg every 4 hours has been used in clinical trials for heroin withdrawal, with careful monitoring of blood pressure.

Because it may be less effective in managing subjective withdrawal symptoms, adjuvant therapy (NSAIDs for myalgia, benzodiazepines for insomnia, and antiemetics for nausea) may be needed.

In a study that examined predictors of successfully completed supervised withdrawal using **clonidine**, patients who completed withdrawal were more likely to be heroin smokers (rather than intravenous users) and to have abstained from opioids for a longer time before presenting for treatment.

Lofexidine and Other α-Adrenergic Agonists Other medications have been sought to replace **clonidine** due its side effect profile, especially hypotension.

The aim is to find a drug that has **clonidine's** capacity to ameliorate the signs and symptoms of opioid withdrawal but with fewer side effects.

Lofexidine, a centrally acting α_2-adrenergic agonist, has, after **clonidine**, been the most used and investigated α_2-adrenergic treatment for opioid withdrawal. Clinical trials are currently underway to secure approval for sale in the United States by the U.S. Food and Drug Administration.

Lofexidine does not reduce blood pressure to the same extent as **clonidine**, but is otherwise similar to **clonidine**.

Medication Combinations, Rapid and Ultrarapid Opioid Detoxification

Rapid protocols use an opioid antagonist (e.g., **naloxone** or **naltrexone**) to cause an accelerated withdrawal response, with the goal of completing withdrawal in shorter periods from 8 days to as little as 2 or 3 days.

In addition to an opioid antagonist, rapid approaches use pharmacotherapies (**clonidine** and sedation) to minimize the acute withdrawal symptoms experienced when opioid antagonists are administered.

Because withdrawal is completed more quickly, the combination rapid approach has been proposed to have the advantage of minimizing the risk for relapse and allowing patients to enter continued treatment with **naltrexone** maintenance more rapidly.

Ultrarapid methods are similar in pharmacologic approach to the rapid method but use general anesthesia and complete the procedure in several hours. This method is not recommended because of the risks of general anesthesia and because the long-term efficacy is not superior to use of **buprenorphine** or **clonidine**.

LONG-TERM TREATMENTS FOR OPIATE DEPENDENCE

Dependence and Protracted Abstinence

In patients with a history of opioid dependence, acute withdrawal and medically supervised withdrawal are only the beginning of treatment.

The concept of PA has been controversial but remains a useful model for scientific hypothesis testing and development of new therapeutic approaches.

Some have recommended **methadone** maintenance treatment (MMT) for PA, even though it establishes physical dependence. Because **methadone** continues physical dependence, PA may remain a problem at a later time when medically supervised withdrawal from **methadone** is undertaken.

In addition to biologic considerations, psychosocial concomitants of opioid dependence also necessitate longer, more specialized adjunct treatments for these and additional problems.

Naltrexone Maintenance Treatment

Naltrexone is a long-acting, orally effective, predominantly opioid antagonist that provides complete blockade of opioid receptors when taken at least three times a week for a total weekly dose of about 350 mg.

Because the reinforcing properties of opioids are completely blocked, **naltrexone** is theoretically an ideal maintenance agent in the rehabilitation of opioid-dependent patients who can successfully complete withdrawal and maintain abstinence from opioids.

However, this optimistic theoretical perspective is contradicted by clinical reality, as reflected in treatment retention rates of only 20% to 30% over 6 months.

Craving for opioids may continue during naltrexone treatment.

A meta-analysis of multiple studies did not provide strong support for **naltrexone** treatment of opioid dependence. Nevertheless, for some patients (such as health care professionals, business executives, or probation referrals) for whom there is an external incentive to comply with **naltrexone** therapy and to remain opioid abstinent, **naltrexone** has been very effective.

A pharmacologic approach to patient noncompliance may be the availability of an injectable, long-acting preparation of **naltrexone**, which would eliminate the need for daily intake.

Clinically, **naltrexone** is initiated after acute withdrawal from opioids. There should be at least a 5- to 7-day opioid-free period for the short-acting opioids and a 7- to 10-day period for the long-acting agents.

The initial dose of **naltrexone** used generally is 25 mg on the 1st day, followed by 50 mg daily or an equivalent of 350 mg weekly, divided into three doses.

The principal reason for the reduced dose on day 1 is the potential for gastrointestinal side effects, such as nausea and vomiting. This occurs in about 10% of patients taking **naltrexone**.

The most serious (but far less frequent) potential side effect of **naltrexone** is liver toxicity; however, 50 mg daily has been given safely to opioid-dependent individuals. Liver toxicity, in the rare instances it occurs, appears to be limited in extent in that it resolves when **naltrexone** is discontinued and does not progress to liver failure.

In summary, though **naltrexone** has not lived up to expectations, for selected, motivated patients who are opioid dependent, it may represent a very effective form of maintenance pharmacotherapy.

Methadone Maintenance Treatment

Rationales for treatment:

1. Relieve the PA syndrome
2. Block heroin euphoria
3. Opportunity it affords for psychosocial stabilization in the context of symptom relief

Good treatment retention, improved psychosocial adjustment, and reduced criminal activity are among the benefits reported.

No serious side effects are associated with continued methadone use with the exception of hypogonadism in men and risk of QT prolongation and exceedingly rare but potential subsequent progression to torsades de pointes.

Minor side effects, such as constipation, excess sweating, drowsiness, and decreased sexual interest and performance.

Neuroendocrine studies have shown normalization of stress hormone responses and reproductive functioning (both of which are significantly disrupted in heroin users) after several months of stabilization on **methadone**.

A series of large-scale studies have demonstrated that patients maintained on doses of 60 mg or more of methadone a day had better treatment outcomes than those maintained on lower doses and that doses below 60 mg appear to be inadequate for most patients.

A recent factor mandating higher doses is the current purity of street heroin: Opioid cross-tolerance implies that the amount of heroin needed to produce euphoria would be prohibitively expensive for someone maintained on a sufficiently high dose of **methadone**.

High doses and pure street drug also may increase the risk of toxicity if patients try to override the cross-tolerance with illicit heroin, as tolerance to respiratory depression may not be as complete as that to euphoria.

Three types of factors that have been shown to significantly modify the metabolic breakdown of **methadone** in the body are as follows:

1. Chronic diseases, (chronic liver disease, chronic renal disease, and possibly other diseases)
2. Medication interactions, including interactions of **methadone** with **rifampin** and **phenytoin**, **carbamazepine** in humans, possibly with ethanol and *disulfuram* and, also, by inference from animal studies, interactions of **methadone** with **phenobarbital**, **diazepam**, **desipramine**, and other drugs, as well as with estrogen steroids, **cimetidine**, and antiviral agents used in treatment of HIV
3. Altered physiologic states, especially pregnancy

In general, for successful rehabilitation, length of treatment with **methadone** is best seen in terms of years rather than months.

The importance of psychosocial treatment as an adjunct to **methadone** pharmacotherapy cannot be over-emphasized.

From an organizational and public health perspective, early treatment termination, illicit use of nonopioid substances (such as cocaine or alcohol), and diversion of the take-home dose of **methadone** to the illicit market remain significant issues for most **methadone** maintenance programs.

Although concurrent substance use also is a problem (initially, 20% to 50% of **methadone** patients use cocaine, and 25% to 40% abuse alcohol), several effective treatment interventions have been developed, including behavioral approaches and pharmacologic interventions.

Diversion of take-home doses is of concern to every **methadone** maintenance program, though its impact on illicit opioid use remains small as **methadone** accounts for about 4% of opioids used on the street.

Buprenorphine Maintenance Treatment

Buprenorphine is a μ opioid partial agonist.

Early on in its development, researchers thought a sublingual tablet of **buprenorphine** should have added to it **naloxone**, an opiate antagonist, that would help fight diversion and injection of the **buprenorphine**.

The **buprenorphine** s.l. tablet is available in two forms. One formulation (**Subutex**) contains only **buprenorphine** (the "mono" tablet). The second formulation (**Suboxone**) contains **buprenorphine** and the opioid antagonist **naloxone** in a 4:1 ratio, which is designed to discourage illicit diversion and intravenous use.

The "mono" form would be employed in the clinical setting under direct observation, whereas the "combo" form would be suitable for take-home use.

Clinical research over the past 15 years has established that **buprenorphine** (and **buprenorphine** with **naloxone**) is a safe and effective alternative to **methadone** for opioid agonist maintenance treatment.

Treatment with **buprenorphine** produces significant and substantial improvements over time in psychosocial functioning.

In particular, **buprenorphine's** ceiling on agonist activity reduces the danger of overdose and may limit its abuse liability.

Buprenorphine has low toxicity even at high intravenous doses.

Buprenorphine appears less likely than **methadone** to prolong the QT interval on the ECG.

Buprenorphine also can produce sufficient tolerance to block the effects of exogenously administered opioids.

A transdermal and a depot formulation of **buprenorphine** have been developed that may provide extended relief from opioid withdrawal, reduce required clinic visits, and improve adherence, while having less potential for diversion and abuse.

Buprenorphine and naloxone in combination and **buprenorphine** alone are safe and reduce the use and craving for opioids in an office-based setting.

Buprenorphine Induction and Stabilization

Buprenorphine can produce withdrawal discomfort among opioid-dependent volunteers under certain conditions:

1. Low **buprenorphine** doses may provide too little agonist effect, that is, insufficient substitution relative to the maintenance opioid (such as heroin). In this case, raising the **buprenorphine** dose may or may not surmount this problem.

2. Alternatively, **buprenorphine** may directly precipitate withdrawal discomfort, in which case higher doses could be expected to aggravate the problem. Individuals maintained on the long-acting, full μ opioid agonist **methadone** can experience withdrawal symptoms, when given the high-affinity partial μ-agonist **buprenorphine**, which abruptly reduces the extent of opioid receptor stimulation.

As a result, it was recommended that the induction dose of **buprenorphine** be administered when patients are beginning to experience opioid withdrawal, so that **buprenorphine** can suppress those symptoms.

Clinical experience with administering initial doses of **buprenorphine** to heroin-dependent patients suggests that an interval of 6 hours probably is sufficient to minimize the risk of precipitated withdrawal. Precipitated withdrawal usually is more sudden and can be more severe and uncomfortable than naturally occurring withdrawal.

The general guidelines for beginning opioid treatment medication are published in the CSAT Treatment Improvement Publications.

The typical first dose of **buprenorphine** is 4 mg, and a sublingual tablet should be observed to have dissolved completely under the tongue.

After the first dose, patients should wait in an observation area and be checked 30 to 60 minutes later for acute adverse effects.

If same-day dosing adjustments must be made, patients should wait 2 to 4 more hours after the additional dosing, for further evaluation when peak effects are achieved.

If withdrawal symptoms persist after 2 to 4 hours, the initial dose can be supplemented with up to 4 mg for a maximum 1st day dose of 8 mg of **buprenorphine**.

The 1st day's dose should be followed by dosage increases over subsequent days until withdrawal symptoms are suppressed within about 2 hours after taking the medication and lasting until the next day's dosing when using once-daily dosing.

For most patients undergoing induction with the combination tablet, the initial target dose after induction should be 12 to 16 mg of **buprenorphine** in a 4-to-1 ratio to **naloxone**.

During dose induction, patients may need to visit their physician's office daily for dose adjustments and clinical monitoring.

SPECIAL ISSUES IN MAINTENANCE TREATMENT

Opioid Maintenance Treatment During Pregnancy

Opioid misuse during pregnancy carries with it risk of adverse consequences for both the mother and her infant including high rates of infection, premature delivery, and low birth weight, which is an important risk factor for later developmental delay.

The pattern of increased nonmedical use of analgesics seen in the general population has also been found for pregnant women, with self-reported nonmedical use increasing from 51,900 in 1993 to an average of 109,000 in 2002 to 2004.

Treatment options studied include **methadone** maintenance, antagonist maintenance (i.e., **naltrexone**), and medication-assisted withdrawal.

Methadone maintenance has been the recommended standard of care over no treatment or medication-assisted withdrawal.

This recommendation is based on longer durations of maternal drug abstinence, better obstetrical care compliance, avoidance of associated risk behaviors, reductions in fetal illicit drug exposure, and enhanced neonatal outcomes.

Methadone is the oldest, most widely used medication prescribed during pregnancy. Infants from heroin-abusing mothers and infants from **methadone**-treated mothers have increased fetal growth, reduced fetal mortality, decreased risk of HIV infection, decreased risk of preeclampsia and fetal exposure to rapid and unpredictable cycles of heroin-induced highs and withdrawal, and an increased likelihood of the infant being discharged to his or her parents.

Prenatal exposure to **methadone** provided as a part of comprehensive treatment does not appear to be associated with developmental or cognitive impairments.

Although newborns of **methadone**-maintained women may experience opioid withdrawal symptoms, these are readily treated without damaging consequences. Generally, 50% to 81% of neonates prenatally exposed to **methadone** show some signs of neonatal abstinence syndrome (NAS).

Maternal **methadone** dosage does not correlate with neonatal withdrawal; therefore, maternal benefits of effective **methadone** dosing are not offset by neonatal harm.

Large, definitive randomized controlled trials of **buprenorphine** in pregnant women have not been conducted.

Interactions of Opioid Maintenance and Human Immunodeficiency Virus and Acquired Immunodeficiency Syndrome Pharmacotherapy

Methadone maintenance thus appears to be extremely effective in reducing injection-related risk factors for HIV.

Preclinical studies of antiretroviral medications and opioids indicate that drug interactions are likely to occur as both **methadone** and **buprenorphine** are primarily metabolized by hepatic cytochrome CYP450 3A4.

Methadone has been associated with several clinically important adverse drug interactions with HIV medications.

- Patients who receive MMT may show a potentially toxic increase in serum levels of AZT: careful clinical monitoring for signs of dose-related AZT toxicity is suggested.
- Antiretroviral medications that can induce **methadone** metabolism, when discontinued, may cause cardiac dysrhythmias due to increased **methadone** exposure after reversal of **methadone** metabolism induction leads to increased **methadone** exposure: It has been recommended that after the medication that is inducing CYP450 3A enzymes is stopped, the **methadone** dose should be tapered over 1 to 2 weeks to reestablish the previous therapeutic dose of **methadone**.

Reductions in **buprenorphine** concentrations resulting from drug interactions have not been associated with opioid withdrawal.

Though pharmacologically buprenorphine may present fewer medication interaction problems, the outpatient office setting may not be the most therapeutic with respect to medication adherence. Drug abuse treatment programs, irrespective of modality, are associated with improved adherence to antiretroviral therapies among drug users.

MMT, in particular, has been shown to be associated with highly active anti-retroviral therapy (HAART) adherence and improved HIV treatment outcomes among HIV/HCV coinfected injection drug users.

Methadone-to-Buprenorphine Transfer

Some patients will be transferred from **methadone** to **buprenorphine** for maintenance or medically supervised withdrawal.
Reasons include

1. Unique pharmacology of **buprenorphine**, leading to its more favorable safety profile and longer duration of action (thus permitting less-frequent dosing) relative to **methadone**
2. Given its status as a novel treatment option (which may differentially attract or retain novelty seeking individuals), **buprenorphine** may engender less fear of stigma than **methadone**.
3. Owing to its availability in office-based primary care—outside the domain of standard opioid treatment program—**buprenorphine** is more accessible over a wide geographic area.

Buprenorphine also may be more appropriate as an early intervention strategy for those with short dependence histories (e.g., adolescents), or with less physical dependence.

A multitude of small clinical studies now show that **methadone** to **buprenorphine** transfer is feasible over a range of starting methadone doses.

Recommendations from CSAT for patients taking **methadone** are to taper **methadone** to 30 mg or less per day for 1 week or more before initiating **buprenorphine**.

Induction should not begin until at least 24 hours after the last dose of **methadone** and should start at 2 mg of the monotherapy formulation.

If signs or symptoms of withdrawal are seen after the first dose, a second dose of 2 mg should be administered and repeated, if necessary, to a maximum of 8 mg **buprenorphine** on day 1.

Larger clinical trials are needed to answer questions concerning short- and long-term clinical outcomes after **methadone** to **buprenorphine** transfer.

Buprenorphine in Agonist-to-Antagonist Treatment

Buprenorphine has been used in several experimental studies as a transitional agent between agonists (such as **methadone** or heroin) and antagonists (such as **naloxone** or **naltrexone**).

The use of **buprenorphine** to stabilize opioid-dependent patients before switching them to **naltrexone** has the advantage of psychosocial stabilization prior to medically supervised withdrawal.

This approach may represent a compromise between acute medically supervised withdrawal and long-term treatment of chronic dependence. The **buprenorphine/naltrexone** may be combined in a clinical protocol that places **methadone** patients or heroin-dependent patients on **buprenorphine** for several weeks to stabilize and engage them in the psychosocial aspects of treatment. This could be followed by rapid transition to **naltrexone**, using clonidine to relieve any withdrawal symptoms caused by stopping the **buprenorphine**.

Summary Author: Ashok Krishnamurthy
Judith Martin • Joan E. Zweben • J. Thomas Payte

Opioid Maintenance Treatment

UNIQUE ASPECTS OF OPIOID DEPENDENCE

Vincent Dole, a pioneer in developing **methadone** treatment, held the view that there is something unique about opioid addiction that makes it difficult for patients to remain free of illicit heroin use for extended periods of time.

> It is postulated that the high rate of relapse of addicts after detoxification from heroin use is due to persistent derangement of the endogenous ligand narcotic receptor system and that **methadone** in an adequate daily dose compensates for this defect.

> Some patients with long histories of heroin use and subsequent rehabilitation on a maintenance program do well when the treatment is terminated. The majority, unfortunately, experience a return of symptoms after maintenance is stopped. The treatment, therefore, is corrective but it is for future research to identify the specific defect in receptor function and to repair it. Meanwhile, **methadone** maintenance provides a safe and effective way to normalize the function of otherwise intractable opiate addict.

Further research is needed to define the metabolic disease process and the respective roles of genetic predisposition and environmental exposure.

PET scans that look at cerebral metabolism in opiate-dependent patients suggest that **methadone** maintenance at least partly normalizes cerebral glucose metabolism, as compared with patients withdrawn from **methadone** and in sustained remission.

CLINICAL ISSUES IN MAINTENANCE PHARMACOTHERAPY

Goals of Pharmacotherapy of Opioid Dependence

1. Prevention or reduction of withdrawal symptoms
2. Prevention or reduction of opioid craving
3. Prevention of relapse to use of addictive opioids
4. Restoration to or toward normalcy of any physiologic function disrupted by chronic opioid use

Profile of Potential Psychotherapeutic Agents

Characteristics of potential psychotherapeutic agents can be defined as follows:

1. Such medications are effective after oral administration.
2. They have a long biologic half-life (≥24 hours).
3. They have minimal side effects during chronic administration.
4. They are safe.
5. They are efficacious for a substantial proportion of persons with the disorder.

Methadone and **buprenorphine** generally demonstrate these characteristics.

MAINTENANCE TREATMENT USING METHADONE

Heroin Versus Methadone

The opioid-dependent person who is actively misusing heroin or other short-acting opioids typically experiences

1. Rapid and wide swings in opiate effects after each use
2. Followed by sedation, fading into a period of normalcy and alertness
3. Followed by the beginnings of *subjective withdrawal*, sometimes called *craving*
4. Develops into the full *objective withdrawal* syndrome typical of opioid addiction

A full cycle from "sick" to "high" to "normal" to "sick" can occur repeatedly throughout the day.

Methadone, regularly administered at steady state, is present at levels sufficient to maintain alertness without craving or drug preoccupation (comfort zone or therapeutic window) throughout the dosing interval—usually 24 hours.

With the next maintenance dose, there is a gradual rise in blood level, *reaching a peak at 3 to 4 hours*.

Typically, the peak level *is less than two times the trough level*.

There is a gradual decline over the rest of the 24-hour period, back to the trough level. When the patient is on the correct dose at steady state, at no time does the rate or extent of change in blood levels cause a sensation of being high or result in withdrawal symptoms.

Induction

The starting dose of **methadone** must be much fairly low, and the eventual steady state is reached slowly, sometimes over weeks.

The first several doses require careful evaluation and adjustment. This phase is usually called *induction* and *is the most critical phase of treatment.*

Even though methadone maintenance has been shown to reduce mortality, including overdose mortality, several studies have reported deaths during the first 10 to 14 days of treatment, particularly when induction doses are high and when the patient is also ingesting sedatives.

Up to 42% of drug-related deaths during treatment have occurred during the 1st week of opioid maintenance treatment (OMT).

Initial Dose

The response to the initial dose of agonist medication provides valuable information about tolerance levels and the target "therapeutic window." Significant relief during peak (2–4 hours) is evidence that the dose is in the range of the established level of tolerance and may not require further escalation.

The absence of relief suggests that the dose is well short of the therapeutic window.

Additional methadone can be provided when significant objective withdrawal persists during peak methadone levels.

Patients who present at the dosing window 24 hours after their very first dose can be expected to be uncomfortable as tissue stores accumulation is still incomplete. If they were comfortable during the first 4 to 12 hours after their dose, they probably need more time at the same dose, and not a higher daily dose.

The initial dose of **methadone** is no >30 mg in most cases and may be lower in patients in whom low tolerance might be expected (e.g., recent relapse after a significant period of abstinence or addiction to lower potency opioids such as **hydrocodone** or **codeine**, or in opium smokers).

Under federal regulations, the first dose is limited to no >30 mg and a total dose of no >40 mg on the first treatment day unless the program physician documents in the patient's record that 40 mg did not suppress opioid abstinence symptoms.

Stabilization and Steady State

The induction phase can be considered to last until the patient has been on a stable dose for 4 to 5 days (half-lives).

In general, steady-state levels are reached after a drug is administered for 4 to 5 half-lives (**methadone** has an average half-life of 24–36 hours). The clinical significance is that, with daily dosing, a significant portion of the previous dose remains in tissue stores, resulting in increased peak and trough **methadone** levels after the second and subsequent doses. Thus, the levels of methadone increase daily, even without an increase in dose. The rate of increase levels off as steady state is achieved at 4 to 5 half-lives, that is, 3 to 7 days.

Dose adjustments can be done in 5- to 10-mg increments for highly tolerant patients, every 3 to 7 days to reestablish steady state between each dose adjustment.

Maintenance

A stable dose occurs when the desired clinical effects arise, cravings are quenched, and withdrawal is prevented. The maintenance phase thereafter begins.

Maintenance continues until such a time that there is a reason to alter the treatment.

Most **methadone**-maintained patients do well on a dose range of 80 to 120 mg/day, though some patients require less and some require more.

Tolerance appears to remain stable with no need to escalate the dose, as would be the case for short-acting opioid analgesics. Endocytosis of μ-opioid receptors and *N*-methyl D-aspartate receptor antagonism are unique characteristics of **methadone** itself, which may contribute to this stabilizing feature.

Duration and Dose

Dose level and duration of treatment are individualized clinical decisions.

There is no scientific or clinical basis for an arbitrary dose ceiling on **methadone**, although QT prolongation has been seen in the electrocardiograms of patients receiving high doses of **methadone**.

Methadone doses of 80 to 100 mg have greater benefits than doses below 50 mg in heroin-dependent patients.

The American Society of Addiction Medicine supports the principle that MMT is most effective as a long-term modality.

The known risks of discontinuing **methadone** treatment, with predictable relapse to injected heroin use, become increasingly critical when viewed in the context of the human immunodeficiency virus (HIV) epidemic. These risks, when compared to the proven safety and efficacy of long-term **methadone** treatment, suggest that long-term—even indefinite—**methadone** treatment is appropriate and even essential for a significant proportion of eligible patients.

Treatment should be continued as long as

1. The patient continues to benefit from treatment.
2. The patient wishes to remain in treatment.
3. The patient remains at risk of relapse to opioid or other substance use.
4. The patient suffers no significant adverse effects from continued MMT.
5. Continued treatment is indicated in the professional judgment of the physician.

Techniques to Ensure Adequacy of Dose

Blood Levels in Dose Determination Mean, random, or trough levels of methadone *do not define an adequate dose.*

The clinical utility of blood levels is based on peak and trough values to define a rate of change or a peak-to-trough ratio.

In the **methadone** clinic setting, patients occasionally experience problems in maintaining stability on a given dose of **methadone**

The same dose may vary in efficacy among individuals and that patients may be doing poorly as a result of inadequate dosing. Under-dosing or rapid metabolism of the dose can be determined by examination of the patient at peak and trough when steady state would be expected, i.e., after 3 to 7 days of regular dosing at a given dose of methadone. Rarely, blood levels are needed to support or clarify the clinical picture and can be valuable in making decisions about divided dosing.

There is growing consensus that in the highly tolerant patient, levels above 400 ng/mL can represent an optimum level in providing adequate cross-tolerance to make ordinary doses of intravenous heroin ineffective (nonreinforcing) during **methadone** treatment. It should be emphasized that *there is no "therapeutic" standard blood level.*

Methadone peak, trough, and mean levels and the rate of elimination (half-life) (24-hour dose response curve) can be influenced by several factors:

1. Individual differences in the metabolism
2. Poor absorption
3. Changes in urinary pH
4. Effects of concomitant medications
5. Diet
6. Vitamins

Pregnancy, particularly during the third trimester, is associated with significant decrease in trough **methadone** levels, suggesting increased rates of metabolism of **methadone**.

Blood levels can help identify patients who may benefit from a divided-dose regimen or demonstrate the effectiveness of a divided-dose regimen.

Procedure for Obtaining Blood Levels
Ideally, peak blood levels should be drawn at 3 hours after a dose and trough levels at 24 hours.

Patients already on a divided dose, such as every 12 hours, should have 2- to 3-hour and 12-hour specimens.

The peak level at 3 hours should be no more than twice the trough level. A peak-to-trough ratio of 2 or less is ideal (peak/trough ratio). *Ratios >2 suggest rapid metabolism.*

Methadone-Drug Interactions
Clinical experience suggests that concomitant medications can either induce or inhibit CYP450 activity on methadone metabolism.

Drugs that stimulate or induce CYP450 activity can precipitate opioid withdrawal by accelerating metabolism, thus shortening duration and diminishing intensity of the effect of **methadone**.

Rifampicin, phenytoin, carbamazepine, phenobarbital, nevirapine, or **efavirenz** may result in onset of withdrawal symptoms and require dose adjustments of the methadone.

Cimetidine, ciprofloxacin, fluconazole, erythromycin, and **fluvoxamine** may inhibit this CYP450 activity, slowing the metabolism and extending the duration of the drug effect.

A 17-fold variability between patients in their **methadone** metabolism is shown, mostly due to activity of various intrinsic enzymes.

Methadone and QT Interval
In vitro study of hERG K+ channels confirms that **methadone** at therapeutic doses can affect cardiac conduction.

In vitro studies suggest that most of this prolongation is due to the nontherapeutic S-methadone enantiomer. Methadone maintenance has been shown to prolong the QT interval and has been associated with torsades de pointes.

Risk-benefit discussion with patients includes a review of other medications that might contribute to additional cardiac risk. In general, it is considered that almost certain relapse to uncontrolled opioid use is more risky than the rare occurrence of and dysrhythmia.

Coordination of care with outside physicians to monitor use of other medications or transfer to **buprenorphine** treatment in some cases may be indicated.

Methadone-Related Deaths of Persons Not in Treatment
There has been a dramatic increase in mortality by ingestion of diverted **methadone** intended for pain treatment since 1995.

Deaths from **methadone** overdoses exceeded deaths from heroin overdoses in some states by 2002.

MAINTENANCE TREATMENT USING BUPRENORPHINE

Buprenorphine is a partial mu-opioid agonist.
The FDA approved two sublingual formulations of **buprenorphine** for treatment of opioid dependence.

1. Combination of **buprenorphine** and **naloxone** in a 4:1 ratio is designed to discourage injected diversion and misuse—this formulation is intended for general outpatient use and is available in sublingual tablet and sublingual film.
2. Sublingual formulation contains only **buprenorphine** and is used in controlled settings, such as inpatient medically supervised withdrawal, or in pregnancy.

Naloxone is an opioid antagonist that is not significantly bioavailable when taken sublingually or when swallowed. When injected into actively using opioid-dependent subjects who are blinded, the combination formulation was not judged to be desirable or to be different from antagonist in the 1st hour after injection.

Pharmacology of Sublingual Buprenorphine
Buprenorphine has slow onset and long duration of action, conferring similar maintenance benefits as discussed earlier for **methadone**.

Its peak effect is 2 to 4 hours after sublingual administration, and its duration is 72 hours.

As a partial mu agonist, **buprenorphine** has a maximal dose-effect ceiling that is well below significant respiratory depression.

Induction and Precipitated Withdrawal

Buprenorphine is a partial agonist with strong receptor attachment.

The first dose should be given when the patient is already in obvious opioid withdrawal.

When opioid withdrawal is already present, the onset of activity will be felt as agonist, with relief of withdrawal.

Contrary to **methadone**, induction doses are not set by regulation, though clinical guidelines and physician training courses recommend 2 to 4 mg of sublingual **buprenorphine/naloxone** as a first dose, with 1st-day maximum of 8 mg.

Buprenorphine Dose Adjustment

The dose can be rapidly titrated over the first 3 days to control withdrawal. Average daily doses are 16 to 20 mg.

Because of the partial agonist ceiling effect, no additional maintenance benefit is expected in doses above 32 mg/day.

Compared to **methadone**, **buprenorphine** may confer advantages when certain HIV medications are used and in cases of QT prolongation with **methadone**.

Federal Regulations and Sublingual Buprenorphine

When dispensed in the OTP, sublingual **buprenorphine/naloxone** is subject to the same regulations as **methadone**.

When prescribed in the office-based setting, there are certain restrictions set forth in the Drug Addiction Act of 2000.

This law provides for a waiver to the 1914 Harrison Act that forbids prescription of a narcotic to an addicted person. The qualifying physician notifies the Secretary of Health and Human Services of his or her intent to prescribe, after which the DEA assigns to the physician a second DEA number that is specifically for use under DATA 2000.

The DATA 2000 restrictions do not apply when **buprenorphine** or **buprenorphine/naloxone** is dispensed at clinics under their OTP license.

Diversion and Abuse of Buprenorphine

No serious adverse events were found by the introduction of sublingual **buprenorphine/naloxone** in the office-based setting.

Wherever **buprenorphine** treatment has been introduced, there have been diversion and abuse of the medication, including injected use.

One study in the United States showed that diverted **buprenorphine/naloxone** is being used mostly for relief of withdrawal and rarely as a primary drug of abuse.

Choice Between Methadone and Buprenorphine

Systematic reviews suggest that **methadone** is superior in retaining patients.

Observed Doses and Take-Home Medication in OMT

Patients who do well and who improve according to specified criteria set out in federal regulations can earn take-home medications for unsupervised dosing.
Eligibility criteria include

1. Adherence to treatment
2. Stability of home environment
3. Involvement in productive activity
4. Abstinence from drugs of abuse
5. Resolution of any legal problems

Monthly observed dosing at the OTP, with carryout of the remaining doses for the month, is as close as most MMT patients come to receiving their medication in a fashion similar to that in other well-controlled medical conditions.

Methadone Medical Maintenance

Methadone medical maintenance, designed for "stable, recovered" patients on **methadone**, is an effort to release the patient from burdensome attendance in an OTP by allowing a physician who is affiliated with the clinic, but in office practice, to prescribe or administer the maintenance medication.

Medical maintenance generally refers to attendance that is reduced to one or two visits per month, with a minimum number of supportive services, and is offered to selected stable patients.

Many patients risk their abstinence and, in an AIDS epidemic, their lives in an effort to withdraw from **methadone** for nonmedical reasons. For those who are attempting to free themselves from OTP constraints rather than from the effects of daily medication, medical maintenance could be an acceptable solution.

Current regulations require a federal waiver for medical maintenance.

A 2001 study randomly assigning patients to either office- or OTP-based **methadone** showed no difference in clinical outcomes and improved patient and physician satisfaction.

PAIN MANAGEMENT

Patients on OMT require special consideration because of their baseline maintenance opioid. They will be tolerant to additional opioids, and if nonopioid approaches are not effective, *they may need unusually high and frequent doses of opioids to manage their pain.*

Acute Pain

In cases of acute pain associated with surgery, trauma, or dental work, the physicians or dentists involved often—incorrectly—assume that the maintenance dose of **methadone** also will relieve any ensuing pain from the injury or procedure.

Several points should be kept in mind:

1. Single daily doses of **methadone** may be effective in controlling addiction, but multiple daily doses may be required for analgesia.
2. Long-term use of **methadone**, and possibly **buprenorphine** as well, is associated with *hyperalgesia*.
3. *Tolerance* and *hyperalgesia* combined means that patients in OMT who require opioids for pain management may need very high doses of opioids.

Mixed agonist-antagonists (**pentazocine**, **butorphanol**, **nalbuphine**) and partial agonists (**buprenorphine**) must not be used in **methadone**-maintained patients, as they will precipitate an opioid withdrawal syndrome.

Meperidine and **propoxyphene** should be avoided because of the risk of seizures at the higher doses required to produce analgesia in **methadone**-maintained patients.

Chronic Pain

More than 30% of OMT patients report chronic, severe pain.

Compared to those who primarily misuse heroin, patients admitted to the OTP for prescription opioid abuse may have higher prevalence of pain.

In a patient with chronic nonmalignant pain who is able to comply with the regulatory criteria for take-home medication, the OTP physician can order a divided dose of **methadone**, and the outside physician can prescribe short-acting rescue medication.

PREGNANCY AND OPIOID AGONIST TREATMENT

Opioid maintenance remains the treatment of choice for pregnant, opioid-dependent patients.

Methadone and **buprenorphine** are category C medications, though there is more experience with the use of methadone in pregnancy.

Except for HIV-positive mothers, breastfeeding by patients on OMT is encouraged.

Maternal medically supervised withdrawal during pregnancy is technically possible.

There is concern that it would result in potentially dangerous intrauterine fetal distress. For this reason, medically supervised withdrawal of pregnant patients is usually done in the hospital with fetal monitoring. The main practical consideration of medically supervised withdrawal during pregnancy is relapse.

NEEDLE-RELATED COMORBIDITY

Of heroin-addicted patients admitted to OMT in 2005, 63% were injection drug users.

Infections related to needle use are a main source of comorbidity and death in the OMT population. Related comorbidities are

1. Acute skin infections (abscesses, cellulitis)
2. Necrotizing fasciitis
3. Botulism
4. Endocarditis

Human Immunodeficiency Virus

Between 15% and 20% of long-term injection drug users are positive for HIV.

Maintenance patients are routinely screened and if necessary treated with antiretrovirals.

Participation in OMT is useful in prevention of HIV.

MMT is associated with fewer high-risk behaviors, such as unsafe injection practices or having multiple sexual partners.

Dose adjustments may become necessary in patients on **methadone** or **buprenorphine** maintenance who begin highly active antiretroviral treatment for HIV.

HIV-related conditions usually require coordination with specialty clinics.

Hepatitis C Virus

The most common presenting symptoms are fatigue, abdominal pain, anorexia, and weight loss. The initial workup indicated 26% had chronic hepatitis, 37% had chronic active hepatitis, 36% had cirrhosis, and 0.8% had hepatocellular carcinoma. Alcohol use increases the severity of the disease.

OTP programs are developing educational interventions to encourage health practices (such as complete elimination of alcohol) that are likely to prolong the period of good health.

Patients with hepatitis C should be vaccinated against hepatitis A and hepatitis B if they are not immune or if serologic status cannot be determined.

When patients need treatment for hepatitis C, the standard care includes a weekly pegylated **interferon** injection and oral ingestion of **ribavirin** several times a day. Most IDUs require a year of treatment, depending on genotype. Patients on OMT can expect excellent results in treatment, with sustained remission in 54%.

PATIENTS WITH CO-OCCURRING PSYCHIATRIC DISORDERS

Depression and dysthymia are common co-occurring disorders in the treatment-seeking population.

Psychosocial stress and the discomforts of withdrawal may contribute to temporarily low mood as well.

Life crises and depressive symptoms pose a substantial risk of relapse, which lessened for those who remained in treatment.

Studies of antidepressants with this population have produced mixed results, indicating a need to determine how to select opiate-dependent patients most likely to benefit.

Anxiety disorders also are common, with symptoms abating with a combination of an adequate **methadone** dose and the provision of counseling or psychotherapy over a period of time.

Posttraumatic stress disorder (PTSD) is common in **methadone** patients, and though it may be associated with greater drug abuse severity, PTSD does not necessarily worsen the outcome of substance abuse treatment. Patients with PTSD received higher doses of medication, attended more psychosocial treatment sessions, and had better treatment retention. However, their PTSD symptoms did not improve with substance abuse treatment alone. *Seeking Safety* represents a manualized intervention for early recovery stabilization of patients with PTSD and substance abuse.

Schizophrenia is relatively uncommon in opioid treatment patients, though most programs have some patients with the disorder.

PSYCHOSOCIAL INTERVENTIONS

Psychosocial interventions are considered integral to good treatment in a methadone program, and requirements for this are written into regulations.

In many OTPs, psychosocial interventions are provided by counselors, who range widely in educational level and professional training.

The counselor's task is to identify and address specific problems in the areas of drug use, physical health, interpersonal relationships (including family interaction), psychologic problems, and educational or vocational goals.

The counselor often serves as a case manager as well, initiating screening for medication and other program services; attending to issues concerning program rules, privileges, and policies; and providing links to other agencies.

Clinics that have access to professionally trained staff may offer psychotherapy to selected patients.

The provision of comprehensive services is supported by recent research. For example, studies have shown that the addition of enhanced onsite professional services led to better results than basic counseling alone.

Quality, quantity, and the match between the patient's specific problem areas (e.g., vocational, family, or psychiatric) and the services offered all led to demonstrably better outcomes in a variety of populations.

A quality assurance process that monitors and encourages a close fit between the patient's needs and the services delivered is likely to produce the best outcome, in contrast to a single approach in which most patients receive a similar mix of services.

OVERSIGHT AND REGULATORY CHALLENGES

A consensus statement issued in 1998 by the National Institutes of Health supported the chronic disease model of opiate addiction and pointed to MMT as the best available treatment.

The Center for Substance Abuse Treatment (CSAT) has published Guidelines for the Accreditation of Opioid Treatment Programs, and facilities providing MMT must be accredited.

An urgent need to increase access to treatment while improving and ensuring the quality of that treatment drives the need for restructuring. However, the rapid rise of **methadone**-associated deaths has created a new context for efforts to reduce barriers. *Although the majority of these deaths are related to pain management rather than clinic practices*, deaths due to poor management of the induction period have been documented. Extensive efforts to train physicians more systematically are underway.

Summary Author: Ashok Krishnamurthy
Andrew J. Saxon

Special Issues in Office-Based Opioid Treatment

EPIDEMIOLOGIC AND REGULATORY ISSUES

Most opioid-dependent individuals cannot access adequate treatment services.

In 2005, approximately 254,000 individuals entered treatment for heroin dependence, but only 30% received medication-assisted treatment.

Similarly, 67,000 entered treatment for dependence on other opioids, but only 20% received medication-assisted treatment. These data reflect a circumstance that has been prevalent throughout the past 100 years.

Thousands of untreated opioid-dependent individuals also worried society in the early part of the 20th century.

Although controversy raged then, as it does now, about how best to handle opioid-dependent individuals, many experts of that generation already had recognized the high likelihood that opioid-dependent patients would resume opioid use after enforced withdrawal. Physicians in many areas of the country thus viewed opioid addiction as a medical disorder; they advocated and practiced the ongoing prescribing of opioids from their offices as a form of harm reduction.

In 1919, the U.S. Supreme Court ruled that the Harrison Act disallowed such prescribing to opioid-dependent individuals for "maintenance" purposes. The decision was largely based on a small number of reports of inappropriate prescribing and increasing concern (from doctors, regulators, and the public) about safety and wisdom of prescribing opioids to opioid-dependent individuals. *This decision effectively ended the first era of office-based treatment for opioid addiction.*

Thus, from the 1920s onward, physicians were actively discouraged from treating heroin-dependent individuals and, indeed, medical school curricula provided no training to physicians in this regard.

Convicted violators of federal narcotics laws caused an overload in the federal penal system, so Congress established federal narcotics hospitals at Lexington, Kentucky, and Fort Worth, Texas, in the 1930s. Despite high recidivism rates, these isolated facilities remained the only treatment option for opioid-dependent individuals until the advent of methadone maintenance 30 years later.

The divergence between mainstream medicine and opioid addiction treatment has had some unfortunate consequences. Licensed opioid agonist treatment programs often lack the resources to provide comprehensive medical care, with the result that comorbid medical disorders may be unattended, delaying care and driving up its ultimate cost.

Similarly, a high prevalence of Axis I psychiatric comorbidity, particularly mood and anxiety disorders, is seen among patients who are addicted to opioids, and licensed programs typically cannot provide the treatment these conditions require.

Many potential patients who need and desire opioid agonist treatment and are willing to enroll in licensed programs cannot overcome the barriers to entry. Three states (North Dakota, South Dakota, and Wyoming) do not offer licensed opioid agonist treatment.

In states that do offer such programs, the licensed clinics, by virtue of economic necessity and neighborhood acceptance, tend to be sited primarily in urban locations.

Even within larger metropolitan areas, specific neighborhoods or communities can bar licensed clinics.

Inadequate treatment capacity creates another barrier for potential patients who do live in reasonable proximity to a licensed clinic: Many clinics have waiting lists that discourage potential patients from even attempting entry.

Many more potential patients lack the financial resources to pay for their treatment.

Finally, the very nature of licensed opioid agonist treatment clinics, with the potential to be recognized and stigmatized by passersby, waiting lines for medication administration, rigid attendance policies, and lack of privacy, deters some potential patients.

Three important developments have now altered the Landscape.

1. Since March 2000, the licensed opioid agonist treatment programs can apply for exceptions so that stable, long-term patients can enter **methadone** medical maintenance and have visits to obtain medication less frequently than once per week.
2. The *Drug Addiction Treatment Act*, passed in 2000, allows qualified physicians to prescribe certain opioid agonist medication in an office-based setting.
3. In October 2002, the FDA approved **buprenorphine** and **buprenorphine/naloxone** for the treatment of opioid dependence. These medications were placed in Schedule III and so are available for use in office-based opioid treatment (OBOT).

RESEARCH ISSUES

Research Related to Stable, Long-Term Patients in Office-Based Practice

The available research regarding methadone patients who have achieved some measure of stability shows fairly convincingly that most *can transfer successfully to office-based care.*

In addition, in virtually all cases, patients who fail in office-based treatment because of substance relapse or rule violations *can be returned from office-based care to methadone clinic care to receive intensified counseling and monitoring without undue harm.*

The controlled studies also suggest that relapse or other problems in previously stable patients in office-based practice occur at rates *no greater than those of similarly stable patients who remain in methadone clinic care.*

Research Related to Patients Entering Directly into Office-Based Practice

In Scotland, most patients who receive **methadone** have it prescribed in general practitioners' offices and ingest it in community pharmacies.

England also has had a policy since the 1980s of encouraging opioid-dependent individuals to get methadone maintenance treatment (MMT) through office-based treatment by general practitioners.

Today, general practitioners in France can prescribe up to 28 days' supply of take-home medications and a maximum daily **buprenorphine** dose of 16 mg. About 65,000 patients per year have received **buprenorphine** in this office-based paradigm.

Multiple studies of direct office-entry opioid maintenance treatment have been conducted in the United States since the 1990s.

All of these early evaluations of direct entry to office-based treatment for opioid addiction support its viability as a treatment option and show its acceptance by patients, physicians, and pharmacists.

Treatment retention in these office-based investigations did not fall markedly below—nor did illicit opiate use rise strikingly above—rates reported in recent clinic-based investigations of opioid agonist treatment.

CLINICAL ISSUES

Patient assessment and appropriate selection of patients for transfer from clinic-based to office-based care obviously are key elements of a comprehensive paradigm.

Studies suggest that more episodes of MMT and longer time in treatment are associated *with a greater likelihood of a good outcome after transfer to office-based care.*

Hair testing studies suggest that many of the patients who relapse after transfer to office-based care had intermittent ongoing use while still in methadone clinic care and that this ongoing use was missed because of infrequent urine toxicology testing. Because hair testing is not routinely available, an alternative might be to obtain weekly or more frequent urine screens for some period before the anticipated transfer of any apparently stable patient from a licensed clinic to office-based care.

How thoroughly one would assess and how stringently one would screen patients for potential transfer to office-based care may depend on how much illicit substance use is to be tolerated in the office-based setting.

Safety concerns would dictate that patients who are using illicit drugs should not have any take-home *methadone* to minimize the potential for overdose.

Patients who use illicit drugs may pose a greater risk of diverting **methadone** to raise cash to buy drugs. Nevertheless, the controlled studies indicate that substance use did not differ on the basis of treatment in office-based versus standard clinic care.

Office-based practitioners vary in their ability to tolerate and manage relapse. Some may feel very uncomfortable and immediately wish to transfer the patient back to standard clinical care, while others may prefer to intensify services in other ways.

A monitoring plan that would be practical in an office-based setting would involve

1. Monthly nonrandom urine specimens at the time of scheduled office visits
2. A few unscheduled callbacks per year, with medication checks and provision of random urine specimens
3. A very quick callback after any positive urine specimen to obtain a repeat specimen within a few days

Psychosocial interventions form another potentially valuable element of office-based treatment for transferred patients.

Such interventions would be brief and might be minimal or unnecessary for the highly stable, long-term patients.

In the context of an office visit, it would be desirable for the physician to ask about the patient's drug and alcohol use and cravings; how the patient is doing at work and/or with family or child care responsibilities, and financial and housing circumstances; about psychiatric and medical status; and about use of leisure time.

To a great extent, patient selection for direct entry into office-based treatment must rely on the specific areas of expertise and clinical skills of the treating physician.

Through thorough assessment, including a complete history and physical examination, the physician should ascertain whether he or she can comfortably manage—either by direct care and/or by adequate referral networks—the combination of substance use problems, general medical problems, psychiatric problems, and life crises likely to arise in the treatment of each patient.

Physicians should exercise caution and refer patients who are not good candidates for their practice settings to licensed treatment programs.

No solid scientific data are available to guide precise techniques or monitoring schedules.

Urine toxicology testing and periodic medication callbacks, coupled with regular clinical evaluation, likely will continue to serve as the mainstays of monitoring.

For newly entering patients, tight control of medication dispensing, when practical, likely enhances the patient's progress toward stability.

Buprenorphine and **buprenorphine/naloxone** are the only agonist medications approved for the treatment of patients directly entering office-based care in the United States.

Although daily observation of medication ingestion would not be practical in most office-based settings, **buprenorphine** can be administered effectively three times a week, a schedule that probably is feasible in some office-based settings and/or their affiliated community pharmacies.

Indicators of ensuing clinical stability include

1. Compliant behavior
2. Regular, timely attendance at scheduled office visits
3. Successful compliance with medication callbacks
4. Negative urine toxicology tests
5. Productive use of time
6. Supportive interpersonal relationships
7. Absence of criminal justice involvement

Careful pharmacotherapy of newly entering patients can contribute to their stability.

The potential for medication diversion plays into decisions about medication dose and frequency of dispensing. Diversion by a patient undermines and endangers the patient's efforts toward achieving a stable recovery from opioid dependence.

Possible signs of diversion: failing a medication callback, request for early refills, sudden unexplained increase in disposable income, and sudden request for a dose increase in a previously stable patient without an apparent explanation for instability.

Diversion can be prevented at the outset by

1. Provider-initiated treatment contract detailing consequences of diversion, preferably by written agreement
2. Loss of take-home medication privileges or medication callbacks
3. Discontinuation of treatment

If patients know that they will have to account for all outstanding medication, diversion will be deterred.

Repeated episodes of diversion clearly indicate that office-based treatment is not an appropriate setting and argue for transfer to a more structured, licensed program.

Psychosocial treatments may be even more important to patients who are newly entering office-based treatment than to stable patients who already have received regular counseling at a licensed program.

Studies of various intensities of psychosocial services in licensed **methadone** programs do offer some illumination on this point: *Patients who receive minimal psychosocial services do not fare as well as do those who receive moderate or high levels of services*; however, the lower cost-effectiveness of more intensive services may nullify any slight advantage they hold over moderate services.

At present, physicians are eligible to practice office-based treatment of opioid addiction on completion of 8 hours of formal training.

Expert consensus suggests that appropriate training should consist of most of the following topics:

1. Overview of opioid dependence and rationale for agonist treatment
2. Legislation permitting office-based treatment general opioid pharmacology
3. General opioid pharmacology
4. Pharmacology of **buprenorphine** and **buprenorphine/naloxone**
5. Efficacy and safety of **buprenorphine**
6. Clinical use of **buprenorphine** including induction, stabilization, and withdrawal
7. Patient assessment and selection
8. Office management, including treatment agreements, urine testing, record keeping, and confidentiality
9. Co-occurring psychiatric and medical disorders
10. Psychosocial treatments
11. Special populations including adolescents, pregnant women, and patients with pain

CHAPTER 51

Summary Author: Ashok Krishnamurthy
David A. Gorelick*

Pharmacologic Interventions for Cocaine, Methamphetamine, and Other Stimulant Addiction

Stimulants such as cocaine and amphetamines are the second most widely used illegal drugs in the United States, surpassed only by cannabis.

There is no well-established, broadly effective pharmacotherapy for stimulant dependence.

COCAINE DEPENDENCE

Goals of Treatment

The behavioral mechanisms by which medication achieves treatment goals are poorly understood and can vary across patients and medications.

Currently available medications are considered to act by one or more of three mechanisms:

1. By reducing or eliminating the positive reinforcement from taking a cocaine dose
2. By reducing or eliminating a subjective state (such as "craving") that predisposes to taking cocaine
3. By reducing or eliminating negative reinforcement from taking a cocaine dose (as by reducing withdrawal-associated dysphoria)

Medication does not address these other mechanisms:

4. By making cocaine-taking aversive
5. By increasing the positive reinforcement obtained from non–cocaine-taking behaviors

The last mechanism (No. 5) is crucial to successful treatment because it ensures that other behaviors are reinforced to replace cocaine taking as the latter is extinguished, but such medications do not exist—as a result, this mechanism is engaged by psychosocial interventions that address issues such as vocational rehabilitation, the patient's social network, and use of leisure time.

Medication almost never is used without some psychosocial treatment component.

The type, intensity, and duration of psychosocial treatment that should accompany pharmacologic treatment are questions with little data to guide clinical decision making.

Pharmacologic Mechanisms

Four pharmacologic approaches are potentially useful in the treatment of cocaine dependence:

1. *Substitution* treatment with *a cross-tolerant stimulant* (analogous to methadone maintenance treatment [MMT]) of opioid dependence
2. Treatment with an *antagonist* medication that blocks the binding of cocaine at its site of action

---

*Dr. Gorelick is supported by the Intramural Research Program, NIH, National Institute on Drug Abuse.

3. Treatment with a medication that *functionally antagonizes* the effects of cocaine (as by reducing the reinforcing effects of or craving for cocaine)
4. *Alteration of cocaine pharmacokinetics* so that less drug reaches or remains at its site(s) of action in the brain

No medication currently is approved by the U.S. Food and Drug Administration (FDA) or any other national health authority for the treatment of cocaine dependence, chiefly because no medication has met the scientifically rigorous standard of consistent, statistically significant efficacy in replicated, controlled clinical trials.

Most current clinical research has focused on the second and third approaches mentioned above: reducing or blocking cocaine's actions, either directly at its neuronal binding site (true pharmacologic antagonism) or indirectly by otherwise reducing its reinforcing effects.

Cocaine's positively reinforcing effects derive from its blockade of the dopamine reuptake pump, causing presynaptically released dopamine to remain in the synapse and enhancing dopaminergic neurotransmission.

Cocaine's local anesthetic effects are believed to contribute to cocaine-induced kindling, the phenomenon by which previous exposure to cocaine sensitizes the individual so that later exposure to low doses produces an enhanced response.

CHOICE OF MEDICATION

Antidepressants

Heterocyclic Antidepressants Tricyclic and other heterocyclic antidepressants *are the most widely used and best-studied class of medications for the treatment of cocaine dependence.*

Their use is based both on the clinical observation of frequent depressive symptoms among cocaine-dependent individuals seeking treatment and on their pharmacologic mechanism of increasing biogenic amine neurotransmitter activity in synapses.

Desipramine is the best-studied of the tricyclic antidepressants. Meta-analysis suggests a non-significant trend towards efficacy.

Typical doses are 150 to 300 mg per day (about 2.5 mg/kg), similar to those used in the treatment of depression. Differences in patient characteristics, concomitant treatment, and **desipramine** plasma concentrations may account for some of the variability in efficacy of **desipramine**.

Some subsets of patients do better on **desipramine**.

Patients with depression and without antisocial personality disorder may respond best to **desipramine**.

Patients dually dependent on cocaine and opiates may do better on **desipramine** if their opioid dependence is treated with **buprenorphine** rather than methadone, or if they receive contingency management.

Experience with other heterocyclic antidepressants has shown limited evidence for efficacy.

No unexpected or medically serious side effects have been reported in published clinical trials of heterocyclic antidepressants. However, patients who relapse to cocaine use while still on antidepressant medications could, in theory, be at increased risk of cardiovascular side effects. Both cocaine and the tricyclics have quinidine-like membrane effects that, when superimposed, could lead to cardiac arrhythmias.

Selective Serotonin Reuptake Inhibitors A recent clinical trial found **citalopram** (20 mg per day) significantly better than placebo. That study, unlike previous studies, used contingency management in addition to cognitive-behavioral therapy, suggesting the important influence of psychosocial treatment on medication efficacy. There is no evidence for efficacy of other SSRIs.

Monoamine Oxidase Inhibitors The rationale for use of monoamine oxidase (MAO) inhibitors lies in their effect of increasing brain levels of biogenic amine neurotransmitters by inhibiting a major catabolic enzyme.

Limited open-label experience with **phenelzine**, at antidepressant doses of 30 to 90 mg per day, suggests that this medication can reduce cocaine and other stimulant use.

However, its clinical usefulness may be *limited by the need for dietary and concomitant medication restrictions* to avoid precipitating a hypertensive crisis, as well as by the theoretical *possibility of potentiating cocaine-induced effects, should the patient relapse to cocaine* use while still taking the medication.

Current research is focusing on selective MAO inhibitors that act only on MAO type B, the predominant type in the brain, while sparing MAO type A, the predominant type in the gastrointestinal tract. It is inhibition of MAO in the gastrointestinal tract that produces a hypertensive crisis.

Selegiline, marketed for the treatment of parkinsonism and, in the transdermal form, for treatment of depression, *is fairly selective for MAO type B at recommended doses* (10 mg per day for parkinsonism, 12 mg per day for depression). A recent multisite controlled clinical trial using **selegiline** administered via a skin patch (**selegiline** transdermal system) found no evidence for efficacy.

Dopamine Agonists (anti-Parkinson Agents)

Dopamine agonists, by stimulating synaptic dopamine activity, would ameliorate the effects of decreased dopamine activity caused by cessation of cocaine use; these include anhedonia, anergia, depression, and cocaine craving.

Bromocriptine, **pergolide**, and **amantadine**, all marketed for the treatment of parkinsonism (another dopamine deficiency condition), have not shown consistent efficacy in clinical trials.

Disulfiram can be considered a *functional dopamine agonist* because it blocks the conversion of dopamine to norepinephrine by the enzyme dopamine-β-hydroxylase, thereby increasing dopamine concentrations.

Interest in **disulfiram** as a treatment for cocaine dependence initially was generated by suggestions of its efficacy in patients with concurrent cocaine and alcohol dependence, a common comorbidity.

Three controlled clinical trials in cocaine-dependent patients without alcohol dependence (but with, in two studies, concurrent opioid dependence treated with **methadone** or **buprenorphine**) found **disulfiram** (250 mg per day) significantly better than placebo in promoting cocaine abstinence.

A more recent human laboratory study also found that **disulfiram** (250 mg daily for 4–6 days) decreased cocaine clearance but found no potentiation of the cardiovascular effects of intravenous cocaine (0.25 or 0.5 mg/kg). **Disulfiram** did significantly reduce the positive subjective response to cocaine. These findings suggest that **disulfiram** may be a promising new treatment for cocaine dependence, although raising a caution about potential adverse drug interactions should patients use cocaine while on the medication.

Stimulants

Several orally active psychomotor stimulants marketed for the treatment of attention deficit/hyperactivity disorder (ADHD) and narcolepsy or as appetite suppressants (anorexiants) have been used to test the substitution approach.

Two small controlled clinical trials with sustained release D-amphetamine found significant reductions in cocaine use at 30 to 60 mg daily, with no difference from placebo at lower doses.

Two controlled clinical trials using **methylphenidate** (90 mg daily) found no significant effect on cocaine use.

None of these studies reported significant adverse effects, suggesting that stimulant substitution treatment might be safe in cocaine-using patients.

Modafinil, used for the treatment of excessive sleepiness in narcolepsy, obstructive sleep apnea, and shift work sleep disorder, can be considered a weak stimulant (CSA schedule IV). A small phase II study found that 400 mg daily reduced cocaine use. A recent multi-site clinical trial found no efficacy overall at 200 mg or 400 mg daily. However, among a subgroup of subjects without alcohol dependence, **modafinil** was associated with an increased percentage of abstinent days.

Antipsychotics

The older antipsychotics, which are potent dopamine receptor antagonists (chiefly D2 [postsynaptic] subtype), do not appear to significantly alter cocaine craving or use.

Newer "second-generation" antipsychotics also have not been confirmed to significantly reduce cocaine craving or use in clinical trials of cocaine users without comorbid psychiatric disorders.

Caution should be exercised when prescribing any antipsychotic to cocaine users because of their potential vulnerability to the neuroleptic malignant syndrome, based on their presumed cocaine-induced dopamine depletion. Cocaine or amphetamine users may also be at elevated risk of antipsychotic-induced movement disorders.

Anticonvulsants

Anticonvulsants have been tried in the treatment of cocaine dependence because they block the development of cocaine-induced kindling in animals.

Kindling (increased neuronal sensitivity to a drug because of prior intermittent exposure) has been hypothesized as a neurophysiologic mediator of cocaine craving in humans.

At the neurotransmitter level, anticonvulsants might be effective because they increase inhibitory γ-aminobutyric acid (GABA) activity and decrease excitatory glutamate activity in the brain, both actions that would decrease the response to cocaine in the dopaminergic corticomesolimbic brain reward circuit.

Carbamazepine, the most-studied anticonvulsant, has not shown efficacy, nor have gabapentin or baclofen. Other anticonvulsants studied in recent trials with some beneficial effects on cocaine use:

Tiagabine, topiramate, vigabatrin

Phenytoin (300 mg daily) significantly reduced cocaine use in one controlled clinical trial, especially at serum concentrations above 6.0 μg/mL.

Nutritional Supplements and Herbal Products

Nutritional Supplements The use of amino acid mixtures, either alone or with other nutritional supplements (vitamins and minerals), has been widely publicized in the drug abuse treatment field, encouraged by their freedom from the regulations imposed on prescription medications and their perceived safety and absence of side effects. The majority of these studies have shown little benefit.

Herbal Products Various herbal and plant-derived products have been touted as treatments for drug abuse, but few have undergone controlled clinical evaluation.

Calcium Channel Blockers

Calcium channel blockers have been suggested as treatment for cocaine dependence. However, **amlodipine** showed no efficacy in a controlled clinical trial.

Other Physical Treatments

Acupuncture of the outer ear (auricular) has enjoyed growing popularity as a treatment for drug withdrawal, especially using five standard locations recommended by the National Acupuncture Detoxification Association (NADA): kidney, liver, lung, shen men, and sympathetic. *Meta-analyses of nine published studies (six using the NADA locations) did not find a significant benefit of active acupuncture over sham treatment.*

Transcranial magnetic stimulation (TMS) involves activation of brain cells by magnetic fields generated by electromagnetic coils placed on the scalp.

Single and multiple sessions of rTMS of the prefrontal cortex (either right or left) have been reported to reduce cocaine craving.

AMPHETAMINE DEPENDENCE

Many of the medications evaluated for the treatment of cocaine dependence have also been studied for the treatment of amphetamine dependence, often for the same pharmacologic rationale. As with cocaine dependence, most controlled clinical trials do not show efficacy.

The most promising approaches to date appear to be agonist substitution with stimulants and enhancement of GABA activity.

Two of three controlled clinical trials with D-**amphetamine** found a significant reduction in amphetamine use compared with placebo.

Slow-release **methylphenidate** (54 mg daily) reduced amphetamine use significantly more than did placebo in one controlled clinical trial.

Modafinil (200 mg twice daily) reduced amphetamine use in a case report and is currently undergoing a controlled clinical trial.

Vigabatrin, an anticonvulsant that increases GABA activity by inhibiting the breakdown of GABA by GABA transaminase, substantially reduced methamphetamine use in two open-label trials.

SPECIAL TREATMENT SITUATIONS

Mixed Dependence

Opioid Dependence Concurrent opioid use, including dependence, is a common clinical problem among cocaine-dependent individuals. Some individuals use cocaine and opioids simultaneously (as in the so-called speedball) to enhance the drugs' subjective effects.

Up to 20% or more of opioid-dependent patients in MMT also use cocaine for a variety of reasons, including continuation of prior polydrug abuse, replacement for the "high" no longer obtained from opioids, self-medication for the sedative effects of high **methadone** doses, or attenuation of opioid withdrawal symptoms.

Three different pharmacologic approaches have been used for the treatment of such dual cocaine and opioid dependence:

1. Adjustment of **methadone** dose
2. Maintenance with another opioid medication, e.g., high-dose buprenorphine (16–32 mg daily)
3. Addition of medication targeting the cocaine dependence

Higher **methadone** doses (usually 60 mg or more daily) generally are associated with less opioid use by patients in **methadone** maintenance. This relationship also holds in general for cocaine use among patients in **methadone** maintenance, although exceptions have been reported.

Increasing the **methadone** dose as a contingency in response to cocaine use can be effective in reducing such use (and more so than decreasing the **methadone** dose in response to a cocaine-positive urine sample).

Alcohol Dependence Alcohol dependence is a common problem among cocaine-dependent individuals, both in the community and in treatment settings, with rates of comorbidity as high as 90%.

Alcohol use by cocaine-dependent patients is associated with poorer treatment outcome.

Due to

1. Production of the toxic psychoactive metabolite cocaethylene
2. Stimulation of cocaine craving by alcohol
3. Alteration of medication metabolism by the hepatic effects of alcohol

Two medications used in the treatment of alcohol dependence have been studied in the treatment of outpatients concurrently dependent on cocaine and alcohol, **disulfiram** and **naltrexone**.

Both separate and combined treatment with **disulfiram** and/or **naltrexone** (100–150 mg daily) significantly improved abstinence from cocaine and alcohol.

Psychiatric Comorbidities

Treatment-seeking, cocaine-dependent individuals have high rates of psychiatric comorbidity (i.e., psychiatric diagnoses other than another substance use disorder), with rates as high as 65% for lifetime disorders and 50% for current disorders.

The most common comorbid disorders tend to be major depression, bipolar spectrum, phobias, and posttraumatic stress disorder.

Personality disorders are common among treatment-seeking, cocaine-dependent individuals, with rates in this population as high as 69%. *The most common of these is antisocial personality disorder.*

Depression **Desipramine**, **imipramine**, and **bupropion** have usually, but not always, been found effective, whereas selective serotonin reuptake inhibitors (e.g., **fluoxetine**) are usually not effective.

Bipolar Disorder Case series and open-label trials suggest that anticonvulsants such as **valproate**, **divalproex**, **lamotrigine**, and **carbamazepine** have some efficacy in reducing cocaine use in dually diagnosed patients.

Combining **lithium** with an anticonvulsant may be helpful in treatment-resistant patients.

The second-generation antipsychotics have generated mixed results in cocaine-dependent patients with comorbid bipolar disorder.

Attention Deficit/Hyperactivity Disorder Up to one fourth of cocaine-dependent adults have either adult ADHD or a history of childhood ADHD.

Stimulant and dopaminergic medications are the mainstay of treatment for ADHD, suggesting that some of these patients may be self-medicating their ADHD with cocaine.

Case series and clinical trials generally find that such medications successfully treat ADHD symptoms and reduce cocaine use in adults: **dextroamphetamine** (up to 60 mg per day), **methamphetamine** (15 mg per day), and **bupropion** (up to 100 mg three times a day).

Schizophrenia Although schizophrenia is not a common comorbid psychiatric disorder among cocaine-dependent individuals, cocaine use and abuse are common among treatment-seeking patients with schizophrenia.

Clinical experience indicates that first-generation antipsychotics, at doses that are effective in the treatment of schizophrenia, do not significantly alter cocaine craving or use.

Depot **flupenthixol** (40 mg of **decanoate** intramuscularly every 2 weeks) reduced cocaine use and improved psychopathology in a small case series of cocaine-using patients with schizophrenia.

Several case series and open-label trials suggest that the second-generation antipsychotics, including **clozapine, olanzapine, quetiapine, risperidone,** and **aripiprazole,** may be more effective in reducing cocaine and other drug use among patients with schizophrenia.

The use of cocaine or amphetamines can exacerbate or provoke antipsychotic-induced movement disorders and increase vulnerability to the neuroleptic malignant syndrome.

Gender-Specific Issues

Women tend to be excluded from or underrepresented in many clinical trials of cocaine dependence pharmacotherapy, in part because of concern, embodied in former FDA regulations, over risk to the fetus and neonate should a female subject become pregnant.

In the absence of directly relevant and systematically collected data, caution should be used when prescribing medications to pregnant women with stimulant dependence and to those with pregnancy potential, keeping in mind both the risks of medication and the risks of continued stimulant use.

Tricyclic antidepressants, **bupropion,** and **buprenorphine** appear to have little potential for morphologic teratogenicity or disruption of pregnancy, although there are little or no data on behavioral teratogenicity.

Amantadine is associated with pregnancy complications, **lithium** with cardiac malformations and neonatal toxicity, anticonvulsants with increased risk of congenital malformations, and antipsychotics with nonspecific congenital anomalies and neonatal withdrawal.

Disulfiram and **naltrexone** may generate different treatment responses in men versus women. The reasons for such gender differences are poorly understood, but may include differences in

1. Medication pharmacokinetics
2. Hormonal interactions
3. Subjects' psychological/socioeconomic status

Age

Although adolescents make up a substantial minority of heavy cocaine users, they have been largely excluded from clinical trials of cocaine pharmacotherapies because of legal and informed consent considerations.

Summary Author: Ashok Krishnamurthy
Richard D. Hurt • Jon O. Ebbert • J. Taylor Hays

Pharmacologic Interventions for Tobacco Dependence

PATHOPHYSIOLOGY OF TOBACCO DEPENDENCE

Nicotine binds to and causes conformational changes in nicotinic acetylcholine receptors (located in all areas of the human brain) → receptor stimulated → release of dopamine, norepinephrine, glutamate, vasopressin, serotonin, γ-aminobutyric acid, β-endorphins, and other neurotransmitters.

High concentrations of nicotinic acetylcholine receptors exist in the mesolimbic dopamine system and locus coeruleus.

Although not completely understood, up-regulation of the high affinity $\alpha_4\beta_2$ nicotinic acetylcholine receptor is critical for the development of tolerance to and dependence on nicotine.

Repeated exposure to high concentrations of nicotine causes up-regulation of the $\alpha_4\beta_2$ nicotinic acetylcholine receptors, leading to an absolute increase in their numbers.

Neuroadaptation of the mesolimbic system in smokers and its target neurons in the nucleus accumbens may be longer lasting than previously thought, which could explain the observation that cravings to smoke last for months after a smoker stops smoking.

The mesolimbic system area is also involved with the positive reinforcing effects of amphetamines, cocaine, and opiates.

Nicotine-induced dose-dependent increases in feelings of pleasure have been observed to occur simultaneously with increases in the functional MRI of neuronal activity in the nucleus accumbens, amygdala, cingulate, and frontal lobes.

In laboratory animals, self-administered intravenous nicotine *increases the sensitivity of brain reward systems and imprints an indelible memory of its effects in reward systems*, an action that appears unique to nicotine among drugs of abuse. This may partially explain the rapid relapse to former levels of smoking that frequently follows a smoker having a few cigarettes after a prolonged period of smoking abstinence.

Tobacco dependence may carry a genetic component as well.

Twin studies have confirmed an inherited component for tobacco use and dependence, and familial transmission of smoking behavior has been observed across three generations of families.

The evidence for a contribution of specific genes to smoking behavior remains modest.

Further work is needed to study the spectrum of heritable traits that influence genetic susceptibility to tobacco dependence.

MEASURING NICOTINE EXPOSURE

One approach to the therapeutic use of nicotine replacement therapy (NRT) for the treatment of tobacco dependence is to determine the patient's level of nicotine exposure. After this exposure is determined, a nicotine replacement dose approximating the dose the individual receives from smoking can be prescribed.

Factors making the above difficult:

1. Smokers exposed to the same amount of nicotine through inhaled tobacco smoke have marked interindividual differences in venous nicotine concentrations.

2. Cigarette smoking produces initial arterial nicotine concentrations that are severalfold higher than concomitant venous nicotine levels.
3. In addition, nicotine has a short half-life (i.e., 120 minutes) and, with smoking, tends to have peaks and troughs in both the venous and the arterial circulation.

Cotinine, the major metabolite of nicotine, has a half-life of 18 to 20 hours and can be used to quantify an individual's exposure to nicotine.

Venous nicotine concentrations (albeit less than arterial levels) reflect acute nicotine exposure, *whereas cotinine reflects nicotine exposure over 2 to 3 days.*

Anabasine is a tobacco alkaloid that is not a metabolic product of nicotine. Anabasine is present in the urine of tobacco users but not in the urine of patients using NRT. *Anabasine thus can be especially useful in distinguishing abstinent tobacco users who are using NRT from those who are continuing to use tobacco.*

NICOTINE REPLACEMENT THERAPY

Every patient who is willing to make an attempt to stop smoking should be offered counseling and medications.

Clinical trials have shown that adding pharmacotherapy to a behavioral intervention generally doubles smoking abstinence rates and that the combination of medication and counseling is more effective than either alone.

NRT remains a mainstay of pharmacotherapy for the treatment of tobacco dependence.

To date, the FDA has approved five nicotine replacement products: *nicotine gum, nicotine patches, nicotine nasal spray, a nicotine vapor inhaler, and nicotine lozenges.* Gum, patches, and lozenges are available over the counter; nasal spray and inhaler are available by prescription only.

The dose and duration of therapy should be based on the patient's subjective need for relief of withdrawal symptoms and support of smoking abstinence.

Nicotine Gum

Nicotine gum is available as an over-the-counter product in both the 2- and 4-mg doses and has been shown to be effective as monotherapy or in combination with other NRT.

Venous nicotine concentrations achieved through the proper use of nicotine gum are relatively low compared with those produced by smoking cigarettes.

The 4-mg dose is indicated for use in smokers who are more dependent and is recommended for those who smoke 25 or more cigarettes per day.

Patients should be instructed to bite into a piece of nicotine gum a few times until a mild tingling or peppery taste indicates nicotine release. Patients then should "park" the gum between the cheek and gum for several minutes before chewing it again.

Because the absorption of nicotine is lowered by a more acidic pH, patients should be instructed not to drink beverages or eat for several minutes before and while using the gum.

When nicotine gum is used as a single agent, most patients should use a minimum of 10 to 15 pieces per day to achieve initial smoking abstinence.

The most common adverse effects of nicotine gum are nausea and indigestion, which can be minimized with the proper "chew-and-park" technique. Other adverse effects reported include gingival soreness and mouth ulcerations.

Nicotine Lozenge

The nicotine lozenge is available in 2- and 4-mg doses.

The 4-mg strength is used in "high" dependence smokers (i.e., time to first cigarette of the day, 30 minutes after arising).

The lozenge is simpler to use than the gum and likely will demonstrate improved patient compliance.

As with the other short-acting NRT products, it can be used alone or in combination with other NRT.

Nicotine Patch

Nicotine patch therapy delivers a steady dose of nicotine for 24 hours after a single application.

The once-daily dosing requires little effort on the part of the patient, which enhances compliance.

Nicotine patches are available without a prescription in doses of 7, 14, and 21 mg, which deliver nicotine over 24 hours.

In almost every randomized clinical trial performed to date, the nicotine patch has been shown to be effective compared with placebo usually with a doubling of the stop rate.

TABLE 52.1	Nicotine Patch Dose Based on Baseline (While Smoking) Blood Cotinine Concentration
Cotinine in ng/mL	**Nicotine patch dose**
<200	14–21 mg/day
200–300	21–42 mg/day
>300	≥42 mg/day

Standard-dose nicotine patch therapy is 21 mg per 24 hours.

However, the standard-dose patch approach is not effective in all smokers. In fact, it has been shown that a standard dose (21 mg per 24 hours) of nicotine patch therapy achieves a median serum cotinine level of only 54% of the cotinine concentrations achieved through smoking.

Uses of high doses of nicotine patch therapy (i.e., doses >21 mg per day) are appropriate for smokers who previously failed single-dose patch therapy or for those whose nicotine withdrawal symptoms are not relieved sufficiently with standard therapy. This approach can be especially important for heavy smokers because they will be significantly underdosed with single-dose patch therapy.

High-dose nicotine patch therapy has been shown to be safe and well tolerated in patients who smoke >20 cigarettes per day.

By employing the concept of therapeutic drug monitoring, clinicians can use serum cotinine concentrations to tailor the nicotine replacement dose so that it approaches 100% replacement.

A baseline cotinine concentration is obtained while the smoker is smoking his or her usual number of cigarettes. An initial nicotine patch dose based on the baseline cotinine concentration (or cigarettes per day) is prescribed.

After the patient reaches steady state, the serum cotinine concentration is rechecked and the replacement dose can be adjusted to achieve a steady-state cotinine level that approaches the baseline level.

For special populations in whom a need to use the lowest possible effective dose exists (e.g., pregnant women), therapeutic drug monitoring with cotinine can be used to maintain nicotine replacement levels close to baseline.

Serum cotinine is the test of choice for calculating the percentage replacement, even though urine nicotine or cotinine can be used. If serum cotinine testing is not available, the replacement dose can be estimated based on the number of cigarettes smoked per day (Tables 52.1 and 52.2).

Abstinence from smoking during the first 2 weeks of patch therapy has been shown to be highly predictive of long-term abstinence. The first 2 weeks of nicotine patch therapy are critical.

If the patient continues to smoke at all during the first 2 weeks, the treatment must be changed by changing the nicotine patch dose, by adding additional pharmacotherapy, or by intensifying behavioral counseling.

Nicotine patch doses should be increased for patients experiencing pronounced withdrawal symptoms such as irritability, anxiety, loss of concentration, or craving, or for patients who do not achieve 100% replacement based on the second serum cotinine concentration.

TABLE 52.2	Recommended Initial Dosing of Nicotine Patch Therapy Based on Number of Cigarettes Smoked Daily
Cigarettes/day	**Patch dose (mg/day)[a]**
<10	7–14
10–20	14–21
21–40	21–42
>40	42+

[a]Nicotine patches are available in the following doses: 7, 14, and 21 mg.

Most patients use the nicotine patch for 4 to 8 weeks, but it is safe to use it longer if needed to maintain abstinence. Optimal length of treatment has not been determined.

Side effects of nicotine patch therapy are relatively mild and include localized skin reactions at the patch site. Such reactions generally begin to occur about 4 weeks after initiation of patch therapy. Lesions vary from erythema to erythema plus vesicles. Rotation of the patches to different sites of the skin helps to reduce the frequency of this side effect.

Although sleep disturbance is another side effect that has been attributed to nicotine patch therapy, it often is difficult to ascertain whether this is attributable to nicotine withdrawal or to the administration of nicotine during the evening hours.

If there is a concern that nicotine patch therapy is causing sleep disturbance, the patch can be removed at night to see if the sleep disturbance resolves.

Some concern was expressed in the lay press that smokers might be at increased risk of myocardial infarction if they continued to smoke while using the patch. *Subsequent studies have shown no adverse effects in smokers with a history of coronary artery disease receiving the 14- or 21-mg patch doses.*

Nicotine patch doses up to 63 mg per day were not associated with short-term adverse cardiovascular effects in smokers.

Nicotine Nasal Spray

This device delivers nicotine more rapidly than other therapeutic nicotine replacement delivery systems and reduces withdrawal symptoms more quickly than nicotine gum.

Each spray contains 0.5 mg of nicotine, and one dose is one spray in each nostril (a total of 1 mg). Recommended dosing is one to two doses per hour, not to exceed five doses per hour or 40 doses per day.

When using the nicotine nasal spray as a single agent, most patients initially use 12 to 16 doses per day. The recommended length of treatment is up to 12 weeks of *ad lib* use, followed by a tapering schedule.

Patients should be instructed to spray against the lower nasal mucosa and not to sniff the spray into the upper nasal passages or to attempt to inhale it.

The most common adverse side effects are rhinorrhea, nasal and throat irritation, watery eyes, and sneezing. These irritant side effects decrease significantly within the 1st week of use.

Nicotine nasal spray should be used with caution in patients with reactive airway disease.

There is no abuse liability with the nicotine spray.

Nicotine Inhaler

This device is a plastic holder into which a cartridge containing a cotton plug impregnated with 10 mg of nicotine is inserted. The device delivers a nicotine vapor that is absorbed across the oral mucosa.

Although the device is called an inhaler, this is a misnomer because little of the nicotine vapor reaches the pulmonary alveoli even with deep inhalations.

When the nicotine inhaler is used as a single therapy, efficacy is increased when more than six cartridges per day are used.

The recommended initial dose of the nicotine inhaler when used alone is 6 to 16 cartridges per day. The recommended length of treatment is approximately 12 weeks followed by a tapering schedule, although the inhaler could be used longer. This device requires frequent puffing to deliver substantial amounts of nicotine and to some smokers the puffing mimics some of the behavior of smoking.

Adverse effects generally are mild and most often involve mouth or throat irritation, with occasional coughing.

NONNICOTINE PRODUCTS

Bupropion SR

Smokers are more likely than nonsmokers to have a history of major depression.

During the course of an attempt to stop smoking, many smokers develop a depressed affect and some become overtly depressed.

The development of a depressed affect during an attempt to stop smoking is associated with relapse to smoking.

Among the antidepressants evaluated, **bupropion** is the first nonnicotine pharmacologic treatment approved for the treatment of tobacco dependence. **Bupropion** is a monocyclic antidepressant that inhibits reuptake of both norepinephrine and dopamine. Dopamine release in the mesolimbic system and the nucleus accumbens is thought to be the basis for the reinforcing properties of nicotine and other drugs of addiction.

The efficacy of **bupropion** in smoking cessation is hypothesized to stem from its dopaminergic activity on the pleasure and reward pathways in the mesolimbic system and nucleus accumbens.

Bupropion also has been shown to have an antagonist effect on nicotinic acetylcholine receptors.

Treatment with **bupropion SR** alone or in combination with the nicotine patch *resulted in a significantly higher long-term rate of abstinence from smoking than did use of either the nicotine patch alone or placebo.*

Treatment with **bupropion SR** should be initiated about 1 week before the patient's stop date at an initial dose of 150 mg per day for 3 days, then 150 mg twice daily. The usual length of treatment is 6 to 12 weeks, but **bupropion SR** can be used safely for much longer. As with other antidepressants, a small risk (0.1%) of seizures is associated with this medication.

Bupropion SR *is contraindicated in patients who have a history of seizures*, serious head trauma with skull fracture or a prolonged loss of consciousness, an eating disorder (i.e., anorexia nervosa or bulimia), or concomitant use of medications that lower the seizure threshold.

The most common adverse side effects are insomnia and dry mouth. Treatment-emergent hypertension can occur rarely during treatment with bupropion SR, especially when it is used in combination with nicotine patch therapy.

However, lower smoking rate, prior abstinence from smoking for brief periods (<24 hours) or long periods (>4 weeks), and male gender all were predictors of better outcome independent of the **bupropion SR** dose.

The extended use of **bupropion SR** for relapse prevention is effective for smokers with or without a history of depression.

Because of the high prevalence of a history of depression in smokers, clinicians often encounter smokers who want to stop smoking but already are being treated with an antidepressant. No drug–drug interactions exist to preclude the use of **bupropion SR** with either selective serotonin reuptake inhibitors (SSRIs) or tricyclic antidepressants. Thus, adding **bupropion SR** to an SSRI is preferable to discontinuing that medication and using **bupropion SR** only.

Varenicline

Varenicline is a partial nicotine agonist/antagonist that selectively binds to the nicotinic $\alpha_4\beta_2$ acetylcholine receptor.

Varenicline both blocks nicotine from binding to the receptor (*antagonist effect*) and stimulates (*agonist effect*) receptor-mediated activity leading to the release of dopamine, which reduces craving and nicotine withdrawal symptoms.

Varenicline:

- Rapidly absorbed after one administration
- Reaches peak serum concentration in 4 hours
- Steady-state serum concentrations after 4 days
- Is not metabolized
- Excreted virtually unchanged in the urine
- Half-life is approximately 17 hours

Varenicline was more effective at achieving smoking abstinence compared to placebo or **bupropion SR**, with end-of-treatment continuous smoking abstinence rates of 44% versus 30% for **bupropion SR** and 18% for placebo, in two key clinical trials.

Varenicline showed better smoking abstinence outcomes compared with NRT and was equally effective and safe in smokers with or without a mental illness.

Varenicline has not been studied systematically in combination with other medications to treat tobacco dependence.

Varenicline *is not recommended for use in combination with NRT*; however, some patients may need short-acting NRT for nicotine withdrawal symptom control, especially in the first few days per weeks of **varenicline** therapy.

Bupropion SR and **varenicline** *have different mechanisms of action and no drug interactions between these drugs are likely.* Clinical trials assessing this combination are ongoing. However, no clinical trial data to support this treatment approach are available.

The most frequent adverse effect of **varenicline** is nausea reported by approximately 30% of the participants. However, the nausea was most often mild to moderate, and participant dropouts related to nausea were infrequent.

In February 2008, the FDA issued a public health advisory because of reports of suicidal thoughts and aggressive and erratic behavior in a patient who have taken **varenicline**. In addition, some case reports have suggested that **varenicline** *could exacerbate psychiatric symptoms in individuals with severe mental illness, so these types of patients should be monitored carefully when on* **varenicline**.

Nortriptyline

Nortriptyline is a tricyclic antidepressant recommended as a second-line drug for treating tobacco dependence.

Systematic reviews demonstrate the efficacy of **nortriptyline** in contrast to SSRIs, which have not been shown to help smokers stop.

Nortriptyline seems to be as efficacious as **bupropion SR** in treating smokers with chronic obstructive pulmonary disease.

The most common adverse effects with **nortriptyline** are sedation and dry mouth. **Nortriptyline** produces higher smoking abstinence rates than placebo, independent of a history of depression.

Nortriptyline *is contraindicated in combination with an MAOI* (monamine oxidase inhibitor) or within 14 days of discontinuing one, **nortriptyline** allergy, or in the acute recovery phase after a myocardial infarction.

Clonidine

Clonidine is a centrally acting alpha-agonist that can be used as a second-line drug. The transdermal form is easier to use with a recommended dose of 0.2 mg per day for 3 to 10 weeks. The **clonidine** patch should be initiated a week before the patient's stop date and changed weekly thereafter. Common side effects include dry mouth and drowsiness. The only contraindication to its use is a **clonidine** allergy.

COMBINATION PHARMACOTHERAPIES

The 2008 United States Public Health Service (USPHS) Guideline states that certain combinations of first-line medications have been shown to be effective. Long-term (>14 weeks) nicotine patch therapy combined with nicotine gum or nicotine nasal spray, nicotine patch therapy plus nicotine inhaler, and nicotine patch therapy plus **bupropion SR** are cited as examples.

Whether the superiority of combination therapy is due to the use of two types of delivery systems or to the fact that two delivery systems tend to produce higher blood nicotine levels remains unclear.

Combination pharmacotherapy or higher than usual doses of NRT effectively relieve withdrawal symptoms especially in more dependent smokers.

Based on the treatment of over 45,000 smokers, the Mayo Clinic's Nicotine Dependence Center offers the following clinical pearls: (1) Nicotine patch therapy, bupropion SR, and/or varenicline are the "foundation medications" on which to begin building a patient's pharmacotherapeutic regimen. (2) Most medication regimens for treating tobacco dependence should contain at least one if not more than one of these medications. (3) Short-acting NRT products (such as nicotine gum, nicotine inhaler, nicotine lozenge, or nicotine nasal spray) are added to "foundation medications" to help control intermittent withdrawal symptoms or cravings. Short-acting NRT should rarely be used alone. (4) Patients with tobacco dependence will usually require combination therapy, and those with more severe dependence often need three or more products simultaneously.

CLINICAL DECISIONS ABOUT PHARMACOTHERAPY

The 2008 USPHS Guideline observes that there is stronger evidence that counseling is an effective tobacco dependence treatment strategy and that counseling adds significantly to the efficacy of the approved medications.

Practical counseling (problem solving/skills training) and social support delivered as part of treatment are especially effective.

Guidelines state that the combination of counseling and medication is more effective than either alone; thus, both should be routinely offered to smokers.

Self-Help Materials and Longer Term Pharmacotherapy for Relapse Prevention

Specific self-help materials, such as the National Cancer Institute's *Forever Free*, have been effective in helping smokers maintain smoking abstinence.

Longer use of pharmacotherapy is useful in some patients to maintain smoking abstinence long enough to stabilize the initial treatment effect. The optimal length of pharmacotherapy has not been established for any of the available medications.

CHAPTER 53

Summary Author: Ashok Krishnamurthy
Jeffery N. Wilkins • Mark Hrymoc • David A. Gorelick*

Pharmacologic Interventions for Other Drug and Multiple Drug Addictions

MARIJUANA

There is no recognized or proven role for pharmacotherapy in the short- or long-term treatment of marijuana abuse or dependence.

The development of specific agonists or antagonists for the cannabinoid CB1 receptor (which mediates the psychoactive effects of marijuana) could lead to a pharmacologic treatment for marijuana abuse.

Agonist substitution with oral synthetic 9-tetrahydrocannabinol (**dronabinol; marinol**) suppresses cannabis withdrawal in human laboratory studies and outpatient settings. A recent case report found that **dronabinol** reduced cannabis use in two outpatients.

The CB1 receptor antagonist **rimonabant** (developed for the treatment of obesity and the metabolic syndrome, but no larger marketed) blocks the physiologic and psychologic effects of marijuana in animals and humans.

ANABOLIC STEROIDS

There is no established medication for the treatment of anabolic steroid abuse.

Two pharmacologic treatment approaches have been suggested:

1. Hormonal treatments to restore hypothalamic-pituitary-gonadal dysfunction caused by use of steroids
2. Medications to relieve specific psychiatric symptoms associated with steroid withdrawal

The first approach could be implemented with tapering doses of a long-acting steroid such as **testosterone enanthate**. This approach could be considered analogous to treating heroin withdrawal with a long-acting opiate such as **methadone**.

The second approach uses standard psychotropic medications to target the depression, irritability, and aggression often associated with anabolic steroid use, although these symptoms often resolve without medication. SSRI antidepressants are most often used.

The use of tricyclic antidepressants has been discouraged on theoretical grounds because their cardiovascular and anticholinergic effects might exacerbate the cardiotoxicity and urinary retention (because of prostatic hypertrophy) associated with anabolic steroid use.

Low-dose neuroleptics (such as **phenothiazine**-equivalent doses of about 200 mg daily) have been reported effective for managing steroid-induced psychosis, hostility, and agitation.

PHENCYCLIDINE

There is little systematic experience with pharmacologic treatment of phencyclidine (PCP) addiction.

Both **desipramine** and the anxiolytic **buspirone** have significantly improved psychologic symptoms such as depression in small outpatient-controlled clinical trials, but neither medication significantly reduced PCP use when compared with a double-blind placebo.

*Dr. Gorelick is supported by the Intramural Research Program, NIH, National Institute on Drug Abuse.

INHALANTS

Inhalants are a heterogeneous group of volatile abused substances that include adhesives, aerosols, solvents, anesthetics (including nitrous oxide), gasoline, cleaning agents, and nitrites.

Many inhalant abusers entering treatment have co-occurring psychiatric and addictive disorders, typically involving alcohol and marijuana that can complicate treatment.

The mainstay of treatment is psychosocial, including techniques such as cognitive-behavioral therapy, multisystem and family therapy, Twelve-Step facilitation, and motivational enhancement.

NICOTINE WITH OTHER DRUGS

Among US adults with current nicotine dependence, 8.2% have a current (nonalcohol) drug use disorder, an odds ratio of 3.2 for having a drug use disorder compared with those without nicotine dependence.

Conversely, 52.4% of those with a current drug use disorder are nicotine dependent. Comorbidity rates may exceed 70% among patients in treatment.

Most studies find that smoking cessation treatment does not adversely influence the outcome of drug abuse treatment.

Limited evidence suggests that polydrug abusers (e.g., alcohol and stimulants and cannabis) may respond better to the combination of nicotine replacement therapy (NRT) and **bupropion** than to either treatment alone.

Nicotine and Alcohol

Among adults with nicotine dependence, 22.8% have an alcohol use disorder (an odds ratio (OR) of 4.4).

Conversely, among adults with an alcohol use disorder, 34.5% have nicotine dependence (OR of 2.7).

Tobacco-related diseases are a greater cause of morbidity and mortality in patients with alcohol use disorders than are alcohol-related medical conditions, highlighting the importance of smoking cessation treatment for this population.

Cigarette smokers with a current alcohol use disorder (but not those in remission) tend to have more severe nicotine dependence, and so may need more intensive treatment, including higher doses of medication.

Most, but not all, studies suggest that nicotine and alcohol dependence can be successfully treated at the same time without adversely affecting outcome.

Nicotine and Opioids

More than three fourths of individuals with opioid dependence (including patients in **methadone** maintenance treatment) smoke cigarettes.

Opiate drugs, including **methadone**, *may acutely increase cigarette smoking.*

Limited evidence suggests that nicotine replacement therapy, with or without **bupropion**, can be effective for smoking cessation in patients on methadone maintenance.

Treatment outcomes are improved with concurrent psychosocial treatment.

OPIOIDS WITH OTHER DRUGS

Opioids and Alcohol

Heavy drinking, alcohol abuse, or alcohol dependence occur in one third or more of opioid-dependent individuals, including those in methadone maintenance treatment (MMT) and is associated with poor treatment outcome.

There does not appear to be a strong association between **methadone** dose and alcohol use.

Buprenorphine, a partial mu-opioid receptor agonist marketed for the treatment of opioid dependence, reduces alcohol intake in animal studies, but has not yet been evaluated for this in clinical trials.

Disulfuram, at typical doses used to treat alcohol dependence, can be effective in reducing alcohol intake among patients in MMT.

Other medications being studied for the treatment of dually dependent patients include **acamprosate** and **memantine**.

Opioids and Cocaine

Cocaine use is common among opioid addicts and is associated with greater opioid use, even among those in MMT.

A popular pattern involves simultaneous use of the two drugs ("speed balling"), which is said to provide a qualitatively better subjective experience ("high") than either drug alone.

For patients already in MMT, increasing the **methadone** dose (usually to >60 mg per day) can reduce both opioid and cocaine use.

Buprenorphine equivalent to 16 to 32 mg per day as sublingual tablet reduces both cocaine and opioid use in dually dependent patients, although lower doses do not.

HALLUCINOGENS

Hallucinogens include compounds that influence serotonergic neurotransmission, such as lysergic acid diethylamide (LSD), psilocybin, and N,N-dimethyltryptamine (DMT), and those that influence catecholaminergic neurotransmission (such as **mescaline** and amphetamine analogues like 3,4-methylenedioxmethamphetamine [MDMA]).

At present, no pharmacologic treatment is available for the treatment of hallucinogen abuse.

Single doses of the selective serotonin reuptake inhibitor (SSRI) antidepressant **citalopram** or the 5-HT$_{2A/C}$ receptor antagonist **ketanserin** attenuated many of the acute psychologic effects of MDMA in human experimental studies.

The mainstay of treatment remains psychosocial intervention, which can require residential treatment in patients with severe personality disorganization.

Prolonged psychotic reactions appear to occur chiefly in individuals who have preexisting psychiatric disorders; these can be difficult to distinguish from hallucinogen-induced precipitation or exacerbation of a preexisting psychotic disorder such as schizophrenia. Low doses of a high-potency neuroleptic have been recommended.

LSD use has been associated with perceptual abnormalities, such as illusions, distortions, and hallucinations, persisting or recurring intermittently for long periods (up to years) after the last LSD use.

When these abnormalities occur after a period of normal perceptual functioning, they are termed *flashbacks.*

Case reports suggest that **sertraline**, **naltrexone**, **clonidine**, or benzodiazepines can be helpful in the treatment of both persisting perceptual abnormalities and flashbacks, while antipsychotics (e.g., **haloperidol**, **risperidone**) and **SSRIs** *have been reported to worsen the condition.*

HALLUCINOGENS AS PHARMACOLOGIC TREATMENT FOR ADDICTION

MDMA

MDMA (3,4-methylenedioxmethamphetamine, "Ecstasy") is an amphetamine analog with stimulant and hallucinogenic properties.

Several controlled clinical trials of MDMA-assisted psychotherapy for posttraumatic stress disorder or anxiety associated with advanced-stage cancer are under way in the United States, Israel, and Switzerland.

LSD

LSD was used clinically as a pharmacologic treatment for a variety of psychiatric disorders, including depression, anxiety, alcoholism, and drug abuse.

LSD was given orally as a psychiatric treatment in two ways: one or two high doses (usually 200–800 mg), with or without formal psychotherapy, to generate a cathartic or transforming emotional experience, or multiple low doses (usually 25–200 mg) as an adjunct to psychotherapy to break down therapeutic resistance and enhance access to unconscious material.

There have been case reports of the beneficial effects of LSD for cluster headaches.

Psilocybin

Psilocybin is one of the psychoactive compounds in hallucinogenic mushrooms of the *Psilocybe* genus.

Psilocybin showed efficacy in a recent open-label study of obsessive-compulsive disorder and in several cases of cluster headaches. Two clinical trials of psilocybin for relief of anxiety in advanced-stage cancer patients are under way.

Ketamine

Ketamine is marketed as a dissociative anesthetic and is also used as an analgesic.

A controlled clinical trial of high-dose ("psychedelic-dose") **ketamine**-assisted psychotherapy found a higher rate of abstinence and less craving for heroin over a 2-year follow-up period compared with low-dose **ketamine**.

A clinical trial in patients with alcohol dependence also had positive results. Intravenous **ketamine** has been shown to produce rapid (within 2 hours) and robust antidepressant effects in patients with treatment-resistant depression.

Ibogaine

Ibogaine is a psychoactive alkaloid derived from the West African plant *Tabernanthe iboga*. In animals, it blocks the drug-induced release of dopamine in the nucleus accumbens caused by cocaine, opioids, and nicotine.

Open-label case series suggest that single high doses (1 g or more) alleviate withdrawal symptoms, reduce drug craving, and produce long-term (>3 months) abstinence in patients with cocaine, heroin, and polydrug dependence. No clinical trials have been conducted because of concern over ibogaine's neurotoxicity.

This has generated interest in the ibogaine metabolite noribogaine and the structural analogue 18-methoxycoronaridine (18-MC), which appear to be less toxic in animals.

CHAPTER

54

Summary Author: John Young
James O. Prochaska

Enhancing Motivation to Change

THE STAGES OF CHANGE

Change is a process that unfolds through a series of stages:

Precontemplation is a stage in which the individual does not intend to take action in the foreseeable future (usually measured as the next 6 months). Such individuals tend to avoid reading, talking, or thinking about their high-risk behaviors. Individuals in the precontemplation stage typically underestimate the benefits of change and overestimate its costs but are unaware that they are making such mistakes. As a result, many remain stuck in the precontemplation stage for years.

Contemplation is a stage in which an individual intends to take action within the ensuing 6 months. Such a person is more aware of the benefits of changing but also is acutely aware of the costs. This balance between the costs and the benefits of change can produce profound ambivalence and thus can keep an individual stuck at the contemplation stage. Such individuals are not ready for traditional action-oriented programs.

Preparation is a stage in which an individual intends to take action in the immediate future (usually measured as the ensuing month). It is these individuals who should be recruited for action-oriented treatment programs.

Action is a stage in which the individual has made specific, overt modifications in his or her lifestyle within the preceding 6 months.

Maintenance is a stage in which the individual is working to prevent relapse, but does not need to apply change processes as frequently as one would in the action stage. Such a person is less tempted to relapse. Maintenance lasts from 6 months to about 5 years.

Termination is a stage at which individuals have zero temptation and 100% self-efficacy. Although the ideal is to be cured or totally recovered, it is important to recognize that, for many patients, a more realistic expectation is a lifetime of maintenance.

USING THE STAGES OF CHANGE MODEL TO MOTIVATE PATIENTS

The stages of change model can be applied to identify ways to motivate more patients at each phase of planned interventions for the addictions. The five phases are (a) recruitment, (b) retention, (c) progress, (d) process, and (e) outcomes.

Recruitment

Fewer than 25% of persons with addictive disorders enter professional treatment in their lifetimes.

How can more people with addictive disorders be motivated to seek the appropriate help? There are two paradigms that need to be changed. The first is an action-oriented paradigm that construes behavior change as an event that can occur quickly, immediately, discretely, and dramatically. Treatment programs that are designed to have patients immediately quit abusing substances are implicitly or explicitly designed for the portion of the population in the preparation stage. The problem is that, with most unhealthy behaviors, fewer than 20% of the affected population is prepared to take action. To meet the needs of the entire addicted population, interventions must meet the needs of the 40% in the precontemplation and the 40% in the contemplation stages.

The second paradigm change that is required is movement from a passive-reactive approach to a proactive approach. The passive-reactive paradigm is designed to serve populations with acute conditions. The pain, distress, or discomfort of such conditions can motivate patients to seek the services of health professionals. But the major killers today are chronic lifestyle disorders such as the addictions. To treat the addictions seriously, professionals must learn how to reach out to entire populations and offer them stage-matched therapies.

Retention

What motivates patients to continue in therapy? At least five studies are available on dropouts from a stage model perspective. These studies found that stage-related variables were more reliable predictors of dropout than demographics, type of problem, severity of problem, and other problem-related variables. Figure 54.1 presents the stage profiles of three groups of patients with a broad spectrum of psychiatric disorders. The before-therapy profile of the entire group who dropped out quickly and prematurely (40%) was a profile of persons in the precontemplation stage. The 20% who finished quickly but appropriately had a profile of patients who were in the action stage at the time they entered therapy. Those who continued in long-term treatment were a mixed group, with most in the contemplation stage.

The lesson is clear: persons in the precontemplation stage cannot be treated as if they are starting in the same place as those in the action stage. With patients who begin therapy in the precontemplation stage, it is useful for the therapist to share key concerns: "I'm concerned that therapy may not have a chance to make a significant difference in your life, because you may be tempted to leave early."

The author and others have conducted four studies with stage-matched interventions in which retention rates of persons entering interventions in the precontemplation stage can be examined. What is clear is that, when treatment is matched to stage, persons in the precontemplation stage will remain in treatment at the same rates as those who start in the preparation stage.

Progress

What moves people to progress in therapy and to continue to progress after therapy? Figure 54.2 presents an example of what is called the stage effect. The stage effect predicts that the amount of successful action taken during and after treatment is directly related to the stage at which the person entered treatment. The stage effect has been found across a variety of problems and populations.

One strategy for applying the stage effect clinically involves setting realistic goals for brief encounters with patients at each stage of change. A realistic goal is to help patients progress one stage in brief therapy. If a patient moves relatively quickly, he or she may be able to progress two stages. One result for health professionals trained in this approach to the addictions can be a dramatic increase in the morale of the health professionals involved.

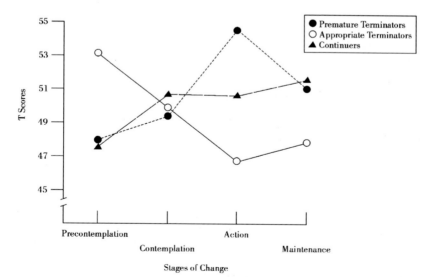

FIGURE 54.1 Pretherapy stage profiles for premature terminators, appropriate terminators, and continuers. (Data from Brogan ME, Prochaska JO, Prochaska JM. Predicting termination and continuation status in psychotherapy using the Transtheoretical Model. *Psychotherapy* 1999;36:105–113.)

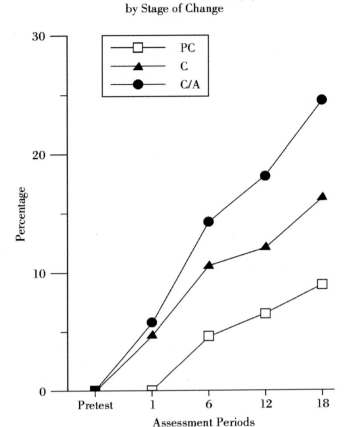

Point-Prevalent Abstinence (%)
by Stage of Change

FIGURE 54.2 Percentage of smokers who maintained abstinence over 18 months. Note: Groups were in the following stages at the time of entry into treatment. PC, precontemplation; C, comtemplation; C/A, preparation ($n = 570$).

They can see progress with most of their patients, where they once saw failure when immediate action was the only criterion for success.

Process
To help motivate patients to progress from one stage to the next, it is necessary to know the principles and processes of change.

Principle 1 The rewards for changing must increase if patients are to progress beyond precontemplation. A technique that can be used in population-based programs involves asking a patient in the precontemplation stage to describe all the benefits of a change such as quitting smoking or starting to exercise. Most persons can list four or five. The therapist can challenge the patient to double or triple the list for the next meeting.

Principle 2 The cons of changing must decrease if patients are to progress from contemplation to action.

Principle 3 The relative weight assigned to benefits and costs must cross over before a patient will be prepared to take action.

Principle 4 The strong principle of progress holds that, to progress from precontemplation to effective action, the rewards for changing must increase by one standard deviation (SD).

Principle 5 The weak principle of progress holds that, to progress from contemplation to effective action, the perceived costs of changing must decrease by one-half SD. Because the perceived rewards for changing

TABLE 54.1	Stages of Change in Which Change Processes are Emphasized				

| | Stages of change | | | | |
Processes	Precontemplation	Contemplation	Preparation	Action	Maintenance
	Consciousness raising				
	Dramatic relief				
	Environmental reevaluation				
		Self-reevaluation			
			Self-liberation		
				Contingency management	
				Helping relationships	
					Counterconditioning
					Stimulus control

must increase twice as much as the perceived costs decrease, twice as much emphasis must be placed on the rewards than the costs of changing. Such principles can produce much more sensitive assessments to guide interventions.

Principle 6 It is important to match particular processes of change with specific stages of change. Table 54.1 presents the empirical integration found between processes and stages of change.

1. Consciousness raising involves increased awareness of the causes, consequences, and responses to a particular problem. Consciousness raising should be designed to increase the perceived rewards for changing.
2. Dramatic relief involves emotional arousal about one's current behavior and the relief that can come from changing. Fear, inspiration, guilt, and hope are some of the emotions that can move persons to contemplate changing. Psychodrama, role playing, grieving, and personal testimonies are examples of techniques that can move people emotionally.
3. Environmental reevaluation combines both affective and cognitive assessments of how an addiction affects one's social environment and how changing would affect that environment. Empathy training, values clarification, and family or network interventions can facilitate such reevaluation.
4. Self-reevaluation combines both cognitive and affective assessments of an image of one's self free from addiction. Imagery, healthier role models, and values clarification are techniques that can move individuals in this type of intervention.
5. Self-liberation involves both the belief that one can change and the commitment and recommitment to act on that belief. Techniques that can enhance such willpower include public rather than private commitments. Motivational research also suggests that individuals who have only one choice are not as motivated as if they have two choices. Three choices are even better, but four choices do not seem to enhance motivation. Wherever possible, then, patients should be given three of the best choices for applying each process.
6. Contingency management involves the systematic use of reinforcements and punishments for taking steps in a particular direction. Because successful self-changers rely much more on reinforcement than punishment, it is useful to emphasize reinforcements for progressing rather than punishments for regressing. Contingency contracts, overt and covert reinforcements, and group recognition are methods of increasing reinforcement and incentives that increase the probability that healthier responses will be repeated.

To prepare patients for the longer term, they should be taught to rely more on self-reinforcements than social reinforcements. Many patients expect much more reinforcement and recognition from others than they actually receive.

7. Helping relationships combine caring, openness, trust, and acceptance, as well as support for changing. Rapport building, a therapeutic alliance, counselor calls, buddy systems, sponsors, and self-help groups can be excellent resources for social support. If patients become dependent on such support to maintain change, the support will need to be carefully faded, lest termination of therapy becomes a condition for relapse.

8. Counterconditioning requires the learning of healthier behaviors that can substitute for addictive behaviors. Counterconditioning techniques tend to be quite specific to a particular behavior. They include desensitization, assertion, and cognitive counters to irrational self-statements that can elicit distress.

9. Stimulus control involves modifying the environment to increase cues that prompt healthy responses and decrease cues that lead to relapse. Avoidance, environmental reengineering (such as removing addictive substances and paraphernalia), and attending self-help groups can provide stimuli that elicit healthy responses.

Outcomes

What is the result when all of these principles and processes of change are combined? A series of clinical trials applying stage-matched interventions offers lessons about the future of behavioral health care generally and treatment of the addictions specifically.

In a large-scale clinical trial, the author and colleagues compared four treatments: (a) a home-based action-oriented cessation program (standardized), (b) stage-matched manuals (individualized), (c) a computerized expert system plus manuals (interactive), and (d) counselors plus an expert system and manuals (personalized). Patients were randomly assigned by stage to one of the four treatments.

Figure 54.3 presents point-prevalence abstinence rates for each of the four treatment groups over 18 months, with treatment ending at 6 months. Results with the two self-help manual conditions were parallel for 12 months, but the stage-matched manuals achieved better results at 18 months.

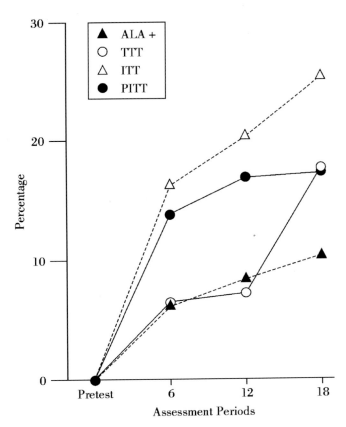

FIGURE 54.3 Point-prevalence abstinence (%) for four treatment groups at pretest and at 6, 12, and 18 months. ALA+, standardized manuals; TTT, individualized stage-matched manuals; ITT, interactive computer reports; PITT, personalized counselor calls.

This is an example of a delayed action effect. It takes time for participants in early stages to progress all the way to action. Therefore, some treatment effects as measured by action will be observed only after considerable time has elapsed.

The next test was to demonstrate the efficacy of the expert system when applied to an entire population recruited proactively. This study demonstrated significant benefits of the expert system at each 6-month follow-up. Moreover, the advantages over proactive assessment alone increased at each follow-up for the full 2 years assessed. The implications here are that expert system interventions in a population can continue to demonstrate benefits long after the intervention has ended.

Multiple Behaviors

A series of studies applied our best practice of tailored expert systems plus a stage-based self-help manual for multiple behaviors. Consistent across all studies was that the treatments produced significant impacts on multiple behaviors. This is the first body of research that has demonstrated that multiple-behavior treatments can be as effective as treating single behaviors. Although it is counterintuitive to suggest that outcomes for groups that are proactively recruited can match those of individuals who reach out for help, that is what informal comparisons strongly suggest.

CHAPTER **55**

Summary Author: John Young
Dennis C. Daley • Antoine Douaihy • Roger D. Weiss • Delinda E. Mercer

Group Therapies

GOALS OF GROUP THERAPIES

The ultimate goal of addiction treatment is to enable an individual to achieve and maintain lasting abstinence, but the immediate goals are to reduce drug or alcohol abuse, improve the individual's ability to function, and minimize the medical and psychosocial complications of addiction. Individuals in treatment for addiction will also need to change their behaviors to adopt a healthier lifestyle. Group therapies help patients achieve these goals by creating a milieu in which members of a group can bond with each other, thus reducing the stigma associated with addiction and the humiliation of having lost control of one's own behavior. Treatment groups provide a context in which addicted persons can gain support, encouragement, feedback, and confrontation from peers who understand from personal experience how addicted individuals think, feel, and act, including the manipulations, schemes, and diversions they sometimes use to rationalize their substance use and other maladaptive behaviors.

ORGANIZATION OF GROUP THERAPIES

Types of Group Therapies

Although many different types and structures of group treatments are available for the treatment of substance use disorders, many of the problems or issues addressed are similar (Table 55.1). Group therapies for substance use disorders generally fall into one of the following categories.

Milieu Groups Milieu groups are offered in residential programs. A group may review the upcoming day's schedule, discuss issues pertinent to the community of patients, ask each patient to state a goal for the day, or have patients listen to and reflect on the reading of the day. A wrap-up group may review the day's activities and provide participants a chance to reflect on experiences and insights from the day's treatment activities.

Psychoeducational Groups Psychoeducational groups provide information about specific topics related to addiction and recovery. These groups use a combination of lectures, discussions, educational videos, behavioral rehearsals, and completion of written assignments.

Skill Groups Skill groups are aimed at helping patients develop or improve their intrapersonal and interpersonal skills. These groups teach problem-solving methods and stress management, cognitive, and relapse prevention strategies.

Therapy or Counseling Groups These groups are less structured and often give the participants an opportunity to create their own agenda. Any of the issues presented in Table 55.1 can be discussed. These groups focus more on insight and raising self-awareness than on education or skill development.

Format of Group Therapy Sessions

Group sessions usually last from 60 to 90 minutes. Groups can be limited to a specific number of sessions or be open ended. Programs vary in the frequency of sessions as well.

TABLE 55.1	Issues Commonly Addressed in Recovery Groups

Physical/Lifestyle Issues

Tolerance, physical withdrawal, and the need for detoxification
Craving management
Medications for addiction and for co-occurring disorders
Medical problems including pain issues
HIV/AIDS, hepatitis C virus, and hepatitis B virus
Sexuality issues
Importance of exercise, rest, relaxation, and nutrition in recovery
Types and purposes of treatment
Defining personal goals/values
Structuring time
Engaging in non–substance-using activities
Achieving balance in life
Regular use of recovery tools in daily life

Psychological/Behavioral/Spiritual Issues

Understanding and identifying feelings and their connections to relapse
Managing anxiety
Managing depression
Managing feelings of emptiness
Managing boredom
Reducing shame and guilt
Grief and loss issues
Self-esteem
Self-defeating and therapy-sabotaging behaviors
Psychiatric comorbidities
Relapse and personal growth
High risk factors or dangerous situations for relapse
Relapse warning signs
Relapse setups
Lapse/relapse interruption
Spirituality
Meditation and prayer

Understanding Addiction and Recovery

Understanding addiction (etiology, symptoms, effects)
Effects of specific substances (e.g., alcohol, cocaine, marijuana)
Acceptance of addiction
Stages of change
Motivation to change and motivational struggles such as ambivalence
Tips for quitting alcohol or drug use
Pros and cons of change
Pros and cons of abstinence
Denial and other defenses
Phases of recovery and domains of recovery (physical, psychologic, family, social, spiritual)
Risky behaviors (such as sharing needles and equipment)
Other nonsubstance addictions

(Continued)

TABLE 55.1	Issues Commonly Addressed in Recovery Groups (*Continued*)

Family/Interpersonal/Social Domains

Effects of addiction on family and interpersonal relationships
Role of the family, concerned significant others in treatment/recovery
Resolving marital or family conflicts
Making amends to family or others
Managing high-risk people, places, and events
Engaging in healthy leisure interests
Addressing social life and relationship conflicts
Resisting social pressures to drink alcohol or use other drugs
Presenting a history of addiction disorders to the employer
Facing versus avoiding interpersonal conflicts
Learning to ask for help and support
Love and intimacy
Self-help programs in recovery
The 12 steps
Recovery clubs

Recovery Group Sessions In the cocaine collaborative study in which the authors participated, patients attended 90-minute Recovery Group sessions each week for 12 weeks. Topics of Phase 1 therapy sessions included the following:

Understanding Addiction
The Process of Recovery
Social and Interpersonal Issues in Recovery
Self-Help Groups and Support
Managing Feelings in Recovery
Relapse Prevention and Maintenance

Phase 2 groups met for 90 minutes weekly for 12 sessions after completing Phase 1 therapy. The goals were to help patients identify, rank, and discuss their problems in recovery and identify strategies to manage these problems. The issues and problems reviewed in the psychoeducational groups were revisited frequently.

Obstacles to Group Therapy Other researchers who have written about group treatments identify problems with group participants who create obstacles to treatment. Because the problems affect the group as a whole, the leader must have strategies to address any that arise in the course of a group session.

Family Psychoeducational Workshops Family psychoeducational workshops (FPWs) and other family programs often are used to educate the family, provide support, help reduce the family's burden, increase helpful behaviors, and decrease unhelpful behaviors. FPWs are semistructured sessions in which specific information is provided to patients and families in the context of a group of families.

EMPIRICAL VALIDATION OF GROUP THERAPIES

Controlled trials of group interventions have been somewhat limited, and many studies report results from programs that involve multiple components (i.e., individual plus group, multiple types of group treatments, or group plus other services). A recent paper reviewed 24 prospective treatment outcome studies comparing group therapy with one or more treatment conditions. The findings showed three important patterns: additional specialized group therapy can enhance the effectiveness of "treatment as usual," no differences were found between group and individual modalities, and no single type of group therapy demonstrated any consistent superiority in efficacy. The content of the group (whether skill based or interpersonal) did not make a difference. The authors concluded that the most notable finding of that study was the paucity of research on this topic.

The interest in researching various models of psychotherapy has led to the development of treatment manuals that describe the various psychotherapeutic approaches. Psychotherapy outcome studies have found that such manuals have an important, positive effect on the quality of both research and clinical practice. In fact, the use of treatment manuals has become a standard practice in research studies because they help ensure that therapists or counselors are providing treatment in a defined, measurable way.

Adherence to Group Sessions and Treatment Dropout

Most randomized clinical trials on addiction treatment showed significant reductions in drug use, improved health, and reduced social pathology. However, two of the major problems in the treatment of addictive disorders and co-occurring psychiatric disorders are poor adherence with session attendance or medications and early termination.

Reasons for Dropping Out of Group Treatment In the National Institute on Drug Abuse Collaborative Cocaine Treatment Study, patients were assessed to learn the reasons for early termination of treatment. The reasons most commonly cited were time problems; the relapse to use or the desire to use; not finding group sessions helpful; wanting a different treatment, such as individual therapy; improvement in the problem; other unspecified reasons; unwillingness to participate in treatment; and need for hospitalization.

Limitations to the research conducted on group treatments arise from two sources: variations in content and differences in process. Very often, group programs are studied rather than a single group intervention. In addition, studies sometimes involve a combination of group and individual treatments, making it difficult to determine how much each intervention contributes to the outcome.

The Need for Physician Support

Physicians and other addiction professionals who do not provide group therapies can play a significant role in supporting and facilitating patients' participation in groups. First, they can educate, encourage, and persuade patients to participate in groups as part of their overall treatment program. It is helpful for all clinical staff members to give patients a consistent message about the value of groups. Second, the physician can monitor and discuss a patient's group participation. Third, the physician can collaborate with group therapists about patients' clinical status or problems with adherence.

COUNSELOR TRAINING AND SUPERVISION

Counselor Training

To provide effective group treatment, it is necessary for counselors or therapists to be familiar with and skillful in addiction treatment and group therapy.

The knowledge base that one should have to provide competent addiction treatment involves knowledge of the effects of the various drugs of abuse and which drugs are commonly used in combination and their interactions, as well as the medical, psychologic, social, family, and spiritual consequences of addiction. It also is necessary to understand the processes of recovery and relapse and the strategies or tools that can help the recovering person to manage the recovery process. The clinician should be familiar with the Twelve-Step self-help approach for addiction recovery and with alternative self-help resources for patients who are not comfortable with Twelve-Step programs. In terms of group counseling or therapy, counselors should have an understanding of counseling theory and experience in counseling individual patients.

"Group process" refers to the attitudes and interaction of the group members and leaders. It also is important for the counselor to be familiar with the stages of groups: the beginning, the middle or working stage, and the ending or closing stage. The group leader should be familiar with the kinds of interventions he or she will use most often and how to deal with problem situations that occur most commonly in groups.

Counselor Supervision

Supervision is a very important, meaningful part of the practice of group treatment, yet it often is overlooked or provided in a less than optimal manner. It also is important to communicate that supervision is not primarily about evaluation of the counselor's work, but rather an opportunity for the counselor to air problems, hone his or her skills, and continue to learn.

Counselor Satisfaction

It is important that counselors feel satisfied with the group approach they are providing. When counselors are dissatisfied, burnout, indifferent treatment and departures from appropriate counseling behavior often result. Dissatisfied counselors also tend to feel less positive about their work and to express less confidence in their patients' ability to achieve recovery; such feelings can undermine the patients' own perception of their ability to recover.

LIMITATIONS OF GROUP THERAPIES

Although group therapies offer many benefits, they also have some limitations with which the clinician should be familiar. One of the most common is an overemphasis on group treatment at the expense of individual treatment. Patients often reported that there were certain types of problems or issues that they would not discuss in group sessions and that they preferred the privacy and confidentiality afforded by an individual counseling or therapy session. As a result of social anxiety, patients may choose to limit participation in therapy or self-help group discussions, miss group sessions, or drop out prematurely. They often do so without discussing their reasons with a therapist, counselor, or sponsor.

Summary Author: John Young
Bruce J. Rounsaville • Kathleen M. Carroll • Sudie E. Back

Individual Psychotherapy

Although always present as an option for the treatment of addictions, individual psychotherapy has not been the predominant treatment modality since the 1960s, when inpatient Twelve-Step–informed milieu therapy, group treatments, methadone maintenance, and therapeutic community approaches came to be the fixtures of treatment programs. In fact, these newer modalities derived their popularity from the failures of individual psychotherapy when it was used as the sole treatment for addictive disorders; such an approach was poorly suited to the needs of addicted patients because the lack of emphasis on symptom control and the lack of structure in the therapist's typical stance allowed the patient's continued drug or alcohol use to undermine the treatment. Also, the anxiety-arousing nature of individual therapy could result in increased drug use.

Individual psychotherapy has become a resurgent approach since the 1980s, and some form of behavioral therapy should now be considered as a treatment option for all patients who seek help for a substance use disorder. It is now standard practice to introduce anxiety-arousing aspects of treatment only after a strong therapeutic alliance has been developed or within the context of other supportive structures.

The alternatives to psychotherapy are either pharmacologic or structural (as through sequestration from access to drugs and alcohol in a residential setting), and both treatments can have limited effectiveness or high rates of premature dropout if not combined with psychotherapy or counseling.

PSYCHOTHERAPY AND PHARMACOTHERAPY

Even when the principal treatment for an addictive disorder is seen as pharmacologic, psychotherapeutic interventions are needed to complement the pharmacotherapy by enhancing the motivation to stop substance use by taking the prescribed medications, providing guidance for the use of prescribed medications and management of side effects, maintaining motivation to continue taking the prescribed medications after the patient achieves an initial period of abstinence, providing relationship elements to prevent premature termination, and helping the patient to develop the skills to adjust to a life without drug and alcohol use. The importance of psychotherapy and psychosocial treatments is reinforced by recognition that the repertoire of pharmacotherapies available for treatment of drug addicts is limited to a handful, with the most effective agents limited in their utility to treatment of opioid dependence and alcohol dependence. Effective pharmacotherapies for dependence on cocaine, marijuana, hallucinogens, sedative-hypnotics, and stimulants have not yet been developed, and behavioral therapies remain the principal approaches for the treatment of these classes of drugs.

Conversely, pharmacotherapy can be important to enhancing the efficacy of psychotherapy. Psychotherapies effect change by psychologic means in psychosocial aspects of drug abuse, such as motivation, coping skills, dysfunctional thoughts, or social relationships; they have limited effects on the physiologic aspects of drug use or withdrawal. Also, the effects of behavioral treatments tend to be delayed, requiring practice, repeated sessions, and a "working through" process. In contrast, the relative strengths of pharmacologic treatments are their rapid actions in reducing immediate or protracted withdrawal symptoms, drug craving, or the rewarding effects of continued drug use. In effect, pharmacotherapies for drug dependence reduce the patient's immediate access to and preoccupation with drugs, freeing the patient to address other concerns such as long-term goals or interpersonal relationships.

Dropout from psychotherapy is reduced because drug urges and relapse are mitigated by the effects of the medication. Greater duration of abstinence can further enhance the effects of psychotherapy because substance-related effects on attention and mental acuity are prevented, maximizing new learning that therapy can induce.

INDIVIDUAL VERSUS GROUP THERAPY

A central advantage of group over individual psychotherapy is economy, which is a major consideration in an era of skyrocketing health care costs and increasingly curtailed third-party payments. There are other aspects of group therapy that can be argued to make this modality more effective than individual treatment of drug addicts:

- Given the social stigma attached to having lost control of substance use, the presence of other group members who acknowledge having similar problems can provide comfort.
- Other group members who are farther along in their recovery can act as models and offer a wide variety of coping strategies that go beyond the repertoire known even by the most skilled individual therapist.
- Group members frequently can act as "buddies" who offer continued support outside of the group sessions in a way that most professional therapists do not.
- The "public" nature of group therapy, with its attendant aspects of confession and forgiveness, coupled with the pressure to publicly confess future slips and transgressions, provides a powerful incentive to avoid relapse.
- Because the group is composed of recovering addicts, members may be better able to detect each other's attempts to conceal relapse or early warning signals for relapse than would an individual therapist who may not have personal experience with an addictive disorder.

Individual therapy, however, has benefits that can justify its greater expense in certain circumstances:

- Participation in group therapy always risks a breach in confidentiality. Public knowledge of drug and alcohol use still can ruin careers and reputations.
- Individual therapy allows the therapist more flexibility to address the patient's problems as they arise.
- Individual therapy allows a much higher percentage of therapy time to concentrate on issues that are uniquely relevant to that individual.
- Individual therapy is more feasible for mental health professionals or medical practitioners who do not have a caseload of addicts large enough to conduct group treatment.
- If group therapy is to be started with a new group, it can be many weeks before enough members are screened to be entered into a new group, resulting in patients' discouragement and high dropout rates while awaiting the onset of treatment. Scheduling can be very difficult for those patients whose employer is not apprised of the need for treatment.
- Individual therapy can be more conducive to the development of a deepening relationship between the patient and therapist over time, which can allow an exploration of issues that is not possible in group therapy.
- Patients with particular personality disorders, such as borderline or schizoid patients, may be unable to get involved with other group members, as with patients who are so shy that they cannot bring themselves to attend group sessions.

SPECIALIZED KNOWLEDGE NECESSARY FOR THERAPY WITH ADDICTED PATIENTS

Pharmacology, Use Patterns, Consequences, and Course of Addiction

For therapy to be effective, it is important not only to obtain the textbook knowledge about frequently abused drugs—pharmacology, use patterns, consequences, and course of addiction—but also to become familiar with street knowledge about drugs (e.g., slang names, favored routes of administration, prices, and availability) and the clinical presentation of individuals when they are intoxicated or experiencing withdrawal. This knowledge is important for several reasons:

- It fosters a therapeutic alliance by allowing the therapist to convey an understanding of the world in which the addict lives.
- The clinician can help the patient anticipate problems that will arise in the course of initiating abstinence—for example, knowing the typical type and duration of withdrawal symptoms, and their transient nature, can help the addict to successfully complete detoxification.
- Knowledge of drug actions and withdrawal states is crucial for helping the addict to understand and manage transient dysphoric affects and for diagnosing comorbid psychopathology.
- The need to distinguish transient substance-induced affects from enduring attitudes and traits also is an important psychotherapy task. Substance-related affective states can greatly color the patient's view of self and

world, and it is important for the therapist to be able to recognize these states so that the associated distorted thoughts can be recognized as such rather than being taken at face value. Similarly, it is important that the patient be taught to distinguish between sober and substance-affected conditions and to recognize when, in the colloquial phrase, it is "the alcohol talking" and not the person's more enduring sentiments.

- Learning about drug and alcohol effects is important in detecting when patients have relapsed or come to sessions intoxicated, as it is rarely useful to conduct psychotherapy sessions when the patient is intoxicated.

Other Treatment and Self-Help Group Philosophies and Techniques

For many addicts, individual psychotherapy is best conceived as a component of a multifaceted program of treatment to help the patient overcome a chronic, relapsing condition. One function of individual psychotherapy can be to help the patient choose which additional therapies to employ in his or her attempt to stop using alcohol or other drugs.

Another major function of knowing about the major alternative treatment modalities for addicts is to be alert to the possibility that different treatments can provide contradictory recommendations that may confuse the patient or foster the patient's attempts to sabotage treatment. It is vital that the therapist attempts to adjust his or her own work to bring the psychotherapy in accord with other treatments.

A commonly occurring set of conflicts arises between the treatment goals and methods employed by professional therapists and those of Twelve-Step self-help movements such as AA, Cocaine Anonymous, and Narcotics Anonymous. For example, the recovery goal for many who use a Twelve-Step approach is a life of complete abstinence from psychotropic medications. This approach may conflict with professional advice when the therapist recommends use of psychopharmacologic treatments for co-occurring psychiatric disorders. Twelve-Step literature supports use of appropriately prescribed medications of all kinds; however, individual members may disagree. One way to approach this issue is to describe the psychiatric condition for which the medications are prescribed as a disease separate from the addictive disorder. In this and similar situations, it may also be helpful to acknowledge that different strategies appear to work for different individuals and that alternative approaches may be employed sequentially if the initial plan fails.

COMMON ISSUES AND STRATEGIES

Even when attempting to explore other issues in depth, the therapist should devote at least a small part of every session to monitoring the patient's substance use and be willing to interrupt other work to address slips and relapses as they occur. Implicit in the need to maintain this focus is the recognition that psychotherapy with these patients entails a more active therapist stance than does treatment of patients with other psychiatric disorders.

Enhancing Motivation

An early task for psychotherapists is to gauge the patient's level of motivation to stop his or her substance use by exploring the patient's treatment goals. Addicts often enter treatment not with the goal to stop but rather to return to the days when drug and alcohol use was enjoyable. One way to approach the patient's likely ambivalence is to attempt an exploration of the patient's perceived benefits from use of alcohol or drugs, or his or her perceived need for them; to obtain a clear picture of the patient's positive attitudes toward substance use, it may be necessary to elicit details of the patient's early involvement with drugs and alcohol.

Although virtually all types of psychotherapy for addiction address the issue of motivation and goal setting to some extent, motivational therapy or interviewing makes this the sole initial focus of treatment. Motivational approaches, which are usually brief (e.g., two to four sessions), are designed to produce rapid change by seeking to maximize patients' motivational resources and commitment to abstinence. Active ingredients of these approaches include objective feedback of personal risk or impairment, emphasis on personal responsibility for change, clear advice to change, a menu of alternative change options, therapist empathy, and facilitation of patient self-efficacy.

One major controversy in this area is whether controlled use can be an acceptable alternative treatment goal to abstinence from all psychoactive drugs. In practice, the therapist cannot force the patient to seek any goal that the patient does not choose, and failure to address a presenting goal of controlled use may result in failure to engage the patient. Frequently, the patient needs to make several failed attempts at controlled use before becoming convinced that a goal of abstinence is more appropriate.

Teaching Coping Skills

The most enduring challenge in treating patients with addiction is to help the patient avoid relapse after achieving an initial period of abstinence. A general tactic is to identify specific circumstances that increase an individual's likelihood of resuming substance use and to help the patient anticipate and practice strategies (e.g., refusal skills, recognizing and avoiding cues for craving) for coping with these high-risk situations.

Changing Reinforcement Contingencies

A key element of deepening dependence on alcohol or other drugs is the rise of substance-related behavior to the top of an individual's list of priorities. As compulsive use becomes a part of every day, previously valued relationships or activities may be given up, so that the rewards available in daily life are narrowed progressively to those derived from use of the substance. When such use is ended, its absence may leave the patient with a need to fill the time that had been spent using drugs or alcohol and to find rewards to substitute for those derived from their use.

The ease with which the patient can rearrange priorities is related to the level of achievement before he or she became involved with alcohol or drugs and the degree to which substance use damaged or replaced valued relationships, jobs, or hobbies. Because the typical course of illicit drug use entails initiation of compulsive use between the ages of 12 and 25 years, many patients come to treatment without having achieved satisfactory adult relationships or vocational skills. In such cases, achieving a drug- and alcohol-free life may require a lengthy process of vocational rehabilitation and development of meaningful relationships. Individual psychotherapy can contribute importantly to this process by helping maintain the patient's motivation throughout the recovery process and by helping the patient to explore factors that have interfered with achievement of rewarding ties to others.

Fostering Management of Painful Affects

Dysphoric affects are the most commonly cited precipitant for relapse, and many have suggested that failure of affect regulation is a central dynamic underlying the development of compulsive alcohol or drug use. In addition, difficulty in differentiating among negative emotional states has been identified as a common characteristic among addicted patients. To foster the development of mastery over dysphoric affects, most psychotherapies emphasize enhancing the patient's ability to identify, tolerate, and respond appropriately to strong affects.

Improving Interpersonal Functioning and Enhancing Social Supports

A consistent finding in the literature on relapse is the protective influence of an adequate network of social supports. Self-help groups offer a fully developed social network of welcoming individuals who are understanding and committed to leading a substance-free life. Moreover, in most urban and suburban settings, self-help meetings are held daily or several times a week, and a sponsor system is available to provide the recovering person with individual guidance and support on a 24-hour basis.

EFFICACY RESEARCH

Individual Psychotherapy for Opioid Dependence

Opioid Agonist Therapy In the landmark study in this area, opiate-addicted patients undergoing methadone maintenance who received professional psychotherapy evidenced greater improvement than the subjects who received drug counseling alone. Although methadone-maintained patients with lower levels of psychopathology tended to improve regardless of whether they received professional psychotherapy or drug counseling, those with higher levels of psychopathology tended to improve only if they received psychotherapy; this can point to the best use of psychotherapy when resources are scarce.

Contingency Management Several studies have evaluated the use of contingency management to reduce the use of illicit drugs in patients who are maintained on methadone. In these studies, a reinforcer (reward) is provided to patients who demonstrate specified target behaviors such as providing drug-free urine specimens, accomplishing specific treatment goals, or attending treatment sessions. For example, offering methadone take-home privileges contingent on reduced drug use is an approach that capitalizes on an inexpensive reinforcer that is potentially available in all methadone maintenance programs. Similarly, the use of a contingency management system in which abstinence is reinforced by patients receiving points redeemable for items consistent with a drug-free lifestyle (e.g., movie tickets and sporting goods) has been shown to be effective in reducing illicit opioid and cocaine use among methadone-maintained opioid-addicted patients.

Opioid antagonist treatment (naltrexone) offers many advantages over methadone maintenance, including the fact that it is nonaddicting and can be prescribed without concerns about diversion, has a benign side effect profile, and can be less costly in terms of demands on professional time and of patient time than the daily or near-daily clinic visits required for methadone maintenance. Yet naltrexone has not fulfilled its promise: Naltrexone treatment programs remain comparatively rare and underutilized, a situation largely due to problems with retention, particularly during the induction phase. Recently, however, strategies to enhance retention and outcome in naltrexone treatment have come from investigations of contingency management approaches such as providing vouchers for naltrexone compliance.

Individual Psychotherapy for Cocaine Dependence

Contingency Management In this approach, abstinence, verified through drug-free urine screens, is reinforced through a voucher system as described above. High acceptance, retention, and rates of abstinence have been demonstrated for patients receiving this approach, as compared with standard counseling oriented toward Twelve-Step programs. Rates of abstinence do not decline substantially when less valuable incentives are substituted for the voucher system, and the voucher system has been shown to have durable effects. These findings are of great importance because contingency management procedures are potentially applicable to a wide range of target behaviors and problems, including treatment retention and compliance with pharmacotherapy. Nevertheless, despite the very compelling evidence of the effectiveness of these procedures, they are rarely used in clinical treatment programs. One major impediment to broader use is the expense associated with the voucher program; average earnings for patients are about $600. Recently developed low-cost contingency management (CM) procedures may be a way to bring these effective approaches into general clinical use; a recently completed study demonstrated that a variable ratio schedule of reinforcement that provides access to large reinforcers but at low probabilities is effective in retaining subjects in treatment and reducing substance use. This system is far less expensive than the standard voucher system, because only a proportion of behaviors are reinforced with a prize.

Cognitive-Behavioral Therapies (CBTs) Another behavioral approach that was shown to be effective in treating cocaine abusers is CBT. Its goal is to foster abstinence by helping the patient master an individualized set of coping strategies as an effective alternative to substance use.

CBT appears to be particularly more effective with more severe cocaine users or those with comorbid disorders. Moreover, CBT appears to be a particularly durable approach, with patients continuing to reduce their cocaine use even after they leave treatment.

Manualized Disease-Model Approaches Randomized clinical trials have demonstrated the effectiveness of manualized disease-model approaches. One such approach is Twelve-Step Facilitation (TSF), a manual-guided, individual approach intended to be similar to widely used approaches that emphasize principles associated with disease models of addiction. Although this treatment has no official relationship with AA or CA, its content is consistent with the 12 steps of AA, with primary emphasis on the concepts of acceptance (e.g., to help the patient accept that he or she has the illness, or disease, of addiction) and surrender (e.g., to help the patient acknowledge that there is hope for sobriety through accepting the need for help from others and a "Higher Power"). In addition to abstinence from all psychoactive substances, a major goal of the treatment is to foster active participation in self-help groups.

TSF has been found to be comparable to CBT in reducing cocaine use. Moreover, there is a strong relationship between the attainment of significant periods of abstinence during treatment and abstinence during follow-up, which emphasizes that the inception of abstinence, even for comparatively brief periods, is an important goal of treatment.

Individual Psychotherapy for Marijuana Dependence

Treatment of marijuana abuse and dependence is a comparatively understudied area to date. No effective pharmacotherapies for marijuana dependence exist, and only a few controlled trials of behavioral approaches have been completed. A recent comparison of a two-session motivational approach with a nine-session combined motivational/coping skills approach suggested that both active treatments were associated with significant reductions in marijuana use through a 9-month follow-up period; moreover, the nine-session intervention was significantly more effective than the two-session intervention, and this effect also was sustained through the 9-month follow-up period. A contingency management approach involving adding voucher-based incentives to coping skills and motivational enhancement has also been shown to improve outcomes in this population.

Summary Author: John Young
Stephen T. Higgins • Jennifer W. Tidey • Randall E. Rogers

Contingency Management and the Community Reinforcement Approach

Contingency management (CM) interventions and community reinforcement approach (CRA) therapy for treating substance use disorders (SUDs) are based in the conceptual framework of learning and conditioning theory. Fundamental to these treatment approaches is operant conditioning, which is the study of how systematically applied environmental consequences increase (reinforce) or decrease (punish) the frequency and patterning of voluntary behavior.

In this model, drug use is considered a normal, learned behavior that falls along a continuum ranging from little use and few problems to excessive use and many untoward effects. The same principles of learning and conditioning are assumed to operate across this continuum. Within this framework, all physically intact humans are considered to possess the necessary neurobiologic systems to experience drug-produced reinforcement and hence to develop drug use and SUDs. Genetic or acquired characteristics (e.g., family history of alcoholism, other psychiatric disorders) are recognized as factors that affect the probability of developing SUDs but are not deemed to be necessary for the problem to emerge.

TREATMENT MODEL

Within an operant conceptual framework, reinforcement derived from drug use and the associated lifestyle is deemed to have monopolized the behavioral repertoire of the user. Treatments developed within this framework are designed to reorganize the user's environment to systematically increase the rate of reinforcement obtained while abstinent from drug use and reduce or eliminate the rate of reinforcement obtained through drug use and associated activities. Primary emphasis is placed on decreasing drug use by systematically increasing the availability and frequency of alternative reinforcing activities, either through relatively contrived sources of reinforcement as in CM interventions or through more naturalistic sources as in CRA therapy: by *contrived*, we mean a set of contingencies that are put in place explicitly and exclusively for therapeutic purposes, for example, earning vouchers exchangeable for retail items contingent on cocaine-negative urine toxicology results; by *naturalistic*, we mean a set of contingencies that are already operating in the natural environment for nontherapeutic purposes but can be used to support the therapeutic process, for example, teaching a spouse to deliver praise when a patient avoids bars and to withhold praise or express disapproval for going to bars. Additionally, arranging the environment so that aversive events or the loss of reinforcing events occur as a consequence of drug use also can decrease drug use. As with reinforcement, such aversive procedures can involve relatively contrived (e.g., forfeiture of a large-value incentive) or more naturalistic (e.g., suspension from work) consequences.

Some treatments, such as the CRA + vouchers treatment for cocaine dependence described below, are designed to deliver contrived consequences during the initial treatment period, with a transition to more naturalistic sources later in treatment. The rationale for this approach is that the lifestyle of the user is often so disrupted upon treatment entry that it is largely devoid of effective alternative sources of reinforcement that can compete with the reinforcement derived from drug use. Contrived sources of alternative reinforcement delivered through CM are designed to promote initial abstinence, thereby allowing time for therapists and patients to work toward reestablishing more naturalistic alternatives that will be needed to sustain long-term abstinence.

Also important to recognize is that some patients may have behavioral repertoires that are too limited to recruit sufficient sources of naturalistic reinforcement to effectively compete with drug use, and as such, these patients will need some form of maintenance treatment involving contrived reinforcement contingencies in order to sustain long-term abstinence. This is widely recognized with opioid-dependent individuals who often need a maintenance pharmacotherapy in order to sustain long-term abstinence from illicit drug use. Others may need lifelong participation in self-help programs in order to succeed; such programs might be regarded as falling somewhere around the midpoint on the continuum of contrived versus naturalistic sources of alternative reinforcement.

TREATMENT PLANNING

First, detailed information is collected on drug use, treatment readiness, psychiatric functioning, employment/vocational status, recreational interests, current social supports, family and social problems, and legal issues. Obtaining a current address and phone number is important, as is a number of someone who will always know the client's whereabouts.

A practical needs assessment questionnaire is then used to determine whether the patient has any pressing needs or crises (e.g., housing, legal, medical, transportation, or childcare) that may interfere with initial treatment. If it appears that a medication is indicated, steps are taken toward implementing the relevant medical protocols.

PRETREATMENT ISSUES

Selection and Preparation of Patients

We know of no particular type of SUD patient for whom CM or CRA is contraindicated. With CM, it is quite common to have patients sign a written contract stipulating all aspects of the CM arrangement so as to avoid any confusion about the contingencies.

Therapist Characteristics

To implement CRA effectively, therapists need to be directive but also flexible. Particularly in the early stages of treatment, therapists try to work around patient schedules and generally make participation in treatment convenient to the patient. Therapists also try to be flexible with regard to tardiness to sessions, early departure from sessions, and the time of day that sessions are scheduled and will meet with patients outside the office if necessary.

Within ethical boundaries, therapists must be committed to doing what it takes to facilitate lifestyle changes on the part of patients. Therapists often accompany patients to appointments or job interviews, initiate recreational activities with patients, and schedule sessions at different times of day to accomplish specific goals; they have patients make phone calls from their office; they search newspapers for job possibilities or ideas for healthy recreational activities for patients.

Therapists typically do not manage CM programs owing to the detailed record keeping involved and the need to biochemically verify abstinence.

TREATMENT AND TECHNIQUE

For illustration purposes, in this section we describe basic elements of CM and CRA interventions using the CRA + vouchers treatment for cocaine dependence.

In the voucher-based CM program, vouchers exchangeable for retail items are earned contingent on cocaine-negative results in thrice-weekly urine toxicology testing. The first cocaine-negative specimen earns a voucher worth $2.50 in purchasing power. The value of each subsequent consecutive cocaine-negative specimen increases by $1.25. The equivalent of a $10 bonus is provided for each three consecutive cocaine-negative specimens. A cocaine-positive specimen or failure to submit a scheduled specimen resets the value of vouchers back to the initial $2.50 value. This reset feature is designed to punish relapse to cocaine use after a period of sustained abstinence, with the intensity of the punishment tied directly to the length of sustained abstinence that would be broken. In order to provide patients with a reason to continue abstaining from drug use after a reset, submission of five consecutive cocaine-negative specimens after a cocaine-positive specimen returns the value of points to where they were prior to the reset.

If someone is continuously abstinent throughout the 12-week intervention, total earnings would be approximately $997.50. However, because most patients are unable to sustain abstinence throughout the intervention, the average earning is usually about half that amount.

The voucher CM intervention contains most of the features that are important to effective CM:

- The details of the intervention are carefully explained to patients in the form of a written contract prior to beginning treatment.
- The response being targeted by the CM intervention (cocaine abstinence) is defined in objective terms (i.e., cocaine-negative urine toxicology results).
- The methods for verifying that the target response occurred are well specified and objective (urine toxicology testing).
- The schedule for monitoring progress is well specified.
- The schedule is designed to include frequent opportunities for patients to experience the programmed consequences.
- The duration of the intervention is stipulated in advance.
- The intervention is focused on a single target. CM interventions that focus on a single target on average produce larger treatment effects than those that target multiple targets (e.g., abstinence from multiple substances).
- The consequences that will follow success and failure to emit the target response are clear.
- There is minimal delay in delivering designated consequences (urine specimens are analyzed on-site, and vouchers earned are delivered immediately after testing). Delivering the consequence on the same day that occurrence of the target response is verified produces larger treatment effects than delivering the consequence at a later time.
- The magnitude of reinforcement that can be earned is relatively substantial. Larger value incentives on average produce larger treatment effects.

Community Reinforcement Approach

The CRA component of the CRA + vouchers treatment has seven elements.

1. Patients are instructed in how to recognize antecedents and consequences of their cocaine use and how to use that information to reduce the probability of using cocaine. A twofold message is conveyed to the patient: (a) His or her cocaine use is orderly behavior that is more likely to occur under certain circumstances than others and (b) By learning to identify the circumstances that affect one's cocaine use, plans can be developed and implemented to reduce the likelihood of future cocaine use.
2. Systematically developing and maintaining a new, "safe" social network that will support a healthier lifestyle and getting involved with recreational activities that are enjoyable and do not involve cocaine or other drug use are given high priority and addressed individually with all patients. For those patients who are willing to participate, self-help groups (Alcoholics or Narcotics Anonymous) can be an effective way to develop a new network of associates who will support a sober lifestyle.
3. Various other forms of individualized skills training are provided, usually to address some specific skill deficit that may influence directly or indirectly a patient's risk for cocaine use (e.g., time management, problem solving, assertiveness training, social skills training, and mood management).
4. Unemployed patients are offered Job Club, which is an efficacious method for assisting chronically unemployed individuals to obtain employment.
5. Patients with romantic partners who are not drug abusers are offered behavioral couples therapy, which is an intervention designed to teach couples positive communication skills and how to negotiate reciprocal contracts for desired changes in each other's behavior.
6. HIV/AIDS education is provided to all clients in the early stages of treatment, along with individual counseling directed at addressing any specific needs or risk behavior. Patients are encouraged to get tested for HIV and hepatitis B and C.
7. All who meet diagnostic criteria for alcohol dependence or report that alcohol use is involved in their use of cocaine are offered disulfiram therapy. Disulfiram therapy is only effective when implemented with procedures to monitor compliance with the recommended dosing regimen.

The use of substances other than caffeine is discouraged as well via CRA therapy, although we never dismiss or refuse to treat a patient owing to other drug use. Anyone who meets criteria for physical dependence on opiates is referred to an adjoining service located within our clinic for methadone or other opioid replacement therapy. We recommend cessation of tobacco use but usually not during the course of treatment for cocaine dependence.

EMPIRICAL SUPPORT

Contingency Management Interventions

Contingency Management as a Treatment for Alcohol Use Disorders
The use of CM to treat primary alcohol use disorders has largely failed to gain a foothold among the alcohol research or clinical communities. One obstacle is that objectively monitoring alcohol intake using blood alcohol levels (BALs) provides evidence about use only during the few hours preceding the test; this difficulty could be surmounted by relying on a combination of observations by individuals in the subject's natural environment and randomly scheduled BALs. Alternatively, reinforcing compliance with disulfiram can reduce drinking when the contingencies are managed systematically.

While the work begun using CM to reinforce disulfiram compliance has not been continued in any programmatic manner, the concept has been successfully extended to reinforcing naltrexone compliance among patients with opioid use disorders, as well as reinforcing adherence to antiretroviral therapies among HIV-positive patients with SUDs.

Developing Contingency Management as a Treatment for Illicit Drug Use Disorders
During the 1970s and 1980s, a concerted body of work emerged on the use of CM to treat illicit drug use, conducted almost exclusively with patients enrolled in methadone treatment for opioid use disorders.

Though methadone and related substitution therapies are effective at reducing the use of illicit opioids, a subset of patients continue abusing other nonopioid drugs. A commonly used reinforcer in this area of CM research is the medication take-home privilege, where the dispensing of extra daily doses of opioid medication gives the patient a break from the grind of having to travel daily to the clinic to ingest the medication under staff supervision.

Other consequences have been investigated as well: for example, increasing the maintenance dose of methadone contingent on drug-free urine testing has been found effective for improving abstinence from other opiate use and from polydrug use.

Voucher-Based Contingency Management as a Treatment for Illicit Drug Use Disorders
Voucher-based interventions garnered significant interest when they were introduced in the 1990s because of their efficacy with cocaine use disorders. At a time when most clinical trials investigating treatments for cocaine use disorders were consistently producing negative outcomes, a series of controlled trials examining voucher-based CM produced reliably positive outcomes.

The first randomized trial designed to isolate the contribution of voucher-based CM to outcome demonstrated that those patients receiving vouchers were more likely to complete treatment and had an improved average duration of continuous cocaine abstinence. In more recent trials further examining the efficacy of contingent vouchers when combined with CRA, positive effects on cocaine abstinence remained discernible through posttreatment follow-up periods extending out to 21 months following discontinuation of the voucher program.

A series of studies conducted in a clinic located in a relatively rural community demonstrated that this approach could be applied to abusers residing outside a large urban area. Another study examined the efficacy of the voucher program with cocaine-abusing methadone maintenance patients; cocaine use was substantially reduced in the group for which CM was added to standard outpatient counseling. Also, use of opiates decreased during the voucher period in the contingent compared to the noncontingent conditions, even though the contingency was exclusively on cocaine use.

Subsequent studies have supported the efficacy of vouchers in the following situations:

- Promoting abstinence from cocaine and heroin use along with participation in vocational training among pregnant and recently postpartum women
- Reducing days of homelessness and promoting abstinence from cocaine and other substance use in homeless individuals seeking work and housing
- In combination with antidepressant treatment to promote abstinence in opioid- and cocaine-dependent patients

With the goal of improving chances that a voucher-based CM approach could be disseminated to community clinics, a variation known as prize-based CM was developed: in this procedure, rather than reinforcing each occurrence of the target response, patients earned the opportunity to draw from an urn that contained vouchers of varying value, including many that are of zero value but offer verbal praise, some that are of relatively low monetary value, still fewer of moderate value, and a very few of high value. Studies have demonstrated this approach to be efficacious for increasing cocaine and other drug abstinence in drug-free and methadone community clinics; it is worth clarifying, however, that there is no evidence that the prize-based arrangement results in better outcomes than a voucher-based program involving lower-than-usual voucher values. As would be expected, effect sizes obtained with the prize-based intervention appear to be smaller than those achieved with more expensive CM interventions in comparable populations.

New Directions

Marijuana Studies have supported the efficacy of abstinence-contingence vouchers and money incentives for increasing abstinence in marijuana users, including those suffering from serious mental illness, although several individuals in a study involving outpatients with schizophrenia were not sensitive to the contingencies. The addition of CBT may enhance outcomes after the vouchers are discontinued.

Cigarette Smoking

Smoking in Pregnancy Voucher-based reinforcement of abstinence has been successfully extended to the treatment of pregnant cigarette smokers. In a recent study, estimated fetal growth also was significantly greater in the contingent compared to the noncontingent conditions.

Smoking in Adolescence A feasibility study indicated that cash reinforcement contingent upon breath CO samples significantly increased smoking abstinence in a group of adolescents; a similar study enrolled college-aged smokers, with similar results. Recently, two studies have extended the duration of these interventions, with similar results. Another study found that contingently reinforcing smoking reductions for several days prior to an abstinence-based CM trial enhanced CM effects.

Smoking and Schizophrenia Schizophrenia is associated with high rates of smoking and low smoking-cessation success. A feasibility study involving outpatients who were not seeking treatment for smoking demonstrated that cash reinforcement of CO reductions significantly reduced smoking. These results were later replicated systematically.

Methamphetamine Patients with methamphetamine use disorders who received CM in addition to usual treatment submitted significantly more negative drug samples and were abstinent for a longer period of time.

Community Reinforcement Approach

Initial Study In the initial study of the effectiveness of CRA with alcoholic patients, CRA was designed to rearrange and improve the quality of the reinforcers obtained by patients through their vocational, family, social, and recreational activities, these reinforcers being available and of high quality when the patient was sober and unavailable when drinking resumed. Patients treated with CRA demonstrated markedly reduced time spent drinking and superior outcomes on a number of other measures, at 6-month follow-up after hospital discharge.

Further Developing the Community Reinforcement Approach After publication of the seminal study described above, CRA was expanded to include disulfiram therapy, with monitoring by a significant other (SO) to ensure medication compliance. Additionally, counseling directed at crises resolution was added, as was a switch from individual to group counseling to reduce cost and a "buddy" system in which individuals in the alcoholic's neighborhood volunteered to be available to give assistance with practical issues. This revised intervention proved superior to standard care in terms of percent time spent drinking, time unemployed, time away from family, and time institutionalized.

Extending the Community Reinforcement Approach to Treatment of Patients with Cocaine and Opioid Use Disorders As described earlier, studies on the use of CRA to treat cocaine use disorders examined a treatment involving CRA in combination with voucher-based CM (CRA + vouchers). Outcomes were significantly better among those treated with the CRA + voucher treatment than standard drug abuse counseling. Two trials have been reported wherein CRA was investigated in the treatment of opioid-dependent patients receiving opioid pharmacotherapy; they provide evidence that CRA delivered alone or in combination with voucher-based CM can improve outcomes.

Extending the Community Reinforcement Approach to Special Populations

Adolescents The first study with adolescents involved individuals randomly assigned to CRA or supportive counseling. Abstinence from drug use in the CRA condition was significantly higher across the 12-month study period as compared to the supportive counseling condition. Measures of attendance at school and employment, family relationships, depression, and time institutionalized were also better in the CRA condition. Follow-up results collected 9 months after completion of the initial study period indicated better outcomes in the CRA compared to the supportive counseling conditions.

Adolescent CRA therapy was compared to motivational enhancement therapy plus CBT (MET/CBT) and multidimensional family therapy (MDFT) in a multisite trial conducted with adolescent cannabis users. Over 1 year of posttreatment follow-up, the overall percent of patients in recovery was somewhat higher among patients treated with CRA than with MET/CBT and MDFT.

The Homeless In a study with adults, alcohol-dependent homeless persons treated with CRA versus standard treatment showed greater improvement on measures of drinking conducted over a 1-year period. In a study with individuals between 14 and 19 years of age, substance use and depression scores decreased during a 6-month study period among a larger proportion of those treated with CRA than with usual care, while measures of social stability increased more among those treated with CRA.

Treatment-Resistant Individuals As part of the original series of studies, CRA was adapted for use with the SOs of treatment-resistant alcoholics. The CRA intervention included education about alcohol problems, information and discussion of the positive consequences of not drinking, assistance in involving the alcoholic in healthy activities, increasing the involvement of the SO in social and recreational activities, and training in how to respond to drinking episodes and to recommend treatment entry. In the control group, none of the alcoholics entered treatment during the 3-month follow-up, and their drinking remained unchanged. In the CRA group, six of seven alcoholics entered treatment, and average drinking decreased from 25 days per month at pretreatment to fewer than 5 days per month after treatment.

Significant Others A series of controlled trials have consistently supported the efficacy of CRA in assisting concerned significant others (CSOs) to get unmotivated individuals with alcohol or illicit drug use disorders to enter treatment. The treatment has come to be referred to as community reinforcement and family training (CRAFT). In the most recent of the trials, CSOs of treatment-refusing illicit drug users were randomly assigned to CRAFT, CRAFT with additional after-care sessions, or Al-Anon and Nar-Anon facilitation therapy (Al-Nar-FT). Percentages of treatment-refusing loved ones who got engaged in treatment after the intervention were 58.6%, 76.7%, and 29.0% in CRAFT alone, CRAFT plus aftecare, and Al-Nar-FT, respectively.

CHAPTER 58

Summary Author: John Young
Christopher W. Kahler • Adam M. Leventhal • Richard A. Brown

Behavioral Interventions in Smoking Cessation

Smoking is the leading cause of preventable death in the United States. Costs of medical care, lost productivity, and forfeited earnings from smoking-related disability are estimated at >$100 billion per year.

Smokers are generally well aware of the possible benefits of quitting; however, multiple attempts are often needed before individuals are successful in quitting. Clinicians play a crucial role in assessing tobacco use, encouraging all patients to quit smoking, and providing ongoing assistance for patients attempting to quit and for those who have relapsed back to smoking.

RELEVANCE FOR ADDICTIONS TREATMENT

Knowledge of assessment, intervention, and treatment of cigarette smoking is especially important for clinicians working with patients who drink alcohol excessively or are dependent on alcohol or other drugs. Approximately 23% of those with nicotine dependence meet criteria for a current alcohol use disorder and 8% meet criteria for a current drug use disorder. Conversely, in the general US adult population, approximately half of alcohol-dependent people use tobacco daily. Rates of smoking are especially high among those in substance abuse treatment.

There are compelling reasons to address tobacco use in individuals seeking treatment for other addictions, the most notable being that patients who have been treated for alcoholism or other nonnicotine drug dependence are more likely to die from tobacco-related than from other substance-related causes. Nonetheless, there has traditionally been limited support from addictions treatment staff for smoking cessation programs, reflecting beliefs that smoking is less harmful than the patients' alcohol or drug use, doubts that alcohol- and drug-dependent patients can mount a serious effort to quit smoking, or concerns that smoking cessation during chemical dependency treatment will jeopardize abstinence from alcohol or drugs. However, studies have found that inclusion of smoking cessation treatment in other addictions programs does not reduce long-term treatment completion. Furthermore, most studies have found that smoking cessation interventions initiated during treatment do not harm treatment outcome and may even be associated with better drinking and other substance use outcomes.

Another barrier to integrating tobacco dependence treatment into addictions treatment programs is that a high proportion of staff members in these programs smoke.

About 50% to 80% of all patients involved in substance abuse treatment indicate an interest or desire to quit smoking. Recent studies have concluded that nicotine replacement therapy results in improved smoking abstinence rates; the use of pharmacotherapy may be especially important given that alcohol- and drug-dependent individuals tend to smoke more per day and to be more nicotine dependent than those without alcohol and drug problems.

Whether to initiate smoking cessation treatment early in the course of substance abuse treatment or to wait until sobriety has been attained for a few months remains a question. Greater lengths of sobriety from alcohol are positively associated with improved smoking cessation outcomes, suggesting that individuals with more prolonged recovery are more capable of quitting smoking successfully. Furthermore, the majority of addiction treatment patients state a preference for treating their alcohol problems before initiating treatment for smoking.

On the other hand, initiating smoking cessation interventions during addictions treatment increases rates of participation in smoking cessation treatment.

We recommend that all smokers in addictions treatment be provided at least a brief smoking cessation intervention, including offering pharmacologic aid to cessation, with encouragement to quit smoking as soon as possible. Especially after smokers in addictions treatment have attained sobriety from alcohol and drugs, it is essential that clinicians clearly advise these patients to quit smoking as soon as possible and provide assistance.

TREATMENT PLANNING

For those who are not ready to quit, methods for moving smokers toward initiating a quit attempt and for continuing to assess readiness to quit are indicated. In Figure 58.1, we provide a general schematic for treatment planning with patients who smoke. The figure provides different steps for those who are willing and those who are not willing to quit smoking in the near future. It also highlights the need for continued assessment of smoking status at each stage of intervention.

- A simple set of procedures for working with patients who smoke is to follow what has been termed the five As of intervention:
- *Ask* patients whether they use tobacco: All patients should be asked whether or not they have ever smoked, when they last smoked a cigarette, and the typical number of cigarettes they currently smoke per day. The enactment of procedures and systems that routinely identify and document smoking status in health care settings is critical, resulting in about three times higher rates of smoking cessation interventions being delivered by clinicians and almost two times higher quit rates among patients who smoke.
- *Advise* all patients to quit: Smokers report that physician advice to quit smoking is often an important factor in their deciding to make a quit attempt, and trials have found that brief advice (<3 minutes) by a clinician to quit smoking increases the odds of abstinence by about 30%. Advice is most effective if it is clear ("It is very important for you to quit smoking."), strong ("Quitting smoking is one of the most important things you can do to improve and protect your health."), and personalized ("Smoking increases the risk of heart attacks, which is especially important for you given your family history of heart disease and your high blood pressure.").
- *Assess* willingness to make a quit attempt: Patients present with differing levels of motivation for quitting smoking, and intervention should be based on patients' readiness to change. Motivation is a state that fluctuates over time; it is, therefore, crucial to continue to assess and monitor readiness to quit smoking with all patients who continue to smoke, so that appropriate assistance can be provided when a smoker expresses a willingness to make a quit attempt. About 20% of smokers who seek medical care are intending to quit smoking in the next month. Many of these patients have made a quit attempt in the past year or have taken steps toward quitting, such as cutting down on the number of cigarettes they smoke. These smokers should be encouraged to set a specific quit day and be offered additional assistance as described in the following sections.
- *Assist* patients in making a quit attempt, as described in the following sections.
- *Arrange* follow-up contacts to help prevent relapse.

TREATMENT AND TECHNIQUE

Preparing for Quitting

We recommend a "preparation" period before quitting smoking, the length of which can vary according to program needs. There are three key objectives for this period:

- Patients' motivation to quit and commitment to the program should be clarified and reinforced.
- Patients should self-monitor their daily smoking behavior to begin to learn about their smoking triggers.
- A target quit day should be clearly established to allow patients the time to "mentally prepare" and develop coping strategies for quitting smoking.

Motivating Smokers to Quit

Smokers may be ambivalent about the prospect of quitting. Although acknowledging rational reasons for quitting, they may dread the potential discomfort of quitting, feel that they are attached to smoking and that they are giving up a friend, lack confidence in their ability to quit, feel hopelessly addicted, and continue to question whether the health risks could ever really impact them. This may be especially true of smokers who may have tried in the past to quit and failed. Acknowledging this ambivalence without directly challenging smokers

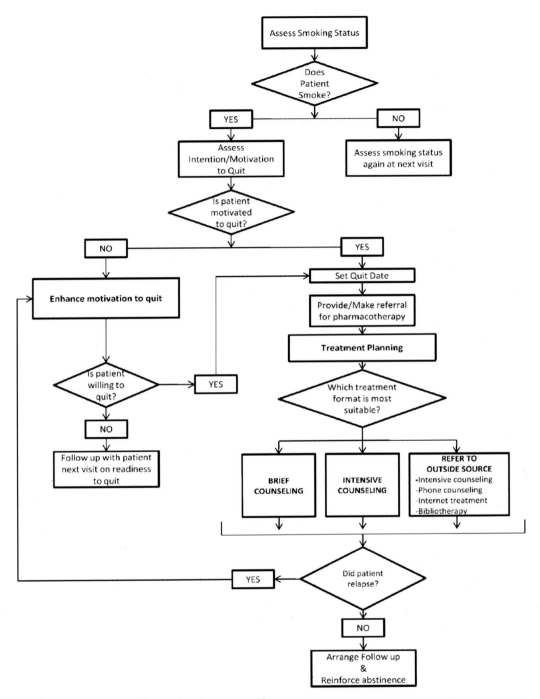

FIGURE 58.1 Schematic for treating cigarette smoking.

can help diffuse some of its power to undermine commitment. For example, clinicians can use double-sided reflective statements to highlight both sides of ambivalence (e.g., "On the one hand you find that smoking helps you relax and serves as a reward for a hard day's work, but on the other hand you know that it is costing you a lot of money, has made it harder for you to be physically active, and is greatly raising your risk of having a heart attack.").

A useful and effective method for exploring readiness to change is to have patients rate on a numeric scale (e.g., from 0 to 10) the importance they place on quitting smoking and the confidence they have in successfully quitting. After a patient has provided these ratings, a clinician can inquire further about factors influencing each rating. For example, a clinician might ask, "What made you give a rating of 4 to the importance of quitting rather than a 0?" In this way, the patient is prompted to generate reasons to quit smoking on his or her own. Similarly, exploration of confidence ratings can reveal roadblocks that may prevent more motivated patients from taking action and help identify potential strategies for overcoming these roadblocks. For example, a clinician might ask, "What would help you to increase your confidence from a 6 to a 7 or an 8?"

The challenge is to move smokers from general acceptance of potential negative consequences ("Smoking is dangerous to health.") to personalized acceptance ("Smoking is dangerous to *my* health."). For patients who have low importance ratings, personalized information and feedback can raise awareness of the ways in which smoking is affecting their health. Feedback can take several forms, including evidence of the effects of smoking on the patient's current physical symptoms (smoker's cough) and laboratory findings, impact of smoking on disease states, and relationship between smoking and risk. When appropriate, exploring the consequences of illness or premature death of a loved one or what they will miss if they themselves die prematurely also can be a powerful motivator. Feedback about the deleterious effects of continued smoking should be paired with feedback about smoking cessation's beneficial effects. After each piece of information, clinicians should elicit patients' reactions and questions and then empathize with and validate their concerns before providing new information. It can also be helpful to have patients write down their specific, self-relevant reasons for wanting to stop smoking and also for wanting to continue smoking: the latter can help patients identify likely barriers to quitting.

For patients who place higher levels of importance on quitting but are not taking action because of a lack of confidence, clinicians can emphasize that it may take several quit attempts before they are finally successful. It is also useful to explore reasons for continued smoking and barriers to quitting so that potential solutions for overcoming barriers can be discussed. Given that the majority of smokers are not willing to quit immediately, it is important that clinicians have modest expectations of whether their patients will make a quit attempt; smokers who are chronically stuck may benefit from encouragement to take small steps toward action, such as cutting down the number of cigarettes they smoke, delaying their first cigarette of the day, or trying to quit for just 24 hours. A commitment to change is unlikely to occur in one brief session; instead, the goal of intervention with a patient who is not committed is to move him or her closer to change. Follow-up visits can allow for continued monitoring of readiness and for repeated interventions to enhance motivation and facilitate quitting.

Motivation for quitting smoking needs to be monitored throughout treatment for potential setbacks.

Self-Monitoring of Smoking Behavior

Keeping a written record of cigarettes smoked can help increase knowledge about the factors cueing and maintaining smoking behavior. Self-monitoring also interrupts the automatic smoking habit, encouraging patients to think about every cigarette they smoke and why they smoke it. Often this procedure reduces the number of cigarettes smoked per day. Preprinted forms can be given to patients to record the time of day and the situation in which each cigarette is smoked (e.g., "talking on the phone"). Assessment of mood at the time of each cigarette also can be useful. The situational notations allow patients to identify antecedents that trigger their smoking.

Patients typically find self-monitoring of their smoking behavior inconvenient. It is important that clinicians present the rationale for self-monitoring clearly and follow through at all sessions by reviewing the self-monitoring information with patients to highlight its relevance in their quitting efforts. For example, it is useful to ask each patient what he or she learned about his or her smoking behavior and its patterns over the course of a typical week, specifically, what moods were common triggers of smoking, during which times of the day did the patient smoke most often, and which people or events typically triggered the smoking.

Choosing a Quit Date

Central to the quit plan is setting a quit date, ideally within 2 weeks. Setting this date allows smokers to plan for quitting and to obtain the necessary support, which may include

- Telling their family and friends about their quit date, perhaps asking those who smoke to refrain from doing so in the house or in front of them
- Making sure that all tobacco products and associated cues, such as ashtrays and cigarette lighters, have been removed
- For those who drink alcohol, avoiding drinking alcohol as much as possible while quitting (alcohol use is involved in about one fourth of all lapses to smoking)

- Thinking about potential triggers for smoking and considering situations in which relapse might be likely to occur. After situations have been identified, the clinician can discuss with the patient's potential strategies for handling those high-risk situations
- Reading self-help materials, available through numerous agencies
- Accessing state-funded quitlines, which offer from three to six sessions of proactive counseling (i.e., the quitline counselor calls the patient to deliver counseling according to the quitline's protocol)
- Pharmacotherapies, including nicotine replacement therapies (gum, inhaler, nasal spray, lozenge, or patch), varenicline (Chantix), and bupropion SR (Zyban)

Patients should be advised to smoke their last cigarette on the night before their quit date so that they wake up a nonsmoker.

Follow-Up

Providers should schedule a specific time to connect immediately after quit day to reinforce successes and troubleshoot difficulties in cessation efforts. Follow-up contacts also provide an opportunity to work with patients who have lapsed to smoking. Clinicians can help patients view a lapse as a learning experience that is part of the normal process of quitting and encourage patients to continue their efforts to quit.

CESSATION STAGE INTERVENTIONS

Self-Management

Self-management (sometimes termed *self-control* or *stimulus control*) procedures are a critical component of behavioral smoking interventions. They refer to strategies intended to rearrange environmental cues that "trigger" smoking or to alter the consequences of smoking. Using their written smoking records, patients develop a list of trigger situations. They then begin to intervene in these situations to break up the smoking behavior chain (situation—urge—smoke) by using one of three general strategies:

- *Avoid* the trigger situation: foregoing a coffee break at work with other smokers, leaving the table after dinner, and avoiding social situations involving alcohol
- *Alter* or change the trigger situation: drinking tea or juice in the morning instead of coffee, watching television in a nonsmoking room, and putting cigarettes in the trunk of the car before driving
- Use an *alternative* or substitute in place of the cigarette, often in conjunction with avoiding or altering trigger situations or in situations that cannot be avoided or altered: chewing gum, sugarless candy or cut up vegetables, toothpicks, relaxation techniques in stressful situations, or activities such as needlework that keep hands busy

Patients should choose strategies they think will work for them and then try out different approaches, rejecting those that are not useful until they have successfully managed all or most trigger situations without smoking.

Social Support Positive social support can be a source of motivation for quitting, has been shown to increase cessation rates, and can provide positive reinforcement for maintaining abstinence as well as a buffer against stressful life events that might precipitate a relapse. Social support outside of treatment might include making specific requests to friends and family members about steps they can take to support patients' abstinence efforts.

Maintenance Because the majority of smokers who initially quit resume smoking within several months of treatment termination, maintenance is a critical issue for smoking cessation programs. The most commonly used behavioral maintenance strategies are based on the relapse prevention model. Preliminary evidence suggests that extending behavioral treatment and pharmacotherapy may improve cessation outcomes.

Identifying and Coping with High-Risk Situations for Relapse Relapse prevention theory proposes that the ability to cope with "high-risk" situations for relapse determines an individual's probability of maintaining abstinence. High-risk situations often involve at least one of the following elements: negative moods, positive moods, social situations involving alcohol, and being in the presence of smokers. To help patients identify high-risk situations, a clinician can ask, "If you were to slip and smoke a cigarette after quit day, in what situation would it be?" For each high-risk situation, patients can develop a set of strategies for managing the situation without smoking. They should be reminded that these high-risk situations are similar to the trigger situations they have previously addressed and that they can apply similar self-management strategies (i.e., avoid, alter, or use an alternative), as well as other problem-solving skills.

Managing Slips When patients experience a slip to smoking, they often progress to further smoking and relapse. In the event that a slip happens, a few steps can be taken to regain abstinence. First, a slip is an important time for clinicians to assess motivation or commitment to quitting. Has motivation changed or is the patient ambivalent about quitting? Does the patient support the goal of quitting completely or does he or she believe that occasional cigarettes are unlikely to be harmful? If motivation is flagging, then use of the motivational interventions described above is appropriate. If motivation remains high, then it is important for the clinician and the patient to review the circumstances of the lapse to figure out what conditions allowed that lapse to occur. The lessons learned from the lapse are reviewed, and plans for avoiding similar lapses in the future can then be made.

Lifestyle Change A negative addiction such as smoking can be replaced with a "positive addiction" by increasing participation in activities that are incompatible with smoking and are a source of pleasure. Patients are encouraged to set aside time as often as possible (ideally, on a daily basis) for this purpose. It is in this context that we strongly encourage patients to engage in some type of regular physical exercise. Exercise may also be a good alternative to dieting for individuals who are concerned about postcessation weight gain.

SPECIAL POPULATIONS

Heavy Drinkers

Alcohol consumption is the third leading cause of death in the United States, and excessive drinking results in numerous well-documented health, mental health, and social problems. The combined effects of excessive drinking and smoking are enormous.

A recent clinical trial found that incorporating a brief alcohol intervention into smoking cessation treatment for heavy drinkers who were not alcohol dependent led to significantly lower levels of drinking and increased the odds of smoking abstinence. Steps for brief alcohol intervention include assessing alcohol use and problems, providing clear advice to reduce drinking to those who are drinking at medically unsafe levels, assessing readiness to change drinking, and helping patients set drinking goals and make plans for achieving those goals.

Psychiatric Patients

More than 50% of psychiatric patients smoke, compared with 25% of individuals without psychiatric problems. Psychotic disorders, mood disorders, anxiety disorders, and attention deficit hyperactivity disorder are among the most common psychiatric problems among smokers. Certain clinical characteristics of psychiatric patients and contextual factors present only in psychiatric settings should be taken into account when applying behavioral treatments for smoking.

Psychiatric patients with tobacco dependence are more likely to have sociodemographic risk factors that could lead to poorer smoking outcomes, including being divorced or separated, disabled, uninsured, and having fewer years of education. Psychiatric patients who are smokers also have more comorbid psychiatric disorders, lower global functioning, and poorer compliance relative to psychiatric comparisons. Thus, smokers in the psychiatric setting may be encountering the most severe and complex psychosocial problems of any population. Despite this, severity and chronicity do not predict whether or not depressed psychiatric patients are willing to accept a combined behavioral-pharmacologic nicotine-dependent treatment program, nor does severity predict current motivation to quit smoking.

Another clinical characteristic that may differ in smokers with versus smokers without psychiatric problems is nicotine withdrawal severity. Evidence suggests that smokers with anxiety, depression, and eating disorder symptoms are more likely to experience greater nicotine withdrawal symptoms when discontinuing tobacco use, which in turn suggests that psychiatric patients may potentially benefit from assessment and treatment to buffer the effects of nicotine withdrawal. Psychiatric patients also are more likely to experience cognitive problems because disorders such as major depression and psychosis often present with disturbance in memory, concentration, and thinking. Nonetheless, studies have demonstrated that skill-building and motivational enhancement techniques can be applied to psychiatric patients, including those with active psychotic disorders, though modifications should be made to meet the needs of this population.

CHAPTER 59

Summary Author: John Young
Marc Galanter

Network Therapy

HISTORICAL PERSPECTIVE

Support for addiction treatment itself has expanded over time, and recognition of the severity of the problem initially led to an increase in resources for inpatient care. The "Minnesota model" for inpatient management, based on a protracted inpatient stay, became a standard of treatment for many middle-class addicts. The imposition of managed care, however, led to a transition to ambulatory care. The decline in inpatient treatment was also fueled by a lack of support in randomized controlled trials for its relative advantage over ambulatory care.

In early studies, no difference in outcome was found when outpatients were offered individual therapy as a treatment added to medical monitoring alone, nor was insight-oriented therapy found to enhance the effectiveness of outpatient milieu treatment for alcoholism. As conventionally practiced, individual therapy did not appear to be an effective tool for addiction rehabilitation.

New perspectives on ambulatory care soon arose. Evidence mounted for both research-based and clinically based support for the importance of securing abstinence for substance-dependent persons as an initial step in addiction treatment, rather than awaiting results of an exploratory therapy. To implement a regimen of abstinence, clinical researchers have developed a number of structured techniques, focusing on cognitive-behavioral change and interpersonal support from family and peers. These approaches can be adapted to an office practice oriented toward individual therapy so as to promote abstinence and effective rehabilitation.

The integrated approach discussed here is called *network therapy* because it draws on the support of a group of family and peers who are introduced into individual therapy sessions.

THE TREATMENT MODEL

Social Support

Social environmental factors are the most robust predictors of long-term positive outcome. Social networks for individuals in treatment can be differentiated into two basic components: the peer-led self-help network, which is inherent in the philosophy of the therapeutic community model, and the natural social network consisting of family and close friends. It has been demonstrated that family involvement in substance abuse treatment is effective in improving outcome, and there are numerous approaches that make use of social network involvement in treatment, including behavioral couples therapy, marital therapy, and the community reinforcement approach. Other approaches involve utilizing the social network to encourage the addict to seek treatment, such as Community Reinforcement and Family Training (CRAFT) and the Johnson Intervention. The philosophy of supportive collaterals and the philosophy of social networks have several underlying similarities, in particular those of affiliation. Both approaches seek to discourage the affiliation of the client with negative social supports or those sources that encourage drug use and encourage the clients' affiliation with positive drug-free networks.

Cognitive-Behavioral Orientation in Treatment

Network therapy makes use of a variety of empirically tested cognitive-behavioral relapse prevention techniques that are delivered with participation by members of the patient's natural support system (i.e., family and friends). Along with the patient, these supportive others are taught to apply a behavioral model of the nature of addiction to understanding the patient's addiction; to participate in the development of relapse prevention strategies; to assist the therapist in securing patient adherence with medication regimens; and to assist the therapist in securing patient adherence with other parts of the treatment plan, such as in the execution of relapse prevention strategies. In these respects, network therapy shares some of the components of both the community reinforcement approach and behavioral marital therapy (e.g., behavioral skills training, medication monitoring by a significant other).

TREATMENT AND TECHNIQUE

Selection of Patients

Network therapy is appropriate for individuals who cannot reliably control their intake of alcohol or drugs once they have taken their first dose, those who have tried to stop and relapsed, and those who have not been willing or able to stop. Individuals whose problems are too severe for the network approach in ambulatory care include those who cannot stop their drug use even for a day or who cannot comply with outpatient detoxification.

The Network's Membership

Networks generally consist of three or four members. Once the patient has come for an appointment, establishment of a network is undertaken with active collaboration between the patient and the therapist. The two, aided by those parties who join the network initially, must search for the right balance of members. The therapist, however, must carefully promote the choice of appropriate network members. The network will be crucial in determining the balance of the therapy.

The Network's Task

The therapist's relationship to the network is one of a task-oriented team leader rather than of a family therapist oriented toward restructuring relationships. The network is established to implement a straightforward task, that of aiding the therapist to sustain the patient's abstinence. Competing and alternative goals must be implicitly suppressed or at least prevented from interfering with the primary task, but the atmosphere must be kept supportive.

Unlike family members involved in traditional family therapy, network members are not led to expect symptom relief or self-realization for themselves. This approach prevents development of competing goals for the network's meetings. It also protects members from having their own motives scrutinized and thereby supports their continuing involvement without the threat of an assault on their psychologic defenses. Because network members have kindly volunteered to participate, their motives must not be impugned. Their constructive behavior should be commended. Network members should be acknowledged for the contribution they are making to the therapy.

Couples

A cohabiting couple provides the first example of how natural affiliative ties can be used to develop a secure basis for rehabilitation. Couples therapy for addiction has been described in both ambulatory and inpatient settings, and good marital adjustment has been found to be associated with a diminished likelihood of dropping out and a positive overall outcome. It is recognized, however, that a spouse must be involved in an appropriate way. Constructive engagement should be distinguished from a codependent relationship or overly involved interaction, which is thought to be a problem in recovery. Indeed, couples managed with a behavioral orientation showed greater improvement in alcoholism than those treated with interactional therapy, where attempts were made to engage them in relational change. Thus, we will consider here a simple, behaviorally oriented device for making use of the marital relationship: working with a couple to enhance the effectiveness of disulfiram therapy.

The use of disulfiram has yielded relatively little benefit overall in controlled trials when patients are responsible for taking their doses on their own. This is largely because this agent is effective only when it is ingested as instructed, typically on a daily basis. Alcoholics who forget to take required doses likely will resume drinking in time. Indeed, such forgetting often reflects the initiation of a sequence of conditioned drug-seeking behaviors.

The involvement of a spouse, however, in observing the patient's consumption of disulfiram has been shown to yield a considerable improvement in outcome. Patients alerted to taking disulfiram each morning by this external reminder are less likely to experience conditioned drug seeking when exposed to addictive cues and are more likely to comply on subsequent days with the dosing regimen. The potential efficacy of this approach is illustrated by the reaction of a patient who experiences a precipitous collapse of psychologic defenses and potentially relapses. If he or she has been taking disulfiram as described here, knowledge of a potential disulfiram reaction can alert him or her to avoid going out to get a drink. Patients who are maintained with disulfiram, as described, for an initial year of recovery thus have the opportunity to deal in therapy with the issues that precipitate craving, without exposing themselves unduly to the threat of relapse.

The technique also helps in clearly defining the roles in therapy of both the alcohol-addicted person and spouse, typically the wife, by avoiding the spouse's need to monitor drinking behaviors she cannot control. The spouse does not actively remind the alcohol addicted to take each disulfiram dose. She merely notifies the therapist if she does not observe the pill being ingested on a given day. Decisions about managing compliance are then shifted to the therapist, and the couple does not become entangled in a dispute over the patient's attitude and the possibility of secret drinking. By means of this technique, a majority of alcohol-addicted patients in one clinical trial experienced marked improvement and sustained abstinence over the period of treatment.

A variety of other behavioral devices shown to improve outcome can be incorporated into this couples format. For example, it has been found that scheduling the first appointment as soon as possible after the initial telephone contact improves outcome by diminishing the possibility of an early loss of motivation. Spouses also can be engaged in history taking at the outset of treatment to minimize the introduction of denial into the patient's representation of the illness.

It is important to clarify certain aspects of engaging a collateral in the treatment, particularly a spouse. Long-standing conflicts between members of an alcohol-misusing couple should not be allowed to interfere with the disulfiram monitoring. For example, the spouse should not be placed in a role in which he or she must demand compliance; his or her role is only to notify the therapist in a telephone message if one does not see the other taking the pill on a given morning. Discussions of compliance per se, therefore, are initiated by the therapist and not by the spouse.

Typical Networks

Members of a network can help to counter the patient's inclination to deny a substance use problem in the initial stages of engagement and during relapse as well; they can also provide the therapist with the means of communicating with a relapsing patient and of assisting in reestablishment of abstinence. An effective intervention need involves no more than the network members' providing advice in the therapy session. The weight of the patient's relationship with his own chosen network members and his ability to respond to their efforts to help him are potent tools in securing compliance.

In the network format, a cognitive framework can be provided for each session by starting out with the patient's recounting events related to cue exposure or substance use since the last meeting. Network members then are expected to comment on this report to ensure that all are engaged in a mutual task with correct, shared information. Their reactions to the patient's report are addressed as well; however, it is important to maintain an appropriate therapeutic milieu in the network sessions. In volunteering to participate, members agree to help the patient but not to subject their own motives to scrutiny. In this, the network format, therefore, differs materially from the systemic family therapy approach, as it avoids subjecting network members to the demands of addressing their own motives. The didactic or intellectualized approach can be helpful in neutralizing excessive anger that may be felt toward the patient, without scrutinizing the reasons for a member's anger.

In addition, the patient himself is expected to help maintain amicable relations with network members to protect the supportive milieu. This is made explicit in both network and individual sessions. For example, if a network member is absent for a few sessions, the patient is expected to discuss the matter with that member and to resolve any outstanding issues in order to promote the member's return. Any difficulty the patient may experience in carrying out this role is viewed as an issue to be addressed in individual sessions. The network, therefore, is conceived of as an active collaboration in which conflicts are minimized to ensure optimal function. When led effectively, members are inclined to be effective team members: they develop a positive transference toward the therapist and are willing to support the therapist's views.

Principles of Network Treatment

The following is a set of guidelines for applying network therapy. It can be adapted to the needs of a given patient and to the relative availability of potential network members.

Begin a Network as Soon as Possible

1. It is important to see the patient promptly, as the window of opportunity for openness to treatment generally is brief.
2. If the patient is married, engage the spouse early on, preferably at the time of the first telephone call. Point out that addiction is a family problem. The spouse generally can be enlisted in ensuring that the patient arrives at the office with a day's sobriety.

3. In the initial interview, frame the exchange so that a good case is built for the grave consequences of the patient's addiction, and do this before the patient can introduce his or her system of denial. This approach avoids putting the spouse or other network members in the awkward position of having to contradict a close relative.
4. Make clear that the patient needs to be abstinent, beginning immediately. (A tapered detoxification may be necessary with some drugs, such as the sedative hypnotics.)
5. An alcoholic patient can be started on disulfiram treatment as soon as possible, in the office at the time of the first visit, if possible. Instruct the patient to continue taking disulfiram under the observation of a network member. Get baseline chemistries concomitantly.
6. Start to build a network for the patient at the first visit, involving the patient's family members and close friends.
7. From the very first meeting, consider how to ensure the patient's sobriety until the next meeting and plan that with the network. Initially, their immediate companionship, a plan for daily AA attendance, and planned activities all may be necessary.

Keep the Network's Agenda Focused

1. *Maintain abstinence*: The patient and the network members should report at the outset of each session any exposure of the patient to alcohol or drugs. The patient and network members should be instructed as to the nature of relapse and should work with the clinician to develop a plan to sustain abstinence. Cues to conditioned drug seeking should be examined.
2. *Support the network's integrity*: Everyone has a role in this: The patient is expected to ensure that network members keep their meeting appointments and stay involved with the treatment. The therapist sets meeting times and summons the network for any emergency, such as relapse. The therapist does whatever is necessary to secure stability of the membership if the patient is having trouble doing so. Members of the network are responsible for attending network sessions and engaging in other supportive activities with the patient.
3. *Secure future behavior*: The therapist should combine any and all modalities necessary to ensure the patient's stability. This may involve establishing a stable, drug-free residence; avoiding substance-abusing friends; attending Twelve-Step meetings; using medications such as disulfiram or blocking agents; observing urinalysis; and obtaining ancillary psychiatric care. Written agreements may be useful. This may involve a mutually acceptable contingency contract, with penalties for violation of understandings.

End Network Therapy Appropriately

1. Network sessions can be terminated after the patient has been stably abstinent for at least 6 months to 1 year. Before network therapy is stopped, the therapist should discuss with the patient and network the patient's readiness to handle sobriety.
2. An understanding is established with the network members that they will contact the therapist at any point in the future if the patient becomes vulnerable to relapse. The network members can also be summoned by the therapist. These points should be made clear to the patient before termination, in the presence of the network, but they also apply throughout treatment.

CHAPTER 60

Summary Author: John Young
Donald J. Kurth

Therapeutic Communities

The modern addiction therapeutic community (TC) is a powerful therapeutic tool that, over the past several decades, has helped addicts and alcoholics achieve abstinence-based recovery, with abstinence rates of >90% for many years after treatment documented in well-established TCs. It is less clear how and why this therapeutic modality is so effective in changing difficult behaviors for which so many other methods are not successful.

Historically, the TC has been used to treat a variety of problems in living, but the modern addiction TC or "concept TC" is a hybrid of self-help and public support geared toward the treatment of addictive and co-occurring psychiatric disorders.

The philosophic foundation of the modern TC is personal responsibility for one's behavior and the belief that change is fully possible if the individual exerts the personal effort to follow the teachings of the program.

Evolving out of Alcoholics Anonymous (AA) in the 1960s, the modern addiction TC still retains many of the underpinnings of the Twelve-Step approach to treatment. Drug addiction is viewed as a "whole person" disorder and, therefore, is treated with a holistic approach. Emotions and feelings are considered important and can be explored in-depth, but change is based on action, and that action is the responsibility of the individual. As in Twelve-Step recovery, the individual is not expected to walk this road alone: The community is available to help the addict at every step of the way.

In the TC philosophy, drug or alcohol use is considered a symptom of a complex disorder involving the whole person. Self-destructive and defeating patterns of behavior and thought processes are thought to disrupt both the individual's lifestyle and society's functioning. Though genetic, environmental, and pharmacologic contributions to addiction are recognized, the individual is held fully responsible for his or her own disorder, behavior, and recovery. Addiction is regarded as the symptom, rather than the disorder. The problem is the behavior of the person, not the drug.

FEATURES OF THE MODERN THERAPEUTIC COMMUNITY

The modern TC rests on a foundation of secular ideology with certain existential assumptions, including the following:

- Self-determination: A core value is self-determination. Each individual is seen as the captain of his or her own ship and the one who determines the path of his or her life.
- Individual responsibility: The TC philosophy holds each individual fully responsible for his or her own behavior. No matter the genetic predisposition or environmental or family influences, each person is seen as fully and completely responsible for his or her own behavior.
- Self-change: The concept of self-change is regarded as possible through personal commitment and adherence to recovery teachings.

Components of a Therapeutic Community Program
Several features characterize TC programs.

Community Separateness TC-oriented programs have their own identities and are housed in a space or locale that is separated from other agency or institutional programs or units or generally from the drug-related environment. In residential settings, clients remain away from outside influences 24 hours a day for several months before earning the privilege of a brief visit to the outside community. In nonresidential "day treatment" settings, the individual spends 4 to 8 hours a day in the TC environment and is monitored by peers and family while outside the TC. Even in the least restrictive outpatient settings, TC-oriented programs and components are in place. This is designed to help members gradually detach from old networks and relate to the drug-free peers in the program.

A Community Environment The TC environment prominently features communal spaces and collective activities. Walls carry signs declaring the philosophy of the program, the messages of right living and recovery. Cork boards and blackboards are used to identify all participants by name, seniority level, and job function in the program. Daily schedules are posted as well. These visuals display an organizational picture of the program that the individual can relate to and comprehend, thus promoting program affiliation.

Community Activities The TC philosophy holds that, to be effective, treatment and educational services must be provided within a context of the peer community. Thus, with the exception of individual counseling, all activities are programmed in collective formats. These activities include at least one daily meal prepared, served, and shared by all members; a daily schedule of groups, meetings, and seminars; jobs performed in teams; organized recreational/leisure time; and ceremonies and rituals to mark birthdays, graduations, and the like.

Staff Rules and Functions Staff members are a mix of self-help professionals who are themselves in recovery and other helping professionals (medical, legal, mental health, and educational), who are integrated through cross-training grounded in the TC perspective and community approach. Professional skills define the function of staff members (e.g., nurse, physician, lawyer, teacher, administrator, case worker, clinical counselor). Regardless of professional discipline or function, however, the generic role of all staff members is that of community members who, rather than treatment providers, are viewed as rational authorities, facilitators, and guides in the self-help community method.

Peers as Role Models Members who demonstrate the expected behaviors and reflect the values and teachings of the community are viewed as role models. Indeed, the strength of the community as a context for social learning relates to the number and quality of its role models. All members of the community are expected to be role models: roommates; older and younger residents; and junior, senior, and directorial staff. TCs require these multiple role models to maintain the integrity of the community and to ensure the spread of social learning effects.

A Structured Day Ordered activities conducted in a regular routine counter the characteristically disordered lives in which clients have lived and distract them from negative thinking and boredom, factors that are thought to predispose individuals to drug use. Structured activities also are regarded as facilitating the acquisition of self-structure (expressed in time management, planning, setting, and meeting goals) and general accountability. Thus, regardless of its length, the day has a formal schedule of therapeutic and educational activities with prescribed formats, fixed times, and routine procedures.

Work as Therapy and Education Consistent with the TC's self-help approach, all clients are responsible for the daily management of the facility (e.g., cleaning, meal preparation and service, maintenance, purchasing, security, scheduling, preparation for group meetings, seminars, activities). In the TC, the various work roles mediate essential educational and therapeutic effects. Job functions strengthen affiliation with the program through participation, provide opportunities for skill development, and foster self-examination and personal growth. The scope and depth of clients' work depends on the program and client resources (levels of psychologic function, social and life skills).

Phase Format The treatment protocol, or plan of therapeutic and educational activities, is organized into phases that reflect a developmental view of the change process. Emphasis is placed on incremental learning at each phase, so as to move the individual to the next stage of recovery.

Therapeutic Community Concepts Formal and informal curricula are focused on teaching the TC perspective, particularly its self-help recovery concepts and view of right living. The concepts, messages, and lessons are repeated in the various groups, meetings, seminars, and peer conversations, as well as in readings, signs, and personal writings.

Peer Encounter Groups The principal community or therapeutic group is the encounter, though other forms of therapeutic, educational, and support groups are employed as needed. The minimal objective of the peer encounter is similar to TC-oriented programs—to heighten the individual's awareness of specific attitudes or behavior patterns that need to be modified. However, the encounter process can differ in degree of staff direction and intensity, depending on the client subgroups (e.g., adolescents, prison inmates, and the dually diagnosed).

Awareness Training All therapeutic and educational interventions involve raising the individual's awareness of the effects of his or her conduct and attitudes on himself or herself and the social environment and, conversely, the effect of the behaviors and attitudes of others on the individual and his or her environment.

Emotional Growth Training Achieving the goals of personal growth and socialization involves teaching individuals how to identify feelings, express them appropriately, and manage them constructively through the interpersonal and social demands of communal life.

Planned Duration of Treatment

How long an individual must be involved in the program depends on his or her phase of recovery, though a minimum period of intensive involvement is required to assure internalization of the TC teachings. The duration of treatment of the traditional TC generally is 12 to 18 months.

Continuity of Care

Completion of primary treatment is a stage in the recovery process. It is followed by aftercare services, which are an essential component of the TC model. Whether implemented within the main program or separately (as in residential or nonresidential halfway houses or ambulatory settings), the perspective and approach guiding aftercare programming must be continuous with the primary treatment in the TC. Thus, the views of right living and self-help recovery and the use of a peer network are essential to enhance the appropriate use of vocational, educational, mental health, social, and other typical aftercare or reentry services.

REFERRAL CRITERIA

For the physician in office-based practice, a question often arises as to which type of treatment is most appropriate for a particular patient. This question may not be easy to answer but may well be the critical step that makes the difference between life and death for that particular human being.

Treatment in a TC is not appropriate for every person with a drug or alcohol problem; the commitment of time, money, and surrender to the program are significant. Although a detailed discussion is beyond the scope of this chapter, any one of four specific characteristics may qualify an addict and/or alcoholic for treatment in a TC (Table 60.1).

Many patients seem to do better with a little external motivation; requirements imposed through probation or parole orders can be helpful as well. Such requirements may sound harsh but are appropriate when balanced with the fact that the patient has a fatal illness and has failed at every other form of therapy. Admission to a TC may be the only defense between the addict and death in the street.

Outcome Studies

Studies have demonstrated that even those who did not achieve complete abstinence showed significant improvement in terms of frequency of drug use, illegal activity, full-time work, and psychiatric factors. It has also been shown that longer lengths of stay in residential treatment resulted in dramatically better outcomes over a variety of parameters.

Application to Specific Population Groups

Those dealing with specific subpopulations have not overlooked the powerful rate of successful outcome of the TC. In particular, prison, adolescent, and dually diagnosed persons all have good recovery rates in TC programs. Broader applications are now being evaluated.

TABLE 60.1	**Indicators of the Presenting Disorder Among Typical TC Clients**

A life in crisis

- Clients have a history of out-of-control behavior with respect to drug use, criminality, and often sexuality.
- Clients evidence suicidal potential through overdose.
- Clients are at risk of injury or death through other drug-related means.
- Clients exhibit a high degree of anxiety and fear concerning violence, jail, illness, or death.
- Clients have a history of profound personal losses (financial, relationships, employment).

Inability to maintain abstinence

- Clients are unable to maintain any significant period of drug abstinence or sobriety on their own; characterized by multiple substance use though often having a primary drug of choice.
- Clients have some previous treatment experiences, self-initiated attempts at abstinence, cycles of short-term medical detoxification, or social and interpersonal dysfunction.
- Clients have a diminished capacity to function responsibly in any social or interpersonal setting.

Social and interpersonal dysfunction

- Clients are involved in the drug lifestyle (friends, places, activities), have a poor record of maintaining employment or school responsibilities, and have minimal or dysfunctional social relations with parents, spouses, and friends outside the drug lifestyle.
- Clients need a TC that focuses on the broad socialization or habilitation of the individual building these basic skills and fostering the individual's progress through developmental stages that previously were missed.

Antisocial lifestyle

- Clients have criminal histories involving illegal activities, incarceration, and court proceedings: Some are involved with the criminal justice system as juveniles; a considerable number are legally referred to treatment.
- Clients have other characteristics that are highly correlated with drug use, including exploitation, abuse, and violence; attitudes of disaffiliation with mainstream society; and the rejection of absence of prosocial values.

CRITICISMS OF THE THERAPEUTIC COMMUNITY MODEL

Critics of TCs generally fall into one of two groups: those who believe that TCs cost too much and those who believe that the treatment is too harsh. The increased cost is one reason why this modality is reserved for those who have failed at lesser forms of treatment, usually on more than one occasion. Also, TC treatment costs just a fraction of incarceration—usually about one-third the price per resident per year. Even that cost is easily recouped by the lower rates of relapse or recidivism in TC programs.

The "rough edges" of TC life have been smoothed over the years in response to public opinion and payer oversight. Still, treatment in the modern addiction TC is the most difficult thing most residents will ever do. Generally, TC treatment is reserved for those who have had multiple treatment failures and who are at high risk of dying of the disease. The goal of the modern addiction TC is to rebuild human lives from the ground up. Some struggle and effort are required to achieve that change.

CHAPTER 61

Summary Author: John Young
P. Joseph Frawley • Matthew O. Howard

Aversion Therapies

AVERSION THERAPY AS PART OF A MULTIMODALITY TREATMENT PROGRAM

Addicts have been conditioned by their drug of choice. Studies have shown that alcoholics increase the number of swallows and amount of salivation in response to the sight of alcohol, as compared to nonalcoholics. Studies of smokers seeking to quit show that those who are least likely to quit have a much larger conditioned drop in pulse (presumably to compensate for the increase in pulse rate caused by smoking) when presented with a cigarette. Cocaine-dependent addicts experience progressively steeper drops in skin temperature and increased galvanic skin response (a sign of arousal) when viewing progressively more intense and explicit pictures of cocaine use. These responses can be shown to decay in strength as time away from the drug increases.

The presence of these phenomena suggests that one of the consequences of addiction is that the body becomes conditioned to drink or use drugs in the presence of certain stimuli. This may contribute to the sensation of physical craving experienced by addicts.

Aversion therapy, or counterconditioning, is a powerful tool in the treatment of alcohol and other drug addiction. Its goal is to reduce or eliminate the "hedonic memory" or craving for a drug and to simultaneously develop a distaste and avoidance response to the substance. Unlike punishments, which often are delayed in time from the use episode, aversion therapy relies on the immediate association of the sight, smell, taste, and act of using the substance with an unpleasant or "aversive" experience. Also, with punishment, it is the individual who receives the negative consequences, whereas in aversion therapy it is the behavior—the negative consequence is only paired with the act of using a drug. This has a very important benefit to self-esteem. While the patient is engaging in positive recovery activities, he or she is receiving immediate positive support for a new way of behaving and thinking. It is only when the patient is engaging in an old behavior—alcohol or drug use—that he or she experiences immediate and consistent discomfort. Hence, self-esteem is rebuilt by separating the drug from the self.

The development of an aversion can be very specific; for example, inadequate treatment can occur when aversion is developed only to one type of alcoholic beverage. Also, repetition is an essential part of training and conditioning; adequate trials are needed to develop an aversion and to maintain and reinforce it to prevent extinction.

Note that, contrary to popular belief, disulfiram (Antabuse) is not an aversion treatment. In aversion therapy for alcohol addiction, alcohol is not absorbed into the system. With disulfiram, alcohol must be absorbed and metabolism begun for it to produce its toxic effect. Aversion relies on safe but uncomfortable experiences that can be repeated, whereas disulfiram reactions can be life threatening, even in healthy persons. For this reason, patients today are not given alcohol at the same time that they are prescribed disulfiram; as a result, they have not actually experienced a disulfiram reaction. Thus, disulfiram does not change the way the addict feels about alcohol. He or she may fear the consequence of drinking, just as he or she fears being arrested for drinking and driving; nevertheless, he or she still retains the euphoric recall of past episodes of drinking alcohol and hence the craving for the alcohol itself. Aversion works to eliminate or reduce euphoric recall by recording new negative experiences with the drug.

USES OF AVERSION THERAPY

Aversion Therapy for Alcohol Addiction

Nausea Aversion Studies in rats suggest that humans and other organisms may be biologically predisposed to form long-lasting conditioned aversions to consumables such as alcohol and foodstuffs whose consumption is followed by nausea and vomiting.

The usual treatment session involves having the patient take nothing except clear liquids by mouth for 6 hours prior to treatment, in order to reduce the likelihood of aspiration. After receiving a full explanation of the treatment procedure, the patient is taken to the treatment room, which has shelves containing all types of alcoholic beverages along the walls, as well as cutouts of various liquor ads on the walls: the intent is to have the majority of the patient's visual stimuli associated with visual cues for drinking. The patient receives an oral dose of emetine and is given water and electrolytes to provide a volume of easily vomited material. Shortly before the expected onset of nausea, the nurse administering the treatment pours a drink of the patient's preferred alcoholic beverage. The patient is instructed to smell the beverage, take a small mouthful, swish it around in the mouth to get the full flavor of it, and then to spit it out into the basin. This ensures that the patient has well-defined visual, olfactory, and gustatory sensations associated with the preferred beverage prior to the onset of the nausea. The nausea and vomiting ensue shortly thereafter and the "sniff, swish, and spit" procedure described above is altered to "sniff, swish, and swallow," with the swallowed alcoholic beverage being returned shortly as emesis so that no significant amount of alcohol is retained to be absorbed. After a session, the patient is returned to the hospital room, where another drink of alcoholic beverage is given containing an oral dose of emetine and tartar emetic, which induces a slower-acting residual nausea lasting up to 3 hours. The average patient receives five treatment sessions, which are given every other day over a 10-day period. In the private sector, Smith and Frawley compared 249 inpatients receiving aversion therapy as part of a multimodality treatment program with 249 inpatients from a large (>9,000 patients) treatment registry of patients receiving multimodality treatment, but without aversion therapy. All were matched on 17 baseline characteristics. Of the patients receiving aversion therapy, 84.7% had total abstinence from alcohol at 6 months, compared with 72.2% in the control group ($p < 0.01$); at 1 year, 79% of those treated with aversion had maintained abstinence, versus 67% of those without such treatment ($p < 0.05$). The group showing the greatest benefit from aversion therapy was the daily drinkers (84% vs. 67%, $p < 0.001$).

Faradic Aversion The treatment paradigm consists of pairing an aversive level of electrostimulation with the sight, smell, and taste of alcoholic beverages. At the direction of the therapist (forced choice trial), the patient reaches for a bottle of alcoholic beverage, pours some of it in a glass, and tastes it without swallowing. Electrostimulus onset occurs randomly throughout the entire behavior continuum, from reaching for the bottle through tasting the alcoholic beverage. The number of electrostimuli with each trial varies. An additional 10 free choice trials are designed so that the patient is negatively reinforced, with removal of the aversive stimulus if he or she selects a nonalcoholic choice such as fruit juice. The patient is instructed not to swallow any alcohol at any time throughout the faradic session, and this behavior is closely monitored by the therapist.

Covert Sensitization Conditioned nausea responses can be trained in alcoholic patients through the use of imagination and verbal suggestion without the use of an emetic drug. In covert sensitization, patients are helped to imagine personally relevant drinking scenes that emphasize the motivational, sensory, and behavioral precursors and concomitants of alcohol ingestion. The drinking scenes then are paired repeatedly with verbally induced nausea. Most cooperative participants can learn to experience genuine and intense nausea reactions by focusing on the therapist's noxious verbal suggestions; these suggestions prompt recipients to remember and recreate prior feelings and thoughts that have been prominent in their former nausea experiences. Such verbally induced nausea is designated as demand nausea. Repeated presentations of the drinking scenes (i.e., conditioned stimulus [CS]) followed by episodes of verbally induced demand nausea (i.e., unconditioned stimulus [US]) can, over extended conditioning trials, produce conditioned aversions to alcohol in a majority of participants. The goal of treatment is for a patient's demand nausea to transition to conditioned nausea, an automatic consequence of the patient's focusing on a drinking scene without any attempted therapist or self-induction of nausea.

In one study of 52 patients, 33 were able to develop verbally induced nausea after imagined drinking scenes; of these, 23 were able to develop conditioned nausea to either the desire for alcohol or other alcohol-related physical stimuli. Those who developed conditioned nausea had an average of 13.74 months of total abstinence as compared to 4.52 months for those who failed to progress beyond the demand nausea stage.

Aversion Therapy in Smoking Cessation

A review of modern smoking cessation treatments concluded that programs that use rapid smoking aversion or satiation had superior outcomes. Rapid smoking involves smoking cigarettes with inhalations every 6 seconds; though nicotine is taken into the system during rapid smoking, the aversion developed to smoking is adequate to prevent relapse. Sessions last an average of 15 minutes, during which the subject smokes an average of five cigarettes. The treatment sessions are usually daily for 5 days with a tapering frequency of booster treatments after that. When compared to the physical effects of normally paced smoking, clients undergoing rapid smoking experience increased burning in the lungs, palpitations, facial flush, headache, and feeling faint or weak. The best results have been reported by programs in which aversion was combined with several other modalities, including relapse prevention, relaxation training, written exercises, contract management, booster sessions of aversion, and group support. A study of patients with cardiopulmonary disease who underwent satiation treatment found no myocardial ischemia or significant arrhythmia in this group; five patients with ischemic changes on the treadmill did not experience the changes during the satiation treatment.

Faradic aversion has also been used for smoking cessation: Each time a patient brings a cigarette toward his or her lips, a mild electrical stimulus is administered automatically by a 9 V battery. With faradic aversion, the smoke is not inhaled but merely puffed; inhaling may lead to early relapse because of maintenance of the nicotine dependence. One advantage of this form of treatment is that less medically sophisticated staff can supervise the administration of the treatment.

In both forms of treatment, patients personally administer the aversive agent to themselves, while the therapist serves as a coach.

Aversion Therapy for Marijuana Dependence

In clinical practice, aversion therapy for marijuana uses faradic aversion. The protocol for faradic aversion is similar to that of the treatment for alcohol, except that it uses a variety of bongs, drug paraphernalia, and visual imagery. An artificial marijuana substitute and marijuana aroma are used in treatment. A 1-year abstinence rate of 84% was reported after 5 days of treatment, combined with three weekly group sessions on self-management techniques.

Aversion Therapy for Cocaine-Amphetamine Dependence

In a study of the use of chemical aversion for the treatment of cocaine dependence, an artificial cocaine substitute called Articaine was developed from tetracaine, mannitol, and quinine. Patients snorted this substance and paired it with nausea induced by emetine. Of those so treated, 56% were continuously abstinent and 78% currently abstinent (i.e., for the prior 30 days) at 6 months after treatment; at 18 months, 38% were continuously abstinent and 75% currently abstinent. For those treated for both alcohol and cocaine, 70% were continuously and currently abstinent from cocaine at 6 months, and 50% were continuously abstinent and 80% currently abstinent at 18 months after treatment.

A well-designed experimental evaluation of aversion therapy treatments for cocaine dependence enlisted volunteer participants from the Augusta VA Medical Center Substance Abuse Treatment Program. The abstinence rate at 6 months posttreatment follow-up was reported as 57.9% for participants who had received emetic therapy, significantly exceeding the 26.5% 6-month abstinence finding for control group participants. Covert sensitization also produced a significant therapeutic benefit, but its effect did not extend beyond 3 months posttreatment. A result unique to participants who received emetic therapy was a total loss of cravings for cocaine by the end of treatment.

Aversion Therapy for Heroin Addiction

One study employed a unique approach to aversion therapy by pairing aversive stimuli with cognitive images of heroin use. Patients were asked to verbalize only after they had conjured up a strong mental image. In the second part of the treatment, addicts were asked to conjure up images of socially appropriate behavior, including employment, education, or nondrug entertainment. Latency to verbalization was measured: at baseline, addicts could rapidly conjure up positive thoughts about heroin use but had significant delays in conjuring up thoughts about rewarding nondrug activities. Subjects were in a halfway house for heroin addicts and received group therapy in conjunction with relaxation therapy, along with aversion treatment. A faradic stimulator was used; once addicts had conjured up drug images, faradic aversion was applied. At other times, addicts were given 15 seconds to conjure up images of nondrug, socially appropriate behavior to prevent aversion from being applied. With this training in an average of 15 sessions, latency for drug-related images increased, while that for socially appropriate images decreased. Thirty of fifty patients completed the treatment and, at 24 months, 80% of these were reported to be drug free.

Use of Reinforcement (Booster) Aversion Treatments

Researchers followed up at 1 year on 437 of 600 patients treated with chemical and faradic aversion for alcohol, marijuana, or cocaine. One-year complete abstinence rate for alcohol for those who did not return for any reinforcements was 29.4%; for one booster aversion treatment, the abstinence rate was 50.5%; the two booster aversions abstinence rate was 68.5%; and for more than two aversions, the abstinence rate was 80%.

Use of Support Programs and Twelve-Step Meetings after Receiving Aversion Therapy

Follow-up studies found that those who used some form of support groups after aversion treatment did better than those who did not use such support, with an additive effect of the use of reinforcement (booster) aversion treatments and support and/or Twelve-Step meetings after completion of a hospital aversion program. Though total abstinence was associated with use of support groups after treatment, for those with urges to drink, increased support use was negatively associated with abstinence. A similar pattern was found for patients going to Schick Shadel Hospital–sponsored support groups.

SAFETY OF AVERSION THERAPY

Faradic aversion has virtually no unsafe side effects and has been found to be safe for patients with pacemakers and pregnant women (because the current only travels between two electrodes on the arm). To be eligible for chemical aversion therapy, patients must be free of medical contraindications such as esophageal varices, serious coronary artery disease, or active GI pathology. There was no increased incidence of medical utilization or hospitalization in the 6 months after treatment in a group treated with aversion therapy, as compared to matched controls treated without aversion.

The contraindications to covert sensitization are similar to those for chemical aversion; however, with this therapy, emesis can be prevented in most cases. The drawback to covert aversion therapy is that the induction of nausea or other aversive state is not as predictable as with medication and requires more patient preparation.

AVERSION THERAPY AS PART OF ESTABLISHED CARE FOR ADDICTIVE DISEASE

Selecting the appropriate treatment for a particular patient involves the patient having full informed consent. The practitioner needs to counsel the patient about the risks of continuing the addiction and the risks, benefits, and expected outcomes of various methods of treatment. Studies of patients who voluntarily received aversion therapy do not show higher rates of leaving against medical advice than is found in patients in Minnesota Model programs. Patients seeking aversion therapy in clinical settings complete treatment at the same rate as patients seeking alternative established treatments.

Aversion therapy has been recognized by both governmental and private agencies as appropriate treatment for patients with addictive disease.

NEED FOR FURTHER RESEARCH

A study of emetic therapy for cocaine dependence, funded by the National Institute on Drug Abuse (NIDA), demonstrated that recipients did more than simply lose their cravings for cocaine; they also developed strong active revulsions for the placebo cocaine materials and for cocaine related cues as detailed in that report. However, the revulsions were not measurable by the 0 to 10 cravings scale that was used in the study. Future studies should incorporate bidirectional scales that measure maximum craving at one extreme and maximum revulsion at the other extreme with a neutral zero-craving midscale region.

Future research should better characterize the physiologic changes that coincide with the transition from cue-induced cravings to cue-induced revulsion within a course of emetic aversion treatments. The dynamically expanding field of brain imaging research is likely to provide the greatest near-term advancements in our basic understanding and possible clinical applications of cue-induced brain changes that occur during the emetic therapy–induced transition from cocaine cravings to revulsions. Recent studies have reported activations of specific brain regions during cue-induced cravings for cocaine. Reliable change in brain activation patterns may be revealed by comparisons of the initial episodes of cue-induced cravings that typify the beginning of treatment with those that accompany the late-treatment cue-induced revulsions of successfully conditioned participants. The landmark positron emission tomography (PET) scan findings of Volkow et al., obtained from cocaine-addicted human volunteers, have shown that dopamine in the dorsal striatum is involved in cocaine craving and addiction. The dorsal striatum is a region that has been implicated in habit learning and in action initiation; the dorsal striatum, therefore, is a high-interest area for studies of possible transitions from cravings to revulsions. Cue-induced craving to revulsion changes also are likely to be found in brain regions that include the amygdala, the right nucleus accumbens, the dorsal anterior cingulate cortex, the ventral anterior cingulate cortex, and the frontal cortex. An obvious clinical application of such information would be to assess the strength of the attained aversion at the end of treatment. Additionally, the findings could support propitious individually tailored timings of booster treatments.

Functional magnetic resonance imaging (fMRI) also may be well suited to studies of emetic therapy–induced changes of cue-induced cravings to revulsions. The fMRI technology, unlike PET scan technology, does not involve the injection of radioactive compounds; it, therefore, can be safely used during repeated measures of the same participants across different time periods.

A variety of researchers have reported that some patients do not seem to develop aversions, leading researchers to develop and study lines of selectively bred taste aversion–prone (TAP) and taste aversion–resistant (TAR) rats. Such studies give promise of leading to identifications of biologic indices to separate conditionable and nonconditionable potential emetic therapy recipients. Additionally, studies of the two lines may support the development of pharmacologic or nutritional interventions to increase the nausea-based conditionability of TAR substance abusers.

A new treatment for OxyContin dependence has been developed in the Schick Shadel Hospital. This treatment capitalizes on the use of naltrexone to negate the psychotropic effects of OxyContin. OxyContin-dependent recipients first are detoxified; they then are started on a daily naltrexone regimen that begins in the morning of the first treatment day. The recipients then use OxyContin in their customary manner during emetic therapy sessions. The treatment has been well received and is being requested by an increasing number of patients.

Summary Author: John Young
Michael R. Liepman • Theodore V. Parran, Jr. • Kathleen J. Farkas • Maritza Lagos-Saez

Family Involvement in Addiction, Treatment, and Recovery

It is vital to address family issues with the patient who has an alcohol or drug use disorder, or a process addiction (e.g., gambling, sex addiction, Internet addiction, overeating) for the following reasons:

- Addiction disorders are very prevalent, produce a significant amount of morbidity and mortality in family members, and often are overlooked by physicians and other treatment providers.
- Patient denial or deception might make it difficult for the clinician to initially discover an addiction disorder and to later stay current on the relapse/recovery status of the patient.
- Addiction can be seen as a prototype for chronic illnesses that affect families.
- Addiction disorders overwhelmingly are familial in origin.
- Family members can have a significant impact on the processes of enabling the addiction to progress and also on recognition and recovery.
- Family education and therapy as part of addiction treatment have been shown to have substantial therapeutic value for the addicted patient as well as the other family members.

FAMILY CONSEQUENCES OF ADDICTION

Transmission of Addictions Across Generations and Within Families

Addictions are among the most familial of disorders, with strong genetic determinants and significant environmental contributions.

Pregnant women who abuse substances are at particular risk of poor pregnancy outcome. Alcohol has been implicated in serious teratologic effects known as fetal alcohol effects and fetal alcohol syndrome, which can produce a child with serious health and mental handicaps.

Children who grow up in a home where alcohol or other drugs are abused, whether in the open or "under wraps," generally are at increased risk of developing addiction problems themselves; this may be related to genetic predisposition. Exposure to substance use in the home provides behavioral role models, tacit approval, and ease of access to the drugs, all of which encourage early experimentation. Substance abuse prevention research suggests that smoking and drinking alcohol are two early steps in an adolescent's progression into illicit drug use.

Social, Psychological, Physical, and Spiritual Harm

Addiction repetitively and unpredictably impairs judgment and disrupts moral values, resulting in erratic and atypical behaviors. As the addicted person becomes progressively more enmeshed in obtaining and using alcohol or other drugs, his or her values are compromised. Sporadic failures to honor religious, civic, and family responsibilities because of intoxication, withdrawal, or trying to obtain drugs may accumulate to such an extent that the individual shirks responsibility altogether.

As the relationship with the drug gradually hypertrophies, it crowds out and severely stresses all other major relationships in the lives of addicts. As the addiction progresses, the amount of time spent impaired increases. Over time, this individual may become convinced that he or she cannot live or function without it, and family members may likewise become convinced that it is hopeless and can never be resolved.

An individual who abuses alcohol or other drugs has a substantially increased risk of illness or disability. Risk of accidents increases, and family members can be harmed in these accidents. The burden on the family increases during times when the alcohol or drug-abusing member is ill or disabled. Interpersonal verbal, physical, and sexual violence often erupts within addicted families.

Active addiction carries with it a sevenfold increase in risk of mortality. Some members may blame themselves or others in the family for the untimely death of the addicted parent, sibling, child, or spouse. Loss of a role model may affect children, and loss of a spouse and sexual partner may lead to more instability, sometimes accompanied by introduction of a new—and often addicted—spouse/partner, whose presence as stepparent or transient surrogate may be resented and resisted by the children. Loss of a parent or sibling may occur in other ways, through institutionalization (in prison, mental hospital, foster or group home, or nursing home), as the result of trauma or emotional problems, or through running away from home, adolescent pregnancy, and premature marriage, divorce, or separation. Family addiction may lead to other family structural changes as various members remove themselves from an increasingly dysfunctional family.

FAMILY ADJUSTMENT TO ADDICTION

Addiction disorders alter family "rules, roles, and rituals." The early onset, gradual progression, and intermittent chronic nature of addiction disorders, coupled with the addict's resistance to the constructive influences exerted by family members, often lead other family members to resigned acceptance of the disordered member's addiction as an unchangeable trait of family life, especially in families where the addiction has persisted for decades or generations. Such families adjust to addiction by evolving self-defeating defensive routines, often so completely that adjusting to recovery may become stressful. Typical defense mechanisms include *classic denial* that there is a problem, *minimization* of the magnitude of the problem, *projection* of the problem (i.e., blaming the problem on others), and *rationalization* or making excuses for the problem. Addicted families tend to employ *isolation* as a defense to shame, minimizing the amount of potential embarrassment to which they are exposed and at the same time limiting the exposure of their own members to other, healthier family systems. If families do not identify addiction as a problem for an individual family member, then they are not able to recognize that addiction also is adversely affecting the family as a system.

The rules in an addicted family have been summarized as "don't talk" (discussing dysfunctional and painful using events is often energetically avoided by the family), "don't feel" (suppressing feelings is common in addiction-affected families, much as it is in addicted individuals), and "don't trust" (repeated episodes of irresponsible and erratic behavior cause frequent disappointments to family members and diminishes their ability to trust in others). Following these rules does not encourage the development of healthy, intimate, nurturing relationships.

Children in families with alcoholism internalize limited and rigid family roles that can stay with them throughout their lives. These roles—enabler, hero, scapegoat, lost child, mascot—are taught in virtually every treatment program. Individuals may move from one role to another over time. *Enablers* typically align themselves with the addiction, sometimes assisting in defensive activities against others who would apply constructive influences against it. *Codependence* refers to the tendency of family members in an addicted family to become harmfully overinvolved with the addiction process in such a manner that reduces the level of well-being of this codependent family member. Family members may neglect to invest in recovery support for their codependence, and they might relapse as well.

THE PHYSICIAN'S ROLE WITH ADDICTED FAMILIES

Screening

Most families affected by addiction are missed by health care teams; this is due in part to family denial and in part to families not having recognized the problem themselves. Emotional factors may play a role in help seeking that does not overtly identify the underlying problem of addiction in the family; for example, frequent visits to emergency rooms for injuries and psychosomatic complaints are typical with children of alcoholics and addicts.

Addiction may be missed if the right questions are not asked. Given their high prevalence rate and significant effect on all family members, addiction disorders should become part of the routine family history. Simply asking all patients if they have a family history of alcohol or drug problems would improve detection considerably, but the optimal approach to the family history of addiction is through the use of the family CAGE (f-CAGE), a clinical tool that permits screening for the symptoms of addiction without requiring that the individuals actually have made the diagnosis themselves.

Questions that identify consequences in the family as a result of an addicted person's disorder and behavior should be asked in order to help the family make a "family diagnosis of addiction"—that is, morbidity, pain, and suffering in their own lives. A tool that can help in this effort is the use of a questionnaire such as the "Family Drinking Survey" (FDS). The FDS identifies issues of family morbidity including self-pity, ruined occasions, arguments, anger or depression, worry, fear for safety, insomnia, and other somatic symptoms. Counseling family members about family addiction is more effective when it incorporates their own responses on the FDS.

The Risk Inventory for Substance Abuse Affected Families is a tool to help physicians and other health professionals who work with children and family services. It assesses the dimensions and consequences of substance abuse that make it difficult for parents to care safely and adequately for children.

Working with the Family to Confront and Motivate the Addicted Persons in the Family to Seek Treatment when Needed

In hospital consultations and in the office, when it becomes apparent that an addiction disorder is active, one may begin by discussing this with the identified patient. Motivational interviewing offers the opportunity to assess barriers and facilitate change via an array of possible stage-specific goals and outcomes. If resistance is met, widening the net to include family members in the discussion is indicated. By mentioning that their involvement would improve treatment outcome for self and for the other members of the family, the addicted patient is more likely to grant permission for a family meeting. During inpatient rounding or office visits involving family members, listening for or asking about family reactions to the addiction behavior and its consequences may lead to the opportunity to invite family members in for a conjoint consultation to discuss the family's concerns. In cases where the addicted person is extremely defensive, family members may independently approach the physician with a desire to get help for this person. The physician can listen and seek out additional information about what is going on at home that may not have been shared during office visits or hospitalizations. The physician can then refer the family to a family therapist with skills in addiction or to an interventionist who may help the family to engage their addicted member and the whole family in treatment and recovery.

The traditional approach often mentioned by members of Alcoholics Anonymous, Narcotics Anonymous, and Al-Anon of waiting until the addicted person hits *rock bottom* before accepting treatment and beginning recovery is suboptimal for several reasons: (a) hitting rock bottom can be very damaging to self and others or, in the worst case, fatal; (b) it may take a very long time for the individual with addiction disorder to lose enough to accept treatment; (c) significant others may have given up on this person by the time stable and lasting recovery is established; (d) losses that accumulate to eventually motivate engagement in recovery also diminish the resources that the person has to apply to recovery; (e) family members who give up on the addicted person often do not address their own issues before (or sometimes after) the addicted person does recover; and (f) resentments or termination of relationships may interfere with willingness to volunteer for family treatment when the addicted person eventually engages in recovery.

A Relational Intervention Sequence for Engagement (ARISE) can be used when someone requests help engaging a person who suffers from an addiction disorder but who is resistant to admitting it is a problem or to getting help. This approach involves a series of visits with the family and significant others, including the addicted person if he or she is willing to participate, beginning with the first caller over the telephone or at a face-to-face visit at the office or hospital.

This approach engages the supporters of the addicted person in resisting further enlistment as enablers and builds a confident, cohesive team to put a firm, healing structure into the life of the addicted person. This team must withstand pleading, lying, threats, rationalizations, and subterfuge and hold the addicted person responsible for his or her behavior, for completing needed treatment, and for sustaining recovery. Even if it is not successful in engaging the index patient into treatment, such an approach usually alters the family system surrounding the index patient in a positive way by helping family members to free themselves from the secrets, isolation, guilt, and fear engendered by the index patient's addiction.

Referring Addicted Persons for Family-Oriented Treatment

Many addiction treatment programs offer some sort of family-oriented care such as:

- Psychoeducational multifamily groups in which information is presented about the disease concept of addiction disorders and recovery, information about genetics and familial transmission of addiction disorders, the impact of growing up in a dysfunctional family with addiction, and how Twelve-Step support groups enhance recovery of the addicted person (e.g., Alcoholics Anonymous, Narcotics Anonymous) and significant others (e.g., Al-Anon, Adult Children of Alcoholics Al-Anon, Families Anonymous)

- Family or couples therapy focusing on either recovery only or on broader issues that trouble the family
- Parenting education, parent-child therapy, or reunification therapy for single parents whose children are symptomatic or who have been removed
- Communication and problem-solving training or anger management for families with domestic violence

Although most alcohol and drug treatment programs offer family-oriented aspects in their services, there can be wide variation in attendance policies and family involvement. Some programs offer variants of empirically tested cognitive-behavioral treatments designed specifically to promote abstinence while improving family function (e.g., communication training).

When the addicted person refuses any involvement in formal treatment, there are unilateral family therapy and community reinforcement and family training, which trains concerned significant others (CSOs) to positively reinforce abstinence, reduced substance use, and recovery behaviors while negatively reinforcing continuing substance abuse.

The community reinforcement and family training procedure when tested in a randomized controlled trial with 130 CSOs of alcoholics found that 64% of their index patients engaged in alcoholism treatment, whereas Al-Anon facilitation found only 13%. These results reflect the dominant themes of Al-Anon: disengage from the alcoholic behavior (i.e., stop enabling), abandon hope of influencing the drinking behavior, and take care of yourself.

Referring the Family Members for the Help They Need

Self-help groups for family members—including Al-Anon, Alateen, Ala-Tot, Tough Love, and Families Anonymous—are widely available. Most such groups are organized on the principles and steps of Alcoholics Anonymous but focus on the recovery tasks of the individual family member who is experiencing pain from another's addiction disorder.

For individuals or families who are willing, referral to individual or family counseling or psychoeducational sessions can be extraordinarily helpful. In making such a referral, the physician needs to communicate with the therapist regarding the family illness and consequences that led to the referral: individuals and even whole families can participate in counseling for long periods without ever disclosing the presence of the underlying addiction disorder.

Identifying the Benefits of the Addiction to the Family

Although there are many negative aspects of addiction, it is the positive aspects that underlie resistance to recovery. Both the individual with the addiction disorder and the family may perceive, often unconsciously, that the addiction somehow makes their lives better. Understanding how families change with substance use versus abstinence sheds light on family resistance to treatment and recovery.

Helping Family Members Identify and Address Enabling Behaviors and Codependency Issues

Several questions on the FDS assess family enabling, covering areas such as making excuses for the individual, avoiding situations that may prove embarrassing, trying to limit the family member's drinking or drug use, joining in the drinking or drug use, and altering schedules or habits to accommodate the family member's addiction behavior. Presenting information to help them understand how their actions may actually be sheltering the addicted person from appropriate consequences can be very helpful for families. It is important to remember that the identification of enabling behaviors is a late step in family treatment and is useful only after families have progressed through the core steps discussed earlier.

Once continuing abstinence is maintained, the focus for the therapy shifts to improving the relationships. Positive feelings and communication are enhanced, and resentments over past mistakes, disloyalties, dishonesties, and the like must be resolved without triggering a relapse.

FAMILY THERAPY FOR ADDICTIONS

Approaches for Adults with Addiction Problems

Behavioral couples therapy (BCT) is the most extensively researched family approach in the treatment of substance abuse and has been shown effective. BCT works with couples who cohabitate where one of the partners suffers from an addiction disorder. It uses a recovery contract to clearly set out the goals of the treatment and conditions that would indicate relapse. Partners go over the recovery contract daily with a discussion about intent to remain sober and verbal reinforcement for doing so. Providing clean urine drug screens and taking medications to assist in maintaining sobriety in the presence of the partner are used, and progress is recorded on a calendar. Urges and triggers are discussed openly. Relapses are identified by either partner and must be interrupted as soon as possible as specified in the contract.

Approaches for Families with Troubled Adolescents

Families with adolescents who require substance abuse treatment present special problems. It is well known that adolescents exposed to group therapy approaches actually get worse as they feed on one another's pathologic attitudes and behaviors, whereas family therapy helps immensely in improving outcome.

The Behavioral Exchange Systems Training program is an 8-week parent group that supports and assists parents in coping with their adolescent's substance use; parents participating in the Behavioral Exchange Systems Training program showed reductions in mental health symptoms and increases in satisfaction and assertive parenting behaviors. A coping skills training program for parents of substance-abusing adolescents was associated with improved parental coping, family communication, and parental reports of their own functioning. Prosocial family therapy integrates specific parent training with nonspecific family therapy and is designed as a preventive intervention for juvenile offenders and their families. Brief strategic family therapy has been developed to address not only drug use behavior but also the host of other behavioral problems that cluster with drug abuse such as oppositional defiance, underachievement and lack of interest and connection with school, aggression and delinquency, sexual risk behaviors, and disinterest in prosocial behaviors.

Another type of family therapy for adolescents is multidimensional family therapy (MDFT). It addresses expectancies about using intoxicants, parental addiction, and prevention of family relapse. This model uses both individual and family sessions to address the myriad of issues within the addiction-affected family. Multisystemic therapy (MST) for juvenile offenders also has been shown effective in reducing substance use. This approach analyzes the symptomatic behavior in its environmental context, maintains an optimistic positive attitude, and empowers parents and caregivers to influence youth to take progressively more responsibility for their behavior. Treatment may occur at home, in schools, and elsewhere in the youth's environment; one goal is to prevent out-of-home placement. Finally, many physicians who treat high-risk families struggle with ways to engage them in treatment interventions. The Youth Support Project was developed especially for high-risk families—those who are difficult to enroll and to retain in addiction treatment.

Given the demographic changes in US society and the expected increase in the number of older adults experiencing problems with alcohol and other drugs, family therapy approaches for adult children and their older, substance-using parents will become increasingly important. Physicians can play a significant role in screening, assessment, and treatment planning for older families because of the increased number of physician services older people use, the greater extent to which they take prescription medications, and gerontologic health models that stress family involvement. Age-appropriate tools, such as the Michigan Alcoholism Screening Test-Geriatric Version, improve accuracy in detection among older adults.

CHAPTER 63

Summary Author: John Young
Kathleen M. Carroll

Twelve-Step Facilitation Approaches

Twelve-Step Facilitation (TSF) therapy is a manual-guided treatment that was originally developed for use in Project MATCH, a major multisite trial of behavioral treatments for alcohol abuse and dependence. Recognizing that self-help programs represent an important, broadly available, and inexpensive resource, the defining feature of TSF is to encourage meaningful, long-term involvement with Alcoholics Anonymous (AA) and other self-help groups.

TREATMENT MODEL

TSF is a highly structured, individual, manual-guided approach delivered over the course of 12 to 24 weeks. It consists of a set of core topics that are to be covered with all patients, a set of elective topics that can be selected to tailor the treatment to different individuals, and guidelines for conjoint sessions with family members.

TSF assumes that alcoholism and addiction are progressive diseases of mind, body, and spirit, for which the only effective remedy is abstinence from mood-altering substances. TSF adheres to the concepts set forth in the 12 Steps and 12 Traditions of Alcoholics Anonymous. Core, essential features of TSF include:

- Taking a thorough substance use history, identifying positive and negative consequences of substance use, and giving feedback as ground work to Step 1 (admitting powerlessness and acknowledging unmanageability)
- Providing education about Steps 1, 2, and 3
- Explanation of the disease concept of alcoholism and addiction
- Exploring discrepancies between the patient's stated goals and actions in terms of denial
- Identifying "people, places, and things" that trigger substance use and that support recovery
- Encouraging patients to actively "work the Steps" as the primary goal of treatment
- Supporting the point of view that the best chance of abstinence and health is to accept loss of control and the need to reach out to the fellowship of AA (or NA or CA)

TREATMENT PLANNING AND EVALUATION

A thorough evaluation of the individual's alcohol and drug use history is an essential feature of TSF. The goal is to begin the breakdown of the patient's denial system. The therapist begins with the age of earliest use and progresses by looking at different time periods. As this is done, patterns usually emerge; this information is used to highlight loss of control over alcohol or drugs, which is the hallmark of addiction in TSF.

The TSF therapist also explores positive and negative consequences of substance use. Typically, the relationship with alcohol and drugs starts out very positively; however, as use increases in amount and frequency, there is invariably an increase in negative consequences. These negative consequences are evidence of the "unmanageability" referred to in Step 1 and can be physical (health problems, accidents, injuries), legal (arrests, civil problems, lawsuits), social (loss of relationships with family and friends, lack of social skills), sexual (changes in sexual functioning, trading sex for drugs), psychological (depression, anxiety, shame, guilt about using despite the intent to stay abstinent), and financial.

After the alcohol and drug use history is completed, the therapist asks the patients to react to what they have observed. For some, this is the first time they have looked at the big picture of how addiction has affected their life.

Finally, the TSF therapist asks about loss of control over alcohol or drug use. This includes behaviors such as repeated failed attempts to stop or control use, using alone, preoccupation with drugs or alcohol, and substance substitution. Using the evidence offered by the patient, usually the only logical conclusion is that the patient is an alcoholic or drug addict.

The TSF therapist then describes addiction as a disease that is lifelong, progressive, and, if left untreated, fatal. Once a person becomes an addict, he or she can never return to safe use of mood-altering substances. The progressive nature of the disease is noted in the patient's history of increasing losses and problems and increasing amounts and frequency of use over time. The therapist emphasizes that alcoholism and drug dependence are treatable and that what has worked best for most is to abstain from all mood-altering substances. To learn how to do this and to gain support with the task, the TSF therapist recommends that the patient makes use of Twelve-Step recovery programs.

THERAPIST CHARACTERISTICS

The goal of TSF treatment is to engage the patient's interest in voluntarily committing to this Twelve-Step facilitation program; approaches that use excessive pressure, threat, or coercion toward this are likely to elicit a false commitment from the patient at best. The therapist takes a direct, nonjudgmental, and educative approach to confrontation of denial. The history is relied on consistently as the basis for directly confronting patients with their current situation in a supportive and empathetic way; the TSF therapist is careful to confront the patient's behavior as it relates to his or her addiction (i.e., denial, avoidance) rather than confronting the person. This means separating the person from the disease and communicating that the patient is a good person who has a disease that leads him or her to act in ways that are hurtful toward himself or herself and others.

In TSF, the therapist also uses his or her therapeutic skills to help the patient overcome barriers to becoming actively involved in Twelve-Step recovery programs. It is critically important for the therapist to be an educator about Twelve-Step programs. The therapist also provides empathy and a sense of hope for the patient through communicating and understanding of the struggles of early recovery.

CHAPTER 64

Summary Author: John Young
Zebulon Taintor • Richard N. Rosenthal

Microprocessor Abuse and Internet Addiction

INTRODUCTION

Microprocessors help us manage many aspects of our lives. Some of us use them too much, lose track of time while getting too involved, and become dependent on the stimulation they provide. Significant negative life consequences can occur as a result of that dependence.

The Internet provides enhanced opportunities for people to do things that would tend to bring them to the attention of a clinician even if they didn't happen to use the Internet (sex, gambling, etc.). Some of these last activities are regarded as addicting in their own right.

"Internet addiction" covers only part of the problems encountered by clinicians in patients who spend too much time using devices built around microprocessors. Consider the accident resulting from instant messaging while driving, too many hours on the Internet using a mobile phone, or a person who finds Second Life more real than his or her real life. The common denominator is the use of microprocessors in an increasingly wide variety of devices.

HISTORICAL PERSPECTIVE

The Internet was established in 1969 at the University of Southern California as a way of linking computers for national defense uses. Even early on, computers offered opportunities to impair functioning. Weitzenbaum described the development of compulsive programmers who had lost the broad view of problem solving, and came to see problems simply as means to interact with the computer. The concept of the impaired computer user was described in 1992 by Kuiper, who called them "space cadets," characterized as spending too much time in front of industrial or commercial computers and having too few other ambitions or interests.

Widespread use of e-mail skyrocketed in the 1990s as e-mail programs became interoperable. The first wave of articles about Internet addiction appeared in the mid 1990s. Text and instant messaging took off as the twenty-first century began with personal digital assistants (PDAs), Blackberrys, and increasingly smart telephones. Currently, it is estimated that 82% of American population has access to the Internet. More than that have cellular telephones, although the number with Internet and e-mail capability is unknown. Most use e-mail, which can be used without the Internet or a computer. E-mail is checked while in bed, in the bathroom, in church, and while driving.

The Internet offers many advantages over other agents with high liability for abuse and dependence, including

- Always available, lending itself to impulsive access and marathon sessions
- Convenient: no need to leave home or work
- Inexpensive
- Rewarding: content-rich, with Web sites consistently present and calculated to please; increasing interactivity; a continuous flow of new sites that offer novelty, all developed and distributed at an ever-increasing pace.
- Controllable: the user can go wherever desired and leave at will.
- Escapist: sites of interest offer a welcoming reality in which all sex partners are attractive and interested, and bets are likely to be won.
- Validating: one can find that which caters to one's interests and tastes, thus verifying that these are legitimate because others feel the same way.

Identity and the Internet is emerging as a separate field of study with the growth of programs such as Second Life (*www.secondlife.com*), a "3-D virtual world entirely created by its Residents [who socialize, create, and chat using voice and text chat]." One creates an identity for one's self, which often is quite opposite from one's regular self. Since opening to the public, Second Life has grown explosively and today is inhabited by millions of Residents from around the globe. Its world is filled with creations of the Residents, often with special powers. Several other sites (Metaverse, Open Life) offer similar fare; all are developing additional features to make their offerings more attractive and enveloping. Some people have reported having more success in Second Life than in their real lives, while other patients have entered therapy because of Second Life relationships gone awry.

DIAGNOSTIC DILEMMAS

In considering whether microprocessors are a bona fide substrate for addictive processes, it is important to present some caveats:

- Using the computer, cell phone, or videogame is not intrinsically illegal.
- Using the computer, cell phone, or videogame is generally normal, prosocial, encouraged behavior.
- There is a learning curve to information acquisition, time management, and social behavior when people experience these new and powerful tools.
- People can be very engaged in microprocessor use without its being pathological.
- Calling maladaptive microprocessor-related behavior pathological rather than, say, a bad habit may medicalize what is in actuality a social problem.

In considering the necessary components that would subtend diagnostically both chemical and behavioral addictions, six necessary domains have been identified based on problem gambling behavior:

- Salience: the drug or behavior has gained primacy in a person's life, which can be a cognitive change dominating the person's mental life or, behaviorally, dominating a person's activity in a compulsive fashion.
- Mood modification: the substance or behavior subjectively gives one a rewarding high or alleviates a negative mood state.
- Tolerance: the person must increase the amount or intensity of the substance or behavior in order to achieve the desired effect.
- Withdrawal symptoms: after stopping or reducing the substance or behavior, the person demonstrates either physical symptoms afterward, or dysphoria characterized by irritability, mood lability, depressive symptoms, and so on.
- Conflict: the person has conflicts regarding the use of the substance or the behavior that manifests as either interpersonal (e.g., marital strife) or intrapsychic (e.g., guilt).
- Relapse: after a period of abstinence, the use or behavior is reinstated with the same intensity.

The symptom of loss of control despite negative consequences, which is one of the hallmarks of the modern concept of addiction, is accounted for as compulsive behavior in the Salience category.

It may be argued that problem Internet use better fits criteria for other *DSM-IV* groups such as impulse control disorder (ICD); for example, as with pathological gambling, hallmarks of problem Internet use include repeated failure to resist impulses that are harmful to self or others and tension or arousal before and pleasure or relief during the act, followed by guilt or self-reproach. Another possible diagnostic category is compulsive disorders such as OCD; however, in OCD the intrusive thoughts or compulsive behaviors are typically ego-dystonic, whereas in pathological Internet use, the preoccupation is ego-syntonic and pleasurable. Also, OCD patients are anxious and full of doubt and tend to avoid risk, whereas patients with problem Internet use often underestimate risk.

TREATMENT PLANNING

Evaluation-Diagnosis

The diagnostic divides are among addiction, impulse control (non–substance-based reward), and compulsive disorders. There remains a population that compulsively uses devices without seeming to get much gratification. Frequently, they meet criteria for a compulsive disorder.

Rating scales serve as diagnostic aids and, in offering objective data for feedback in motivational approaches, can help patients to realize the extent of their problems. Several are available, but that from the Center for Recovery from Internet Addiction, the Internet Addiction Test (IAT) (*http://netaddiction.com/resources/internet_addiction_test.htm*)

is best established. Many of the items in the IAT correspond to similar items in the *DSM-IV* diagnostic categories of substance abuse and substance dependence. The scale can be used by significant others, who usually insist on treatment for reasons common to other addictions: a sense of losing the loved one whose life has been taken over by the addiction and significant impairment in activities and relationships.

INDICATIONS FOR TREATMENT

Morbidity occurs at several levels. The amount of time spent with microprocessors results in necessary tasks going undone. Real-life social relationships get less time as what may be thought to be more satisfying relationships are developed on the Internet. The patient is not necessarily a recluse and can document that hours spent in his room involve communicating with "friends" around the world; objective observers may rate these relationships less favorably, often reminiscent of an alcoholic's drinking buddies. Some patients present as having lost touch with what is the "true" reality. Physical impairment may result from prolonged sitting in front of screens, with increased obesity and less exercise; however, inactivity is preferable to accidents that can occur while multitasking.

PRETREATMENT ISSUES

Motivation-Rationale for Choice of Treatment

As with most addictions, motivation prior to engagement in treatment may be scant or absent. Problems are minimized, rationalized, or denied. A nonconfrontational discussion of impairment often helps the patient to gain perspective. This can be done using the principles of motivational interviewing (MI), where the facts about the impact of microprocessor overuse are carefully elicited and then fed back to the patient in a nonjudgmental manner.

Selection and Preparation of Patients/Suitability Unlike the subpopulations that comprise the sufferers of many chemical addictions, microprocessor abusers are technically competent, often innovative, and well-educated. However, the subpopulation has also been shown to have high rates of current and lifetime co-occurring mental disorders that tend to have a negative impact upon recovery. Retreat into cyberspace may mask co-occurring social phobia and/or other anxiety disorders.

Treatment and Technique

Complete abstinence is usually not a feasible long-term treatment goal, as use of microprocessors is unavoidable in today's world, and nonuse is associated with significant vocational and social disadvantage.

The general plan is reintroduction into the real world, which must be done in stages to ease transitions. Where identity issues predominate, the successful elements of the Internet identity should be characterized, and there should be an open discussion of integrating these into the real-world persona. Therapy should be seen as a rewarding process that helps the patient get in real life what had once been available only on the Internet. Medication treatment for co-occurring obsessive-compulsive disorders and/or anxiety can be helpful. Clearly, treating co-occurring mood, anxiety, psychotic, and substance use disorders is likely to be helpful in supporting recovery; the involvement of significant others is key to supporting recovery and reintegration into the real world. Social skills training may also be helpful.

CHAPTER 65

Summary Author: John Young
Antoine Douaihy • Dennis C. Daley • G. Alan Marlatt • Crystal R. Spotts

Relapse Prevention: Clinical Models and Intervention Strategies

Epidemiologic studies of people with lifetime substance dependence suggest that 58% eventually enter sustained recovery (i.e., no symptoms for the past year). Although most people with a substance use disorder (SUD) eventually abstain or manage to control their use without professional help, many will suffer from a long-lasting chronic condition, whereby they cycle through episodes of lapse, relapse, treatment reentry, and recovery. High rates of relapse have led many researchers to conceptualize addiction as a "chronic relapsing illness" and to understand relapse prevention (RP) as an iterative process of change rather than as a full inoculation against relapse. Focusing on the relapse process helps us better understand the challenges of posttreatment change and identify RP interventions targeting the various pathways in the addiction-recovery cycle.

LAPSE, RELAPSE, AND RECOVERY

The lack of consensus regarding the conceptualization of relapse has made it difficult to assess treatment outcomes and different estimates of relapse rates. Relapse has been described both as a discrete phenomenon and as a process of behavior change; the term holds meaning that goes beyond the dichotomous outcome of abstinence versus continued use. A lapse has been defined as the initial episode of use of a substance after a period of abstinence, whereas relapse refers to continued use after the initial slip, a "breakdown or set-back in the person's attempt to change or modify any target behavior."

The definition of relapse has a significant impact on the conceptual and clinical approach to assessment. The ways in which clinicians quantify and qualify relapse determine how they will respond to patient's behaviors. If a patient is involved in a treatment program that identifies any drinking behavior such as one drink after a period of abstinence as a relapse, it is more probable for him or her to engage in heavier drinking behavior, which is explained by the phenomenon of the "abstinence violation effect": self-blame and loss of perceived control that individuals often experience after the violation of self-imposed rules. If the same behavior occurs with a patient receiving treatment in a program that does not convey that this behavior is a relapse, it is more probable for him or her to have an increased awareness of his or her reactions to drinking and he or she may be less vulnerable to the abstinence violation effect. Lapse and relapse may also be defined according to the individual's goals for change. If abstinence is a goal, then a drink may be considered as a lapse; but if the individual maintains harm reduction goals, then a lapse may be defined as a harmful consequence of drinking behavior. Also, it should be noted that, at least with regard to tobacco and cocaine, studies have shown that a lapse does not necessarily herald a full-blown relapse.

Different rates of relapse vary between studies and across substances, but "relapse is the rule" not the exception.

As with relapse, recovery can be defined as a long-term and ongoing process rather than an end point, with the road being anything but linear and smooth, and the outcome anything but predictable. Recovery tasks and areas of clinical focus are contingent on the stage or phase of recovery the individual is in. Individuals who achieve only partial recovery are at risk for multiple relapses over time, yet still can benefit from the cumulative effects of multiple treatments.

DETERMINANTS OF RELAPSE

Intrapersonal Determinants

Self-efficacy *Self-efficacy* refers to individuals' beliefs in their capabilities to organize and carry out specific courses of action to attain some goal or situation-specific task. These beliefs have great influence on self-regulation and the quality of human functioning, because they shape the goals individuals set for themselves, the persistence in reaching those goals, and the effectiveness of problem-solving activities. Individuals' sense of efficacy is the result of their cognitive processing from many sources of efficacy information. This construct is intimately related to the individual's coping abilities and reflects the degree of confidence that the individual has about being confronted with a high-risk situation and successfully avoiding a lapse. The patient's personal belief in his or her ability to control his or her substance use is a reliable predictor of lapses immediately after treatment and over long-term outcomes, and low levels of self-efficacy are predictive of relapse. Given the relationship between self-efficacy and relapse, self-efficacy should be thoroughly assessed during treatment and appropriately targeted for interventions.

Outcome Expectancies One factor enhancing the likelihood of relapse is the set of expectancies that individuals develop about the expected outcomes associated with addictive behaviors. Individuals who develop an addiction typically have developed a set of expectancies that anticipate positive outcomes from engaging in the behavior, such as changing one's mood or increasing sociability. Such outcome expectancies are shaped by an individual's past direct and indirect experience with the behaviors related to the addiction, including vicarious learning through the modeling they see early on displayed by parents and later by peers.

Expectancies are strongly related to outcome, *although there is little evidence that targeting expectancies in treatment leads to changes in posttreatment consumption*. There is a possibility that expectancies influence outcome via their relationship with other relapse predictors, such as negative emotional states and beliefs about substances relieving negative affect, particularly among treatment-seeking individuals. Individuals endorsing positive outcome expectancies at the beginning of treatment may benefit from an intervention challenging their expectancies.

Craving Multiple and often conflicting theories, definitions, and measurements have plagued the study of craving. Craving has been described as a cognitive experience focused on the desire to use a substance and is often highly related to expectancies for the desired effect of the substance, whereas an urge has been defined as the behavioral intention or impulse to use a substance. Although craving has been implicated in general in the relapse process, its role in alcohol relapse remains controversial; craving has generally been found to be a poor predictor of relapse.

It has been proposed that the subjective experience of craving may not directly predict substance use and that relapse may be predicted from the correlates and underlying mechanisms of craving. A recent study assessing the usefulness of craving as a predictor of relapse in alcohol-dependent adults admitted to residential treatment programs showed that the number of days in which cravings were reported in the week before discharge predicted alcohol use at 3-month follow-up. Admission spirituality, alcohol-refusal self-efficacy, and depression levels differentiated cravers from noncravers. Another study demonstrated that stress-induced cocaine craving is predictive of cocaine relapse outcomes. Mindfulness and meditation may provide a useful antidote to the experience of craving. The heightened state of present-focused awareness that is encouraged by these techniques may directly counteract the conditioned automatic response to use substances in response to cravings and urges. In addition, the use of anticraving medications can pharmacologically reduce the experience of craving.

Motivation An important element in determining the likelihood of relapse is the individual's commitment to or motivation for self-improvement. Motivation may relate to the relapse process in two distinct ways: the motivation for positive behavior change and the motivation to engage in the problematic behavior. Motivation is judged with regard to a particular action or outcome. For example, a person might be quite motivated for change but not for treatment, and polysubstance users commonly show levels of motivation that are different depending on the drug.

The most common motivational obstacle to early help seeking is ambivalence. The ambivalence toward change is highly related to self-efficacy and outcome expectancies. It has also been suggested that any analysis of relapse needs to examine the interaction between commitment and coping skills: even well-developed coping abilities will not prevent relapse if the individual's commitment to stay clean is low, and strong commitment may be insufficient in the absence of adequate coping skills. Interventions that focus on addressing ambivalence (decisional balance) may increase intrinsic motivation by allowing patients to explore their own values and how they differ from their actual behavioral choices. Motivational interviewing (MI) is a person-centered, goal-oriented approach for facilitating change through exploring and resolving ambivalence. MI has demonstrated efficacy for reducing alcohol consumption and frequency of drinking in this population.

It is important to assess commitment and motivation to change and understand that motivation for change is comprised of multiple dimensions that are at best modestly intercorrelated. Interventions designed to enhance commitment to change should be a component of any RP approach.

Coping Based on the cognitive-behavioral model of relapse, the most critical predictor of relapse is the individual's ability to utilize adequate coping strategies in dealing with high-risk situations. Coping has been shown to be a critical predictor of substance use treatment outcomes and is often the strongest predictor of behavioral lapses in the moment. There is a distinction between approach and avoidance coping: approach coping may involve attempts to accept, confront, and reframe, whereas avoidance coping may include distraction from cues or engaging in other activities. One study demonstrated that treatment outcomes in alcoholic patients could be predicted by focusing on this distinction: results suggested that avoidance coping, particularly cognitive (as opposed to behavioral) avoidance coping, was predictive of fewer alcohol, interpersonal, and psychologic problems at the 12-month follow-up. Approach coping also predicted decreased alcohol problem severity at 12-month follow-up when it was behavioral rather than cognitive in nature.

Coping may be also experienced as inaction. Inaction has been understood as the acceptance of substance cues, which can be described as "letting go" and not acting on an urge. An example of this is the use of "urge surfing." In this strategy, the patient is first taught to label internal sensations and cognitive preoccupation as an urge and to foster an attitude of detachment from the urge. The focus is on identifying and accepting the urge, not attempting to fight it. In a recent study on the effectiveness of a mindfulness meditation technique of the Vipassana tradition in reducing substance use in an incarcerated population, participants reported that accepting the "here and now," "staying in the moment," and being mindful of the urges were helpful coping strategies.

Emotional States Excessive substance use may be motivated by an attempt at affective regulation, whether to reproduce a positive emotional state (positive reinforcement) or to ameliorate a negative state such as withdrawal (negative reinforcement). Several studies have reported a strong link between negative affect and relapse to substance use; clinicians should therefore incorporate strategies to decrease and manage negative emotional states as a part of the RP approach.

Interpersonal Determinants

Functional social support or the level of emotional support is highly predictive of long-term abstinence across several addictions. Negative social support in the form of interpersonal conflict and social pressure to use substances has been related to an increased risk of relapse. Behavioral marital therapy, which incorporates partner support in treatment goals, has been described as one of the top three empirically supported treatment methods for alcohol problems.

Clinical RP Interventions to Reduce Lapse and Relapse Risk

Strategy 1: Help Patients Understand Relapse as a Process and Event and Learn to Identify Warning Signs
The understanding of addiction as a chronic cyclical condition helps the patient to look at relapse as a process occurring in a certain context and to understand that early warning signs often precede an actual lapse. Attitudinal, emotional, cognitive, and behavioral changes seem to occur days, weeks, and even longer before resuming the use of substances.

Patients in treatment for the first time can benefit from reviewing common relapse warning signs identified by others in recovery. For the patient who has relapsed, a review of the relapse history is essential: the clinician should ask the patient to review the experience in detail to learn the connections between thoughts, feelings, events, or situations and relapse to substance use. *A survey found that "Understanding the Relapse Process" was the topic rated most useful by patients participating in a residential addiction treatment program.*

Strategy 2: Help Patients Identify their High-Risk Situations and Develop Effective Cognitive and Behavioral Coping

The need to recognize and manage high-risk factors is an essential component of RP. Relapse is more likely to occur as the result of lack of coping skills than the high-risk situation itself, so the clinician should assess the patient's coping style to identify targets for an intervention. A person heading for a relapse usually makes a number of mini-decisions over time, each of which brings the person closer to creating a high-risk situation or giving in. These choices are called "apparently irrelevant decisions" and they need to be identified and addressed with patients to decrease lapse risk.

It has also been suggested that in addition to teaching patients "specific" RP skills to deal with high-risk factors, the clinician should use "global" approaches such as problem-solving or skills-training strategies (such as behavioral rehearsal, covert modeling, and assertiveness training), cognitive reframing (such as coping imagery and reframing reactions to lapse/relapse), and lifestyle interventions (such as meditation, exercise, and relaxation).

Strategy 3: Help Patients Enhance Their Communication Skills and Interpersonal Relationships and Develop a Recovery Social Network

Family members, sponsors, other recovering members of self-help groups, personal friends, and employers can become part of an individual's RP network; the patient then can determine how and when to ask for support or help. Behavioral rehearsal can increase confidence, help the patient practice ways to make specific requests for support, understand his or her ambivalence about asking for help, and prepare for potentially negative responses.

Strategy 4: Help Patients Reduce, Identify, and Manage Negative Emotional States

Negative affective states, such as depression, anger, boredom, and anxiety, are factors in a substantial number of relapses. The acronym HALT, frequently cited by members of Twelve-Step programs, speaks to this important issue of negative affect when it warns not to become too Hungry, too Angry, too Lonely, or too Tired.

Strategy 5: Help Patients Identify and Manage Cravings and Cues that Precede Cravings

A craving for a substance can be triggered by exposure to environmental or internal cues associated with prior use. Cue exposure (CE) treatment is one method used to help patients identify drug use triggers and learn to control the conditioned response to those triggers. This treatment differs from the traditional focus on "avoiding people, places, and things" and instead involves exposing the patient to specific cues associated with substance use. CE aims to enhance behavioral and cognitive coping skills as well as the patient's confidence in his or her ability to resist the desire to use. Systematic relaxation, behavioral alternatives, visual imagery, and cognitive interventions are used in CE. Monitoring and recording cravings, associated thoughts, and outcomes in a daily log or journal can help patients become more vigilant. Cognitive interventions include changing thoughts about the craving or desire to use, challenging euphoric recall, talking oneself through the craving, thinking beyond the high by identifying negative consequences of using (immediate and delayed) and positive benefits of not using, using Twelve-Step recovery slogans, and delaying the decision to use. Behavioral interventions include avoiding, leaving, or changing situations that trigger or worsen a craving; redirecting activities or becoming involved in pleasant activities; obtaining help or support from others by admitting and talking about cravings and hearing how others have survived them; attending self-help support group meetings; or taking medications that reduce craving and increase confidence in the ability to cope.

A new cognitive-behavioral treatment program, Mindfulness-Based Relapse Prevention, uses the practice of mindfulness meditation to develop awareness and nonjudgmental acceptance of thoughts, sensations, and emotional states as a coping strategy in the face of trigger situations for relapse. One mindfulness technique is known as "urge surfing": the patient is instructed to detach from his or her craving by externalizing and labeling it, then to imagine "riding the crest" of the craving until it breaks and the wave of feeling subsides.

Strategy 6: Help Patients Identify and Challenge Cognitive Distortions

It has been observed that a patient's cognitive errors and distortions can increase the probability that an initial slip will develop into a total relapse. Patients can be taught to identify their negative thinking patterns or cognitive errors (black-and-white thinking, overgeneralizing, catastrophizing, jumping to conclusions, etc.), and to use counter-thoughts to challenge them. One way to achieve this is to have the patient discuss or write down specific relapse-related thoughts, what is wrong with such thinking in terms of potential effect on relapse, and new self-statements or thoughts that counteract this thinking. Many of the Twelve-Step slogans were devised to help alcoholics and drug addicts alter their thinking and survive desires to use substances: slogans such as "this too will pass," "let go and let God," and "one day at a time" have helped many patients counter "stinking thinking" that can lead to thoughts of using.

Strategy 7: Help Patients Work Toward a More Balanced Lifestyle
In addition to identifying and managing intrapersonal and interpersonal high-risk relapse factors, patients can benefit from global changes to restore or achieve balance in their lives. Development of a healthy lifestyle is seen as important in reducing stress that makes the patient more vulnerable to relapse. Lifestyle can be assessed by evaluating patterns of daily activities, sources of stress, the balance between activities engaged in for pleasure or self-fulfillment and external demands, health, exercise and relaxation patterns, interpersonal activities, and religious beliefs. Working with patients to develop positive habits (such as relaxation, meditation, exercise, hobbies, or creative tasks) can help balance their lifestyles.

Strategy 8: Consider the Use of Medications in Combination with Psychosocial Treatments
There is now a range of medications used for their anticraving effect available for each of the major classes of addictive substances. None of the medications approved for treating alcohol dependence has proved effective without some form of concurrent behavioral therapy. The best use of medications may be in combination with one another and with psychosocial interventions.

Strategy 9: Facilitate the Transition Between Levels of Care for Patients Completing Residential or Hospital-Based Inpatient Treatment (IPT) Programs, or Structured Partial Hospital or Intensive Outpatient Programs
Patients can make significant gains in residential or day treatment programs only to have the gains negated because of failure to adhere to ongoing outpatient or aftercare treatment. *Interventions used to enhance treatment entry and adherence that also lower the risk of relapse include providing a single session of motivational therapy before discharge from IPT, using telephone or mail reminders of initial treatment appointments, and providing reinforcers for appropriate participation in treatment activities or for providing drug-free urine tests.*

Strategy 10: Incorporate Strategies to Improve Adherence to Treatment and Medications
Numerous studies and reports show that patients who are retained in treatment show better outcomes, including lower relapse rates, than those who drop out early.

66

Summary Author: John Young
Richard N. Rosenthal • Richard K. Ries

Integrating Pharmacological and Behavioral Treatments

Independent of the impact of pharmacotherapies, several types of brief psychosocial interventions have been established as effective in the treatment of drug use disorders. The term *brief* in this context most usually refers to the total number of sessions, but in this chapter, it may also refer to the relatively brief amount of time that a prescribing clinician has in the context of a 15- to 30-minute medication management session. This chapter also presents principles for integrating brief behavioral interventions into medication management sessions.

CLINICAL SKILLS ANY CLINICIAN SHOULD USE

Because the outcome of addiction treatment has been shown to be related to the time spent in treatment, techniques that maximize treatment engagement and retention are likely to promote better outcomes. One such technique is to facilitate the therapeutic alliance through psychologic support, using straightforward approaches accessible to clinicians who may not have had any formal psychotherapy training:

- Expression of interest: Interest is expressed by the clinician's bringing in his or her knowledge of the patient into the conversation. In assessing primary care quality, more whole-person knowledge (medical history, home/work/school responsibilities, health concerns, and values and beliefs) of the patient by the clinician has been shown to predict lower drug and alcohol addiction severity and lower odds of subsequent substance use in recently detoxified primary care patients. It is also important that the clinician is aware that asking too many questions of some patients, especially "why?" questions, can be experienced as intrusive or even an attack, which reduces the likelihood of engagement. Information is best garnered by what, when, where, and how questions, all the while monitoring patient comfort in this process.
- Expression of empathy: Expression of accurate empathy has a long history as an important psychotherapeutic technique and corresponds to the concept of *reflective listening* used in motivational interviewing. Empathy, which is more than simple care or concern, is expressed by the clinician relating his or her own internal emotional experience to corroborate that of the patient's.
- Expression of understanding: The clinician can express his or her understanding by simply stating that he or she "gets" what the patient is communicating and sometimes paraphrasing what the patient has said.
- Repairing a misalliance: Misalliances occur in all human relationships; however, when patients in substance abuse treatment get frustrated or resentful about the treatment, they frequently drop out of treatment, relapse, or both. The willingness of the clinician to entertain a patient's grievances, whether factually based or the result of misconstrual, is a powerful interpersonal reinforcer for patients who may have relatively little experience of a nonjudgmental person willing to listen. Trust, including the experience of the clinician as the patient's agent, is also a factor. The clinician can clarify the facts or address incorrect assumptions to help support the patient having more accurate perceptions and assumptions.

BEHAVIORAL THERAPIES IN THE CONTEXT OF DETOXIFICATION

Rates of relapse to drug dependence after detoxification are quite high. Only about 20% to 50% of patients receive postdetoxification treatment for substance dependence, yet engagement in follow-up treatment increases the time to a second admission for detoxification. Systematic review has demonstrated that psychosocial treatments offered in addition to pharmacologic detoxification for opioid dependence demonstrate beneficial effects in terms of completion of treatment, use of opiate, follow-up abstinence, and compliance with clinic visits. Given that the exposure to treatment during inpatient detoxification is relatively brief and the most important outcome for those in detoxification programs is continued engagement in treatment, motivational interviewing is probably the modality of therapy that best matches the needs of the patient during this interval of treatment. With outpatient detoxification, given the generally longer interval of treatment, motivational interviewing with boosters to support continued motivation for treatment engagement, plus some form of CM, is a sensible approach to treatment.

MEDICATION ADHERENCE

It is estimated that the overall adherence to medication regimens for general medical disorders such as hypertension, diabetes, and asthma is between 40% and 60%, with factors such as low socioeconomic status, lack of family and social supports, or significant psychiatric comorbidity associated with the lowest percentages. It would be surprising if adherence rates for unsupervised addiction medications were higher, and they are not. Thus, it makes sense to propose behavioral interventions that might foster improved medication adherence.

Various factors have been identified that adversely affect patients' adherence to a medication regimen. Some of these factors, both intrinsic to patients and external to them, are co-occurring mental disorders, medication side effects, long waiting times, and inadequate understanding of the proposed treatment. For short-term pharmacotherapeutic interventions, counseling, written materials, and personal phone support may be helpful. In general, interventions that are effective in increasing long-term medication adherence include providing information, counseling, reminders, self-monitoring, reinforcement, family therapy, additional supervision or attention, and higher convenience of care. One of the main objectives of network therapy is to enlist the aid of the patient's supportive others to assist in optimizing patient adherence with medications.

MEDICAL MANAGEMENT

Medical Management (MM) is a manualized intervention that is a composite of several different psychosocial interventions focusing on medication compliance and psychosocial treatment engagement and adherence, all of which were integrated for use in the Project Combining Medications and Behavioral Interventions (COMBINE) study. The MM intervention is semistructured, brief in both duration (about nine sessions) and for each session (about 20 minutes after the initial 40-minute session), suitable for delivery in a primary care environment by a medical professional and, with some adaptation, could focus on medications other than that used in COMBINE and on SUDs other than alcohol dependence. The manual is available for hard copy order or online (http://pubs.niaaa.nih.gov/publications/COMBINE.htm) and is highly recommended by the authors as probably the most clinically useful, evidence-based practice manual available to the addictions clinician. The initial intervention has several components, each of which has evidence supporting its use: Using targeted feedback of medical information and individualized advice, the intervention motivates the patient toward medication adherence and reduction in harmful substance use, educates the patient about the need for medication, and offers referral to support groups such as AA. In evaluating the effect of both psychosocial interventions and medications (acamprosate and naltrexone), it was concluded that this relatively brief, but well-rounded biopsychosocial therapy alone accounted for the bulk of positive treatment outcome whether the patients took active or placebo medications. Thus, MM is a model that the busy clinician can use, whether using medications as part of treatment or not.

The intrinsic themes of MM are educating the patient about the disorder and its specific personal impact; advising the patient about the nature of the treatment, the specific rationale for the medication, and the importance of medication adherence; and recovery support in the form of discussion and advice for implementing medication adherence and alcohol or drug abstinence strategies. The initial MM visit takes place after comprehensive clinical evaluation and lasts 40 to 60 minutes. In many cases in clinical practice, this may be shortly after the initial evaluation, but it is optimal to have an interval within which the clinician can compile the relevant medical information necessary for the initial feedback to the patient. In the case of alcohol problems, these data will typically include blood pressure, liver enzymes, other significant labs (e.g., urine or blood), findings on physical exam, recent alcohol intake (days, amount per day), self-reported alcohol problems, and description of specific alcohol dependence or abuse symptoms. The clinician reviews the results of the evaluation with the patient, first focusing on the medical data and then moving to a review of the symptoms of alcohol dependence that the patient endorsed. The intent is to link the patient's use of alcohol to each biopsychosocial consequence that has been identified. Having done so, and answering his or her questions, the patient is then given information about alcohol dependence in a clear, nonthreatening, and supportive manner, and advised to stop drinking.

Framing the problem as a routine medical one and offering a friendly "can-do" attitude about treatment and recovery support the patient in not feeling impugned by the clinician. The clinician advises the patient about the rationale and use of pharmacotherapy as an important medical strategy in assisting in recovery. The patient is then instructed about how to take the medicine, and potential side effects are discussed in advance to minimize their contribution to nonadherence. The patient's past patterns of medication adherence are evaluated and discussed, so that the patient and the clinician together can elaborate a specific plan to assist the patient in remaining adherent with the regimen. Finally, the patient is given education and encouragement for attendance at support groups such as AA and is given brochures and other written materials that have source information on medications, alcohol dependence, and recovery groups.

In each of the subsequent visits, which typically range from 15 to 25 minutes, the clinician checks the patient in terms of medical status, appropriate laboratory data, and vital signs and weight, and evaluates the blood alcohol concentration. Then the drinking status is asked about, focusing on how the patient coped with not drinking or, in the case of continued drinking, what was the context of use. Other problems, such as an increase in other drug use, are evaluated. Because patients often stop medications when they feel better, it is important that the patient is instructed that even if he or she is doing well in treatment and is abstinent, it is not the time to stop the medication.

- If the desire to drink has reduced but the patient is still drinking, that reduction is reinforced as a first step toward change. A nonjudgmental attitude is the key in supporting that change may occur slowly, that there may be ups and downs along the way, and that continuing attempts are associated with success.
- If it is earlier in treatment, and the patient is continuing to drink but adherent to the medication, it is important that the patient be told that the medication has not yet had sufficient time to work completely.
- The patient who is abstinent but not taking medications as prescribed is given positive feedback for not drinking and the general benefits of abstinence are reinforced. The reasons for the nonadherence (e.g., side effects, forgetting, misinformation) are explored with the patient, and the clinician reinforces that over time the risks of relapse are reduced on the medication. The compliance plan is amended with strategies addressing the reasons for nonadherence.
- The patient, who is nonadherent to medications and is drinking but motivated to stop, is encouraged to engage in treatment more fully.

STRATEGIES TO INTEGRATE MEDICATION TREATMENT AND BEHAVIORAL THERAPIES

In attempting to prevent relapse to substance use, it is sensible to have an approach that places as many barriers as practicable of differing content and strategy in the way of the addict struggling with craving and relapse opportunities. Both physiologic and pharmacologic interventions can be brought to bear in this process. Behavioral therapies have a range of possible targets, including enhancing medication adherence, reducing attrition, addressing co-occurring problems, promoting abstinence, and targeting specific weaknesses of the pharmacologic agent. Pharmacotherapy for substance use disorders can be regarded as biologically enhancing mechanisms of either external or internal control. For example, medications that purportedly affect the endogenous reward system, such as neuromodulators like acamprosate, or inhibitors of substance-induced reward like naltrexone would be considered enhancers of mechanisms of internal control.

A combination of different interventions may have *convergent* or *complementary* effects on the inhibition of relapse; for example, in constructing a combination medication and psychosocial intervention for alcohol dependence, one could consider aligning psychosocial interventions that either augment the control impact of the medication (convergent) or offer a different control locus (complementary).

Convergent Strategies

Naltrexone has been demonstrated in meta-analyses to be a medication effective in the treatment of alcohol dependence with the greatest effect on reduction in relapse to heavy drinking. Therefore, with naltrexone therapy in alcohol dependence, one could use a complementary behavioral intervention strategy that supported noninitiation of drinking or a convergent one that increased the likelihood of a slip remaining a slip rather than becoming a full relapse.

Similarly, the craving reduction aspect of naltrexone could be paired as a convergent strategy with the craving attenuating effects of cognitive behavioral therapy (CBT) or cue extinction therapy. Studies have shown that subjects receiving CBT and naltrexone had significantly fewer relapses to heavy drinking than the groups receiving motivational enhancement therapy (MET) and placebo, and those who did drink had a longer time to subsequent relapses. It is hypothesized that CBT offers specific skills to deal with craving, high-risk situations, and family conflict that may be a more complete adjunct to the effects of naltrexone than those that MET provides. Thus, taken together, it is reasonable to provide CBT and naltrexone in combination as a convergent strategy to decrease relapse to heavy drinking in alcohol-dependent patients.

Complementary Strategies

Behavioral couples therapy (BCT), a well-researched and effective behavioral intervention, can provide elements of increased social support for the patient's efforts to change and contingency for sobriety, whereas disulfiram can assist the maintenance of sobriety through deterrence. As one part of BCT, the couple enters into a disulfiram contract, an agreement that stipulates that the spouse observes and records on a calendar the patient is taking the daily disulfiram dose and the patient and spouse then thank each other for their efforts and refrain from arguments or discussions about the patient's drinking behavior. The structured way of relating around the patient's use of sobriety-supporting medications helps to reduce relationship dysfunction in the couple, which is seen as a major driver of substance use.

In a variant of BCT, contracting around naltrexone was used with opioid-dependent men and the family members they lived with in a randomized 24-week trial of behavioral family contracting and individual therapy versus individual therapy alone. In this example of complementary strategies, behavioral family contracting increased medication adherence and provided social support for continuing opioid abstinence, whereas naltrexone blocked the rewarding effects of opioids.

The interaction of bupropion and CM is another complimentary strategy, where the bupropion may affect subjective negative mood and cognitive symptoms post cocaine withdrawal, and the CM reinforces retention in treatment and rewards abstinence.

CHAPTER

67

Summary Authors: Christopher A. Cavacuiti and Aleksandra Vasic
Jerome E. Schulz • Vern Williams • Joseph E. Galligan

Twelve-Step Programs in Recovery

This discussion of recovery groups emphasizes Alcoholics Anonymous (AA) and its basic philosophy. Other programs—including Al-Anon, Alateen, Narcotics Anonymous, Cocaine Anonymous, and Adult Children of Alcoholics—also are described. While Mutual Help and Twelve-Step programs are led by peers, not health professionals, it is nonetheless important that addiction medicine professionals understand the basic principles of Twelve-Step programs as these programs are an important part of addiction recovery for many individuals.

ALCOHOLICS ANONYMOUS

History
AA began in 1935 when recovering alcoholic Bill Wilson met fellow alcoholic Dr. Bob Smith. During their talks together, Wilson and Smith became convinced that the support of fellow alcoholics could help in recovery.

Overview and Philosophy
The preamble of *AA*, which is often read at the start of meetings, points out many important facts about how AA works:

> *Alcoholics Anonymous is a fellowship of men and women who share their experience, strength and hope with each other that they may solve their common problem and help others to recover from alcoholism. The only requirement for membership is a desire to stop drinking. There are no dues or fees for AA membership; we are self supporting through our own contributions. AA is not allied with any sect, denomination, politics, organization or institution; does not wish to engage in any controversy; neither endorses nor opposes any causes. Our primary purpose is to stay sober and help other alcoholics to achieve sobriety.*

The 12 steps of AA are listed in Table 67.1. The 12 steps have been applied effectively to many other problems in life, such as narcotics, cocaine, gambling, sex, emotions, shopping, and eating disorders.

The 12 traditions (Table 67.2), which were formulated in 1945 after conflicts threatened AA's early existence, are the guidelines that help AA groups survive and function smoothly.

Membership and Structure
More than 105,000 AA groups with >2.0 million members exist in 182 countries worldwide. No individual or group is "in charge." The General Service Office in New York City serves as a clearinghouse for AA information and publications and hosts a Web site www.aa.org, under the direction of the General Service Board, composed of both alcoholics and nonalcoholics. Neither the Office nor the Board has any authority over AA members or groups. AA groups are expected to follow the 12 traditions. Becoming a member in AA is simple: All that is required is to attend a meeting and "have a desire to stop drinking." There is no formal application process.

Meetings
AA holds both open and closed meetings. Anyone may attend an open meeting, whereas closed meetings are restricted to alcoholics with a desire to stop drinking. Meetings usually open with the Serenity Prayer:

> *God grant me the serenity to accept the things I cannot change, the courage to change the things that I can, and the wisdom to know the difference.*

TABLE 67.1	**The 12 Steps of Alcoholics Anonymous**

1. We admitted we were powerless over alcohol—that our lives had become unmanageable.
2. Came to believe that a Power greater than ourselves could restore us to sanity.
3. Made a decision to turn our will and our lives over to the care of God as we understood Him.
4. Made a searching and fearless moral inventory of ourselves.
5. Admitted to God, to ourselves, and to another human being the exact nature of our wrongs.
6. Were entirely ready to have God remove all these defects of character.
7. Humbly asked Him to remove our shortcomings.
8. Made a list of all persons we had harmed, and became willing to make amends to them all.
9. Made direct amends to such people wherever possible, except when to do so would injure them or others.
10. Continued to take personal inventory and when we were wrong promptly admitted it.
11. Sought through prayer and meditation to improve our conscious contact with God as we understood Him, praying only for knowledge of His will for us and the power to carry that out.
12. Having had a spiritual experience (awakening) as the result of these steps, we tried to carry this message to alcoholics, and to practice these principles in all our affairs.

Reprinted with permission from Alcoholics Anonymous World Service, Inc. Permission to reprint this material does not mean that AA has reviewed or approved the contents of this publication, not that AA agrees with the views expressed herein.

At most open meetings, a speaker gives the classic AA talk about "how it was, what happened, and how it is now." Speakers may talk for an hour or less and usually do not use notes or scripts, so that they "talk from the heart and not the head." Closed meetings are usually focused on a step, tradition, topic, or reading from the Big Book or the *Twelve Steps and Twelve Traditions*, the "12 by 12," which describes the important aspects of each of the steps and traditions.

TABLE 67.2	**The 12 Traditions of Alcoholics Anonymous**

1. Our common welfare should come first; personal recovery depends on AA unity.
2. For our group purpose there is but one ultimate authority—a loving God as He may express Himself in our group conscience. Our leaders are but trusted servants; they do not govern.
3. The only requirement for AA membership is a desire to stop drinking.
4. Each group should be autonomous except in matters affecting other groups or AA as a whole.
5. Each group has but one primary purpose—to carry its message to the alcoholic who still suffers.
6. An AA group ought never endorse, finance, or lend the AA name to any related facility or outside enterprise, lest problems of money, property, and prestige divert us from our primary purpose.
7. Every AA group ought to be fully self-supporting, declining outside contributions.
8. Alcoholics Anonymous should remain forever nonprofessional, but our service centers may employ special workers.
9. AA, as such, ought never be organized; but we may create service boards or committees directly responsible to those they serve.
10. Alcoholics Anonymous has no opinion on outside issues; hence the AA name ought never be drawn into public controversy.
11. Our public relations policy is based on attraction rather than promotion; we need always maintain personal anonymity at the level of press, radio, and films.
12. Anonymity is the spiritual foundation of all our traditions, ever reminding us to place principles before personalities.

The Twelve Steps and the Twelve Traditions and a brief excerpt from *Alcoholics Anonymous* are reprinted with permission of Alcoholics Anonymous World Services, Inc. ("AAWS").

Note: Permission to reprint a brief excerpt from *Alcoholics Anonymous*, the Twelve Steps, and Twelve Traditions does not mean that AAWS has reviewed or approved the contents of this publication or that AAWS necessarily agrees with the views expressed herein. AA is a program of recovery from alcoholism *only*—use of the Twelve Steps and the Twelve Traditions in connection with programs and activities that are patterned after AA but address other problems, or in any other non-AA context, does not imply otherwise.

Types of Groups

As AA has grown, many special groups have developed. If patients report that they feel uncomfortable at an AA meeting, a referral to a specialized group may be helpful, such as groups for women, young people, older adults, gays and lesbians, African Americans and other racial/ethnic groups, and groups for professionals such as nurses, physicians, attorneys, and clergy. Nonsmoking meetings are also becoming common. Of note is the International Doctors in AA (IDAA), the AA-based group for physicians, psychologists, dentists, veterinarians, educators, and anyone with a doctoral degree.

Sponsorship

Sponsorship is a core AA concept. A sponsor is typically someone of the same gender who has been in AA for at least a year, who acts as a guide to the 12 Steps and role mentor for a newcomer. Newcomers are asked to call their sponsors whenever they are thinking about drinking or are having problems. Newcomers may also talk with sponsors between meetings by phone or in person to discuss progress. Newcomers are urged to find a sponsor as soon as possible, and groups often appoint temporary sponsors. Sponsorship is often a lifelong relationship. After some time in recovery, a member may be asked to sponsor a new member. In one 10-year follow-up, 91% of alcoholics who became sponsors were in stable sobriety.

Anniversaries

Sobriety anniversaries are important milestones in AA. Many groups give newcomers (or returning members following relapse) a "white chip" (a poker chip) that signifies surrender and a willingness to try something new. The chip can also serve as a reminder not to drink. Members may be given a new chip of different colors at specific month anniversaries, signifying their continuing sobriety and commitment to recovery. Other groups may use medallions instead of chips, which can indicate the number of months or years of sobriety on it. Another important date is the "dry date," which is the first drug- or alcohol-free day. Physicians can show support and interest in their patients' recovery by acknowledging anniversaries and dry dates, and noting them in the patients' medical charts.

Alcoholics Anonymous Slogans

AA has many simple slogans and sayings used frequently at meetings. It may be helpful in communicating with patients who attend AA for health professionals to become familiar with some of these sayings.

"One day at a time" is one of the oldest slogans. This slogan emphasizes a basic AA philosophy—that the alcoholic has to be concerned only with today's recovery, not the overwhelming task of a lifetime of recovery.

"Easy does it" helps recovering alcoholics realize they need to go slowly rather than unrealistically expecting years of problems to be resolved the moment they become sober.

"Let go and let God" emphasizes the spiritual aspect of AA and is related to the Serenity Prayer. For alcoholics, attempts to control their drinking can cause them to overcontrol or overanalyze other areas of their lives.

"Keep it simple" reminds members to focus on priorities: not to drink, to go to meetings, to read the Big Book, to work the Steps, and to reach out to other suffering alcoholics.

HOW is an acronym for **H**onesty, **O**penness, and **W**illingness. AA requests that members be honest with themselves, their higher power, and those around them. Openness helps alcoholics overcome their entrenched attitudes. AA encourages members to be willing to listen to new ideas, to share feelings, and to try uncomfortable, new behaviors.

HALT is an acronym that warns alcoholics not to allow themselves to become too **H**ungry, too **A**ngry, too **L**onely, or too **T**ired, because an excess of any of these can lead to relapse.

NARCOTICS ANONYMOUS

History

In 1953, a group of AA members, who also were addicts, started a group in Sun Valley, California, from which narcotics anonymous (NA) grew, due to the discomfort many narcotic and other drug addicts felt when attending AA meetings. At NA meetings, members are able to share problems related to drugs other than alcohol. The 12 Steps are the same, except for Step 1, which in NA is changed from "alcohol" to "addiction," and the 12th Step, which in NA is changed from "alcoholic" to "addict." By refocusing from a specific substance (alcohol) to addiction, NA was able to include all drugs.

NA's philosophy is that drug addiction is a disease that is progressive and lifelong and involves more than the use of drugs. Recovery is based on abstinence from all mood-altering drugs, including alcohol, and the goal of recovery is to live life so that mood-altering chemicals are no longer needed to experience positive feelings.

Structure and Meetings

The structure of NA is almost identical to that of AA. The basic unit is the "group." A World Service Office is NA's information center. There is a Web site (*www.na.org*). NA meetings are similar to those of AA and generally can be classified as discussion, Step, or speaker meetings. Sponsorship is an integral part of the NA program. AA slogans are also used in NA. NA estimates that there are weekly NA meetings in >127 countries and "hundreds of thousands" of members.

Literature

NA has its own "Big Book," entitled *Narcotics Anonymous*, which outlines the principles of NA and contains the personal stories of early NA members. *Welcome to Narcotics Anonymous* is an excellent NA pamphlet that explains the principles of NA to the interested newcomer. For people in communities without an NA group, the World Service Office provides an *NA Group Starter Kit* that describes how to start an NA group.

COCAINE ANONYMOUS

Cocaine Anonymous (CA) groups exist in many urban areas of the country. CA was founded in Hollywood, California, in 1982 and has a World Service Office in Los Angeles, which hosts a Web site (*www.ca.org*). CA is based on the 12 Steps. Its groups are open to anyone who is suffering from addiction to cocaine.

FAMILY SUPPORT GROUPS

It is estimated that the alcoholism of one individual profoundly affects the lives of an average of four other people (often family). The findings of a Gallup poll support this view: 24% of persons interviewed said that their life had been affected by an alcoholic in some way. As the field of alcohol and drug addiction has become more sophisticated, the concept of addiction as a family disease has emerged. Based on this understanding, Twelve-Step support groups for the family members of alcoholics have grown rapidly. The emphasis is on helping the family member, not the drug- or alcohol-addicted person.

Al-Anon

The oldest family program is Al-Anon, which was started by Lois W (wife of Bill W). Early in the history of AA, wives frequently would accompany their husbands to AA meetings and would get together to talk and support each other. They recognized that they also were affected by alcoholism and the value of applying the 12 Steps to their own lives. In 1951, Lois W and several other spouses started their own Clearinghouse, which later became known as Al-Anon Family Group Headquarters and the World Services Office.

Philosophy

Two main ideas are stressed by Al-Anon: The first is that alcoholism is a disease. The second major Al-Anon principle emphasizes that the program is for the relative or friend, not the alcoholic. The Al-Anon program teaches people to look at what they can do to feel better about themselves and to apply the concept of "tough love" and caringly "letting go" of the alcoholics by stopping "enabling behaviors" and making the alcoholic responsible for the consequences of his or her drinking and alcoholism.

Membership and Meetings

The third tradition of Al-Anon states: "The only requirement for membership is that there be a problem of alcoholism in a relative or friend." There are >24,000 Al-Anon groups in 115 countries.

Alateen

Alateen was started by a California teenager in 1957. Alateen is a part of Al-Anon Family Groups specifically for teenagers and follows the Al-Anon Steps and Traditions. Every Alateen group has an active Al-Anon member who serves as a sponsor, provides guidance and stability to the group, and helps the group focus on the 12 Steps and 12 traditions.

Alateen meetings frequently are held at the same place as Al-Anon meetings but in different rooms. Many schools host Alateen meetings. A referral to Alateen can be made through the local Al-Anon office.

Adult Children of Alcoholics

Adult Children of Alcoholics (ACOA) has developed rapidly over the past 35 years. In the late 1970s, a small group of previous Alateen members started an Al-Anon group called "Hope for Adult Children of Alcoholics."

In early days, some Twelve-Step advocates were concerned that some ACOA groups were placing too much emphasis on therapy over support and relying on confrontation instead of the 12 Steps and 12 traditions. Most ACOA groups are now much more closely aligned to the Twelve-Step model.

THE PHYSICIAN'S ROLE

To be able to help patients with addiction, physicians need to be familiar with recovery support groups, including Twelve-Step programs. Project MATCH showed that trained professionals who support meeting attendance in a positive noncoercive way could improve their patient's acceptance of Twelve-Step programs. There are several potential benefits to referring patients to Twelve-Step programs:

- Meetings are free of cost. (AA's preamble states, "There are no dues or fees for AA membership.")
- Meetings are accessible even in the smallest of towns.
- No records are kept of attendance, and anonymity is assured.
- AA accepts members in various stages of recovery. (The only requirement for membership is a desire to stop drinking.)
- Persons from all racial and ethnic backgrounds and socioeconomic groups are welcome.
- Attending group meetings helps overcome the patient's feelings of "terminal uniqueness" and isolation.
- Groups educate patients about the disease process of addiction and hold out the hope of recovery.
- Group members and sponsors can offer newcomers support as they struggle with recovery issues.
- Groups help members constructively use the time formerly occupied by alcohol and drug use.

Making Referrals to Twelve-Step Programs

In the 1996 triennial AA member survey, only 8% of newcomers reported coming to meetings through a physician's referral. Giving the patient the telephone number with a recommendation to call usually is not successful. In one study, investigators randomly assigned newly diagnosed alcoholics to two types of referral. The first group was told to call AA and go to a meeting. The second group was put in direct contact with an AA member while in the physician's office. None of the first group attended a meeting; the entire second group attended a meeting. AA has a listed phone number in most cities and will provide volunteers to contact the patient and explain AA. Physicians may find it helpful to keep a list of AA members willing to do "Twelfth Step" work.

Other Twelve-Step Groups

Referrals to other Twelve-Step groups are similar to those for AA. In most cities, these groups have listed phone numbers and Web sites. The local AA office may also have information about other Twelve-Step groups.

Making the Referral Work

The following suggestions may assist health professionals in making Twelve-Step referrals work:

1. Know the meetings in your area and refer each patient to a meeting that will meet his or her needs. If they are unhappy with a meeting, help them find another.
2. Help patients make direct contact with members of the group.
3. Give patients a "prescription" to attend a meeting.
4. Tell them what is going to happen at the meeting and how meetings are structured.
5. Encourage them to socialize by arriving early and staying late after the meeting.
6. Encourage patients to pick a *temporary* sponsor early to increase their chances of staying clean and sober. Tell them to pick someone of the same gender with at least 1 year of sobriety. Tell them it is okay to change sponsors if necessary.
7. Talk about their fears and apprehensions about attending a meeting and dispel any inaccurate myths or beliefs they may have.
8. Encourage them to attend frequent meetings, but initially do not push or coerce them.
9. Schedule them for a follow-up visit to discuss their experience at meetings. If they have been attending regularly, encourage them to pick a "home" group and become more active. Being actively involved in the program is a better predictor of a successful outcome than the number of meetings attended.

Potential Problems with Referrals

Patient objections to AA and other mutual help groups typically are expressed in the following ways.

"I don't believe in God." There are many atheists and agnostics in AA. *Alcoholics Anonymous* (the Big Book) contains an entire chapter for agnostics.

"I don't like to talk in a group." There is no requirement to talk at an AA meeting. Members can say they "pass" if they do not wish to talk in front of the group.

"I can't stand all the smoke." Nonsmoking group meetings are available in most geographic areas. In others, large groups divide into smoking and nonsmoking sections.

"I don't have a way to get there." Transportation usually can be arranged for an interested newcomer by calling AA.

"I don't want anyone to know about my drinking." Anonymity is a basic concept of AA.

"I can't stay sober." The third tradition of AA clearly states, "The only requirement for AA membership is a *desire* to stop drinking."

Group Problems

The patient may have difficulty identifying with the members of his or her self-help group. If the patient has attended a meeting several times and still has this feeling, he or she should be referred to a different group. In large metropolitan areas, there are many varieties of groups (involving, e.g., young people, senior citizens, gays/lesbians, etc.).

Twelve-Step "Docs"

Though AA as an organization encourages members to cooperate with their physicians, individual AA members may give patients inappropriate advice about stopping essential drugs, such as methadone, antidepressants, antipsychotics, and other medications. If patients are using these medications, physicians should caution them about this possibility, suggesting that patients do not discuss their medication at meetings.

Gender Orientation

Women sometimes have a problem with AA because of the masculine perspective of most AA literature. However, AA groups now are very receptive to women, who do well in the program. There also are AA meetings exclusively for women.

THE 12 STEPS IN TREATMENT PROGRAMS

Twelve-Step Facilitation (TSF) in the inpatient setting should be considered part of a continuum of care, not a free-standing, one-time intervention. After patients are discharged from a residential treatment, Twelve-Step membership can be a useful adjunct to other aftercare interventions.

Because most inpatients are in early recovery and the treatment programs are relatively brief, most TSF generally focuses only on the first three to five steps.

Summary Authors: Christopher A. Cavacuiti and Aleksandra Vasic
Barbara S. McCrady • J. Scott Tonigan

Recent Research into Twelve-Step Programs

Alcoholics Anonymous (AA) is ubiquitous, both in the United States and around the world. Most addiction professionals have some familiarity with AA and the Twelve-Step principles. However, formal scientific knowledge about AA often is more limited. Since the 1990s, much more research on AA and on treatments designed to facilitate involvement in AA has been conducted. Researchers have used a range of methodologies, including ethnographic methods, epidemiologic studies, longitudinal studies of treatment seeking and non–treatment-seeking populations, controlled clinical trials, and meta-analyses to develop a body of new research about AA that has some coherence, confirms some previous findings and beliefs, and challenges others.

UTILIZATION OF AA

AA members enter the program by a number of routes, including self-referral or referral by family or friends, referral from treatment centers, or through coercion from the legal system, employers, or the social welfare system.

Population Studies
Household surveys of US adults show that approximately 10% of men and 8% of women have attended AA at some point.

Help-Seeking Populations
Studies suggest that over two thirds of both inpatient and outpatient treatment seekers attend AA. Most individuals combine AA with other treatment services. According to one study, 78.5% of individuals with alcohol dependence who sought treatment used AA. The majority (66.8%) of individuals who sought help used AA in combination with other formal treatment. Only 11.7% used AA exclusively.

Mandated Populations
Though there has been considerable controversy about the current criminal justice practice of mandating individuals to attend AA, little research has examined the actual process. Rates of referral to AA vary considerably from jurisdiction to jurisdiction and also vary according to the nature and severity of the alcohol-related offense. Mandating attendance at AA requires the cooperation of the groups that the offender attends. AA has no set procedure for providing the courts with proof of mandated attendance. Some AA groups have the group secretary sign a slip that has been furnished by the court; other groups use different procedures.

Patterns of Utilization of AA
Both cross-sectional and longitudinal studies provide information about patterns of utilization of AA. Studies suggest that individuals who attend AA or other self-help groups make an average of about one visit a week to AA and one visit every 2 weeks to professional treatment. Other researchers have looked at varying levels of AA "affiliation." High-level affiliation (e.g., those individuals who attend frequently, use AA supports regularly, and accept AA core principles including the concept of a Higher Power) tends to be associated with better long-term abstinence outcomes than low-level affiliation, declining affiliation, or no affiliation.

FACTORS ASSOCIATED WITH SUCCESSFUL AFFILIATION WITH AA

Characteristics that are predictive of AA affiliation include:

- Male gender
- More serious alcohol problems
- Greater commitment to abstinence
- More social support to stop drinking
- Less support from and more stress in marriage/intimate relationships
- Fewer psychologic problems such as depression or poor self-esteem
- Use of a more avoidant style for coping with problems
- Having a greater desire to find meaning in life

Most of these findings, however, are supported by only one recent study, with the exception of severity of alcohol dependence and commitment to abstinence, which seem to be stable predictors of affiliation across multiple studies.

The impact of personal spirituality or religiosity on AA affiliation has been examined in a series of recent studies. Current evidence suggests that individuals who are less spiritual/religious are less likely to attend AA and are less likely to be referred to AA by clinicians. However, it is worth noting that AA attendance is associated with better outcomes regardless of religiosity. It is also important for health professionals to know that clinician referral to such groups increased attendance regardless of religiosity.

AA AND POPULATION SUBGROUPS

The issue of AA's relevance of AA to various subgroups continues to be controversial. On the one hand, it has been asserted that because AA was developed by educated, middle-aged, white, Christian, heterosexual males, its relevance to less-educated, young, or older persons, persons of color, non-Christians, gays and lesbians, or women is suspect. On the other hand, it has been argued that AA is a program of recovery for a person with alcohol use disorders and that the common experience of alcoholism supersedes "superficial" individual differences.

Studies examining AA outcomes in special subpopulations are limited though increasing.

Women

In one AA member survey, 35% of respondents were women, which is a rate comparable to the rate of women with alcohol dependence in the general population. Likewise, no substantive gender difference was found in Twelve-Step treatment compliance and engagement in Project MATCH. While many female AA members cite AA a crucial element in staying sober, many women nonetheless express serious reservations about not fitting into a male-dominated AA culture, and half the women in one survey had experienced "thirteenth stepping," in which they felt sexually targeted by men in the program. These experiences may help explain why a greater proportion of women than men dropped out of their self-help groups.

Cultural, Racial, and Ethnic Subgroups

Data in this area remain limited. Very few studies have been done and existing studies have only looked at three ethnic groups—Whites, Hispanics, and African Americans. Hispanics, African Americans, and whites tended to endorse equally the basic tenet of AA that "alcoholism is a disease." All groups also held fairly positive views of AA (meaning that they would be more likely to recommend it than any other treatment modality). While Hispanics and African Americans did not differ from whites in AA attendance at the beginning of the follow-up period, the two groups differed significantly from whites in having less AA attendance later in follow-up. Self-help group participation also was found to improve outcomes for both Hispanics and African Americans.

Age-Specific Groups

There is some hesitancy about involving adolescents in AA because of their developmental status and concerns about exposing them to adults with more entrenched substance use prodisorders. However, several studies have suggested a strong association between AA/NA involvement and abstinence in adolescents, similar to that found in adults.

Dually Diagnosed Individuals

An important implication of the presence of comorbid disorders is the need for prescription medications. The subject of medication use by AA members is a particularly important one, given that the AA literature includes cautions about the use of medication, yet psychoactive medications play a large role in mental health treatment today. About 30% of dually diagnosed individuals said they had been encouraged by an AA member to stop taking their psychiatric medication, and an additional 30% had heard of others who had been encouraged to discontinue use. Of those who were encouraged to stop medication use, about 30% actually stopped.

Gay, Lesbian, Bisexual, and Transgender (GLBT) Experience with AA

Research on the experience of the GLBT community in relation to AA is quite limited. The only research on GLBT populations in AA studied lesbians in recovery. They saw AA as a white, male, heterosexist organization, saw AA as providing tools for recovery rather than a prescription for sobriety, and experienced tension between the strongly individual focus of AA and their perception of the importance of examining issues in a cultural context.

THE EFFECTIVENESS OF AA AND TREATMENTS BASED ON AA

Answering the apparently simple question "Does AA work?" is a challenge. Certainly, AA as an organization has been successful, both in terms of number of groups and the number of people involved around the world. More difficult questions, however, have less clear-cut answers: "Is AA *the most effective* approach to alcohol dependence?" "Is AA involvement *necessary* to successful resolution of alcohol problems?" "Does AA *lead to* better outcomes or is it simply a correlate? "What are the most effective strategies to *engage* individuals with AA?" Research to answer these questions has used several different methodologies: (a) randomized clinical trials (RCTs) comparing AA or treatments designed to involve individuals in AA to different forms of alcoholism treatment, (b) naturalistic studies of treatments designed to engage individuals with AA, (c) studies examining the unique contribution of AA to the prediction of outcomes in clinical and nonclinical samples, and (d) studies of effective approaches to engaging patients in AA.

Randomized Clinical Trials

RCTs in which persons are randomly assigned to different treatment conditions are considered the most rigorous experimental tests of therapeutic effectiveness. Early RCTs compared AA alone to different types of formal treatment. None of these studies found better outcomes for AA than the comparison treatment, but all had serious methodological problems, and all used populations mandated to treatment, so it is difficult to draw specific conclusions about the effectiveness of AA from these studies. In contrast, several important RCTs of treatments based on Twelve-Step principles have been reported over the past several years. The most prominent of these is Project MATCH, designed to study the interactions between specific patient characteristics and one of three structured 12-week outpatient individual treatments: Twelve-Step Facilitation (TSF), motivational enhancement therapy (MET), or cognitive-behavior therapy (CBT). Over 1,500 people with diagnosed alcohol abuse or dependence participated (roughly half being outpatients and the rest aftercare patients).

Though Project MATCH was not designed specifically to study the main effects of the three study treatments, some treatment effects did emerge. During treatment, outpatient participants were more likely to maintain abstinence or moderate drinking if they received CBT or TSF rather than MET. One year after treatment, patients in the three treatments had comparable outcomes in the percentage of days that they were abstinent and the mean number of drinks consumed per day. Patients given TSF treatment were more likely to have maintained continuous abstinence and were less likely to have relapsed to heavy drinking. At the 3-year follow-up, few significant differences among the three treatment conditions were noted, but, as at the 1-year follow-up, patients who had received the TSF treatment were more likely to have been abstinent during the 3 months prior to the 3-year follow-up. Also, compared to patients who had participated in CBT, TSF subjects had a significantly greater percentage of abstinent days during the preceding 3 months. The other noteworthy finding is that 1st year after treatment, patients who had low levels of psychiatric symptoms had more days of abstinence if they had received the TSF rather than the CBT treatment. Aftercare patients with higher levels of alcohol dependence also had better outcomes with TSF. In contrast, patients who were low in alcohol dependence had better outcomes with CBT. At 3 years, outpatients whose social networks were highly supportive of their drinking had better outcomes if they received TSF rather than MET treatment.

Naturalistic Studies of Treatments Based on Twelve-Step Principles

In contrast to RCTs, naturalistic study designs evaluate existing treatment programs and patient populations. Information gleaned from such studies is consistent with that obtained from RCTs. In the largest comparative study of Twelve-Step–based treatments, researchers studied 3,698 male veterans being treated at 15 VA treatment units. The treatment units were classified as Twelve-Step oriented, cognitive-behavioral therapy oriented, or eclectic. Overall, patients showed significant decreases in drinking, symptoms of alcohol dependence, and psychological problems and improved in social functioning. Patients who participated in Twelve-Step–oriented treatment were about 1.5 times as likely to be abstinent as patients whose treatment was cognitive behavioral in orientation. Patients from both types of programs, however, were more likely to be employed than patients whose treatment was more eclectic in focus. In the year after treatment, patients from the Twelve-Step–oriented programs attended significantly more self-help groups than patients from the cognitive-behavioral programs and had significantly fewer outpatient visits and inpatient treatment days, and subsequent costs of treatment were 64% higher for patients who had not participated in a Twelve-Step–oriented treatment unit.

Outcomes

One of the most consistent findings of studies examining the contribution of AA attendance and involvement to the prediction of successful outcomes is that there is a positive correlation between AA attendance and drinking outcomes. Studies of treatment populations in the 1990s found that patients who attended AA were significantly more likely to be abstinent 1 year after treatment than were those who did not attend AA. Similar results have now been reported with drug-dependent patients. Other studies have examined the causal relationship between AA attendance and outcomes and found that AA attendance predicted subsequent abstinence but that abstinence did not predict AA attendance, thus suggesting a causal relationship between AA attendance and positive outcomes of treatment.

Studies of non–treatment-seeking populations have likewise found that AA involvement and attendance were one of a handful of significant predictors of long-term (5 years +) abstinence. AA attendance was significantly though weakly correlated with less alcohol consumption, less intoxication, more abstinence, and fewer symptoms of alcohol dependence or alcohol-related problems.

Summary

The research literature suggests that involvement with AA clearly is associated with positive outcomes and that AA involvement leads to positive outcomes, rather than simply being a correlate. Data simply do not exist to determine whether AA itself is more effective than different kinds of treatment, but an accumulating body of literature suggests that treatment programs (inpatient and outpatient) based on Twelve-Step principles may be more successful in effecting total abstinence over time and may be more cost-effective than other treatment models.

MECHANISMS OF CHANGE IN AA

Investigators are now seeking to understand why AA is beneficial. This line of research involves three aims:

1. To identify which of the "active ingredients" of AA result in behavior change (possible active ingredients include sponsorship, reading core AA literature, and AA Twelve-Step work and the frequency and nature of social support offered through AA participation)
2. To determine which elements of behavior and cognition these active ingredients influence
3. To determine the probability that these cognitive and behavioral changes will result in reduced drinking

Investigators have focused most directly on identifying the active ingredients of AA. Historically, the AA meeting has been considered the "dose," and frequency of attendance indicated the intensity of the dose. More recent studies have distinguished AA *attendance* from AA *involvement*, which included, in addition to attendance, the degree of involvement with various aspects of AA—such as participation during meetings, having a sponsor, leading meetings, or doing Twelve-Step work. They reported that AA involvement and attendance were moderately correlated; however, involvement, not attendance, correlated with post-treatment alcohol consumption.

In terms of specific AA-prescribed behaviors, a survey of AA members' views of the relative importance of different aspects of the AA program found that working the Steps, having a sponsor, telling their story at a meeting, and daily meditations were seen as most important. Research tends to confirm the importance of several of these AA-related behaviors for abstinence. Being an AA sponsor can lead to a significant reduction in relapse rates. Another investigation looking at different types of substance use disorders found that of seven specific AA behaviors, only having a sponsor predicted positive outcome across substance abuse categories. Another study reported that sponsorship and frequency of AA attendance were positively associated.

Another body of research has focused on the benefits of social support and network support for abstinence provided through AA participation. In a study of male inpatient substance abusers, results showed that increased group participation predicted both better quality of general friendship and less support of substance use by friends at follow-up. Individuals involved significantly in Twelve-Step groups actually increased the size of their friendship networks by an average of 16%; those *not* significantly involved in Twelve-Step groups showed no change in the size of their friendship networks. The greater increase in social network size was attributable to the fact that those significantly more involved in Twelve-Step groups increased their numbers of friends in the programs and not because those less involved with Twelve-Step groups lost friends.

Given the importance of social network variables in alcohol treatment outcome in general and AA in particular, recent studies have focused on the role formal treatment can play in facilitating AA-related social network benefit. One treatment was designed to enhance network support through either AA or other social resources such as families and social activities. The network support therapy significantly increased AA involvement and more general support for abstinence from members of their social network. Similar to other studies, both network support and AA involvement correlated positively with treatment outcomes.

WHAT DO THE AA ACTIVE INGREDIENTS INFLUENCE?

Spirituality

The core AA literature specifically posits that as a result of working the Twelve Steps one will have a spiritual awakening, with benefits including sobriety and increased sense of well-being. In cross-sectional and longitudinal studies that have employed dozens of different psychometrically validated measures of spirituality and religiosity, two findings have been reported consistently: (a) AA program and fellowship behaviors are significantly and positively associated with measures of spirituality and religiosity and (b) the endorsement of spiritual and religious practices increases in amplitude with longer periods of AA affiliation.

Evidence is mixed about the relative importance of spiritual/religious changes for explaining increased abstinence among AA members. Spirituality may offer secondary benefit. Specifically, one study found that, though neither spiritual beliefs nor believing in addiction as a disease predicted drug use outcomes, both predicted NA attendance, which was related to reduced drug use. Evidence indicates that self-reported atheists are less likely to attend Twelve-Step programs, but those atheists who do affiliate report similar rates of benefit at 1- and 3-year follow-ups relative to self-described spiritual and religious AA members.

Cognitive Shifts

Investigations of the types of cognitive and behavioral processes used by AA members to facilitate change find that current members of AA were more likely to use helping relationships, stimulus control ("people, places, and things"), and behavioral management strategies to maintain sobriety. Those who attended more frequently used more behavioral processes of change.

Several studies have investigated "AA-specific" cognitive mechanisms in Twelve-Step therapy, arguably replicating the mechanisms of change in community-based AA. In general, cognitive shifts congruent with AA ideology can be successfully mobilized in Twelve-Step therapy, but the relative importance of these shifts is mixed, at best, in accounting for increased abstinence.

Summary

AA-related benefit occurs through the interplay of social interactions, prescribed behaviors, and mobilized psychological processes. There is strong evidence that social support for abstinence is an important element accounting for Twelve-Step–related benefit. Consistent support is also found for the benefit of two AA-prescribed behaviors: AA meeting attendance and engagement in the program by having, and being, an AA sponsor. Because sponsorship is a vital prerequisite for working the 12 Steps, an important outstanding question is whether sponsorship per se predicts positive outcome or, alternatively, whether being guided through the 12 Steps by a sponsor accounts for AA-related benefit. Contrary to conventional wisdom, cognitive shifts that appear to account for AA-related benefit, such as increased commitment to abstinence or increased self-efficacy, are not AA specific.

FUTURE DIRECTIONS

AA as a Single Entity

The program of AA is relatively consistent across groups, but evidence suggests that there is substantial variation in the practice of the AA program. Typically, AA-focused research treats AA as a monolithic entity. This research practice makes several assumptions that may not be valid:

1. The "dose" of AA is fixed and invariant across meetings regardless of meeting type (e.g., speaker, closed, open discussion), size, and membership characteristics.
2. AA group social dynamics do not influence the generation, transmission, or reception of the "dose" of AA.
3. AA social context itself does not account for drinking outcome, directly or indirectly.
4. AA social context and individual characteristics do not interact in accounting for sustaining AA membership or drinking outcome.
5. The importance of AA social context in accounting for AA-related benefit is temporally invariant (e.g., "unit benefit" of one AA meeting was the same for AA members regardless of length of membership).

Though these assumptions are useful in facilitating prospective demonstrations of general short- and long-term AA-related benefit, they may also hinder the development of AA-related research and the application of evidence-based findings in clinical settings.

Understanding Utilization of and Affiliation with AA

Many studies indicate that the majority of individuals who try AA do not continue or affiliate. Despite research to understand what drives initial and sustained involvement with AA, we still have a very incomplete picture of why some individuals affiliate with AA while others do not. Given that there are few individual characteristics that are consistent predictors of AA involvement and affiliation, research needs to look elsewhere. One untapped area of research is the possibility of key events or experiences that define affiliation or disaffiliation with AA. Qualitative and narrative analysis methodologies could be brought to bear in understanding these processes.

Population Subgroups

The population of the United States is racially and ethnically diverse but that diversity is not well represented in AA. The research literature provides little information about the experience, utilization, and barriers to use of AA for different groups, in particular young people, older adults, gays and lesbians, persons of color, and persons mandated to attend AA. Culturally informed research methodologies, such as community-based participatory research, may be needed to access populations with limited involvement with AA.

Effectiveness of AA

RCTs of AA as a stand-alone program of recovery (separate from treatment) are simply not being conducted. The barriers to conducting such research are considerable, and it may be appropriate to use methodologies other than RCTs to study the effectiveness of AA. However, as AA is the most recommended program of recovery by both lay persons and professionals, it would be useful to have a stronger empirical base to draw upon in making a decision to refer a patient to AA and/or some form of professional treatment.

CONCLUSION

This chapter has reviewed a substantial body of research on AA and other Twelve-Step groups. AA is used widely in the United States, and 6% to 10% of the population has attended an AA meeting, with that rate doubling or tripling among those with drinking problems. Initially, individuals become actively involved in AA for several months, but there is much variability in patterns of affiliation, with some individuals becoming increasingly committed over time, while others gradually slip away. Longer term involvement is less common, but those who stay with AA for more than a year are very likely to continue their involvement for many years. AA is such a heterogeneous organization that it is difficult to draw generalizations about who is most or least likely to affiliate. Concerns about aspects of the AA program have been documented, particularly among women, but it may be that special interest groups within AA and modifications of the program at the local level can effectively address these concerns. Overall, data suggest that individuals who have more severe problems, more concern about their drinking, a greater commitment to staying abstinent, less support from a spouse, a social network supportive of drinking, a history of turning to others for support, and a greater desire to find meaning in their lives may be most likely to affiliate with AA. Substantial research on mechanisms of change and outcomes associated with AA involvement has been reported. Overall, the more active AA members are in the program, the better are their outcomes in terms of reduced drinking, improved psychologic functioning, and better social support, which seems at least partially attributable to the clear cognitive and behavioral changes that members make and to improved social supports. With more sophisticated and creative research, more varied populations of problem drinkers are being examined, including subpopulations that differ in age, race/ethnicity, and the presence of comorbid psychiatric disorders. Diverse and complementary methodologies have contributed to a richer, data-based understanding of AA, which should continue to expand over the next decade.

CHAPTER 69

Summary Author: Christopher A. Cavacuiti and Aleksandra Vasic
Marc Galanter

Spirituality in the Recovery Process

WHAT IS SPIRITUALITY?

Spirituality broadly consists of the nonmaterial issues that give a person meaning and purpose in life. These can be found in a person's religious orientation but can also be seen in his or her ethnic heritage, altruism, humanism, or naturalism. Spirituality infuses some alternative medical therapies that are not grounded in empirical science but have gained popularity because they address symptoms such as anxiety or depression. Given the prominence of Alcoholics Anonymous and related Twelve-Step groups, it can play an important role in the rehabilitation of substance-dependent people.

The issue of spirituality is prominent within contemporary culture: in a sampling of American adults, 95% of respondents reply positively when asked whether they believe in God or a universal spirit.

UNDERSTANDING THE PHENOMENON

Constructs such as spirituality, personality, culture, and cognition are not observed directly but inferred from observations of their component dimensions. Such constructs are typically multidimensional and can only be understood from the vantage point of more than one discipline. As such, spirituality should be examined from perspectives as diverse as physiology, psychology, and cross-cultural studies.

Some researchers have drawn distinctions between the two concepts of spirituality and religiosity. The fellowship of Alcoholics Anonymous is often described as a spiritual program for living but one in which there is no dogma, theology, or creed to be learned, which is considered to be associated more with religion than with spirituality. When considered from the perspective of its role in organized religion, the nature of spirituality in a given society is culture-bound.

AA AS A SPIRITUAL RECOVERY MOVEMENT

How does spirituality relate to recovery from addiction? There is a parallel between the way in which attitudes are transformed in intensely zealous groups and the way in which the denial of illness and the self-defeating behaviors of alcoholics and drug addicts may be reversed through induction into AA.

AA can be considered as a highly successful example of a spiritual recovery movement, and all such movements have three primary characteristics. They (a) claim to provide relief from disease, (b) operate outside the modalities of established empirical medicine, and (c) ascribe their effectiveness to higher metaphysical powers. The appeal of such movements in the contemporary period is due in part to the fact that physicians tend not to attend to the spiritual or emotional concerns of their patients.

Clearly, the attitudes and behavioral norms that AA espouses are much more in conformity with the values of the larger culture than those of zealous religious sects. The expectation of avoiding drunkenness in AA is also a cultural norm. People who are highly distressed over the consequences of their addiction are therefore candidates to respond to the strong ideological orientation of AA toward recovery and are strongly reinforced by the relief produced by affiliation with the group's ideology and behavioral norms, all related to abstinence and a spiritually grounded lifestyle. AA generates distress in its members by pressing them to give up their addictive behaviors, but the distress associated with this conflict is relieved if they maintain affiliation to the group.

SPIRITUALITY AS A PSYCHOLOGICAL CONSTRUCT

Two empirically grounded perspectives have played a role in how we conceptualize recovery. One is derived from a model of psychopathology modeled on the work of Emil Kraeplin, who framed what became the basis of the contemporary medical model for mental disorders, categorizing disease entities diagnosed on the basis of explicit and discrete symptoms. This approach is evident in the development of criteria for substance use disorders employed in recent editions of the *Diagnostic and Statistical Manual of Mental Disorders*. From this perspective, a state of remission, or *recovery* in rehabilitation circles, can take place with the resolution of the specific symptoms listed as diagnostic criteria.

A second perspective on recovery derives from behavioral psychology, whose model of stimulus-response sequences has led to the ordering of experience around discrete phenomena that can be observed by a researcher or clinician. From this perspective, recovery is defined in terms of observable, measurable responses to substance use. Both the biomedical and behaviorist perspectives are well suited to the study of psychopathology and have allowed the addiction field to study addiction as a disorder, one that is compatible with the use of experimental controls. Both approaches have yielded many advances in addiction treatment.

Another perspective, however, is defined on the basis of addicts' reports of their own subjective experience. This approach is inherent in the psychology of Carl Jung who had a direct influence on Bill W's framing of the Alcoholics Anonymous ethos. Others such as William James (often described as the father of American psychology) and Viktor Frankl (who wrote *Man's Search for Meaning*) also discussed mental phenomena in terms of subjectively experienced mystical or spiritual experience. Research on this third approach would typically rely on self-report scales. In this respect, recovery can be seen as a process whereby an abstinent addicted person moves toward a positive adaptation in life. This movement can take place with varying degrees of success, depending on the person's own innate capacities and the circumstances in which he or she finds himself or herself.

SPIRITUALLY GROUNDED RECOVERY IN AA

The AA program of recovery is mentioned in numerous places in the Big Book, *Alcoholics Anonymous*, and is associated with such terms as *spiritual experience* and *spiritual awakening* and with working AA's 12 Steps. Four of the Steps include the word God, which is qualified "as we understood Him" and also as "a Power greater than ourselves." Moreover, the text points out that even "Agnostics…had to face the fact that we must find a spiritual basis for life" in order to achieve recovery, which shows the AA's distinction between spirituality and theistic religion. In a 5-year follow-up of recovering cocaine-dependent patients, the strength derived from religion and spirituality significantly distinguished those who had a highly favorable outcome from those who did not. Additionally, attendance at religious services distinguished significantly between criminal justice clients referred for substance abuse treatment who had a positive outcome and those who did not.

In the clinical context, recovery is based on a person's behavioral and physiologic status, which can be assessed by recourse to criteria employed in the DSM. Some of these criteria are also embodied in the Addiction Severity Index, which is employed widely in research to evaluate recovery. These items can be evaluated relatively easily, as they are based on observable behavior or symptoms described by the patient, family member, or clinician. A spiritually grounded and more subjective definition of recovery can be useful as well, based on quality of life issues, which can include the following criteria:

- Loss of sense of purpose due to excessive substance use
- A feeling of inadequate social support because of one's addiction
- Continued use of a substance while experiencing moral qualms over its consumption
- Loss of the will to resist temptation when the substance is available

The DSM also stipulates "course specifiers" of remission, such as "on agonist therapy" and "in a controlled environment." To these could be added, "fully engaged in a program of Twelve-Step recovery," which would be equally explanatory to many clinicians. But are spiritually grounded criteria measurable? Recently, methodologies that have been developed and validated could be used to assess outcome based on such subjectively experienced criteria and can be used to describe spiritually related states:

A. Affective state

1. A sense of well-being, measured by the General Well-Being Schedule or the Subjective Happiness Scale
2. Contentment with one's life circumstances, measured by the Satisfaction with Life Scale

3. Positive affect, assessed with the Positive and Negative Affect Schedule, dealing with both variables as separate dimensions rather than bipolar ends of the same scale

4. Feelings of support, employing a scale for Perceived Social Support

B. Existential variables: Meaningfulness in one's life; assessed by the Purpose in Life Test

C. Flow (the experience associated with engaging one's highest strengths and talents to meet achievable challenges), as measured by Experience Sampling or the Flow Scale

D. Spirituality: The Spirituality Self-Rating Scale, which applies to both substance-abusing and non–substance-abusing populations, as well as other such scales

E. Personality Assessment: The Classification of Strengths, a series of characteristics based on categories of moral excellence drawn from observations across different cultures

F. AA Involvement: Measures of the degree of affiliation and commitment to the AA fellowship

A methodology for defining recovery based on measurements such as these may not have the same appeal to biomedically oriented clinicians as does the conventional symptom-based approach, as these measurements are based on self-report of the person's subjective state.

AA IN THE PROFESSIONAL CONTEXT

The spiritually oriented Twelve-Step approach has been integrated into professional treatment in some settings wherein it serves as the overriding philosophy of an entire program, or in others, where it is one aspect of a multimodal eclectic approach. The Minnesota Model for treatment, typically located in an isolated institutional setting, involves an intensive inpatient stay during which a primary goal of treatment is to acculturate patients to acceptance of the philosophy of AA and to continue with AA attendance after discharge.

This approach has been criticized as dogmatic because of its sole reliance on the Twelve-Step approach. The outcome of this model, however, has been shown to yield positive results in a survey of patients discharged from one center, but random assignment of patients treated in Minnesota Model facilities with those treated by means of an alternative approach is needed. In one study of patients in a psychiatric facility that integrates Twelve-Step groups for the treatment of dual diagnosis of mental illness and substance abuse, patients ranked spiritual issues such as belief in God and inner peace higher than tangible benefits such as social service support and outpatient treatment. Clearly such an inspirational approach benefits patients who have become degraded by stigmatization owing to their psychiatric disorders.

In summary, spirituality is a matter of personal meaning that is widely accepted. It is also central to the recovery process from addiction for many AA members. The fellowship of AA, in fact, can be considered a movement developed in relation to people's spiritual needs.

CHAPTER

70

Summary Author: Agnes Kwasnicka
Richard Saitz

Medical and Surgical Complications of Addiction

Medical care for acute and chronic conditions in persons with addictive disorders can be fragmented and inefficient, and opportunities for preventive health care are often missed. In addition to the direct effects of intoxication, overdose, and withdrawal, abused substances can affect every body system. Individuals with substance use disorders are also at risk of health consequences that are not directly related to use of the substance as a result of high-risk behaviors that are associated with these disorders. Yet, regular health care can lead to improved health for persons with addictive disorders. This section addresses the wide range of health consequences of alcohol and other drug use, focusing on the most common and most serious illnesses, mainly by organ system. Preventive care issues specific to persons with addictive disorders are presented because any health care contact is an opportunity for persons with addictive disorders or dependence to obtain such care. Preventive care interventions for the general population should also be offered to these patients but these are beyond the scope of this text and can be found elsewhere (see below).

ROUTINE AND PREVENTIVE CARE

Over the past several decades, preventive care has evolved from "one-size-fits-all" approach in which doing more tests was believed to be indicative of better care to what are now evidence-based, targeted evaluations based on age and other risk factors. The approach to routine and preventative care of patients with substance use disorders presented here follows a targeted strategy based on the known effectiveness of interventions. Ongoing updates of recommendations by the U.S. Preventive Services Task Force can be accessed at *http://www.ahrq.gov/clinic/uspstfix.htm*.

Medical History

The medical history in a person with addiction should include, in addition to a thorough alcohol and drug use history, the categories of assessment employed for all patients (including, but not limited to, *current complaints, present illness, allergies, systems review, medication, past medical and surgical history, social and family history*). Questions regarding past history should address hospitalizations and any medical conditions that might be related to substance use and might not be volunteered by the patient without direct questioning. For persons with addictive disorders, screening for depression and anxiety, assessment of sexual practices, intention to conceive a child, and behavior that might lead to injury (including being alert for signs of interpersonal violence) are particularly important. Such patients should be asked specifically about substance use before operating a motor vehicle, riding with intoxicated drivers, sex without contraception, and sex while intoxicated. In an asymptomatic person with an addictive disorder, items relevant to preventive care can become a greater focus. Additional history is needed to determine if the patient belongs to a high-risk group that would indicate additional preventive interventions. For example, a history of folate deficiency in patients with alcohol use disorders is of particular importance for women of childbearing age due to the associated risk of fetal neural tube defects.

Physical Examination

System	Recommended maneuvers	Clinical clues
Vital signs and measurements	Height, weight, blood pressure, and body mass index	• Assess nutritional status
Skin	Look for signs of injection drug use, tobacco and alcohol use	• Tobacco users may have stained fingers • Palmar erythema may be seen with alcohol dependence • Track marks suggest injection
Head, eyes, ears, nose, and throat	Focus on oral cavity examination	• Look for premalignant and malignant lesions in smokers and alcohol, as these substances have synergistic carcinogenic effects • Extreme tooth decay is associated with methamphetamine use
Chest/ cardiovascular	Cardiac auscultation	• Cardiac murmurs may be evidence of valvular damage from injection drug use
Abdominal	Liver exam	• Small hard liver may indicate cirrhosis • Enlarged liver may indicate chronic viral or alcohol-related hepatitis
Breast examination	Preventive screening evidence for benefit is absent until age 40	• Risk of breast cancer is increased by alcohol consumption
Male genital	Consider testicular examination for young men, rectal and prostate examinations	• Risk of prostate and colorectal cancer may be increased by alcohol consumption
Female genital	Consider pelvic examination with testing for sexually transmitted diseases and cervical cancer screening	• Addicted persons are at risk of sexually transmitted diseases
Lymph node	Examine cervical, axillary, supra-clavicular, and inguinal lymph node regions for lymphadenopathy	• Lymphadenopathy may suggest tuberculosis, chancroid, syphilis, or HIV • Supraclavicular nodes can be the presenting sign of lung cancer in tobacco users

Tests

Reasonable, inexpensive tests that all patients should undergo at least once include

- Complete blood count
- Blood sugar
- Liver enzymes
- Serum creatinine and urinalysis (to assess for the presence of silent renal disease)

Screening for hypercholesterolemia for *cardiovascular risk* assessment can be done by the addiction specialist or the family physician. Of particular importance in heavy drinkers is identifying hypertriglyceridemia, which is associated with and can be a cause of pancreatitis. An unsuspected anemia or pancytopenia can be found in persons with alcohol use disorders or HIV.

Sexually Transmitted Diseases Persons with addictive disorders who have been sexually active or who use injection drugs should be screened routinely for sexually transmitted diseases. Test for syphilis, HIV, and chlamydia (using the ligase chain reaction in a urine or cervical specimen). The serologic test for syphilis (rapid plasma reagin or Venereal Disease Research Laboratory) frequently is falsely positive in injection drug users; thus, should be confirmed by a treponemal test such as the microhemagglutination test for *Treponema pallidum* or the fluorescent treponemal antibody tests.

Other Infectious Diseases Persons with alcohol and other drug use disorders without past known *tuberculosis* should be screened for asymptomatic infection (provided a previous test result is not known to have been positive). If screening is positive and provided the radiograph is not consistent with active tuberculosis, prophylactic pharmacotherapy should be considered regardless of age.

As screening tests for chronic hepatitis and cirrhosis, users of injection drugs, those with alcohol abuse, and persons with multiple sexual partners or high-risk sexual activity should also have to take following tests:

- International normalized ratio (INR)
- Serum bilirubin
- Transaminases (aspartate aminotransferase [AST] and alanine aminotransferase [ALT])
- Serum albumin
- Alkaline phosphatase

If any of the first three are abnormal, perform tests for hepatitis B (surface antigen and core antibody) and hepatitis C antibody. Previously vaccinated individuals should have the antisurface hepatitis B antibody determined to assess current immunoprotection. Consider testing for immunity to hepatitis A in injection drug users, those who practice anal intercourse and who are not from endemic areas.

Cancer Screening and Testing for Other Conditions Smokers are at higher risk of cervical cancer; thus, cervical cytology (Papanicolaou smears) should be performed to detect the premalignant lesions of cervical cancer. Bone mineral density (BMD) testing is of particular importance for persons with inadequate calcium intake, excessive alcohol use, physical inactivity, smoking, and a family history of osteoporosis. Persons with addictive disorders can have poor diets, little sun exposure, and minimal intake of milk products; screening for vitamin D deficiency with a 25-hydroxyvitamin D should be considered.

Preventive Counseling

In addition to specific counseling related to addiction, preventive health counseling for these patients should include that which is provided to all patients. A few general recommendations may be particularly important for patients with substance use disorders as a result of their lifestyle. These include

- Healthy dietary habits
- Safer sexual practices
- Contraceptive options for women of childbearing age and their partners
- Gun safety for those persons who store or carry weapons
- Seat belt and helmet use
- Safe lifting to prevent low-back injury

Counseling specific to the addiction patient:

- Injection drug users should be educated about sterile injection practices
- Encourage engaging in regular primary and preventive health care with a primary care physician in addition to their addiction specialty care
- Linkage to mental health care should be offered when appropriate

Immunizations

Immunizations for adults should include

Vaccine	Specific indication for substance users
Tetanus, diphtheria, and acellular pertussis (TDaP)	Injection drug users can expose themselves to tetanus
Hepatitis B	Injection drug users, persons with hepatitis C, sexually active individuals not in long-term monogamous relationships
Hepatitis A	With any chronic liver disease and injection drug users
Pneumococcal	Sixty-five years and older and those with chronic cardiopulmonary disease and reactive airway diseases—more common in smokers and users of inhaled drugs; alcoholism is a specific recognized indication for the vaccine
Influenza	Particularly for those living in group settings

Other recommended vaccines including varicella, zoster, and human papilloma virus can be considered on an individual basis.

When childhood vaccinations are unknown, consideration should be given to a primary series for routine vaccination. Many adults will have immunity to these diseases but, if unknown, testing is warranted, given that many persons with addictive disorders may be in group living situations, sometimes with children and young adults, in which measles and varicella infections can spread easily.

Chemoprophylaxis

Aspirin

- The benefits of aspirin for cardiovascular protection may not outweigh the risks of serious central nervous system or gastrointestinal bleeding in people with alcohol use disorders without symptoms of coronary disease.

Folate

- As folate deficiency is not uncommon in patients with alcohol use disorder, 400 mcg daily for women of childbearing age to prevent fetal neural tube defects should be emphasized.

Other Vitamins and Minerals

- Recommend daily multivitamin for people with alcohol use disorders and those with deficient diets as they are at risk of thiamine, vitamin D, pyridoxine, niacin, riboflavin, zinc, and folic acid deficiency.
- In people with alcohol use disorders, encourage use of foods with a high magnesium content (such as peanuts) or a magnesium supplement (magnesium oxide tablets or magnesium hydroxide-containing antacids) to prevent magnesium deficiency, which is common in this population.
- Consider vitamin K if the INR is known to be elevated, though generally the INR elevation in addicted persons will be due to liver disease and not to vitamin deficiency.

Osteoporosis

- Risks for osteoporosis are higher in people with alcohol use disorders and other addicted persons.
- The interaction between estrogen and alcohol on breast cancer is not clear, and the side effects of the hormonal medications in people who drink heavily and those with liver disease are not well characterized.

CARE DURING HOSPITALIZATION

Withdrawal

When a history of alcohol dependence and recent use is obtained, withdrawal should be anticipated. Persons not yet symptomatic with withdrawal but with past alcohol-related seizures or concomitant acute medical or surgical conditions (which increase the risk of withdrawal) should be treated with adequate doses of a benzodiazepine to prevent convulsions or delirium. Symptom-triggered therapy results in best outcomes. The use of standardized withdrawal scales generally is encouraged, but their lack of specificity requires that the information they provide be considered in the context of the coexisting medical illness, especially in the hospitalized patient when symptoms of withdrawal may not be distinguishable from the underlying medical condition.

Similarly, opiate and other drug withdrawal should be identified and managed pharmacologically, both for patient comfort and to prevent complications of the medical disorder for which the patient was hospitalized. Patients who already are in treatment for opiate or long-acting sedative dependence should have their prescribed treatment continued (e.g., methadone maintenance). At hospital admission, when deciding on the best treatment for the patient not already in opioid replacement treatment, the patient's disposition at discharge should be anticipated. If the patient plans to abstain from the substance at hospital discharge, the substituted opioid can be tapered if symptoms allow. Alternatively, a dose sufficient to avoid withdrawal can be maintained during the hospitalization for those who intend to continue drug use or to enter a maintenance treatment program.

In addition to providing comfort and helping to prevent the more serious complications of withdrawal, specific treatment of withdrawal controls the autonomic symptoms that can worsen a patient's medical condition and helps the patient cooperate with treatment for the medical condition that prompted hospitalization.

Pain

Pain management often becomes an issue during medical hospitalization of addicted patients due to fear that providing pain control with opioids when a patient is addicted to them will worsen addiction. Patients with addictive disorders, including those on opioid replacement treatment, usually are very tolerant to the substance they use; thus, pain control can be achieved only with substantially higher doses of opioids. Once a dose is determined, pain medications should be given on a regular schedule rather than as needed, to avoid making the patient demand medication to relieve uncontrolled symptoms.

Comorbidities

Finally, while patients are hospitalized, several comorbidities should be considered. As psychiatric comorbidity is common attention to behavioral issues is important. Patients should be assured that their medical, psychiatric, and addiction-related symptoms and pain will be attended to. Discussing withdrawal and pain treatment regimens can help allay their fears.

Screening for coexisting medical disorders (such as HIV, hepatitis, and tuberculosis) during a medical hospitalization should be considered because the acute care setting may provide the only medical care received by the patient. Consideration should be given to the patient's readiness to hear and handle the results and to arranging follow-up medical care for the condition.

MEDICAL CONSEQUENCES OF ALCOHOL, TOBACCO, AND OTHER DRUG USE

Medical consequences of addiction may be due to drug-specific effects, methods of administration, contaminants in or vehicles for drugs used, behavioral habits associated with substance use, or common comorbidities (Table 70.1).

Alcohol

Women are more susceptible to many of the effects of alcohol at lower doses because of less gastric mucosal metabolism of alcohol and lower body weights on average.

Withdrawal, Seizures, and Delirium Tremens Though the direct medical consequences of alcohol withdrawal are covered in detail elsewhere in this book, mention is made here because they are common, often are managed in acute care general medical hospitals, and can lead to death. Benzodiazepines are the only medications proven to ameliorate symptoms of withdrawal, to decrease the risk of seizures and delirium and to speed achievement of a calm but awake state in patients experiencing delirium. Seizures, when they occur, almost always resolve spontaneously. They can recur and generally do so within 6 hours of the first seizure. Benzodiazepines prevent further seizures and progression to *delirium tremens* (DTs). Phenytoin and other anticonvulsants are not indicated unless there is another cause or suspected cause for the seizures in addition to alcohol. DTs should be managed in a setting where frequent and intensive monitoring is possible because of the risk of death from the condition and its treatment. Other medications can be used as adjunctive therapies include β-blockers for tachycardia, clonidine for hypertension, and haloperidol for psychosis or agitation, when these signs and symptoms fail to respond to benzodiazepines. The tachycardia can complicate underlying medical conditions such as coronary artery disease by precipitating angina or myocardial infarction.

Neurologic Consequences Alcohol intoxication can lead to head trauma, but signs and symptoms of intracranial hemorrhage—particularly subdural hematoma—can be confused with intoxication. In addition, heavy drinking (in men one to two or more drinks a day and in women more than one drink per day) increases the risk for ischemic and hemorrhagic stroke. Imaging of the brain is indicated when there are signs of significant head trauma and abnormal mental status, when focal neurologic deficits are present, or when neurologic symptoms do not resolve with declining alcohol levels. Alcohol can lower the seizure threshold in epileptics, and seizures may be the presenting sign of an intracranial hemorrhage.

Cognitive impairment may be caused acutely by Wernicke-Korsakoff disease because of thiamine deficiency, presenting with confusion, ataxia, or nystagmus. Parenteral thiamine, 100 mg administered before glucose, is the initial treatment. Chronically, Wernicke-Korsakoff disease can develop into Korsakoff syndrome, a memory impairment classically characterized by confabulation. More commonly, chronic alcohol dependence is associated with a nonspecific dementia. Alcoholic cerebellar dysfunction results in ataxia and incoordination and is often is irreversible.

People with alcohol dependence can suffer from peripheral neuropathy, usually from vitamin deficiency, pressure on a nerve, or ethanol toxicity. The classic presentation of alcoholic polyneuropathy is of sensory disturbance, including burning, pain, and numbness in a stocking glove distribution.

| **TABLE 70.1** | **Selected Medical Disorders Related to Alcohol and Other Drug Use** |

Cardiovascular

Alcohol: Cardiomyopathy, atrial fibrillation (holiday heart), hypertension, dysrhythmia, masks angina symptoms, coronary artery spasm, myocardial ischemia, high-output states, coronary artery disease, sudden death

Cocaine: Hypertension, myocardial infarction, angina, chest pain, supraventricular tachycardia, ventricular dysrhythmias, cardiomyopathy, cardiovascular collapse from bodypacking rupture, moyamoya vasculopathy, left ventricular hypertrophy, myocarditis, sudden death, aortic dissection

Tobacco: Atherosclerosis, stroke, myocardial infarction, peripheral vascular disease, cor pulmonale, erectile dysfunction, worse control of hypertension, angina, dysrhythmia

Infection: Endocarditis, septic thrombophlebitis

Cancer

Alcohol: Aerodigestive (lip, oral cavity, tongue, pharynx, larynx, esophagus, stomach, colon), breast, hepatocellular and bile duct cancers

Tobacco: Oral cavity, larynx, lung, cervix, esophagus, pancreas, kidney, stomach, bladder

Injection or high-risk sexual behavior: Hepatocellular carcinoma related to hepatitis C

Endocrine/Reproductive

Alcohol: Hypoglycemia and hyperglycemia, diabetes, ketoacidosis, hypertriglyceridemia, hyperuricemia and gout, testicular atrophy, gynecomastia, hypocalcemia and hypomagnesemia because of reversible hypoparathyroidism, hypercortisolemia, osteopenia, infertility, sexual dysfunction

Opiates: Osteopenia, alteration in gonadotropins, decreased sperm motility, menstrual irregularities

Cocaine: Diabetic ketoacidosis

Tobacco: Graves disease, azoospermia, erectile dysfunction, osteopenia, osteoporosis, fractures, estrogen alterations, insulin resistance

Any addiction: Amenorrhea

Hepatic

Alcohol: Steatosis (fatty liver), acute and chronic hepatitis (infectious [i.e., B or C] or toxic [i.e., acetaminophen]), alcoholic hepatitis, cirrhosis, portal hypertension and varices, spontaneous bacterial peritonitis

Opiates: Granulamatosis

Cocaine: Ischemic necrosis, hepatitis

Injection or high-risk sexual behavior: Infectious hepatitis B and C (acute and chronic) and delta

Hematologic

Alcohol: Macrocytic anemia, pancytopenia because of marrow toxicity and/or splenic sequestration, leukopenia, thrombocytopenia, coagulopathy because of liver disease, iron deficiency, folate deficiency, spur cell anemia, burr cell anemia

Tobacco: Hypercoagulability

Injection or high-risk sexual behavior: Hematologic consequences of liver disease, hepatitis C–related cryoglobulinemia and purpura

Infectious

Alcohol: Hepatitis C, pneumonia, tuberculosis (including meningitis), HIV, sexually transmitted diseases, spontaneous bacterial peritonitis, brain abscess, meningitis

Opiates: Aspiration pneumonia

Tobacco: Bronchitis, pneumonia, upper–respiratory tract infections

Injection: Endocarditis, cellulitis, pneumonia, septic thrombophlebitis, septic arthritis (unusual joints, i.e., sternoclavicular), osteomyelitis (including vertebral), epidural and brain abscess, mycotic aneurysm, abscesses and soft tissue infections, mediastinitis, malaria, tetanus

Injection or high-risk sexual behavior: Hepatitis B, C, and delta; HIV; sexually transmitted diseases

(Continued)

TABLE 70.1	Selected Medical Disorders Related to Alcohol and Other Drug Use (*Continued*)

Neurologic

Alcohol: Peripheral and autonomic neuropathy, seizure, hepatic encephalopathy, Korsakoff dementia, Wernicke syndrome, cerebellar dysfunction, Marchiafava-Bignami syndrome, central pontine myelinolysis, myopathy, amblyopia, stroke, withdrawal delirium, hallucinations, toxic leukoencephalopathy, subdural hematoma, intracranial hemorrhage

Opiates: Seizure (overdose and hypoxia), compression neuropathy

Cocaine: Stroke, seizure, status epilepticus, headache, delirium, depression, hypersomnia, cognitive deficits

Tobacco: Stroke, small-vessel ischemia, and cognitive deficits

Any addiction: Compression neuropathy.

Nutritional

Alcohol: Vitamin and mineral deficiencies (B_1, B_6, riboflavin, niacin, vitamin D, magnesium, calcium, folate, phosphate, zinc)

Any addiction: Protein malnutrition

Other Gastrointestinal

Alcohol: Gastritis, esophagitis, pancreatitis, diarrhea, malabsorption (because of pancreatic exocrine insufficiency, or folate or lactase deficiency), parotid enlargement, malignancy, colitis, Barrett esophagus, gastroesophageal reflux, Mallory-Weiss syndrome, gastrointestinal bleeding

Opiates: Constipation, ileus, intestinal pseudoobstruction

Cocaine: Ischemic bowel and colitis

Tobacco: Peptic ulcers, gastroesophageal reflex, malignancy (pancreas, stomach)

Any addiction: Overdose from bodypacking

Prenatal and perinatal

Alcohol: Fetal alcohol effects and syndrome

Opiates: Neonatal abstinence syndrome, including seizures

Cocaine: Placental abruption, teratogenesis, neonatal irritability

Tobacco: Teratogenesis, low birth weight, spontaneous abortion, abruptio placentae, placenta previa, perinatal mortality, sudden infant death syndrome, neurodevelopmental impairment

Perioperative

Alcohol: Withdrawal, perioperative complications (delirium, infection, bleeding, pneumonia, delayed wound healing, dysrhythmia), hepatic decompensation, hepatorenal syndrome, death

Opiates: Withdrawal, inadequate analgesia

Cocaine: Hypersomnia and depression in withdrawal, mimicking of postoperative neurologic complications, complications from underlying drug-induced cardiopulmonary disease

Tobacco: Pulmonary infection, difficulty weaning, respiratory failure, reactive airways exacerbations

Pulmonary

Alcohol: Aspiration, sleep apnea, respiratory depression, apnea, chemical or infectious pneumonitis

Opiates: Respiratory depression/failure, emphysema, bronchospasm, exacerbation of sleep apnea, pulmonary edema

Cocaine: Nasal septum perforation, gingival ulceration, perennial rhinitis, sinusitis, hemoptysis, upper airway obstruction, fibrosis, hypersensitivity pneumonitis, epiglottitis, pulmonary hemorrhage, pulmonary hypertension, pulmonary edema, emphysema, interstitial fibrosis, hypersensitivity pneumonia

Tobacco: Lung cancer, COPD, reactive airways, pneumonia, bronchitis, pulmonary hypertension, interstitial lung disease, pneumothorax

Injection: Pulmonary hypertension, talc granulomatosis, septic pulmonary embolism, pneumothorax, emphysema, needle embolization

Inhalation: Pulmonary edema, bronchospasm, bronchitis, granulomatosis, airway burns

(*Continued*)

TABLE 70.1	Selected Medical Disorders Related to Alcohol and Other Drug Use (*Continued*)

Renal
Alcohol: Hepatorenal syndrome, rhabdomyolysis and acute renal failure, volume depletion and prerenal failure, acidosis, hypokalemia, hypophosphatemia
Opiates: Rhabdomyolysis, acute renal failure, factitious hematuria
Cocaine: Rhabdomyolysis and acute renal failure, vasculitis, necrotizing angiitis, accelerated hypertension, nephrosclerosis, ischemia
Tobacco: Renal failure, hypertension
Injection or high-risk sexual behavior: focal glomerular sclerosis (HIV, heroin), glomerulonephritis from hepatitis or endocarditis, chronic renal failure, amyloidosis, nephrotic syndrome (hepatitis C)

Sleep
Alcohol: Apnea, periodic limb movements of sleep, insomnia, disrupted sleep, daytime fatigue
Opiates: Insomnia
Cocaine: Hypersomnia in withdrawal
Tobacco: Insomnia, increased sleep latency

Trauma
Alcohol: Motor vehicle crash, fatal and nonfatal injury, physical and sexual abuse
Cocaine: Death during "Russian Roulette"
Opiates: Motor vehicle crash, other violent injury
Tobacco: Burns, smoke inhalation
Any addiction: Sexual and physical abuse

Musculoskeletal
Alcohol: Rhabdomyolysis, compartment syndromes, gout, saturnine gout, fracture, osteopenia, osteonecrosis
Opiates: Osteopenia
Cocaine: Rhabdomyolysis
Any addiction: Compartment syndromes, fractures

Gastrointestinal Consequences Alcohol is directly toxic to the gastric mucosa and can lead to asymptomatic or symptomatic gastritis. Vomiting can lead to a Mallory-Weiss tear and hematemesis. Alcohol can lead to stomatitis, esophagitis, duodenitis, esophageal cancer, and gastric cancer. Endoscopy is warranted for persistent reflux symptoms or epigastric pain, particularly if weight loss is present or if patients are aged 40 years and older.

In alcoholic hepatitis, AST usually is higher than ALT; thus, a higher ALT concentration suggests another or a concomitant etiology, such as hepatitis C. Though steatohepatitis is best diagnosed by liver biopsy, clinically it often is diagnosed when serology for hepatitis B and C is negative, the abnormality persists with abstinence, and an ultrasound examination is consistent with the diagnosis. Classic alcoholic hepatitis presents with fever, leukocytosis, right upper-quadrant pain and tenderness, and elevations of the AST concentration out of proportion to ALT elevations. Management consists of abstinence from alcohol as well as supportive care, with attention to fluid and electrolyte balance, vitamin K for coagulopathy, clotting factor replacement when there is active bleeding and coagulopathy, and attention to volume and mental status. Cirrhosis, and associated hypoalbuminemia, coagulopathy, and hyperbilirubinemia, can develop in chronic alcohol users either as a consequence of hepatitis C, recurrent alcoholic hepatitis or, simply, chronic heavy use (40–60 g per day of ethanol for men and 20 g for women). Hepatocellular carcinoma can occur, particularly when hepatitis C is present. Surgical treatment may be hampered by complications of cirrhosis, which include hepatic encephalopathy, esophageal or gastric variceal bleeding, ascites and spontaneous bacterial peritonitis, volume overload and edema, and hepatorenal syndrome. End-stage liver disease of many etiologies can be addressed with liver transplantation with similar survival in those transplanted because of alcoholic liver disease compared with other causes of liver failure. Most transplant recipients do not return to drinking (22% in the 1st year), and few return to heavy drinking (5% to frequent heavy use in 1 year, 20% at 5 years).

In people with alcohol dependence, amylase often is elevated because of chronic parotitis, rather than due to pancreatitis. Abdominal computed tomography is the most sensitive and specific test for pancreatitis, but it is not indicated unless the presentation is atypical, fever is present, or the patient does not improve as expected. Severity can range from mild symptoms to a mortal condition complicated by acidosis, adult respiratory distress syndrome, and hypovolemia. Standard therapy for acute pancreatitis should be instituted early. The only treatment proven to decrease mortality is volume repletion, best accomplished with intravenous normal saline. When the acute episodes resolve, a return to drinking can lead to recurrent episodes and ultimately to constant pain and chronic pancreatitis, loss of pancreatic exocrine function with greasy stools and malabsorption, and even loss of pancreatic endocrine function manifested by hyperglycemia and diabetes.

Hematologic Consequences
In addition to the iron deficiency anemia that can result from gastrointestinal hemorrhage or chronic blood loss, people with alcohol use disorders can develop a pancytopenia (leukopenia, thrombocytopenia, and anemia) from alcohol's direct toxic effects on the bone marrow or splenic sequestration as a result of the splenomegaly associated with cirrhosis and portal hypertension.

- In addition to leukopenia, there may be impaired quantitative and qualitative white blood cell response to infection
- Thrombocytopenia can lead to serious bleeding when the platelet count is below 50,000
- Megaloblastic anemia may be as a result of folate deficiency
- If there is iron deficiency lowering the mean corpuscular volume (MCV) and hemolytic anemias related to liver disease with reticulocytosis or megaloblastic processes simultaneously increasing it, MCV may be noncontributory in differentiating the cause of anemia; the red cell distribution width should be elevated in this situation.

The treatment for bone marrow suppression is abstinence, for iron deficiency it is identification of the cause and iron replacement, and for folate deficiency it is folate (after testing for concomitant vitamin B_{12} deficiency and giving treatment, as needed). Coagulopathy usually is a result of chronic liver disease, though a trial of vitamin K replacement is warranted at least once.

Cardiovascular Consequences
Hypertension can occur as a transient symptom of withdrawal or become chronic with heavy drinking (about two or more standard drinks per day) or even low levels of regular consumption of alcohol. Chronic heavy drinking can lead to alcoholic cardiomyopathy and congestive heart failure and its potential complications such as left ventricular thrombosis and embolic stroke. Treatment consists of alcohol abstinence and standard treatments for congestive heart failure, ventricular clot, and antiarrhythmias.

Atrial fibrillation ("holiday heart") can occur as a consequence of alcohol use or withdrawal and usually resolves spontaneously or after treatment for withdrawal (with benzodiazepines and β-blockers) and abstinence.

The association between moderate drinking (fewer than two standard drinks per day) and fewer cardiovascular events and decreased mortality in men (but not in average-risk women) remains controversial. The epidemiologic findings of benefit for moderate drinking can be confounded by alternative explanations, such as differences in social characteristics that remain unaccounted for. Studies have suggested that if there is a benefit, it may be most pronounced in patients who have the same alcohol dehydrogenase genotype that may predispose them to alcohol dependence.

Renal and Metabolic Consequences
Hepatic disease can lead to renal consequences as seen in the nephrotic syndrome and glomerulonephritis from chronic Hepatitis C and hepatorenal syndrome in severe cirrhosis.

Serious fluid and electrolyte abnormalities may be minimized and overlooked in people with heavy alcohol use who present for acute medical care. Acute renal failure can occur from rhabdomyolysis after alcohol intoxication, seizure, or from volume-depleted from vomiting, diarrhea, and diuresis. Volume repletion should continue at least until the patient no longer manifests postural changes in blood pressure and heart rate and excess losses are not continuing.

Both metabolic acidosis and alkalosis can occur as a result of heavy drinking. In acidosis it is important to determine if an anion or osmolar gap is present to rule out ingestion of substances other than ethanol (ethylene glycol or methanol ingestions if an osmolar gap is present). These ingestions require prompt treatment to prevent blindness or death. If an anion gap is not present, diarrhea is the most common cause of acidosis. If an anion gap is present, the differential diagnosis is broad but, in the people with heavy alcohol use, lactic acidosis (from sepsis, injury, severe pancreatitis, or after convulsion), ketoacidosis, and ingestion should be considered first. Alkalemia can occur as a result of respiratory alkalosis related to liver disease and hyperventilation or metabolic alkalosis from vomiting. Treatment for withdrawal can help speed the resolution of the alkalemia, which is important because it can be associated with hypokalemia and hypomagnesemia; deficiencies common in people with heavy alcohol use. In addition, severe hypophosphatemia (unmasked when dextrose is given to malnourished people with heavy alcohol use), hypokalemia, and hypocalcemia are seen in these patients and will not correct until magnesium is replaced. Consider empiric replacement of magnesium as serum levels do not reflect total body magnesium stores. Oral replacement of magnesium and phosphate is usually possible but intravenous replacement, with cardiac monitoring in the case of severe hypophosphatemia, may be necessary.

Hyperglycemia or hypoglycemia can be seen in people with alcohol use disorders as a result of pancreatic insufficiency or in end-stage cirrhosis.

Trauma Trauma, including physical and sexual abuse, can lead to poorer addiction treatment outcomes. Addiction specialists should be attuned to the high rates of injury (both past trauma and the risk of future injury) when counseling people with alcohol use disorders.

Alcohol can interfere with balance and coordination as well as judgment, thus predisposing to injury. Heavy episodic drinking poses a particular risk of injury and accidents. As these patients often present to emergency departments and trauma centers, these facilities should routinely screen for alcohol problems and refer patients with alcohol-related disorders for treatment.

Infectious Diseases People with alcohol dependence can have impaired defense because of undernutrition, splenic dysfunction, leukopenia, and impaired granulocyte function as well as suppression of the gag reflex during intoxication and overdose. Fever in people with alcohol use disorders must not automatically be attributed to a minor viral syndrome or withdrawal. Pneumonia is more common in people with alcohol use disorders and is associated with increases in the risk of mortality. Tuberculosis must also be considered in this population. Because HIV is more common in people with alcohol use disorders than in the general population, *Pneumocystis carinii* pneumonia and other opportunistic infections must be considered when pneumonia is diagnosed. Meningitis in people with alcohol use disorders has a broader differential diagnosis than in the general population. Brain abscess can result from poor dentition, leading to transient bacteremia and local infection, for example, in a preexisting subdural hematoma. Spontaneous bacterial peritonitis occurs in patients with cirrhosis and ascites. Abdominal tenderness may be minimal or absent. Diagnosis is made by paracentesis. Spontaneous bacterial empyema can occur when pleural effusion is present. Sexually transmitted diseases, including HIV, are more common in people who drink heavily, in part because of sexual risk-taking behavior and potential sexual abuse.

Musculoskeletal Consequences Intoxication to the point of overdose may result in the individual's remaining in one position for prolonged periods of time, predisposing the individual to compression nerve palsies, rhabdomyolysis, and compartment syndrome. Surgical consultation is required for the latter.

Hyperuricemia and gout are more common in alcohol use disorders. Treatment is with colchicine, using caution in renal or hepatic insufficiency, or indomethacin, using caution in the presence of gastritis or renal insufficiency. A brief course of corticosteroids and a single injection of adrenocorticotropic hormone may be safer choices for the person with an alcohol use disorder. Chronic treatment in the setting of renal disease, tophaceous gout, or polyarticular gout should be with allopurinol or probenecid.

Excessive regular alcohol use or heavy episodic drinking increases the risk of skeletal fracture, through higher risk of trauma or alcohol-related osteopenia or both. Heavy alcohol use can lead to osteonecrosis of bone, such as that at the femoral head.

Oncologic Risks Alcohol is a risk factor for several malignancies including of the lip, oral cavity, pharynx, larynx, esophagus, stomach, breast, liver, intrahepatic bile ducts, prostate, and colon. The risk is amplified with concurrent tobacco use. Even moderate levels of alcohol use may increase risk of certain cancers. For example, breast cancer risk increases with consumption of one to two standard drinks per day.

Pulmonary Consequences Alcohol intoxication can lead to respiratory depression and aspiration, leading to a chemical or infectious pneumonia. Tachypnea can be the result of pulmonary infection, respiratory alkalosis of liver disease, alcohol withdrawal, or compensation for a metabolic acidosis.

Endocrinologic Consequences

Alcohol causes sexual dysfunction and hypogonadism in men, both through direct effects on the testes and through secondary effects in chronic liver disease, in which gynecomastia may be seen. In women, alcohol delays menopause and is associated with menstrual disorder and decreased fertility. It increases high-density lipoprotein but also increases serum triglycerides, which can lead to heart disease, hepatic steatosis, and pancreatitis. Moderate drinking can decrease the incidence of diabetes mellitus, but more than three drinks a day increase the risk.

Consequences in the Perioperative Patient Heavy alcohol consumption is a risk factor for postoperative complications and in the perioperative period withdrawal is a concern. Attempting to achieve abstinence prior to elective surgery has been shown to reduce morbidity, as has been demonstrated in at least one randomized trial.

Vitamin Deficiencies Malabsorption and poor dietary intake can lead to deficiencies of thiamine, pyridoxine, niacin, riboflavin, vitamin D, zinc, and fat-soluble vitamins when there is malabsorption because of pancreatic disease. Vitamin replacement is safe and should be done empirically.

Sleep Though alcohol can help people fall asleep, it also can be stimulating and lead to disrupted sleep and daytime fatigue. Alcohol increases the risk of obstructive sleep apnea and worsens the disease (because of its depressant effects on respiration and relaxation of the upper airway) and can increase the risk of periodic limb movements of sleep. Treatment should include attention to sleep hygiene and pharmacotherapy with drugs with a low or no risk of dependence (e.g., trazodone).

Fetal, Neonatal, and Infant Consequences The fetal alcohol syndrome involves craniofacial abnormalities, neurologic abnormalities, and growth retardation and neurologic disabilities persist into adulthood. Because no safe amount of alcohol during pregnancy has been identified and there is no treatment for the effects of alcohol on the fetus, abstinence is recommended during pregnancy.

Tobacco

There is widespread consensus that tobacco use increases the risk of death.

Withdrawal Nicotine replacement, bupropion or varenicline, if appropriate, should be provided for medically ill patients who are hospitalized as nicotine withdrawal and craving can complicate treatment for other medical illnesses. Nicotine replacement can precipitate myocardial ischemia, but the alternative, smoking a cigarette, also can do so. Therefore, in general, even smokers with coronary artery disease can use nicotine replacement, unless they are experiencing unstable angina or myocardial infarction.

Neurologic Consequences Tobacco use is associated with atherosclerosis, peripheral vascular disease and, therefore, cerebrovascular disease and ischemic and hemorrhagic stroke, which can lead to cognitive deficits.

Gastrointestinal Consequences Smoking is a cause of gastric and duodenal ulcers and can exacerbate gastroesophageal reflux disease. Smoking cessation, in addition to pharmacotherapy, is usually necessary for effective treatment.

Hematologic Consequences Though data are conflicting, smoking is known to have hypercoagulable effects and it can be a risk factor for deep vein thrombosis.

Cardiovascular Consequences Smokers are at higher risk of myocardial infarction and sudden death due to poorer control of hypertension and atherosclerosis. Smoking can precipitate angina by causing vasospasm and hypercoagulability, and it can precipitate dysrhythmia. Furthermore, it lowers the beneficial serum high-density lipoprotein subfraction of cholesterol. Smokers are at higher risk of cerebrovascular disease and stroke and peripheral vascular disease as well.

Renal Consequences The renal consequences of tobacco dependence are limited primarily to the effects of atherosclerosis of the renal arteries, which can lead to ischemic renal failure and hypertension from renal artery stenosis.

Injury Tobacco dependence can lead to house fires, smoke inhalation, and death, as well as other accidental death.

Infectious Consequences Because of its pulmonary effects, smoking increases the risk of acute and chronic bronchitis and pneumonia. Smokers have more frequent upper respiratory infections.

Oncologic Risks Smoking is associated with cancer of the oral cavity, larynx, lung, esophagus, bladder, kidney, pancreas, stomach, and cervix. In addition, smokers with one smoking-related cancer are at higher risk for a second one. These risks decrease with cessation.

Pulmonary Consequences Smoking leads to chronic bronchitis and emphysema, collectively referred to as "chronic obstructive pulmonary disease" (COPD). Smoking is the leading cause of both COPD and broncho-genic carcinoma. The risks of both of these mortal diagnoses can be lowered with smoking cessation. Smoking cessation can slow the steady decline in pulmonary function. Smoking leads to pulmonary hypertension, interstitial lung disease, and pneumothorax.

Endocrinologic Consequences Smoking is known to increase the risk of Graves disease (hyperthyroidism) and hypothyroidism, increase insulin resistance and the risk of diabetes, decrease estrogen in both genders and is associated with decreased BMD, osteoporosis, and fractures. In men, it is one of the leading causes of erectile dysfunction and decreases sperm number and function.

Consequences in the Perioperative Patient Smoking increases the risk of postoperative pneumonia, atelectasis, reactive airways exacerbations, and respiratory failure. If possible, smoking cessation at least 2 months before elective surgery is advisable.

Sleep Nicotine increases sleep latency and tobacco withdrawal increases daytime sleepiness.

Fetal, Neonatal, and Infant Consequences Tobacco use during pregnancy causes low birth weight, spontaneous abortion, and perinatal mortality and may increase risks of sudden infant death syndrome and neurodevelopmental impairment.

Opiates, Cocaine, and Other Drugs

The complications of other drugs often are related to route of administration; in particular, injection and inhalation.

Injection Drug Use Skin and soft-tissue infections (e.g., cellulitis, abscess) are common in injection drug users. One must be aware of local epidemiology and practices because there have been reports of unusual pathogens (e.g., *Pseudomonas aeruginosa* and *Serratia* species) and polymicrobial infections from use of saliva to prepare the injection. Soft-tissue infections can progress to become serious and life threatening if fasciitis develops or if there is significant local ischemia, as with cocaine injection. Intravenous injection can result in septic thrombophlebitis, arterial injection with embolus and digital ischemia and infection or venous valvular damage in the extremities, marked by leg ulcers, edema, and a propensity to develop deep vein thrombosis. Rarely, tetanus can develop as a result of nonsterile injection.

Blood-borne pathogens spread by injection or risky behaviors and often result in serous sequelea. Hepatitis B can develop into a chronic infection, and HIV and hepatitis C almost invariably are chronic illnesses. HIV can lead to a variety of opportunistic infections and death. False-positive screening tests for syphilis often are found in injection drug users so treponemal specific tests are needed to determine the diagnosis.

Injection drug users can have septic arthritis in unusual locations (sternoclavicular or sacroiliac joints), spinal epidural or vertebral infections, osteomyelitis, or meningitis. One of the most serious infectious consequences of injection drug use is bacterial endocarditis; thus, in an injection drug user, fever cannot be taken lightly as cardiac murmur and other "textbook" signs of subacute bacterial endocarditis may not be present. Many authorities recommend empiric antibiotic treatment while awaiting blood culture results. Mycotic aneurysms, endophthalmitis, congestive heart failure, brain, spleen, or myocardial abscesses and emboli, renal failure from interstitial nephritis, pulmonary septic emboli with effusions, stroke, and heart block can complicate the course.

In addition to infectious complications, injection of drugs can lead to pulmonary and hepatic talc granulomatosis from injected crushed tablets containing talc, pulmonary hypertension from granulomatous disease or drug-related vasoconstriction, needle embolization, pneumothorax or hemothorax from injection into large central veins gone awry, and pulmonary emphysema related or unrelated to talc granulomatosis.

Nephropathy related specifically to injection drug use, primarily because of HIV infection, is a common renal complication. Amyloidosis and nephrotic syndrome can occur because of chronic skin infections. Hepatitis C infection can lead to glomerulonephritis. The coagulopathy that results from liver and kidney disease in injection drug users can lead to neurologic complications—namely, hemorrhagic stroke. Cerebral infarction has resulted from injection of crushed tablets and even of a melted suppository (intravenously and via inadvertent intra-arterial injection).

Inhalation of Drugs Inhalation of drugs has effects related to the size of the particles: larger particles affect the airways, whereas smaller ones reach the alveoli. In addition to the granulomatous complications listed above, chronic bronchitis from inhaled smoke, bronchospasm, barotrauma with resultant pneumothorax or pneumomediastinum from prolonged breath holding or stimulant use, hemoptysis from airway irritation, and emphysema from inhaled tobacco, marijuana, or opiates can occur. Freebasing can lead to upper airway and facial burns.

Withdrawal Though the withdrawal is not fatal in an otherwise healthy person, in the acutely ill or hospitalized patient it should be treated for symptomatic relief to prevent hyperadrenergic states that complicate treatment of the acute medical problems (e.g., coronary syndromes).

Neurologic Consequences Seizures can occur as a result of sedative withdrawal, stimulant use, or proconvulsant metabolites (meperidine). Similarly, hemorrhagic stroke can occur with use of methamphetamines, phenylpropanolamine, lysergic acid diethylamide, and phencyclidine from hypertension, vasculitis, or other vascular mechanisms. Cocaine use can lead to both hemorrhagic and ischemic strokes. Anabolic steroids can cause stroke by promoting hypercoagulability. Though classic syndromes of dementia have not been described for users of drugs other than alcohol, chronic cognitive deficits can be seen in users of cocaine, sedatives (barbiturate), and toluene. Neuropathy (including plexopathies and Guillain-Barré syndrome) may be caused by heroin use, compression neuropathy in any drug user, quadriplegia in glue sniffers, and combined systems degeneration from vitamin B_{12} deficiency induced by nitrous oxide use. Parkinsonism can develop from the use of a meperidine analogue, MPTP.

Gastrointestinal Consequences In addition to viral hepatitis, which is almost universal in injection drug users, cocaine itself can cause hepatic necrosis, probably because of ischemia. Ecstasy and phencyclidine use has been reported to cause liver failure. Androgenic steroids can cause hepatic toxicity. Anticholinergic and opiate abuse will cause constipation. "Bodypacking" (transporting cocaine, heroin, or other drugs in bags that are swallowed) can lead to mechanical obstruction of the intestines. Rupture can lead to overdose and death from respiratory arrest or cardiovascular collapse.

Hematologic Consequences Amyl nitrate, isobutyl nitrate, and other "poppers" can cause methemoglobinemia.

Cardiovascular Consequences In addition to the infectious complications of drug abuse that are related to route of administration (endocarditis and myocardial abscess), drugs of abuse can directly affect the heart and blood vessels. Cocaine can cause severe hypertension, cardiomyopathy cardiac dysrhythmias, angina, myocardial infarction, sudden death, and stroke. Chest pain often occurs during or after cocaine use, but most persons evaluated in emergency departments with chest pain and cocaine use do not have myocardial infarction. Nonetheless, heart attacks do occur and are thought to be related to coronary vasospasm, in situ thrombosis, or the accelerated development of atherosclerosis. Other stimulants can also produce cardiac complications. Anabolic steroids can lead to coronary artery disease as well as cardiomyopathy. Drugs with anticholinergic effects (muscle relaxants, antihistamines, and antidepressants) cause tachycardia and can cause dysrhythmias in intoxication or overdose. Inhalants (volatile fluorocarbons) can cause dysrhythmias.

Renal and Metabolic Consequences Any drug that leads to sedation with intoxication or overdose can lead to muscle compression and rhabdomyolysis and to acute renal failure. Rhabdomyolysis can also be seen with amphetamine, cocaine, and phencyclidine use. Cocaine can lead to accelerated hypertension and renal failure, hypertensive nephrosclerosis, thrombotic microangiopathy, and renal infarction. Amphetamines can result in a drug-related polyarteritis nodosa. Ecstasy use can lead to hyponatremia when users drink excess water to prevent the hypovolemia associated with its use. Toluene inhalation can lead to metabolic acidosis.

Injury Though much of the literature focuses on alcohol as a risk factor for injury, cocaine and other drugs also have been associated with an increased risk of motor vehicle crash and other violent injuries, including fatal shootings.

Infectious Consequences of Drug Use Most of the infectious complications of drug use are related to injection or risky sexual practices, as discussed previously. Similarly, drug users are at risk of pneumonia from aspiration related to overdose and tuberculosis.

Oncologic Risks Though the magnitude of risk remains unclear, marijuana, when smoked, can lead to squamous cell carcinoma of the oral cavity and to lung cancer.

Pulmonary Consequences Drugs that produce sedation with use or overdose can lead to respiratory depression and death. Atelectasis can develop, as can aspiration and chemical pneumonitis. Opiate use can lead to bronchospasm, as a result of its stimulation of histamine release, and pulmonary edema in the setting of overdose. The pulmonary consequences of sedatives are limited primarily to respiratory depression and arrest from overdose, worsening of sleep-disordered breathing, as well as tachypnea, hyperventilation, and respiratory alkalosis from withdrawal syndromes.

Marijuana use can lead to obstructive lung disease and fungal infection from contamination. Cocaine use can lead to nasal septal perforation, sinusitis, epiglottitis, upper airway obstruction, and hemoptysis, primarily from irritant and vasoconstrictive effects. Cocaine use can lead to pulmonary hemorrhage, edema, hypertension, emphysema, interstitial fibrosis, and hypersensitivity pneumonitis. The treatment for most of these diseases is withdrawal of the cocaine and supportive care, though corticosteroids and bronchodilators are warranted in some cases. Pulmonary hypertension and edema can result from use of stimulants (specifically amphetamines).

Inhalants can lead to methemoglobinemia, tracheobronchitis, asphyxiation, and hypersensitivity pneumonitis. Nitrous oxide can cause respiratory depression and hypoxemia. Anabolic steroids can induce prothrombotic states and lead to pulmonary embolism.

Endocrinologic Consequences Most drugs of abuse can affect a variety of hormone levels. Opiates can impair gonadotropin release, which may lead to impaired sperm motility in men, and women may have menstrual and ovulatory irregularities. This mechanism may explain the reduced BMD seen in heroin addicts, though etiology is likely multifactorial. Cocaine is a risk factor for the more frequent occurrence of diabetic ketoacidosis, in part because of adrenergic effects. Barbiturate use can lead to osteomalacia from vitamin D deficiency. Clinical metabolic consequences have been clearly linked to use of anabolic steroids. Women develop androgenization, and lipids are adversely affected.

Consequences in the Perioperative Patient As with other substances, attention to and treatment of withdrawal symptoms can avert development of tachycardia and hypertension, which may complicate interpretation of assessments and operative and anesthetic treatments. The anesthesiologist must be informed of any recent drug use because of potential interactions between β-blockers and cocaine and because of the potentiation of sedative and anesthetic drugs. Finally, anesthesia and pain management generally require much higher doses than usual in the opiate-dependent patient. Nutritional issues often require attention in addicted persons undergoing surgery, as wound healing may be impaired.

Vitamin Deficiencies Nitrous oxide abuse is a well-known cause of vitamin B12 deficiency.

Sleep Many persons with addictive disorders experience sleep disturbances, because of the effect of the drug used, lifestyles, or comorbid psychiatric conditions. Sleep problems can contribute to the desire to use drugs for self-medication. Stimulants can suppress sleep, whereas opioids and nicotine tend to reduce sleep. The management of sleep disorders, particularly insomnia, therefore, is difficult but important in addicted persons. Attention to sleep hygiene (i.e., a quiet location, using the bed only for sleep and sex, and elimination of napping) and judicious use of drugs less likely to lead to misuse, such as trazodone, are the best approaches.

Fetal, Neonatal, and Infant Consequences No clear teratogenic effects of opiates are known but opiate exposure in utero can lead to the neonatal abstinence syndrome, including seizures. Benzodiazepines have been associated with cleft lip and palate, but the studies of benzodiazepines, like other studies of teratogenesis in drug users, may have been confounded by alcohol use. Toluene and other inhalants use can cause an embryopathy, preterm labor, and intrauterine growth retardation. The effects of caffeine in pregnancy are controversial. It probably is relatively safe, although some reports of increased fetal loss suggest minimizing its use during pregnancy. Dextroamphetamine and cocaine are associated with teratogenesis. Cocaine can induce neonatal irritability and also may cause behavioral and learning disorders.

COMMON MEDICAL PROBLEMS IN PERSONS WITH ADDICTIVE DISORDERS

Persons with addictive disorders suffer from the same medical conditions as nonaddicted persons, but several points specific to addiction and common medical problems are discussed here.

Coronary artery disease is particularly common in persons with alcohol and other drug abuse because of concomitant tobacco dependence. The person with addiction and anginal chest pain must be taken seriously. Angina can be complicated by alcohol, opiate, and sedative withdrawal, as well as cocaine and other stimulant use when the hyperadrenergic states precipitate anginal attacks. β-Blockers are drugs of choice as they also decrease sympathetic outflow associated with drug withdrawal. However, simultaneous use of β-blockers and cocaine should be avoided because of the unopposed vasoconstriction that can result. Aspirin and other treatments for acute coronary events (heparin, tissue plasminogen activator, and similar anticoagulants) can be problematic in persons who have a potential site for internal bleeding, such as people with alcohol dependence with gastritis or liver disease, or intracranial bleeding that is unrecognized.

The diagnosis of hypertension can be problematic in persons with addictive disorders as elevation can be a product of pain, withdrawal, or intoxication, depending on the substance used. Ideally, hypertension should be diagnosed after at least three blood pressure measurements during prolonged abstinence. Treatment of hypertension is the same as in persons without addictive disorders, but diuretics can be somewhat riskier in people with alcohol dependence because of the adverse effects on potassium balance. β-Blockers are excellent alternatives; however, cocaine users should avoid β-blockers.

Diabetes is more difficult to manage in persons with addictive disorders, not only because of difficulty with adherence and more erratic eating habits but also because of the effects of alcohol on glucose metabolism. Heavy alcohol users are more prone to prolonged and more severe hypoglycemia from the sulfonylurea agents often used to treat type 2 diabetes. Choices for the management of diabetes in alcohol dependence are difficult. Thiazolidinediones are relatively contraindicated because of the possibility that they may cause hepatic damage. Metformin should not be given to patients with hepatic impairment or those at risk for lactic acidosis. Insulin injections are preferred, though use of sulfonylureas with careful monitoring is reasonable.

In addition to having etiologic roles in cancers, addiction can lead to difficulties in cancer management. First, any renal, hepatic, or cardiac consequences of addiction can limit the choice of chemotherapeutic agents. Pulmonary consequences of tobacco use may limit surgical options. Finally, pain management can be complicated by ongoing or past addiction.

CONSEQUENCES IN OLDER ADULTS

In older adults, lower amounts of alcohol are associated with adverse consequences because of lower lean body mass and body water, less alcohol dehydrogenase, and impaired ability to develop tolerance. Hip fracture, a leading cause of death in older adults, can result from an increased propensity to fall related to alcohol use and to osteopenia. Older adults are more susceptible to injury from motor vehicle crashes and even more so when alcohol is used. Certain medications are less effective or can be harmful when taken with alcohol. Older adults are more susceptible than younger individuals to alcohol's chronic brain-damaging effects, including cognitive deficits, and are less likely to recover completely from those effects.

In addition to greater susceptibility, alcohol can cause many consequences in older adults that may be misdiagnosed as other common medical problems. For example, the tremor of withdrawal may be diagnosed as Parkinson disease or an essential tremor. The potential contribution of alcohol as cause of conditions common in the elderly (dementia, malnutrition, self-neglect, functional decline, sleep problems, anxiety or depression, cardiovascular disease, cardiomyopathy, congestive heart failure, incontinence, fatigue, neuropathy, sexual dysfunction, pneumonia, fractures, seizures, and cerebellar degeneration) maybe overlooked.

Alcohol and other drug abuse can contribute to the occurrence of falls, worsening of chronic illness (such as hypertension), interference with medication adherence, and side effects. The effects of smoking are of great significance in older adults because smoking-related diseases often appear with aging and can be exacerbated by continued smoking.

CONCLUSIONS

Routine health care of the addicted person differs in that the patient almost certainly is at higher risk of disease than are those without addiction. During hospitalization for medical reasons, special attention must be directed toward management of withdrawal and adequate pain control. Management of common medical illnesses is complicated by addiction, its effect on medication adherence, and the direct consequences of the abused substances. The subsequent chapters in this section delve into the medical consequences of addiction in greater detail.

Summary Author: Agnes Kwasnicka
Howard S. Friedman

Cardiovascular Consequences of Alcohol and Other Drug Use

Because coronary artery disease and stroke are the leading causes of death and disability in most of the world, the effects of addictive psychoactive substances on vasomotion, coagulation, and blood lipids may have serious implications (Table 71.1). Drug abuse may also be the vehicle by which various contaminating cardiotoxins and microorganisms injure or infect the heart.

ALCOHOL

Hemodynamic Effects

There is evidence to suggest that moderate use of alcohol (defined as no more than two drinks per day in men and no more than one drink in women) may have some cardiovascular benefits. However, even these amounts could have adverse effects in some individuals with heart disease, and the consumption of larger amounts can result in serious cardiovascular consequences in many individuals.

Although alcohol depresses myocardial contractility, this may be obscured as a result of the adrenergic and vasodilatory effects of its metabolites, acetaldehyde and acetate. Cardiac output usually increases after alcohol ingestion in healthy subjects, reflecting the changes in heart rate and peripheral resistance that ensue. By contrast, a more sensitive index of cardiac function, such as left ventricular ejection fraction, generally worsens. Alcohol appears to depress myocardial contractility by direct reduction in contractile force; both metabolic changes and abnormalities in the contractile process seem to play a role. The factor (or factors) producing these changes appears so far to have eluded investigators.

Ethanol has regional circulatory effects. It decreases pancreatic blood flow, resulting in reduction in pancreatic oxygenation, suggesting that alcohol may produce pancreatitis by an ischemic mechanism. The opposing effects of ethanol (cerebrovascular constrictor) and its metabolite, acetate (cerebrovascular dilator), are likely why various studies show decreased, increased, or no change in brain flow. Older patients (older than 62 years) seem to be especially sensitive to the cerebral vasoconstrictor actions of alcohol, which may pose an added risk of cerebral circulatory injury in elderly individuals who drink excessively.

Ethanol and its metabolites are coronary vasodilators and have been found to increase coronary blood flow through increases in heart rate, blood pressure, and cardiac dimensions. Despite these changes, alcohol exerts an unfavorable effect on myocardial ischemia. Individuals with coronary artery disease are more inclined to demonstrate evidence of myocardial ischemia after ingesting alcohol; moreover, alcohol may mask angina pectoris, thereby making the occurrences of myocardial ischemia silent and potentially more dangerous. Also, alcohol may precipitate coronary spasms; these spasms often occur several hours after imbibing alcohol, suggesting a "rebound" phenomenon to the vasodilating actions of alcohol and its metabolites.

Alcoholic Heart Disease

Excessive alcohol use can result in an array of cardiac abnormalities. Functionally, these abnormalities range from a heart that is hypocontractile, has a reduced output, and is associated with an increased systemic vascular resistance (the findings of alcoholic cardiomyopathy), to one that is hyperdynamic, has an increased output, and is associated with a reduced systemic vascular resistance (the findings of decompensated

TABLE 71.1	**Salient Cardiovascular Effects of Alcohol and other Drugs**

Alcohol

Hemodynamics

Myocardial depression

Increased cardiac output (heart rate increases and/or peripheral resistance decreases)

Increased skin and splanchnic blood flow

Decreased brain and pancreatic blood flow

Increased coronary flow in normal vasculature but decreased flow to ischemic myocardium

Disorders

Dilated cardiomyopathy (sometimes with marked increase of left ventricular wall thickness)

Arrhythmias, especially atrial fibrillation

Hypertension, systemic

May attenuate (light to moderate use) or promote atherogenesis (heavy use)

Sudden death

Nicotine

Hemodynamics

Increased heart rate and blood pressure

Vasoconstriction

Promotes myocardial ischemia by increasing myocardial demand and decreasing O_2 delivery

Promotes thrombosis

Disorders

Worsens angina pectoris

Promotes acute coronary syndromes

Promotes atherogenesis

Cannabis

Hemodynamics

Increases heart rate

Variable effect on blood pressure

Vasodilation

Increases cardiac output (heart rate increases and/or peripheral resistance decreases)

Promotes myocardial ischemia by increasing myocardial demand and decreasing O_2 delivery (increases carboxyhemoglobin)

Disorder

Worsens angina pectoris and promotes acute coronary syndromes

Opioids

Hemodynamics

Lowers heart rate

Lowers blood pressure

Vasodilation

Promotes "ischemic preconditioning"

Disorder

Heroin-related pulmonary edema

Cocaine

Hemodynamics

Increases heart rate

Increases blood pressure

Myocardial depressant

Vasoconstrictor

Promotes thrombosis

Promotes atherogenesis

Disorders

Atypical chest pain syndrome

Worsens angina pectoris

Promotes acute myocardial infarction

Aortic rupture and dissection

Left ventricular hypertrophy and dilatation (myocarditis/cardiomyopathy)

Arrhythmias

Hypertension, systemic

Stroke

Sudden death

Amphetamines

Hemodynamics

Increases blood pressure

Increases heart rate (with sharp increases of blood pressure may have reflex slowing)

Promotes thrombosis

Disorders

Promotes acute myocardial infarction

Aortic dissection

Left ventricular hypertrophy and dilation (myocarditis/cardiomyopathy)

Arrhythmias

Hypertension, pulmonary

Stroke

Sudden death

cirrhosis). Subclinical cardiac dysfunction can be detected and alcohol-related myocardial disease may be present when no obvious heart disease is evident. Excessive alcohol use leads to myocardial hypertrophy, four-chamber dilation, myocardial necrosis, and interstitial and perivascular fibrosis, leading to alcoholic cardiomyopathy.

Cirrhosis does not preclude cardiomyopathy and the associated hyperdynamic circulation may make detection difficult by standard clinical measures. The salient cardiovascular feature of decompensated cirrhosis is a reduction of systemic vascular resistance, a consequence of a generalized vasodilatory response, which results in a high cardiac output state. Reduced systemic vascular resistance may be evident even before ascites can be detected by abdominal ultrasound; however, tense ascites, by impeding venous return, can elicit counterregulatory responses that antagonize the vasodilatory effects of cirrhosis.

Although some people may have a predisposition to developing alcoholic cardiomyopathy (e.g., African American), people with alcoholism who develop this disorder tend on the average to be 10 years older, have had alcoholism 10 years longer, and drink considerably more than people with alcoholism who maintain normal cardiac dimensions and function. Although other conditions besides alcoholism may be necessary to produce this disorder, the relationship between prolonged heavy alcohol use and the occurrence of a dilated, hypocontractile heart is sufficiently strong to suggest that alcohol, acetaldehyde, or some compound formed from these substances, is toxic to the heart.

Hypertension, seen in heavy drinkers, may contribute to the development of cardiac disease through increased left ventricular wall stress and higher heart rates and resultant increase in myocardial oxygen consumption. Alcohol-associated heart failure might ensue as a consequence of the combination of increased myocardial oxygen requirements and the abnormalities of myocardial metabolism and energetics caused by many years of drinking. Moreover, the occurrence of atrial fibrillation, as seen in "holiday heart" or as a complication of alcoholic cardiomyopathy, might produce or worsen myocardial dysfunction. Abstinence, especially in the early phases of alcoholic cardiomyopathy, may reverse the abnormalities, whereas continuance of alcohol use will lead inexorably to an unfavorable outcome.

Holiday Heart

Often occurring after an episode of binge drinking, "holiday heart" is the term that has been coined to denote an alcohol-associated arrhythmia in the absence of any electrolyte abnormality or evidence of clinical heart disease. Though various atrial and ventricular arrhythmias may be seen, people with alcoholism appear to be particularly at risk for atrial fibrillation.

Possible mechanism of these arrhythmias includes alcoholism-associated hypokalemia, hypomagnesemia, or autonomic neuropathy; a condition that might produce arrhythmia by creating cardiac electrical instability. The epidemiological observation that alcoholics who died suddenly (presumed to be arrhythmic deaths) had low blood ethanol concentrations, however, suggests reactions to alcohol withdrawal rather than to alcohol per se as the cause. Possible mechanisms might include an arrhythmia from an intense sympathoadrenal reaction, postvasodilatory coronary artery spasm, and small coronary artery thromboses due to rebound hypercoagulability.

In some instances, an arrhythmia may be the first manifestation of subclinical alcoholic cardiomyopathy. Heavy alcohol use must, therefore, always be considered in individuals with unexplained arrhythmias, especially those having paroxysmal atrial fibrillation.

Hypertension

Alcohol use elevates blood pressure, and heavy alcohol use produces systemic hypertension; an effect that may be intensified during periods of withdrawal. An increase in blood pressure is evident with one or two drinks per day in men, whereas this effect requires three drinks per day in women. With menopause, the hypertensive effect of alcohol intensifies. The effects of alcohol on blood pressure have been found to be related to baseline blood pressure and to the quantity customarily used, that is, little effect on normotensive, *light* drinkers but significantly increased blood pressure in hypertensive, *moderate* drinkers.

Alcohol, in fact, has a dual effect on blood pressure. Ethanol and its metabolites acetaldehyde and acetate, by their vasodilatory actions on the systemic circulation, lower blood pressure. However, alcohol also stimulates the sympathetic nervous system (with participation of corticotrophin-releasing hormone and through α-adrenergic mechanisms) and attenuates the baroreceptor reflex, actions that would elevate blood pressure. Though the elevations of blood pressure associated with habitual use of alcohol disappear after several days of abstinence, people with alcoholism have a proclivity for an exaggerated response of their blood pressure to stressors that may persist for at least several weeks after withdrawal.

Coronary Heart Disease and Stroke

Heavy alcohol use is associated with an increased risk of coronary artery disease and stroke. In contrast to the cardioprotective effects of limited alcohol use in those with no apparent cardiovascular disease, heavy alcohol use has been associated with sudden death in individuals who have underlying coronary artery disease. The relationships between alcohol consumption and coronary and cerebrovascular diseases can be described as U- or J-shaped, initially favorable, with benefit augmenting as use increases, and then unfavorable, with detriment augmenting as use increases.

The adverse effects of alcohol on atherothrombotic diseases can be related to the blood pressure elevations and perhaps blood homocysteine elevations. Favorable effects appear to be related mostly to the changes alcohol produces on the blood lipid profile with about 50% of the benefit attributed to an increase in high density lipoprotein (HDL) cholesterol. Alcohol's overall antithrombotic actions would also impact favorably on atherothrombotic events, doing so at a cost of an increased chance of hemorrhagic stroke. Alcohol use reduces plasma fibrinogen, reduces platelet aggregability, and enhances the antiplatelet actions of aspirin. Its use is also positively related to plasma tissue-type plasminogen activator (t-PA), suggesting an alcohol-induced enhancement of fibrinolysis.

Though the reduced risk of coronary heart disease associated with moderate alcohol use is not related to any specific alcoholic beverage, there may be some selective differences. For instance, the tannins in red wine and the vitamin B$_6$ (an antagonist of the homocysteine-elevating effects of alcohol) in beer, may provide some additional protective advantages for these beverages. However, the beneficial effects of alcohol use can be related to ethanol per se. This is supported by the observation that individuals who have a genetic variation of alcohol dehydrogenase that results in slow metabolism of ethanol have the most protection against myocardial infarction with moderate alcohol use.

Though the evidence for some benefit of moderate alcohol use is persuasive, the actual value may be less than has been suggested. For instance, a reported 21% decrease in the 12-year incidence of stroke attributable to alcohol use is actually a benefit of only 5.6 per 10,000 per year. Moreover, because the evidence of benefit is based on cohort data, not randomized controlled studies, there are always concerns about a hidden confounder. In addition, even moderate alcohol use may increase heart rate and blood pressure and depress left ventricular function, or produce a "coronary steal," changes that might aggravate congestive heart failure or worsen myocardial ischemia. Thus, encouraging the use of alcohol as a cardiac medicinal would seem to be unwarranted, especially for people with heart disease.

NICOTINE

Cigarette smoking is a leading risk factor for developing cardiovascular diseases. During smoking, heart rate and blood pressure increase and remain above baseline for at least 30 minutes after stopping. Nicotine exerts its adrenergic actions mainly by release of norepinephrine from nerve terminals and by release of epinephrine from the adrenal medulla. Smoking also attenuates baroreceptor responses to blood pressure elevations and the heart rate fluctuations that occur with normal respiration. It exerts a vasoconstrictive effect on most regional circulations. In individuals with symptomatic obstructive peripheral arterial disease, smoking would be expected to diminish blood flow and reduce walking distance before calf pain.

Cigarette smoking causes myocardial ischemia to occur at lower levels of exertion and even at rest in individuals with coronary artery disease by increasing myocardial oxygen requirements, causing vasospasms and adversely affecting "downstream" collaterals and compensatory arteriolar dilatation, diminishing coronary flow reserve, and interfering with myocardial oxygen delivery (via the increases in carboxyhemoglobin). Smoking may also cause an acute coronary thrombosis and promote coagulation through

- Increased platelet activation
- Increase in platelet aggregatory prostaglandin thromboxane A2
- Increasing plasma fibrinogen (thereby increasing blood viscosity)
- Inhibiting fibrinolysis by reducing tissue t-PA activity

The associations between smoking cigarettes and thrombogenesis may be of particular concern in women, especially for those using oral contraceptives or receiving hormonal replacement therapy; the risks of thrombotic events in women smokers using oral contraceptives increases sharply after age 35.

Smokers have more extensive atherosclerosis in the coronary arteries, aorta, and peripheral arteries than nonsmokers. Smoking promotes atherogenesis through several mechanisms: by promoting hemostasis and contributing to atherosclerotic plaque growth, producing an unfavorable lipid profile through reduction in HDL cholesterol, and adversely affecting endothelial function.

Though there have been a few reports of cardiovascular events associated with the use of nicotine replacement products, controlled studies have failed to demonstrate a significant risk of use of these products. Given the hazards of smoking, whatever small risks may be related to continued nicotine exposure are offset by the benefits of cessation: a 50% decrease in risk of having a coronary event after 1 to 2 years of abstinence and a continued decline thereafter so that, after 20 years, ex-smokers have a risk comparable to that of nonsmokers.

CANNABIS

The cardiac excitatory effects of cannabis have been related to the major active compound present in the drug, delta-9-tetrahydrocannabinol (Δ-9-THC). Heart rate increases may last for 2 to 3 hours following smoking and isolated premature ventricular impulses has been observed. Some tolerance develops over time but after 48 hours of abstinence, tolerance is no longer evident. Cannabis' effects on blood pressure are more variable. It may increase, have no change, or even decrease systemic blood pressure. Orthostatic changes in blood pressure with hypotension, and even bradycardia, consistent with a vasovagal reaction may ensue after several days of drug use. Cardiac output generally increases after the administration of cannabis as a result of increases in heart rate and a reduction of total peripheral resistance (vasodilation), not by improvement in cardiac performance.

The hemodynamic changes after cannabis use may have adverse effects for persons with heart disease through increased heart rate, blood pressure, and myocardial oxygen requirements and reduced myocardial oxygen delivery via increased carboxyhemoglobin; together resulting in myocardial ischemia at reduced levels of exertion. Individuals with heart failure might experience deterioration of their condition after cannabis use. Moreover, in a study of patients with an acute myocardial infarction, users of cannabis had almost five times the incidence of the event during the 1 hour after their use of cannabis than at other times, suggesting that smoking cannabis might also be a "trigger" of myocardial infarction. Thus, even though the explanations for their cardiovascular effects have not yet been clearly elucidated, at least for individuals with heart disease, use of cannabis is harmful.

OPIOIDS

Opiates, especially morphine, are important therapeutic agents for their use for pain relief in acute myocardial infarction and for treatment of cardiogenic pulmonary edema. Whereas at therapeutic dosages, these drugs have a modest effect on lowering blood pressure and reducing heart rate, in amounts used by addicts, opiates can evoke intense sympathomimetic effects, manifested by an increased heart rate and blood pressure and an improvement in cardiac performance.

Opiates may have favorable effects on myocardial ischemia. In patients with coronary artery disease, opiates improve myocardial energetics and coronary blood flow and have a direct protective effect against myocardial ischemia at the cellular level. They may exert antiarrhythmic effects on catecholamine-mediated and ischemia-related arrhythmias and may increase the threshold for ventricular fibrillation. Thus, the overall favorable actions of opioids on the heart may explain why abnormalities of cardiac dimensions and function are generally not found in heroin addicts.

Despite the benefits of opiates in the treatment of pulmonary edema, paradoxically, heroin overdose may produce a pulmonary condition resembling cardiogenic pulmonary edema; likely a defect in capillary permeability rather than an elevation of pulmonary capillary pressure. This disorder is probably caused by an unusually high opioid-induced release of histamine from pulmonary mast cells.

The major cardiac hazard of injection drug use (IDU), apart from an accidental overdose, is infective endocarditis. Endocarditis in IDUs, however, differs from that seen in the nonaddict by the frequent occurrence on normal valves, the high incidence of virulent microorganisms, such as *Staphylococcus aureus*, *Pseudomonas* species, and fungus, and the increased involvement of right-sided valves (especially the tricuspid). A high suspicion in any IV drug user presenting with fever, especially when associated with repeated rigors, should prompt treatment with broad-spectrum antibiotics that include an antibiotic against methicillin-resistant *Staphylococcus aureus*, and treatment should be initiated even before a positive blood culture or a confirmation of valvular vegetations by echocardiography is available. The risk of an infection is higher and the consequences of endocarditis are more dire with a prosthetic rather than native valve; thus, the threshold for valve replacement should be higher in this population.

COCAINE

Cocaine may produce seemingly contradictory effects, whether its sympathomimetic or the local anesthetic actions are predominant. Sympathomimetic effects are the result of blocking presynaptic norepinephrine and dopamine reuptake, thereby making more catecholamines available at postsynaptic receptors and enhancing the effects of endogenous catecholamines. As a local anesthetic, cocaine inhibits transmembrane sodium flux during electrical excitation, producing a delay in the upstroke and amplitude of the myocardial action potential, blocks calcium entry into the myocyte, inhibits the release of calcium from the sarcoplasmic reticulum, and makes the contractile proteins less responsive to available calcium. With cocaine use, blood pressure and heart rate increase, and in most vascular distributions, arteries constrict. It may cause angina pectoris and acute myocardial infarction, aortic dissection and rupture, ischemic and hemorrhagic stroke, and left ventricular dilation and hypertrophy. Related in part to cocaine's arrhythmogenic actions, even a single use of cocaine can result in sudden cardiac death.

Hemodynamic Effects

When administered systemically, cocaine is a potent vasoconstrictor, elevating systemic vascular resistance, heart rate, and blood pressure in a dose-related fashion. In contrast, as a consequence of its direct local anesthetic actions, cocaine depresses myocardial function and attenuates vasoconstriction, and under certain conditions, it might even cause vasodilatation. Contrary to the anticipated autoregulatory properties of the coronary circulation, after the administration of cocaine coronary blood flow is reduced.

The coronary vasoconstrictive actions of cocaine (intensified in the presence of coronary artery disease) are attenuated by α-adrenergic blockers, enhanced by noncardioselective β-adrenergic blockers, and are not changed by drugs with both α-adrenergic and β-adrenergic blocker effects. The hemodynamic responses of cocaine follow a bimodal time course; the maximal effects at peak plasma cocaine concentration and a later secondary effect when its metabolites benzoylecgonine and ethyl methylecgonine are high.

When cocaine use is combined with alcohol, cigarettes, or other drugs, the increase in myocardial oxygen requirements, increase in systemic blood pressure, heart rate, or both, is exaggerated (Table 71.2). Smoking cigarettes intensifies the ischemic consequences of cocaine by its vasoconstrictive effects on the coronary circulation. Alcohol intensifies the myocardial depressant actions of cocaine and a metabolite of their interaction, cocaethylene, also has myocardial depressant actions and may continue to exert detrimental effects after cocaine has been metabolized. When cocaine is used with cannabis, heart rate and myocardial oxygen requirements are increased to an extent greater than with the same amount of either drug used alone. Thus, cocaine use, alone or in combination with these other addictive substances, creates an imbalance between myocardial oxygen requirements and oxygen delivery, making cocaine a potent agent for producing myocardial ischemia.

Acute Coronary Syndromes

Habitual and occasional cocaine users, some young and having no known predisposition, are at risk for coronary events, with the hour after cocaine use the time of greatest hazard. At autopsy in those who died or within a few hours of the onset symptoms in those that survived, an acute coronary thrombosis has been found in some but not all individuals. Those that survive generally have patent coronary arteries and no evidence of plaque rupture. The coronary vasoconstrictive actions of cocaine, especially when intensified by smoking, appear to be a pivotal condition.

Cocaine use also appears to promote thrombosis. Taken intranasally, it causes platelet activation, platelet microaggregation, increased plasma concentrations of platelet factor 4 and β-thromboglobulin, and inhibition of fibrinolysis as a result of increased plasminogen activator inhibitor (PAI-1) activity.

TABLE 71.2	Drug Effects on Myocardial Oxygen Demand and Coronary Blood Flow					
Drug	**Rate**	**SBP**	**Rate × SBP**	**CBF**	**CAD-N**	**CAD-AB**
Ethanol	↑	↑/NC/↓	↑	↑	↑	↓[a]
Cocaine	↑	↑	↑	↓	↓	↓
Nicotine	↑	↑	↑	↑/NC/↓	↑/NC/↓	↓
Cannabis	↑↑	↑/NC/↓	↑	↑	↑	UK
Ethanol-cocaine	↑↑	↑↑	↑↑	↑	↑	↓[b]
Nicotine-cocaine	↑↑	↑↑	↑↑	↓	↓	↓↓
Cannabis-cocaine	↑↑	↑	↑↑	↓	↓	↓

[a]Diminishes blood flow by a "coronary steal."
[b]"Coronary steal" expected.
SBP, systolic blood pressure; CBF, coronary blood flow; CAD, coronary artery dimensions; N, normal arteries; AB, stenosed arteries; NC, no change; UK, unknown.

In diagnosing acute myocardial infarction related to cocaine use, the predictive accuracy of the electrocardiogram (ECG) diminished and the confounding effects of rhabdomyolysis increasing creatine kinase make significance of this marker questionable.

Benzodiazepine use has been recommended by the American Heart Association for the management of cocaine-related acute coronary syndromes to reduce seizures and the mortality of cocaine toxicity. In addition to its analgesic action, morphine attenuates cocaine-induced vasospasm and, therefore, may be considered for unremitting chest pains. β-Blockers should be deferred at least until after the effects of cocaine and its congeners have dissipated or coronary patency has been established. Consensus recommendations caution against the use of calcium channel blockers because of their concomitant sympathomimetic actions.

Although most cocaine users who are observed for chest pains do not go on to have a myocardial infarction, chest pains must initially be perceived as a symptom of acute myocardial in these patients. The predilection for myocardial ischemia and for an acute myocardial infarction may persist for days to weeks, after cocaine withdrawal. Counseling people who use cocaine and experience chest pains and those who have had an acute coronary event, that they remain at jeopardy for additional heart attacks and even for sudden death, is therefore especially important.

Chronic Cardiovascular Effects

Cocaine use has also been associated with acceleration of atherosclerosis, myocardial injury and thickening, and vascular complications related to hypertension. Cocaine may increase vascular endothelium permeability, allowing more atherogenic lipoproteins to diffuse into the intima, though coronary vasospasm, catecholamine toxicity, and activation of inflammatory cells may also contribute to these findings.

Demand and Coronary Blood Flow

Focal myocarditis has been reported in 20% of autopsies of cocaine users. Cardiac changes associated with catecholamine excess (focal necrosis with inflammatory cells, myocyte contraction band necrosis) are sometimes found with cocaine-associated deaths. Left ventricular hypertrophy has also been found both in autopsies and in clinical echocardiographic studies of chronic cocaine abusers. Though cases of acute pulmonary edema and dilated cardiomyopathy have been reported, it is not clear whether any of these occurrences are related to the abnormalities that have been reported at autopsy.

The finding of increased left ventricular wall thickness, increased heart weight, and, in some studies, stroke, in habitual users of cocaine may be in part related to the association between cocaine use and systemic hypertension. Aortic dissection and rupture, also complications of hypertension, have been reported in people who use cocaine. Continued use of cocaine after an aortic dissection may result in recurrences. Unlike methamphetamine-associated aortic dissection, crack cocaine–related acute aortic dissection may be less likely to result in an immediate death.

Arrhythmogenesis

Cocaine can cause sudden unexpected cardiac death in individuals not having apparent coronary or myocardial abnormalities, which may be related to the direct and indirect arrhythmogenic effects of the drug. Neurohumoral properties of cocaine including its sympathomimetic effects, its peripheral adrenergic reuptake inhibitory actions, and its vagolytic actions may explain not only cocaine's effect on heart rate but also various atrial and ventricular tachyarrhythmias that might result from enhancing the activity of normal and abnormal pacemaker cells.

Cocaine has remarkable electrophysiologic effects that can produce serious cardiac arrhythmias and even sudden death. Cocaine delays myocardial electrical conduction, which could promote reentrant arrhythmias that might develop around scar tissue or occur as the result of acute myocardial ischemia. Prolongation of the QT interval and Brugada syndrome have also been reported on ECGs of cocaine users. Wide QRS complex tachycardias have been observed with cocaine overdose, especially in the presence of acidemia.

AMPHETAMINES AND RELATED COMPOUNDS

Amphetamines are sympathomimetic drugs *without* local anesthetic actions. These substances act by stimulating the sympathetic nervous system, by displacing catecholamines or interfering with reuptake from their storage sites, by blocking the actions of monoamine oxidase inhibition, and/or by direct adrenergic actions. Amphetamines produce a dose-dependent elevation of blood pressure and an increase of heart rate.

- MDMA and methylphenidate: increase in heart rate parallels blood pressure changes
- Amphetamine and methamphetamine: modest heart rate changes initially; the magnitude of the heart rate changes has an inverse relation to the blood pressure changes

These changes (and accompanying body temperature elevations) may be exaggerated by intense, repetitive activities, and crowded conditions, which may account for the adverse effects observed when these drugs have been used at discos and "raves."

Though not amphetamines, phencyclidine and lysergic acid diethylamide (LSD) also generally increase heart rate and blood pressure. The mechanisms of actions of LSD are sufficiently different from that of amphetamines that cross-tolerance does not develop.

All of these drugs, by their sympathomimetic actions, would also be expected to enhance thrombosis, at least by promoting platelet activation and aggregation, and to produce vasospasms. Ischemic and hemorrhagic stroke, acute myocardial infarction, aortic dissection, and sudden cardiac death have all been related to amphetamine use. Methamphetamine, in particular, has been related to acute aortic dissection. Ventricular tachycardia and fibrillation have also been observed after IV administration of amphetamines. Myocardial injury, likely caused by catecholamine excess, has been reported at autopsy in amphetamine abusers and may be related to the occurrence of dilated cardiomyopathy IV amphetamine abusers.

ANABOLIC STEROIDS

Anabolic steroids are linked to reports of marked cardiac hypertrophy, acute myocardial infarction (sometimes with patent coronary arteries), stroke, and unexpected sudden cardiac death in young athletes. Diastolic dysfunction, that is, severe hypertrophy and evidence of abnormal left ventricular filling, has been observed on autopsy of steroid user, but cardiomegaly alone maybe a nonspecific finding and related to the generalized organ-enlarging effect of these substances.

These drugs can elevate blood pressure (possibly by promoting fluid retention) and may have unfavorable effects on blood coagulation and lipids (decrease HDL cholesterol and increase low-density lipoprotein cholesterol), especially when taken orally. Despite case reports of thrombotic complications in young athletes using anabolic steroids and experimental data demonstrating steroid-induced increased platelet aggregability, studies in humans have not demonstrated that androgens promote a hypercoagulable state. In fact, the evidence suggests that athletes using anabolic steroids have increased levels of plasma proteins with anticoagulant actions. The occurrence of an acute myocardial infarction in a young athlete with patent coronary arteries who used anabolic steroids suggests that vasospasm may play a role in anabolic steroid–related cardiovascular toxicity.

Summary Author: Agnes Kwasnicka
Paul S. Haber • Robert Gordon Batey

Liver Disorders Related to Alcohol and Other Drug Use

The liver is a major target for the toxicity of alcohol and other drugs of abuse (Table 72.1).

ALCOHOLIC LIVER DISEASE

Epidemiology

Cirrhosis of the liver is the 12th most common cause of death in America, and in 2003, 44% of deaths from cirrhosis were alcohol-related. Epidemiological research has demonstrated that the population risk of alcohol-related cirrhosis is related to the population level of alcohol consumption.

Risk Factors for Alcoholic Liver Disease

Risk factors for alcoholic liver disease include the amount of alcohol consumed, gender, genetic factors, obesity, chronic viral hepatitis, ingestion of other hepatotoxins, and nutrition.

Amount of Alcohol Consumed Population studies demonstrate an increasing risk of cirrhosis above 40 g per day for men and 20 g per day for women, but the majority of those with cirrhosis have drunk >100 g per day. Among very heavy drinkers, the risk rises to approximately 50% but does not reach 100% even at the highest levels of alcohol consumption.

Gender Women appear to be at greater risk of alcoholic liver disease, with that risk rising at lower average levels of alcohol consumption than in men (20 vs. 40 g per day in men). Differences in body composition, average weight, gastric alcohol dehydrogenase (ADH) activity (accounting, in part, for first pass, gastric alcohol metabolism), hepatic alcohol metabolic rate, and liver mass per kilogram of body weight between men and women result in a higher relative alcohol dose in women compared to men drinking the same amount. An alternative explanation for a greater female susceptibility to alcohol-mediated liver damage may relate to gender differences in endotoxin-induced Kupffer cell activation in alcoholic liver injury.

Genetic Factors Twin studies suggest that genetic factors contribute to the risk of liver disease among those who abuse alcohol. Studies examining classic genetic markers (such as blood groups and HLA antigens), genes relevant to the disease process (such as neurotransmitter metabolism, enzymes involved in alcohol metabolism, collagen metabolism, and, more recently, the wide variety of proteins involved in the inflammatory process) support genetic links to both susceptibility to dependence and to tissue injury from alcohol ingestion.

Polymorphisms in ADH genotypes coding for highly active isoenzyme and aldehyde dehydrogenase (ALDH) coding for a less active isoenzyme may lead to accumulation of acetaldehyde after alcohol consumption, but the significance of this finding with respect to alcoholic liver disease (ALD) remains unclear. Other gene polymorphisms (c2 promoter polymorphism of CYP2E1, TNFα, interleukin [IL]-10) have been associated with ALD, but not consistently and reproducibly, suggesting that the mechanisms underlying tissue injury are complex.

Obesity

There is both experimental and clinical evidence of an alcohol-obesity interaction in the development of liver disease. Alcoholics with a high body mass index for at least 10 years are at increased risk of liver disease.

TABLE 72.1	Associations Between Drugs of Abuse and Liver Disease
Hepatic drug toxicity	• Alcohol • MDMA • Cocaine • Heroin • Phencyclidine • Androgenic steroids
Toxic interactions with other drugs of abuse	• Alcohol plus MDMA • Alcohol plus cocaine • Alcohol plus acetaminophen
Systemic effect of drugs leading to liver injury	• Hyperthermia and hypothermia • Shock • Rhabdomyolysis
Infectious complications	• Viral hepatitis: A to D, particularly B and C • Bacteria: SBE, septicemia
Coinjected material	• Talc (hepatic granulomas) • Lead (by-product of metamphetamine synthesis)
Lifestyle related	• Fatty liver

MDMA, 3,4-methylenedioxymethamphetamine.

Chronic Viral Hepatitis Heavy alcohol use is widely recognized as a factor that is associated with advanced liver fibrosis in patients with chronic viral hepatitis, particularly hepatitis C. Hepatitis C has been reported to be more common in alcoholics than in the general community—an observation attributed to but not entirely explained by the increased prevalence of injection drug use. A similar but less marked interaction between the hepatitis B virus (HBV) and the effect of alcohol on the liver has been ascribed to chronic hepatitis B infection in alcoholics.

Ingestion of Hepatotoxins Chronic ethanol consumption increases the hepatotoxicity of a number of compounds including acetaminophen, industrial solvents, anesthetic gases, isoniazid, phenylbutazone, and illicit drugs (e.g., cocaine). The induction of cytochrome P450 2E1 (CYP2E1) explains the increased vulnerability of the person who drinks heavily to these substances.

Among patients with alcoholism, hepatic injury associated with acetaminophen has been described after repetitive intake in amounts well within the accepted rate for the general community (2.5–4 g). It is likely that the enhanced hepatotoxicity of acetaminophen after chronic ethanol consumption is caused, at least in part, by an increased microsomal production of reactive metabolite(s) of acetaminophen, Thus, maximal vulnerability to the toxicity of acetaminophen occurs immediately after cessation of drinking, at which time production of the toxic metabolite may be at its peak as competition by ethanol for a common microsomal pathway has been withdrawn.

Nutrition Nutritional impairment is universally present in patients with ALD. It correlates with the severity of the disease and nutritional disorders may accelerate progression of ALD. Protein deficiency is a recognized cause for fatty liver owing to impaired apoprotein synthesis required to export lipid from hepatocytes. Choline deficiency and vitamin A excess are associated with hepatic fibrosis. Heavy alcohol use is associated with low serum levels of vitamin A, and, if supplements are inappropriately given, vitamin A toxicity may result even with normal serum levels.

Clinical Features

Symptoms and signs are not reliable indicators of the presence or severity of ALD, and there may be no symptoms even in the presence of cirrhosis. Alcoholic liver disease comprises three clinicopathologic entities that frequently coexist: alcoholic fatty liver, alcoholic hepatitis, and alcoholic cirrhosis.

Alcoholic fatty liver manifests with anorexia, nausea, right upper quadrant discomfort, and an enlarged, firm and possibly tender liver. *Alcoholic hepatitis* can present as mild to severe cases; the latter carries a high short-term mortality (30%–65%). These cases present with anorexia, nausea and abdominal pain, impaired liver function with jaundice, bruising, and encephalopathy. Ascites and systemic disturbances including fever and neutrophilic leukocytosis may be present. *Alcoholic cirrhosis* may present with nausea or weight loss but typically presents with complications such as portal hypertension leading to variceal bleeding and/or ascites, liver failure, and hepatocellular carcinoma. Alcoholic cirrhosis is a recognized risk factor for hepatocellular carcinoma.

Diagnosis of Alcoholic Liver Disease

Although the liver tests are a sensitive marker for ALD, similar findings may be observed in nonalcoholic steatohepatitis and in patients treated with medications such as anticonvulsants. The aspartate aminotransferase (AST) exceeds the alanine aminotransferase (ALT) level in most alcohol-related cases, and a ratio of 2:1 AST:ALT is commonly quoted as highly suggestive of ALD. Usually, the transaminases are only moderately elevated, but the gamma glutamyl transpeptidase (GGT) level is almost always raised and often exceeds 1,000 U/L. The diagnosis of ALD rests on the history of prolonged heavy alcohol ingestion with a compatible clinical and laboratory picture. Additional investigations are restricted to atypical cases or those that fail to resolve with abstinence from alcohol. Other explanations for liver disease, including autoimmune hepatitis, Wilson disease, alpha-1-antitrypsin deficiency, and cholestatic liver disease including primary biliary cirrhosis, may need to be considered in specific cases.

Role of Liver Biopsy

The practice of biopsying the majority of patients with any form of significant liver injury has changed in the past 5 years As a result of improvements in noninvasive imaging and diagnostic testing, and as patients have become more resistant to the procedure knowing its complications and shortfalls, liver biopsy is commonly now restricted to those patients with complex or incompletely understood disease and in those being considered for liver transplantation. The morbidity (0.5%) and mortality (0.01%) generally outweigh the benefit of obtaining tissue pathology. Where clinical uncertainty despite non-invasive testing persists, biopsy should always be considered.

Pathogenesis

Recent studies demonstrate clearly that alcohol abuse leads to liver injury via oxidative stress. This in association with endotoxin-mediated activation of cytokine production by several cell populations within and beyond the liver leads to progressive fibrogenesis.

Ethanol metabolism within the liver leads to the generation of hepatotoxic metabolites, namely acetaldehyde and acetate via ADH and ALDH enzymes, respectively. Acetaldehyde has been shown to affect many aspects of normal cellular functioning, including DNA repair, microtubule assembly, mitochondrial respiration, fatty acid oxidation, and activation of fibrogenesis. High levels of acetaldehyde have been measured in patients with ALD, in part owing to impaired mitochondrial ALDH function, and impact liver function and disease processes in a variety of ways. A second pathway for alcohol metabolism involves cytochrome P450 2E1 (CYP2E1), induced by chronic ethanol consumption.

Oxidative Stress in Alcoholic Liver Disease

The induction of CYP2E1 generates reactive oxygen species (ROS) during oxidation of alcohol and chronic alcohol use diminishes cellular defenses against oxidative stress. Acetaldehyde, a highly reactive metabolite, binds covalently to normally occurring materials in blood to form compounds known as adducts (such as acetaldehydeprotein adducts and malondialdehyde-acetaldehyde [MAA] adducts). Blood levels of adducts correlate with liver injury in alcoholics and add to ROS in evolving ALD.

A toxic lipopolysaccharide endotoxin, derived from the cell wall of Gram-negative bacteria gut flora, is thought to enter the circulation where it binds to a serum protein (lipopolysaccharide-binding protein). This complex enters Kupffer cells and leads to up-regulation of proinflammatory cytokines. Circulating levels of gut-derived endotoxin in alcoholics are increased and this endotoxin pathway has been implicated in human ALD. Ethanol itself also contributes to liver injury by affecting intracellular signaling pathways.

Other contributors to liver injury observed in experimental and clinical ALD and to alcoholic hepatitis include

- Tissue damage due to increased proinflammtory cytokines levels of IL-1, IL-6, IL-8, and IL-12
- Increased levels of IL-18 (interferon[IFN]-γ-inducing factor) and therefore IFN-γ and TNFα
- Decreased levels of anti-inflammatory cytokine IL-10

Long-term ethanol consumption is known to inhibit the regenerative capacity of the liver. Fibrosis is seen as a potentially reversible lesion. Factors that may be important for liver regeneration and repair include

- IL-6
- Platelet-derived growth factor

Progressive liver fibrosis characterized by accumulation of collagen underlies advanced ALD. The major source of hepatic collagen is now known to be the hepatic stellate cell (HSC). HSCs are activated to secrete collagen and contribute to matrix degradation during resolution of liver injury.

Treatment of Alcoholic Liver Disease

There is considerable evidence that survival is increased by maintaining abstinence; thus, the treatment of ALD rests upon avoidance of further alcohol consumption. Other interventions are reserved for those with particularly severe disease or who are unable to maintain abstinence. Compliance with abstinence can be monitored with GGT. Although advanced cirrhosis does not resolve with abstinence, very ill patients may make striking improvements; therefore, it is never too late to stop drinking.

Defining what level of alcohol consumption to recommend for the patient with only minor abnormalities in liver function tests without clinical evidence of cirrhosis depends partly on the effect of a 6-week period of abstinence followed by repeat liver tests. If these normalize and the patient wishes to resume drinking, consumption within recommended levels may be guided by the results of further liver tests in those who can control their alcohol use.

Pharmacotherapies to address alcohol dependence must be used with particular caution in the presence of serious liver disease. Disulfiram is contraindicated in advanced liver disease owing to recognized hepatotoxicity. Naltrexone is associated with dose-dependent hepatotoxicity (typically at doses of 300 mg per day), but reactions are most unusual at the standard dose of 50 mg per day. In two studies, liver function tests improved in alcoholics, with no cases of clinically evident hepatotoxicity, indicating that the therapeutic effect to reduce alcohol consumption exceeded the potential hepatotoxic effect.

Acamprosate does not accumulate even in severe liver disease, as the drug is excreted unchanged in the urine and is not metabolized. According to the manufacturers, acamprosate is contraindicated in severe decompensated (Child's C) liver disease, but as there are no published reports of an adverse effect on liver function, the risks of treatment should be balanced against the risks of continuing alcohol consumption. Other medications without reported hepatotoxicity include nalmefene, a second-generation orally active opiate receptor antagonist with similar efficacy to naltrexone, and baclofen. Although studies of the use of baclofen in the treatment of alcohol dependence have provided positive evidence, further studies are required to replicate the findings.

Selected cases of alcoholic hepatitis may respond to corticosteroids, but this treatment remains controversial as it may exacerbate sepsis, a common complication of severe liver disease. Pentoxifylline, an inhibitor of TNFα, possibly improves hepatic perfusion and reduces the mortality of alcoholic hepatitis. Preliminary evidence shows that interleukin-10 (IL-10), an anti-inflammatory cytokine, may be effective in severe alcoholic hepatitis.

The management of the complications of cirrhosis, such as ascites and bleeding, lies outside the scope of this chapter. Patients who present with signs of hepatocellular insufficiency or portal hypertension should be evaluated by a gastroenterologist or hepatologist.

Liver transplantation is now an accepted treatment option for individuals with advanced liver disease who have stopped drinking, but only 5% of patients with end-stage ALD receive transplants. The procedure has been controversial because of concerns about allocation of precious donor livers to individuals with a behaviorally mediated disease, the chance of a successful outcome in this cohort after transplantation, and potential resumption of drinking after a successful transplant. The 5-year survival after transplantation for ALD is comparable to that of nonalcoholics in series from the United States, Europe, and Australia. Whereas alcoholics may be at higher risk of some posttransplant problems, there is evidence that the rate of rejection may be lower than for non-ALD. Careful individualized assessment and patient selection are key to favorable outcomes with respect to continued abstinence after transplant.

VIRAL HEPATITIS

Hepatitis A

Hepatitis A is an RNA virus that is transmitted by fecal-oral contamination but does not persist as a chronic infection. The prevalence of hepatitis A IgG antibodies, indicating a history of exposure, is high among injection drug users (IDUs) and prison inmates in California and Australia. Hepatitis A correlated more closely with institutionalization than sharing of injecting equipment. Although acute infection leads to a mild or even clinically inapparent hepatitis, seronegative IDUs should be vaccinated.

Hepatitis B

HBV is the most prevalent chronic viral infection of humans. It is readily transmitted among IDUs. Serologic evidence of past hepatitis B infection increases in prevalence with the duration of injecting drug use, which is now the commonest association of hepatitis B infection acquired in adults. Other risk groups include people who have more than one sexual partner (heterosexual and sexual contact between men), people from certain ethnic groups (e.g., Asia, Southern European, Mediterranean countries), indigenous people, children of infected parents, and health care workers. The incubation period is 6 weeks to 6 months.

Acute hepatitis B may be preceded by a transient serum-sickness prodrome, with polyarthralgia, fever, malaise, urticaria, and proteinuria. The acute illness is characterized by anorexia, nausea, and sometimes vomiting with malaise, jaundice, pale stools, and dark urine, but the infection is frequently subclinical. Hepatitis B persists as chronic hepatitis B infection in about 5% of adults. Acute and chronic hepatitis B is diagnosed by serologic tests, and HBV DNA testing is now used to define the state of infectivity, risk of hepatocellular carcinoma (HCC), and suitability for treatment (Table 72.2). People who remain HBsAg-positive for 6 months have chronic hepatitis B. Severity of inflammation is affected by immune status, viral load and genotype, coinfection with other hepatitis viruses or HIV, male sex, ethnic origin, alcohol ingestion or other illicit drug use, and duration of infection. Chronic active hepatitis B is associated with chronic hepatitis, cirrhosis, and hepatocellular carcinoma in a significant minority. Patients with chronic HBV should be initially assessed with regard to the replication status of the virus and the presence of active liver disease. Patients with persistently abnormal ALT levels or clinical evidence of liver disease should be referred for consideration of antiviral therapy. Patients with chronic HBV should be offered regular screening for HCC, particularly if they have cirrhosis.

Treatment of active chronic hepatitis B is of value in those patients with active liver inflammation (ALT more than twice normal), but it offers no benefit in those with no active liver inflammation. Compared to spontaneous seroconversion from eAg to eAb status of 15%, treatment with standard and now pegylated IFNα leads to seroconversion of 30% to 40% and is associated with suppression of viral replication and decreasing hepatic inflammation. Loss of HBeAg has been associated with improvements in liver histology and clinical outcome, but patients remain infected and infectious. The best response to IFNα is seen in white patients who have had the disease for a short time and who have biochemical hepatitis and a low viral load (low HBV-DNA titers).

There are now a number of oral antiviral agents available for use in the treatment of HBV-infected patients, including lamivudine, adefovir, entecavir, and tenofovir. Combination therapy with two or more antiviral agents may prove more effective than serial monotherapy, but optimal combinations are yet to be defined. Lamivudine and adefovir were used extensively in the past, but drug resistance has become a major problem.

Hepatitis C

Hepatitis C virus (HCV) infection is the most frequently reported notifiable infection in adults. HCV is the leading indication for liver transplantation and is transmitted by blood to blood contact, and the most common risk factor is injecting drug use (Table 72.3).

Virology

HCV is an RNA virus from the flavivirus family. HCV antibodies in the blood reliably indicate exposure to the virus, but the protective significance of these antibodies remains to be fully defined. Recent studies in active IDUs suggest they are at reduced risk of reinfection when HCV antibodies are present.

There are six genotypes of the virus. The most common genotypes in the United States are types 1 and 3. Reinfection after clearance and coinfection with more than one genotype can occur. Patients with genotypes 2 or 3 respond better to current antiviral therapies than those with other genotypes. Continual alteration in genetic structure by mutation is thought to allow HCV to evade immune clearance, leading to chronic infection, but also makes the development of a preventative vaccine difficult.

Transmission

Injecting Drug Use HCV prevalence is strongly associated with duration of injecting with an incidence of approximately 20% for each year of IDU. The continuing high incidence appears to be related to the continuing high prevalence of sharing some component of injecting equipment including mixing spoons, filters, swabs, or tourniquets or even on the hands.

TABLE 72.2	Interpretation of Serological Markers for Viral Hepatitis	
	Interpretation	**Comments**
Hepatitis A		
IgG	Past infection	Persists for life
IgM	Recent infection	Generally indicates acute hepatitis, but may persist after recovery for 18 mo
Hepatitis B		
Hepatitis B surface antigen (HBsAg)	Current infection	Positive in both acute and chronic hepatitis B Marker of infectivity
Antibody to hepatitis B surface antigen (HbsAb; anti-HBs)	Immunity (either after infection or vaccination)	Antibody titers >10 IU/L correlate with protection
Hepatitis B core antigen	Not found in peripheral blood	Present in liver tissue
Antibody to hepatitis B core (HbcAb; anti-HBc)	IgG: past exposure to HBV IgM: (high titer) acute Hepatitis B (low titer)–active chronic hepatitis B	Anti-HBc + anti-HBs = past infection with recovery; anti-HBc + Hbs Ag = chronic HBV infection Distinguishes acute from chronic HBV In chronic HBV, low level titer correlates with ALT level and immune response (some laboratories report all low titer antibodies as negative)
Hepatitis Be antigen (HBeAg) Hepatitis B viral DNA (HBV-DNA)	Acute hepatitis B Chronic active hepatitis B Infectivity, active viral replication	Marker of infectivity in variety of settings Correlates with HBV-DNA Detection by PCR is most sensitive marker of HBV infection HBV-DNA without HbeAg indicates infection with mutant HBV Levels useful to monitor antiviral therapy
Antibody to hepatitis Be antigen (HbeAb; anti-HBe)	Convalescence after acute HBV Marker of lower infectivity	May be associated with active disease, usually with a lower viral load. Less responsive to antiviral therapy
Hepatitis C	Positive: indicates exposure to HCV	Positive result in subject without any risk factor for HCV is more likely to be a false-positive test (confirm this by negative PCR or recombinant immunoblot assay (RIBA))
Hepatitis C antibody	Negative: does not exclude infection if transmission within 3 mo; in rare cases HCV infections occur without antibody response	Positive HCV antibody does not distinguish past infection from current infection Transplacental passage of HCV antibody makes antibody test unreliable marker of infantile infection for 18 mo.
HCV-RNA	Positive: confirms antibody result indicating HCV infection	
Hepatitis C viral load	High: >2 × 10^6 copies/mL	High viral load associated with poorer response to therapy
Hepatitis C genotype	I–VI	Type I associated with poorer response to therapy

(Continued)

TABLE 72.2	Interpretation of Serological Markers for Viral Hepatitis (*Continued*)
Hepatitis D (Delta)	Defective virus that requires HBsAg to be viable
HDV-IgG	Indicates past and/or present infection
HDV-IgM	Indicates recent or chronic infection
HDV-RNA	Indicates current viremia

HAV, hepatitis A virus; HBV, hepatitis B virus; HCV, hepatitis C virus; PCR, polymerase chain reaction (sensitive molecular diagnostic procedure that can detect minute amounts of specific DNA or RNA).

Other Modes of Transmission

- The risk of hepatitis C transmission through *blood products* was mainly before 1990 and was related to the volume of blood products transfused.
- Estimates for the risk of transmission from a needlestick injury in *health care workers* range from 0 to 10%. *Nosocomial* transmission of hepatitis C has been reported in plasmapheresis units, a hematology ward, hemodialysis units, after colonoscopy, and after cardiothoracic surgery.
- Several studies have demonstrated an association between *tattooing* and hepatitis C infection.
- *Sexual transmission* rates are generally thought to be very low. The *vertical transmission* rate from mother to baby is approximately 5%, can be as high as 9.5% from mothers with viremia, or no transmission if the mother was hepatitis C-RNA-negative at the time of delivery. There is no evidence for transmission through breast milk.

TABLE 72.3	Risk Factors for Hepatitis C

High risk

- Sharing contaminated drug injecting equipment: 90% are infected after 10 years of injecting.
- Regular or large volume transfusions of blood products prior to 1990: 85%–90% of haemophiliacs are hepatitis C antibody–positive.
- Incarceration: due to the high prevalence of injecting drug use among prisoners and possibly other high-risk events in prisons

Moderate risk

- Body piercing and tattooing: using contaminated equipment
- Mother to baby at birth: occurs in about 10% if mother is RNA-positive
- Recent outbreaks in HIV-positive men who have sex with men

Low risk

- Small-volume blood transfusion prior to 1990
- Sharing toothbrushes, razors, etc.
- Health care worker, needlestick, or sharps injury
- Birth or medical procedure in a country of high HCV prevalence

Very low risk

- Sexual activity: few well-documented cases. The presence of genital ulcerative STDs and/or traumatic sexual practices may increase the risk.
- Drug use via snorting straws
- Blood transfusion/blood products after 1990
- No evidence of increased risk: household and casual contacts of people with hepatitis C

Hepatitis C in Special Populations

Prisoners The prevalence of hepatitis C in prisoners is high, largely owing to the high proportion of IDUs, though other modes of transmission may occur in prisons due to poor hygiene and frequent physical violence. Tattooing using unsterilized equipment may also play a role.

People Born in Countries of High Hepatitis C Prevalence In Mediterranean, Eastern European, Asian, South American, and African countries, the prevalence of hepatitis C is much higher than in the United States.

Primary Infection Primary infection with HCV is typically subclinical but mild hepatitis may occur and fulminant hepatitis is rare. Clinically evident hepatitis may be associated with a higher rate of viral clearance than subclinical infection (up to 40%). Peak viremia occurs in the preacute or early in the acute phase (weeks 2–3), and antibodies appear as early as 4 weeks (average 6–8 weeks).

Chronic Infection Between 60% and 75% of patients infected with hepatitis C will develop persistent chronic infection (Fig. 72.1). After an average of 20 years, approximately 8% of people will develop cirrhosis, rising to 20% after 40 years. Progression to cirrhosis is associated with duration of disease, age older than 40 at the time of infection, average alcohol consumption of >50 g per day, coinfection with HBV and/or HIV, and male gender. The majority of HCV-infected individuals will not die of their HCV disease. Symptoms of chronic infection (fatigue, with nausea, muscle aches, right upper-quadrant pain, and weight loss) tend to be mild and intermittent.

Diagnosis

The enzyme immunoassay for antibodies to hepatitis C does not differentiate between current and resolved infection, as the antibody typically takes >10 years to disappear after viral clearance. A positive hepatitis C RNA test indicates the presence of active infection. Approximately 50% of antibody-positive patients with normal liver function tests are HCV-RNA-negative. The test should be repeated 3 to 6 months later and, if again negative, the patient can be reassured that the virus has been cleared.

Hepatitis C genotyping and viral load determination should be carried out on all patients considering antiviral therapy for HCV infection as both of these measures provide information about the likely outcome of therapy and thus assist patient and doctor in determining whether to proceed with treatment.

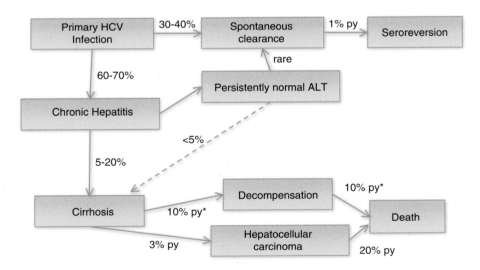

* Progression is accelerated by alcohol, male gender, age >40 at infection, co-infection with HIV and/or HBV. py; person-year.

FIGURE 72.1   The natural history of HCV infection. (Adapted from Di Bisceglie AM. Natural history of hepatitis C: its impact on clinical management. *Hepatology* 2000;31:1014–1018.)

Management Issues

Access to Health Care and Hepatitis C Information for IDUs with Hepatitis C
Specialized outreach clinics held in needle syringe services, opioid treatment programs, and in prisons help reach IUDs infected with hepatitis C who may otherwise lack access to health care.

Assessing the Severity of the Disease
Plasma ALT is the best laboratory indicator of active viral hepatitis, but the level commonly fluctuates and does not correlate well with the stage of liver disease. A normal ALT level does not exclude cirrhosis. Although newer approaches using blood tests or devices such as the Fibroscan are being used, liver biosy is the best established investigation for assessing the extent of fibrosis and the likelihood of serious long-term consequences.

Hepatitis A and B Vaccination
Chronic coinfection with other hepatitis viruses is associated with accelerated progression to cirrhosis. Hepatitis B vaccination should be offered, and patients with hepatitis C respond well, albeit with lower titers, compared to uninfected controls. Vaccination for hepatitis A is appropriate if available.

Alcohol
There is now a consensus that daily consumption of alcohol above 40 g has an additive effect on liver inflammation and accelerates the progression of hepatic fibrosis. The National Institutes of Health (NIH) consensus conference in 1997 recommended a maximum of 10 g alcohol per day for all people with chronic hepatitis C and abstinence for those with significant disease and those contemplating antiviral therapy. Heavy alcohol use is also associated with increased viral load, reduced adherence to therapy, increased risk of progression to HCC, and exacerbation of the skin lesions of porphyria cutanea tarda.

Dietary Guidelines
As a result of hepatic steatosis, obesity and type 2 diabetes mellitus are associated with hepatitis C and accelerated progression of fibrosis. The potential for dietary interventions in selected subjects to control the activity of hepatitis is under investigation.

Antiviral Treatment
The main indication for treatment is active hepatitis with elevated ALT levels and, if performed, biopsy evidence of fibrosis. The main goal of antiviral therapy is sustained virologic response (SVR), defined by a continued normal ALT level and negative hepatitis C polymerase chain reaction (PCR) on more than one occasion at least 6 months after completion of treatment. Several studies have found significant improvements in general health and specific hepatitis C–related symptoms in patients who achieve a sustained response to antiviral therapy. Those who achieve a sustained response and have no cirrhosis should expect to remain free of cirrhosis and its complications.

The combination of pegylated IFNα 2a or 2b and ribavirin is now the standard that is offered to those without contraindications. The duration of treatment varies from 6 months for those with genotype 2 or 3 and noncirrhotic disease to 12 months for those with genotypes 1, 4, 5, or 6 and those with cirrhotic genotype 3 disease. SVR rates of 75% to 80% are achieved in genotype 2, 3, and possibly 6 infections and 45% to 50% in genotypes 1, 4, and 5 infections.

Treatment of Special Groups

Human Immunodeficiency Virus Coinfection
The progression of chronic hepatitis C is accelerated in HIV coinfected patients, and the treatment response rates reported to date have been lower than in monoinfected groups. Consideration must be given to possible drug interactions and to additive blood abnormalities when treating these coinfected patients.

Patients with Compensated Cirrhosis
Treatment of patients with compensated cirrhosis may reduce the risk of hepatocellular carcinoma and decompensation.

Persistently Normal Aminotransferases
In these patients response rates to treatment have been variable. Most patients can be encouraged not to undergo treatment at this stage, but they should be followed up every 4 to 6 months and treated if the ALT becomes abnormal or if signs of progressive liver disease appear.

Patients with Ongoing Substance Abuse
The NIH consensus meeting recommended against treating patients with ongoing substance abuse. A number of 1997 papers have now demonstrated that patients who continue to use drugs in a controlled fashion and those on methadone or buprenorphine programs can be

successfully treated. Most IDUs provided all the information about HCV treatment chose to defer treatment until they have stabilized their drug use and social situations.

Contraindications for Treatment

Decompensated cirrhosis, pregnancy, lactation, active psychiatric illness, and those who drink more than seven standard drinks a week are at higher risk of side effects and lower chance of response and are generally not treated. Depression may worsen during therapy, and suicide has been reported. Contraindications to ribavirin include end-stage renal failure due to drug accumulation, chronic anemias, a history of cardiovascular dysfunction, and inadequate contraception.

Other Treatments

A variety of drugs and some alternative medications have been investigated alone or in combination with IFNα. None of these agents has contributed to improved SVRs. Symptomatic improvement and modest ALT reductions have been reported in studies using silymarin or combination Chinese herbal medicine.

Newer Anti-HCV Agents

This is a rapidly evolving area with new drugs entering clinical evaluation every year. A number of agents designed to impair viral replication have been developed, and some are now being studied in phase 3 clinical trials.

Advanced Hepatitis C

Hepatocellular Carcinoma HCV cirrhosis progresses to HCC at an annual rate of 3% to 5%, and hepatitis C is among the commonest underlying associations of HCC. Depending on size and number of tumors, extrahepatic spread or vascular invasion, resection or consideration for transplantation may be appropriate.

Liver Transplantation Once hepatic decompensation occurs, the 5-year survival falls to 50%, and transplantation should be considered rather than antiviral treatment. The 3-year posttransplantation survival is 84%, equivalent to survival in patients transplanted with other forms of liver disease.

Hepatitis D

The delta agent is a defective viral RNA particle that cannot replicate without coinfection with hepatitis B. Outbreaks of delta virus coinfection with hepatitis B have occurred among IDUs and were associated with high mortality. It responds poorly to IFN unless high doses are given for long periods.

Cocaine Hepatitis Cocaine hepatic injury appears to be uncommon in humans and contributes about 1% to fulminant hepatic failure in several series. Most cases occur in association with systemic heat-shock–like features of cocaine toxicity such as hyperthermia, rhabdomyolysis, hypoxia, and hypotension. The clinical presentation is characterized by a marked increase in serum aminotransferases and begins within a few hours of drug ingestion. The mechanism of hepatic injury is thought to involve *hepatic ischemia* and/or *toxic oxidative metabolites*. No specific therapy has been shown to be effective, but *N*-acetylcysteine may be considered.

Ecstasy An increasing number of cases of severe liver failure are being reported leading to fatalities and liver transplantation. Two clinical syndromes are emerging. One syndrome is similar to cocaine hepatitis and presents shortly after ingestion with systemic toxicity accompanied by severe liver injury. The other presents days to weeks after ingestion with jaundice and pruritus and may proceed to fulminant liver failure. Biochemically, marked hyperbilirubinemia is noted with a disproportionate increase in AST as compared to ALT. The severity of hepatic dysfunction does not appear to be dose-related.

The drug is often taken at parties where participants dance for hours, predisposing to hyperthermia and volume depletion. Those who suffer from hepatic dysfunction with rhabdomyolysis and hyperpraxia may have an abnormality of muscle metabolism similar to that seen in malignant hyperthermia syndrome. Other individuals may be susceptible on the basis of delayed drug elimination as a result of low CYP2D6 activity mutations.

TOXICITY FROM COINJECTED MATERIALS

It is often suspected that other materials may contribute substantially to toxicity after injecting of illicit drugs, but this problem appears to be uncommon. Injection of drugs intended for oral ingestion may lead to accumulation of talc in a dose-dependent fashion at several sites, particularly the lung and liver. Although talc is strongly fibrogenic in the lung, talc liver is inconsequential clinically. Lead acetate used in the synthesis of methamphetamine may contaminate the final product, and sporadic cases of lead poisoning have been reported in patients after amphetamine injecting.

Phencyclidine

A few cases of liver failure associated with malignant hyperthermia have been reported after phencyclidine use.

Cannabis

Regular cannabis use may lead to liver injury either directly or by acceleration of other causes of liver injury. The cannabinoid receptor CB1 is linked to profibrogenic activity, and is upregulated in regular users who may therefore be more at risk of fibrotic complications of diseases such as HCV and ALD. Cannabis use is associated with more severe steatosis in HCV-infected individuals.

Opioids

Currently, there are no studies that demonstrate hepatotoxicity from pure preparations of opioid agonists.

Benzodiazepines

Regular prescribed benzodiazepine use is not associated with liver damage.

ANDROGENIC/ANABOLIC STEROIDS

Steroids can produce cholestasis, toxic hepatitis, and hepatic adenomas and carcinomas. Products purchased via the Internet may contain a range of contaminants that complicate the picture of organ and specifically liver damage.

Summary Author: Agnes Kwasnicka
Jose Carlos T. DaSilva • Derya Bora Hazar

Renal and Metabolic Disorders Related to Alcohol and Other Drug Use

Drug abuse and renal disease are closely intertwined. The causal links are apparent in some cases, but with certain diseases, such as accelerated hypertension or subtypes of focal and segmental focal glomerulosclerosis, the relationship, even if strongly suspected, has not been proven definitively.

Harmful effects of illicit drug use are generally related to

1. Infectious agents inoculated during drug use
2. Infectious diseases acquired through high-risk behavior exposures
3. Direct pharmacologic effects of drugs (e.g., repeated bouts of intense vasoconstriction with cocaine use)

A list of the renal problems thought to be associated with common drugs of abuse presented by drug of abuse or renal syndromes (as often it is difficult to define etiologic agents) is found in Tables 73.1 and 73.2, respectively.

TABLE 73.1   Common Drugs of Abuse Associated with Renal Problem

Opiates

- HIV nephropathy
- Hepatitis C–associated glomerulopathies
- Hepatitis B–associated polyarteritis nodosa
- Bacterial endocarditis and acute glomerulonephritis
- Subcutaneous injection ("skin-popping") amyloidosis
- Nontraumatic rhabdomyolysis (muscle compression) and acute renal failure
- Heroin nephropathy

Cocaine

- Rhabdomyolysis and acute renal failure
- Accelerated hypertension and renal failure
- HIV nephropathy
- Hypertensive nephrosclerosis
- Renal infarction
- Thrombotic microangiopathy and renal failure

Alcohol

- Hepatorenal syndrome
- Rhabdomyolysis and acute renal failure
- Increased incidence and severity of postinfectious glomerulonephritis
- Electrolyte disorders

TABLE 73.2	Renal Syndromes Commonly Associated with Drug and Excessive Alcohol Use

Nephrotic syndrome

- Hepatitis B– or hepatitis C–related membranous nephropathy
- HIV nephropathy (IDU)
- Amyloidosis (subcutaneous IDU ["skin-popping"])
- Focal and segmental glomerulosclerosis (IDU)

Nephritic-nephrotic syndrome

- Hepatitis C–related membranoproliferative glomerulonephritis (IDU)
- Hepatitis C–related cryoglobulinemia (IDU)

Nephritic syndrome

- Bacterial endocarditis and acute glomerulonephritis (IDU)
- Postinfectious glomerulonephritis (IDU)

Acute renal failure

- Rhabdomyolysis (alcohol, cocaine, MDMA [ecstasy], opiates)
- Crystal-induced renal failure (indinavir, acyclovir, sulfonamides)
- Thrombotic microangiopathy (cocaine)

Hypertension

- Hepatitis B– or amphetamine-associated polyarteritis nodosa (IDU, amphetamine)
- Accelerated hypertension (cocaine)

MEASUREMENT OF RENAL FUNCTION

For patients with current or past drug abuse or dependence, tests to perform on a regular and frequent basis include

- Measurement of renal function (creatinine or eGFR)
- Serum electrolytes
- Urinalysis
- Urine protein excretion and/or 24-hour urine quantification of proteinuria
- Twenty-four–hour urine creatinine excretion and calculated glomerular filtration rate (GFR = urinary creatinine concentration × urinary volume/plasma creatinine concentration/1.73 m^2)

Patients with cachexia and cirrhosis often have a serum creatinine values within the "normal range," yet their GFR is markedly diminished. GFR is also important in determining medication dose adjustments. If it is not possible to obtain a 24-hour collection, proteinuria can be estimated by using a spot urine protein-to-creatinine ratio, but this ratio will overestimate actual protein excretion in patients with reduced muscle mass.

NEPHROTIC SYNDROME

Nephrotic syndrome is narrowly defined as heavy proteinuria (>3.5 g per day), hypoalbuminemia, hyperlipidemia, lipiduria, and edema.

HIV-Associated Nephropathy

HIV-associated nephropathy (HIVAN) can occur at any stage of HIV disease, with presentation in patients who already have an AIDS-defining condition or as the presenting manifestation of AIDS in patients who otherwise are asymptomatic. Commonly *collapsing nephropathy*, a form of focal and segmental glomerular sclerosis with collapse of the glomerular tufts, is seen. Proteinuria is not usually accompanied by edema or serosal effusions and there is absence of hypertension, even with advanced renal insufficiency. Ultrasonic evaluation reveals normal-sized or enlarged kidneys that are hyperechoic. African American race (suggesting a genetic predisposition), low CD4 counts, and positive family history of renal disease are risk factors for the development of HIVAN.

The pathogenesis of HIVAN is incompletely understood, but data suggest a direct role of viral infection rather than the indirect effects of modulation of different cytokines and associated infective agents, which often are encountered in the later stages of AIDS.

Renal insufficiency appears very early in the disease and is rapidly progressive, leading to end-stage renal disease (ESRD) in a matter of weeks or months. The use of highly-active anti-retroviral therapy (HAART) at earlier stages of HIV infection is associated with a more benign and protracted course. The use of angiotensin-converting enzyme inhibitors appears to decrease the magnitude of proteinuria and postpone progression.

With longer survival of HIV patients on renal replacement therapy and the better outlook for patients who respond and are adherent to HAART, more often dialysis is provided to these patients, and centers are offering stable HIV patients on dialysis the opportunity for renal transplantation.

Hepatitis Virus–Associated Nephrotic Syndrome

Hepatitis B– and C–associated nephropathies are frequently found among injection drug users (IDUs). The association between hepatitis B and membranous nephropathy is well established. Whereas antiviral therapy may prove beneficial, immunosuppressive treatment used in the idiopathic form of nephrotic syndrome actually may enhance ongoing hepatitis B viral replication.

The most common presentation of renal disease in patients with hepatitis C is a combination of nephritic and nephrotic syndromes (described below). Less often, membranous nephropathy has been described in association with hepatitis C in IDUs.

Heroin Nephropathy

Heroin nephropathy has been considered a secondary cause of focal and segmental glomerulosclerosis, often associated with hypertension and slow progression to ESRD. Its rarity may reflect more purified forms of heroin and/or the removal of contaminants that were, in fact, responsible for "heroin nephropathy."

Subcutaneous Drug Use–Associated Amyloidosis

Chronic suppurative skin infections related to subcutaneous illicit drug injection are known to be associated with secondary amyloidosis with renal involvement. Clinically, these patients may be very difficult to distinguish from those with HIVAN or hepatitis-related renal disease because they present with nephritic range proteinuria, renal insufficiency, and normal-sized or enlarged kidneys. Tubular dysfunction, including nephrogenic diabetes insipidus and proximal or distal renal tubular acidosis, may also be present.

NEPHRITIC-NEPHROTIC SYNDROME

This syndrome is characterized by significant proteinuria, the presence of hematuria, hypertension, and variable degrees of renal insufficiency. Cases with mixed cryoglobulinemia are distinguished by detectable serum cryoglobulins, decreased C4 and normal C3 levels, and characteristic histological findings. Palpable purpura, arthralgias, peripheral neuropathy, and nonspecific systemic complaints may be present.

In the setting of past or present IDU, hepatitis C–related glomerular disease should be considered. In many of these cases, signs of liver dysfunction are not yet present. The course of nephropathy associated with dual infection with HIV and hepatitis C has been reported as aggressive, with rapid progression to ESRD.

The use of combination therapy with interferon and ribavirin is accepted even in the absence of specific indications to treat the liver disease but its use is contraindicated when the creatinine clearance is <50 mL per minute because of increased side effects, including severe hemolytic anemia.

NEPHRITIC SYNDROME

The presence of nephritic urinary sediment (proteinuria, hematuria, and often red blood cell casts), variable degrees of hypertension, and renal insufficiency in the setting of IDU should raise the suspicion of immune complex–mediated glomerulonephritis. In this circumstance, bacterial sepsis and acute bacterial endocarditis are common and the most frequent pathogen is *Staphylococcus aureus*. Hypertension and low complement levels (C3) are present less consistently than in poststreptococcal glomerulonephritis. Recovery of renal function usually occurs with treatment of the underlying infection.

A higher incidence and more severe course of postinfectious glomerulonephritis in people with alcohol dependence have been reported. Patients with bacterial endocarditis who develop renal failure days to weeks after the onset of antibiotic therapy should raise the suspicion of acute interstitial nephritis.

ISOLATED HEMATURIA

The presence of hematuria should not be assumed to be glomerular in origin, especially in the absence of proteinuria, and other urological causes should be ruled out. Hematuria may be the only manifestation of immunoglobulin A (IgA) nephropathy, and there appears to be an association between IgA nephropathy and alcoholic cirrhosis, possibly related to a decreased clearance of IgA molecules because of arteriovenous shunting away from the reticuloendothelial system. In patients with HIV infection treated with certain medications, crystalluria is another possible explanation for hematuria (described below). Such hematuria sometimes is associated with impaired renal function, which usually is reversible after volume expansion and discontinuation of the offending agent.

HYPERTENSION AND RENAL DISEASE

The development of acute hypertension in connection with cocaine use is well recognized. Presentations of cocaine or MDMA intoxication with accelerated hypertension and renal failure have been documented by some. Hypertension and progressive renal failure are also associated with the ingestion of homemade whiskey (so-called moonshine) as a result of lead ingestion from car radiators used to distill the whiskey.

Polyarteritis nodosa has been associated with hepatitis B and drugs of abuse, especially amphetamines. Patients may present with accelerated hypertension, systemic symptoms, and necrotizing vasculitis, which can affect medium-sized arteries, including renal, mesenteric, coronary, and (rarely) cerebral circulation. Treatment usually is with steroids and cytotoxic agents but antivirals such as lamivudine or telbivudine may prove to be effective, without the risk of enhanced viral replication with immunosuppression.

ACUTE RENAL FAILURE

Rhabdomyolysis

A common presentation of rhabdomyolysis is a patient who presents to the emergency department with agitation, confusion, hyperthermia, and brownish red urine positive for blood but without red blood cells on microscopy. A history of use of drugs associated with this condition (phencyclidine, methamphetamines, MDMA, cocaine, heroin, and alcohol) maybe elicited. If tonic-clonic seizures have occurred (as in alcohol withdrawal), markedly elevated serum creatine kinase levels are seen. The presence of volume depletion, hypotension, acidosis, and hypoxemia increases the likelihood of acute tubular necrosis.

Malnourished patients (especially those with alcohol dependence) may be predisposed to ischemic muscular injury as a result of hypokalemia and hypophosphatemia. In addition to hyperactivity, compression of muscle (crush injury) because of drug-induced stupor or coma and immobilization for prolonged periods of time can result in rhabdomyolysis. In this case, hypocalcemia (secondary to deposition of calcium in necrotic muscle cells or precipitation with phosphate released from destroyed muscle cells), hyperkalemia, and hyperuricemia also may be present.

Treatment includes volume expansion with isotonic saline, sodium bicarbonate (in the absence of hypocalcemia) to alkalinize the urine and decrease the toxicity of myoglobin and possibly mannitol. Most patients recover renal function with aggressive treatment.

Crystal-Induced Tubular Injury

Acute renal failure has been described with the use of antiviral agents, including acyclovir, indinavir, ritonavir, and sulfonamide, usually when they are used in large doses in patients who also are volume depleted. Recovery of renal function is the rule when the patient is given adequate hydration and is withdrawn from the offending agent or the dose is reduced.

Hepatorenal Syndrome

Chronic alcohol ingestion can lead to hepatorenal syndrome. This almost uniformly fatal complication is thought to reflect a state of profound renal vasoconstriction and splanchnic vasodilatation associated with severely impaired liver function, often with portal hypertension and ascites. A slow rise in serum creatinine (which may be masked by malnutrition and decreased muscle mass) and oliguria, accompanied by low urinary sodium concentration—usually <10 mEq/L—are characteristic of presentation. Inciting events such as gastrointestinal bleeding, diuresis, or spontaneous bacterial peritonitis can sometimes, but not always, be identified. The prognosis almost always involves the demise of the patient without liver transplantation.

Hemolytic Uremic Syndrome: Thrombotic Microangiopathy

Acute renal insufficiency associated with thrombocytopenic microangiopathic hemolytic anemia has been described in connection with cocaine use and possibly with HIV infection. This syndrome can have catastrophic consequences with renal cortical necrosis and permanent loss of renal function, central nervous system involvement with seizures, and the permanent sequelae of ischemic or hemorrhagic strokes.

The pathogenesis of this syndrome is not known but may involve both immunologic and nonimmunologic mechanisms. Direct endothelial injury, vasoconstriction, and procoagulant effects of cocaine may play a part. Renal biopsy can assist the diagnosis.

Early recognition is important because prompt treatment with plasmapheresis and infusion of fresh frozen plasma can prevent serious complications.

TOBACCO USE AND RENAL DISEASE

Cigarette smoking is related to proteinuria, accelerated atherosclerotic vascular disease, ischemic nephropathy, an increased risk of progression to renal insufficiency in patients with diabetes mellitus and severe essential hypertension, increased risk of sustained proteinuria, and poorer prognosis of renal disease.

OTHER CAUSES OF RENAL INJURY

Opiates can cause urinary retention, especially in older men who have underlying prostatic hyperplasia.

Fluid and Electrolyte Abnormalities among Patients with Drug Abuse

Patients who use illicit drugs may present with myriad fluid and electrolyte abnormalities, but few are specifically associated with a particular drug. People with chronic alcohol dependence are the most frequently seen among this group.

Alcohol-dependent patients, especially if they have been binge drinking and acutely stop, may present with severe anion gap acidosis. This condition is ketoacidosis induced by poor dietary intake, especially carbohydrates, and the inhibition of gluconeogenesis and acceleration of lipolysis by alcohol. Other acid-base disturbances, including nonanion gap acidosis secondary to diarrhea and renal tubular acidosis, seen in alcoholics usually are not life threatening. The finding of reduced serum bicarbonate can represent compensation for respiratory alkalosis.

Hypokalemias, seen in connection with gastrointestinal losses and secondary hyperaldosteronism, can accelerate or worsen hepatic encephalopathy.

One of the most frequent electrolyte abnormalities among people with alcohol dependence is hypomagnesemia. The etiology probably is a combination of poor nutrition and gastrointestinal losses, coupled with direct renal tubular alcohol toxicity, which decreases renal magnesium absorption. Hypocalcemia is often associated. Hypokalemia is worsened by concomitant hypomagnesemia, which promotes kaliuresis and, like hypocalcemia, is refractory to correction unless the magnesium deficit is replaced. The correction of hypomagnesemia is critical to allow repair of any renal potassium wasting. Severe hypomagnesemia should be treated with slow intravenous infusion, whereas oral replacement can be used for therapy of milder forms of hypomagnesemia.

Hypophosphatemia often is seen in alcoholism and may contribute to rhabdomyolysis and encephalopathy. Again, dietary deficiency, increased gastrointestinal losses, and increased renal excretion contribute to this deficit.

Toxic Alcohols

The ingestion of a toxic alcohol—methanol, ethylene glycol, or isopropyl alcohol—is occasionally seen in an alcohol-dependent patient. The metabolic products of these alcohols are severely toxic and produce organ damage and anion gap acidosis. Anion gap acidosis and the presence of an osmolal gap are usually the first clue to toxic alcohol ingestion.

Treatment used to be intravenous ethanol to compete for alcohol dehydrogenase and thus reduces the production of the toxic organic acid metabolites. Currently, fomepizole, an intravenous medication that competitively inhibits alcohol dehydrogenase more than ethanol, is very effective and safer than an ethanol infusion. As long as kidney function is maintained, the alcohol will be removed by renal excretion but with severe intoxication, hemodialysis is used. Failure to recognize and promptly treat these alcohol intoxications can lead to multiple organ damage and, for methanol, to blindness.

Isopropyl alcohol, found in rubbing alcohol and other solvents, is metabolized to acetone and excreted by the kidneys and the lung. Here, the alcohol itself rather than the products of alcohol metabolism is the toxic agent. Patients may appear inebriated but without an odor of ethanol on the breath. There is usually no anion gap acidosis but gastritis, ketonuria, and an osmolal gap are often present.

Inhalants

An unusual cause of metabolic acidosis and hypokalemia involves toluene intoxication from glue sniffing. Distal renal tubular acidosis has been described in this setting, but the principal mechanism producing the acidosis seems to involve increased hippuric acid derived from toluene metabolism. The hippuric acid is rapidly excreted, leading to a normal anion gap metabolic acidosis.

MDMA ("ECSTASY")

Often used in venues where ambient temperature is high and vigorous physical activity occurs, MDMA use can lead to agitation, high fever, hyperventilation, and impaired sensorium. This condition leads to increased insensible fluid losses and sets the stage for dehydration (hypernatremia) and volume depletion. The results, unless treated promptly, can include hypotension, shock, brain damage, and rhabdomyolysis with renal failure. The priority in treatment is to reestablish intravascular volume and restore organ perfusion followed by restoration of isotonicity.

Summary Author: Agnes Kwasnicka
Paul S. Haber

Gastrointestinal Disorders Related to Alcohol and Other Drug Use

GASTROINTESTINAL PROBLEMS RELATED TO ALCOHOL

The relative risk of alcohol-related gastrointestinal (GI) toxicity is not well defined and appears to differ between affected tissues and between benign and neoplastic disorders. Similarly, the pattern and type of beverage has not been consistently shown to predispose to any specific GI effects of alcohol.

Parotids

Painless symmetrical enlargement of the parotid glands (termed *sialosis* or *sialadenitis*) is common in patients with alcoholic liver injury and may contribute to decreased salivary secretions and progressive dental caries and poor oral mucosal health.

Esophagus

Both acute and chronic alcohol consumption are associated with symptomatic gastroesophageal reflux disease (GERD). A number of mechanisms that have been identified may contribute to these effects of alcohol including injury to the esophageal mucosa, reduced lower esophageal sphincter pressure (LESP), and reduced maximal LESP stimulated by a meal. These effects resolve with a month of abstinence. Excessive alcohol may be associated with Barrett esophagus and is strongly associated with carcinoma.

Alcoholic Gastritis

Exposure of the gastric mucosa to high concentrations of alcohol induces gastric mucosal injury characterized by subepithelial hemorrhages and epithelial erosions. Upper GI bleeding is very common among people with alcoholism and may be due to a wide range of pathology, most commonly hemorrhagic gastritis.

One study found that gastritis was not more common in patients with cirrhosis than in healthy controls. The causal relationship between alcohol and gastritis is complicated by the role of *Helicobacter pylori* in the pathology. In one study, gastritis in people with alcohol dependence was strongly associated with *H. pylori* infection, with histologic and symptomatic relief after eradication of the organism but no improvement with abstinence from alcohol. Healing of established ulcers is not retarded by moderate alcohol consumption but heavier drinking is associated with reduced medication compliance and delayed healing.

The clinical term *alcoholic gastritis* is nonspecific and refers to a broad range of upper GI symptoms. Given the uncertainty surrounding the etiologic role of excessive alcohol use in gastritis and the broad range of potential explanations for these symptoms, it is appropriate to evaluate patients on an individual basis for specific causes.

Alcoholic Pancreatitis

Alcoholic pancreatitis remains a major cause of morbidity among people with alcohol dependence. The rise in incidence of pancreatitis correlates with total community alcohol consumption.

Definitions Pancreatitis can be acute or chronic, with the latter characterized by chronic inflammation, glandular atrophy, and fibrosis manifesting as pain with exocrine or endocrine insufficiency. Other terms used to describe specific associating findings include

- *Acute fluid collections*: a collection lacking a defined wall, which is common early in the course of the disease and tends to regress spontaneously.
- *Pseudocyst*: a collection of pancreatic juice enclosed by a connective tissue wall arising from disruption of pancreatic ducts and frequently communicating with the duct system.
- *Pancreatic necrosis*: diffuse or focal areas of nonviable pancreatic parenchyma typically associated with peripancreatic fat necrosis and which may be *sterile* or *infected*.
- *Pancreatic abscess*: a circumscribed collection of pus in or near the pancreas following pancreatitis or pancreatic trauma.

Predisposing Factors Only a minority (fewer than 5%) of people who drink heavily develop clinically evident pancreatic disease, though a postmortem study has shown that pathologic changes in the pancreas are common among those with alcoholism. Attempts to account for this individual susceptibility have not revealed a definitive correlation, though genetic factors appear to play a role in some cases.

Etiology Pancreatitis typically occurs in subjects who have consumed >100 g alcohol (five to six drinks) per day for at least 5 to 10 years and rarely if ever follows an isolated episode of heavy drinking. Once the disease is established, episodic heavy drinking often precipitates relapses. Pancreatitis is common among people with HIV, particularly in association with heavy alcohol use. Though alcohol abuse is a known cause of hypertriglyceridemia and severe hypertriglyceridemia can cause pancreatitis, the majority of cases of alcoholic pancreatitis are not associated with marked hyperlipidemia.

Pathogenesis Two important factors leading to tissue injury in pancreatitis are *autodigestion* and *oxidant stress*. Several lines of evidence indicate that activated digestive enzymes play an important role in pancreatitis. Oxidant stress is characterized by the production of reactive oxygen species (free radicals) that are highly reactive and bind to lipids, proteins, and nucleic acids leading to cellular injury. Free radicals are generated during experimental pancreatitis from infiltrating leukocytes or possibly within acinar cells. Once autodigestion has been activated, progression of the disease involves local inflammation and, when severe, systemic inflammation involving a range of cytokines. Inhibition of these mediators of inflammation has the potential to limit the progression of pancreatitis and prevent serious complications or death but cannot prevent the initial attack. The proposed cascade of events is illustrated in Figure 74.1.

Diagnosis A confident diagnosis of pancreatitis can often be made on the basis of an attack of severe abdominal pain and tenderness with elevation of the serum amylase more than three times the upper limit of normal and with imaging studies suggestive of inflammation in and around the pancreas.

The amylase level does not rise significantly in approximately 10% of cases of acute pancreatitis, including many with alcoholic pancreatitis or in those with delayed presentation. Determination of serum lipase, which remains elevated longer than the serum amylase, may be helpful. Perforated peptic ulcer, ischemic bowel, bulimia, gynecologic conditions (tuboovarian abscess/rupture), renal failure, salivary gland disease, and minor elevations of the serum amylase (less than threefold) due to administration of morphine with secondary spasm of the sphincter of Oddi must be ruled out. Painless pancreatitis generally only occurs in the setting of a comatose or postoperative patient in whom pain is not appreciated.

Assessment of Severity Severe pancreatitis carries a risk of mortality and is characterized by the presence of organ failure (renal, respiratory, circulatory, GI bleeding), local complications, (necrosis, abscess, or pseudocyst) or systemic alterations (falling hematocrit, rising urea, hypocalcaemia, acidosis, significant fluid sequestration). Enzyme levels do not correlate well with disease severity. The contrast-enhanced CT scan is now widely performed to detect pancreatic necrosis and complications of severe pancreatitis but its use is controversial. CT scanning without contrast can detect most diagnostic features of pancreatitis.

Treatment Severe cases, particularly those associated with respiratory or renal failure, require treatment in an intensive care unit. Initially, patients are treated with bed rest, analgesics, intravenous fluids, fasting, and opioid analgesia. Intravenous fluids are given aggressively to restore vascular volume and renal perfusion and

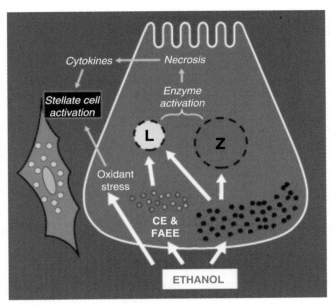

FIGURE 74.1   Overview of the pathogenesis of alcoholic pancreatitis. Ethanol increases pancreatic protein synthesis (•) and pancreatic lipids (o) including cholesteryl esters (CE) and fatty acid ethyl esters (FAEE) and generates oxidant stress. These processes increase the protein content of lysosomes (L) and zymogen granules (z) and destabilize their membranes (*dotted lines*). As a consequence, intracellular activation of digestive enzymes is facilitated, leading to autodigestion. Cellular injury occurs by necrosis and stimulates release of cytokines, which promote inflammation, activation of stellate cells and in turn pancreatic fibrosis.

hour-by-hour monitoring is required. Early refeeding seems to cause clinical relapse; thus, nutritional support is required if oral intake is not likely to be restored within several days. Enteral feeding is safer and less expensive, and there is some evidence that states it may be more effective than total parenteral nutrition (TPN).

Surgery is uncommonly required, the main indication being necrotizing pancreatitis. Infected necrosis carries a high morbidity and mortality and requires surgical debridement followed by postoperative lavage. By contrast, sterile necrosis often improves with conservative therapy alone. Pancreatic abscess carries a very high mortality and is an absolute indication for drainage by open surgery or percutaneous techniques. Small pseudocysts may resolve spontaneously, but large or symptomatic ones usually require drainage via endoscopic, percutaneous, or operative techniques.

Chronic Pancreatitis

Recurrent episodes of acute pancreatitis may lead to chronic pancreatitis. Chronic excessive consumption of alcohol is the most common cause.

Clinical Features

The main problem is usually pain and is typically diffusely located in the upper abdomen, may radiate to the back when severe, increases with meals, decreases appetite and food consumption, and often results in weight loss. The other manifestations are diabetes mellitus and steatorrhea. Investigations of vitamin deficiency reveal malabsorption of fat soluble vitamins and osteopenia.

Treatment   Complete abstinence from alcohol is essential to minimize progression of the disease and to help control pain. Opioid analgesics are often required and should not be unreasonably withheld. Pancreatic enzyme supplements have been evaluated for the treatment of pain, but the evidence is mixed. A trial of 1 month is sufficient to determine whether this works in practice. There is now evidence from a small placebo-controlled trial that antioxidant therapy (a combination preparation that contained selenium, β-carotene, vitamin C, vitamin E, and L-methionine) may reduce pain and improve quality of life in chronic pancreatitis. The relationship between pancreatic duct obstruction and pain is not clear, but relief of obstruction is clinically associated with relief of pain, with better long-term analgesia and improved quality of life.

Exocrine failure is treated by dietary modification and pancreatic enzyme replacement. Reduction of dietary fat intake reduces steatorrhea. Pancreatic enzymes are required with each meal and snack. Histamine-2 receptor antagonists or proton pump inhibitors also limit lipase inactivation. In those that develop diabetes mellitus oral hypoglycemic agents may be used, but most require insulin. The diabetes is "brittle" in that the patient is susceptible to hypoglycemia due to loss of both insulin and glucagon secretion.

Small Intestine

Diarrhea is common among those who drink alcohol excessively, both acutely and chronically. Multiple factors contribute to this problem, including altered motility, permeability, and nutritional disorders. Small intestinal mucosal injury can occur after acute or chronic administration of alcohol.

Acute administration of alcohol leads to increased gut permeability, resulting both in abnormal absorption of luminal content (such as endotoxin, which contributes to the pathogenesis of alcoholic liver disease) and abnormal leakage of mucosal contents (such as albumin). Ethanol also inhibits absorption of actively transported sugars, dipeptides, amino acids, water, lipids, vitamins (notably thiamine, folate), and minerals (calcium, iron, zinc, and selenium). Folate deficiency, common among people with alcohol problems, causes intestinal injury, leading to malabsorption and diarrhea and further loss of folate. Ethanol may exacerbate lactase deficiency, especially in nonwhites.

Colon

Portal hypertension may manifest uncommonly with hemorrhoids and rarely with colonic varices. Alcohol has also been reported to cause nonulcerative inflammatory changes unrelated to folate deficiency in human colonic epithelium.

Alcohol and Gastrointestinal Cancer

Alcohol use is a recognized risk factor for several GI neoplasms, including tumors of the tongue, mouth, pharynx, larynx, esophagus, stomach, pancreas, colon, and liver. Alcohol use has been repeatedly associated with an increased incidence of esophageal (and oropharyngeal) cancer, especially in those who also smoke. The effect of alcohol on cancer risk appears to be dose related but even relatively modest average daily consumption, 25 g per day, within the guidelines for men in many countries is associated with increased risk of GI cancer.

In general, the experimental studies have not shown that alcohol is in itself a complete carcinogen. Rather, ethanol is a cocarcinogen that increases the cancer risk after exposure to another compound. The effect of ethanol may occur at the initiation, induction, or progression stages of tumor development. Ethanol-induced induction of CYP2E1 increases carcinogen activation, potentiation of oxidant stress, diminished DNA repair, suppression of immune responses, and nutritional depletion such as folate deficiency.

The association between alcohol use and hepatocellular carcinoma (HCC) is described in an earlier chapter. There is insufficient experimental evidence to conclude that alcohol is a complete hepatic carcinogen and most patients who develop HCC have cirrhosis, a condition known to predispose to HCC.

GASTROINTESTINAL SYMPTOMS ASSOCIATED WITH ABUSE OF PRESCRIPTION DRUGS

Opioids

Opioids act on gut function in a complex fashion via all three receptor classes in the brain, spinal cord, and enteric nervous systems. Opioids alter both motility and electrolyte absorption, leading to constipation that may be severe. The motility effects, more prominent for the clinically available opioids, decrease the frequency of contractions in, and propulsion along, the small bowel and colon. Among methadone maintenance patients, constipation is common and tends to be worse early in treatment. Fecal impaction and even stercoral perforation have been described and usually respond to increased fluid intake and fiber supplementation to correct for poor dietary intake. Laxatives are not often required, but osmotic agents such as lactulose are the laxatives of choice. The narcotic bowel syndrome is characterized by a picture similar to intestinal pseudo-obstruction. The syndrome is characterized by chronic or frequently recurring abdominal pain that worsens with continued or escalating dosages of narcotics (Fig. 74.2). It is attributed to the effects of opioid drugs on bowel function and opioid-induced hyperalgesia. This syndrome responds to withdrawal of opioids and administration of the α_2-agonist clonidine.

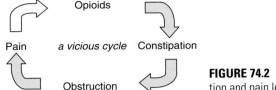

FIGURE 74.2   Opioids increase constipation and in turn obstruction and pain leading to further increase in opioid medication.

Anticholinergics

In high doses, anticholinergic drugs alter mood and are occasionally misused, particularly when prescribed to relieve extrapyramidal symptoms in the mentally ill and among those with limited access to other drugs of abuse. Clonidine and Buscopan prescribed for opioid withdrawal may also be misused. Patients develop marked constipation and abdominal pain as well as dry mouth and blurred vision.

EFFECTS OF TOBACCO ON GASTROINTESTINAL FUNCTION

Gastroesophageal Reflux

Although smoking has been linked to exacerbations of reflux symptoms, on a practical level, smoking cessation is difficult to achieve and has not been shown to induce remission of reflux or healing of esophagitis. Nicotine has been shown to reduce LESP and promote gastroesophageal reflux in response to straining during coughing and deep breathing. People who smoke cigarettes have also been shown to have delayed acid clearance from the esophagus.

Peptic Ulceration

Smoking increases risk of ulcer according to the number of cigarettes smoked and heavy smoking is associated with delayed ulcer healing, increased risk of recurrence, complications, and ulcer-related mortality. The mechanism by which smoking exacerbates peptic ulcer disease remains unclear.

Pancreatic Disease

The finding that smoking moderately increased risk (about threefold) of pancreatic cancer has not been replicated in all studies of this association. In general, most people with alcohol dependence smoke, so it is difficult to separate the effects of tobacco from those of alcohol, which is the major cause for pancreatitis.

Inflammatory Bowel Disease

A curious relationship exists between smoking and inflammatory bowel disease. Smoking has been consistently shown to increase the risk of Crohn disease and to *decrease* the risk of ulcerative colitis. Somewhat provocatively, smoking may also reduce the severity of established ulcerative colitis, suggesting that nicotine has therapeutic potential for this disease. Nicotine influences immune cellular function, increases mucin production, relaxes colonic smooth muscle, increases endogenous glucocorticoids, and influences rectal blood flow and intestinal permeability.

Gastrointestinal Malignancy

Smoking has been strongly linked to cancers of the upper aerodigestive tract and pancreas, as discussed earlier. The link between smoking and stomach cancer is weaker but is present in most studies.

BODY PACKING

Persons smuggling illicit drugs may ingest large amounts of cocaine, heroin, or other drugs aiming to retrieve the packages after reaching their destination. This is referred to as *body packing, cocaine packing,* or *body stuffing syndrome*. Multiple packages made from latex condoms, wax, or plastic bags are used and may also be placed retrogradely into the rectum or vagina. Lethal drug absorption through rubber condoms may occur without rupture. The body packer may present with life-threatening symptoms of intoxication, including seizures and cardiorespiratory collapse, and mechanical obstruction from the ingested drug packets.

Clinical monitoring constitutes frequent clinical and neurologic assessment and abdominal examination daily to detect complications of acute drug intoxication, bowel obstruction, or perforation. The patient should be kept in hospital until all drug packages have cleared owing to the risk of life-threatening overdose if any rupture. Oily or polyethylene glycol laxatives can be given repeatedly to accelerate passage of packages. Plain abdominal x-rays are helpful and can be repeated daily until the gut is cleared, typically 3 to 6 days. Symptomatic cases may require early surgery, but endoscopic removal of packages is not recommended owing to the risk of rupture during manipulation.

Psychostimulants (Cocaine and Amphetamines)

Cocaine may lead to ischemic injury to the gut leading to intestinal perforation, infarction, or ischemic colitis. These uncommon injuries typically present with abdominal pain and peritonitis but may be occult in a critically ill and unconscious person.

Cannabis

Cannabinoid receptors are widely expressed throughout both the upper and lower GI tracts and are also expressed on hepatic stellate cells owing to their influence on a range of GI functions in health and disease. Cannabis (marijuana) and other cannabinoids appear to be effective antiemetics and are involved in inhibition of gastric emptying and gastric acid secretion. Cannabis has also been linked to a series of cases with a cyclical pattern of hyperemesis after several years of cannabis abuse. The mechanism was not understood and the existence of this syndrome remains controversial.

CHAPTER 75

Summary Author: Agnes Kwasnicka
Kevin C. Wilson • Elizabeth Mirabile Levins • Jussi J. Saukkonen

Respiratory Tract Disorders Related to Alcohol and Other Drug Use

RESPIRATORY FUNCTION

Receptors within the lung and in the brain are responsive to a number of addictive substances. Addictive drugs may perturb the active processes within the lung, resulting in local inflammation, infections, airway reactivity, impairment of pulmonary vascular integrity, acute lung injury, structural injury, or derangements of gas exchange. The use of numerous substances at the same time is often associated with a variety of injuries, making it difficult to ascribe a particular respiratory complication to a single agent. Furthermore, coexisting pulmonary pathology may worsen the acute physiologic effects of an addictive drug on the lungs.

COMMON PULMONARY COMPLICATIONS

Respiratory Depression

Nearly all of the drugs discussed here may directly inhibit respiration or induce seizures. With overdose, lethargy may progress rapidly to stupor, severe respiratory depression, coma, and respiratory arrest. Airway protection is paramount, and patients with known or suspected overdose should be admitted to an intensive care unit for monitoring of their respiratory, neurologic, and hemodynamic status.

Atelectasis

In patients with respiratory depression, shallow respirations may result in airway collapse. Ineffective cough and aspirated oral and gastric secretions, with loss of surfactant, lead to atelectasis. This can cause shunting and significant hypoxemia. Incentive spirometry, chest physiotherapy, respiratory suctioning, and supplemental oxygen generally are indicated. Bronchoscopy may be needed for refractory atelectasis.

Aspiration Pneumonitis

Respiratory depression or seizures may cause aspiration of oral secretions or gastric contents. Often the event is only chemical pneumonitis, but this condition may lead to noncardiogenic pulmonary edema and respiratory failure, with or without bacterial superinfection. Preventive care should be directed toward airway control, maintenance of at least a 45-degree angle, avoidance of oral intake while lethargic, pulmonary toilet, supplemental oxygen, and antibiotics as indicated.

Respiratory Infections

Many drugs have adverse effects on leukocyte function, contribute to malnutrition with resultant immune dysfunction, are injected under septic conditions, or may be contaminated with pathogens. In addition, infectious complications may be related to coexisting disease (e.g., HIV, cirrhosis, smoking) or their treatment (e.g., chronic obstructive pulmonary disease (COPD) may require on-going therapy with a corticosteroid, which is immunosuppressive and thus may contribute to infections). Patients often present with typical symptoms but general ill health in this population and polymicrobial infections make atypical or subacute presentations common. Blood cultures are warranted in many patients, especially those who are toxic, ill-appearing, immunocompromised, or otherwise high-risk (e.g., alcohol abuse, intravenous drug abuse).

Respiratory Complications of Contaminants

Illicit drugs vary greatly in purity, as they often are adulterated with various substances. The lungs act as filters, trapping inhaled or injected foreign substances, which may incite local inflammatory or fibrotic responses. Contaminating microorganisms also may lead to pulmonary infection or to hypersensitivity responses.

Respiratory Complications of Injected Drugs

Opiates, stimulants, and combinations thereof are commonly injected into the veins. Acute pulmonary complications are likely to be severe, including respiratory failure and acute pulmonary edema. Chronic pulmonary problems include the development of interstitial and bullous lung disease, endovascular and respiratory infections, and tuberculosis.

Talc Granulomatosis   Talc (magnesium silicate) is widely used as a filler in oral medications, which may be crushed and injected, and it is used to adulterate inhaled and injected drugs. A syndrome similar to sarcoidosis may result, with insidious onset of granulomatous interstitial fibrosis. Dyspnea, particularly with exertion, and cough are the most common symptoms and may present in association with talc retinopathy. The chest radiograph is normal in up to half of patients, but diffuse micronodular interstitial opacity may be evident. High-resolution computed tomography (CT) may be necessary for diagnosis. Pulmonary function tests may show a low-diffusion capacity, and bronchoalveolar lavage may demonstrate local lymphocytosis and birefringent intracellular crystals or free talc. Lung biopsy may be required to establish the diagnosis. In advanced stages or if there is associated granulomatous pulmonary arterial occlusion, pulmonary hypertension and right ventricular failure can occur.

Pulmonary Hypertension   Intravenous drug users may develop chronic pulmonary hypertension from multiple mechanisms, including chronic hypoxemia related to interstitial lung disease and vasoconstriction, or pulmonary arterial thrombosis at sites of foreign body granulomatosis, with subsequent occlusion (angiothrombotic pulmonary hypertension). Primary pulmonary hypertension also may occur as a result of HIV-1 infection. Patients may complain of dyspnea on exertion, and ECG may show evidence of right ventricular enlargement and failure. Treatment options include supplemental oxygen for patients who are hypoxemic, anticoagulation for patients at increased risk for venous thromboembolism, and diuretics for patients with pulmonary or peripheral edema.

Septic Thromboemboli   Septic pulmonary embolism, usually involving *Staphylococcus aureus,* is the most common pulmonary complication among intravenous heroin users and may result from tricuspid endocarditis or from infected injection-site thrombophlebitis. The patient typically presents in an acute toxic state, with fever, dyspnea, chest pain, and leukocytosis. Radiographic examination of the chest may reveal bilateral necrotizing infiltrates or single or multiple pulmonary lesions, which frequently cavitate. Infection may be complicated by bronchopleural fistulas, empyema, or pneumothorax, and antibiotic therapy usually is prolonged. Residual pleural thickening and fibrosis are common.

Needle Embolization   Occasionally, needles, especially those used multiple times, may be broken off inadvertently during or after injection. Chest radiographs aid diagnosis but specific therapy or removal is not necessary.

Pneumothorax   Pneumothorax—unilateral or bilateral—may develop from inadvertent puncture of the lung during attempted needle injection into a jugular or subclavian vessel or from cavitating septic thromboemboli. Depending on the size and complications, tube thoracostomy and antibiotics maybe required.

Empyema   Cavitating infections from septic emboli, pneumonia, or unclean needles may contaminate the pleural space and lead to empyema.

Mycotic Aneurysms   Patients with this endovascular infection, caused by septic emboli, may present with or without hemoptysis. Contrast-enhanced CT demonstrates nodular lesions. Despite surgical intervention, massive hemoptysis may be fatal. Patients without hemoptysis may experience resolution of this condition with antibiotic therapy.

Pulmonary Emphysema   Bullous emphysema may develop in intravenous drug injectors, either in association with talc granulomatosis or in its absence.

Respiratory Complications of Inhaled Drugs

Inhalation has become a preferred route for the consumption of many addictive drugs. Delivery of a drug through the lung affords ease of administration, rapid onset of action, dose minimization, avoidance of intravenous injection, and avoidance of the hepatic first-pass effect. Inhaled drugs vary considerably in size and may be absorbed by impacting proximally against convoluted upper airway walls and bifurcating large airways of the lung (>6 μm particles) or may settle in distal airways (1–5 μm particles). Smoke consists of gas and particulate phases, including inorganic and organic substances that may cause mucosal injury and inflammation.

Chronic Bronchitis   This condition is commonly associated with smoking tobacco, marijuana, cocaine, and other drugs. Cough, dyspnea, mucus hypersecretion, and a propensity to airway reactivity and acute bacterial bronchitis may be seen.

Bronchospasm   Airway reactivity often is seen with inhaled heroin, cocaine, tobacco, and marijuana. Patients typically present with dyspnea, tachypnea, wheezing, and tachycardia within minutes to hours after inhalation. Blood gases may demonstrate respiratory alkalosis (early in presentation) or respiratory acidosis (later), but the chest radiograph typically is clear. Treatment is with supplemental oxygen, bronchodilators, steroids, and, if severe, mechanical ventilation.

Barotrauma   Inhalation of cocaine, heroin, MDMA, marijuana, tobacco, and volatile substances is associated with barotrauma, including pneumothorax and pneumomediastinum. The cause is either extreme breath-holding against a closed glottis (a prolonged Valsalva maneuver) in an attempt to increase the drug's effect or spontaneous rupture of a bleb in those who have developed bullous emphysema. The presentation maybe acute chest or back pain and dyspnea, with or without hypoxemia.

Hemoptysis   Hemoptysis may result from mucosal irritation or ulceration anywhere within the respiratory tract (as in epistaxis, sinusitis, or bronchitis), from pulmonary infarct, or from diffuse alveolar hemorrhage.

Pulmonary Emphysema   Destruction of lung parenchyma, with resultant pulmonary emphysema, may occur with inhaled tobacco, marijuana, and chronic opium use.

TOBACCO AND NICOTINE

Smoking has profound effects on the lung, altering the immunologic and structural milieu. The factors that determine whether these effects will lead to lung cancer, emphysema, bronchitis, and airway reactivity include individual genetic susceptibility, quantity of cigarettes smoked, the years spent smoking, the manner in which they were smoked (e.g., the depth of inhalation) and perhaps heterozygosity for the gene that causes α-1-antitrypsin deficiency.

Tobacco smoke induces the elaboration of chemotactic agents for neutrophils and monocytes, as well as mediators that cause epithelial injury leading to loss of pulmonary architecture, loss of functional gas-exchanging units, and permeability changes.

Smokers display a more rapid decline in FEV1 than do nonsmokers. Tobacco use is associated with clinical syndromes described below and increases the risk of developing cor pulmonale, pulmonary hypertension, lung cancer, and lower respiratory tract infections. Fortunately cessation can slow lung function decline and decrease these risks.

Environmental tobacco smoke contributes to lower respiratory illnesses, chronic respiratory symptoms, middle ear disease, reduced lung function, asthma, and wheezing in children and increased risk of lung cancer, cardiovascular diseases, and acute respiratory symptoms and illnesses in adults.

Chronic Bronchitis

Chronic bronchitis is defined as sputum production for at least 3 months in two successive years in the absence of other causes of chronic cough and maybe associated with airway reactivity. Mucous gland hypertrophy of intermediate-sized airways causes overproduction of mucus, overwhelming the mucociliary escalator already compromised by tobacco smoke.

Airway Reactivity

Smoking exacerbates preexisting asthma and promotes bronchial hyperreactivity even in patients without obstructive lung disease. Bronchoconstriction appears to be caused by nicotine and nonnicotinic components of tobacco. An increased number of activated leukocytes may also contribute to asthmatic symptoms.

Pulmonary Emphysema

Pulmonary emphysema is characterized by irreversible enlargement of the airspaces distal to the terminal bronchiole with destruction of the alveolar walls and septa. This results in hyperinflation and flattening of the diaphragm, decreased ability to oxygenate blood, suboptimal ventilation–perfusion relationships, and carbon dioxide retention. Pneumothorax may develop from rupture of a subpleural emphysematous bleb.

Interstitial Lung Disease

Two forms of idiopathic interstitial pneumonia are associated with smoking: desquamative interstitial pneumonia, which presents with insidiously developing dyspnea, interstitial infiltrates, and restrictive physiology and respiratory bronchiolitis-associated interstitial lung disease, which has radiologic and histopathologic overlap with the former. Open lung biopsy is needed for reliable diagnosis, but both diseases are usually treated with a trial of systemic corticosteroids.

Smoking also is a risk factor for the development of pulmonary histiocytosis X (eosinophilic granuloma) and may precipitate exacerbations of Goodpasture disease.

Pulmonary Hypertension and Cor Pulmonale

Chronic hypoxic vasoconstriction of the pulmonary vasculature leads to pulmonary arterial hypertension and right heart strain. Primary therapy consists of optimizing treatment of the cause of the hypoxemia, for example, inhaled bronchodilators for obstructive lung disease and immunosuppressive therapy for interstitial lung disease. The increased risk for venous thromboembolism and pulmonary or peripheral edema may need to be managed. Supplemental oxygen for at least 18 hours per day prolongs survival and improves symptoms but advanced therapy is often needed.

Pneumothorax

Spontaneous pneumothorax may occur as a result of bullous emphysema, with rupture of a subpleural bleb.

Hemoptysis

Most often, hemoptysis results from acute bacterial bronchitis, but it may betray the presence of other airway pathology, including bronchogenic carcinoma.

Bronchogenic Carcinoma

The cumulative risk of lung cancer among heavy smokers may be as high as 30%, compared to only 1% in lifetime nonsmokers. Inhalation of tobacco, both through direct smoking or second-hand smoke, can lead to bronchogenic carcinoma but smokeless tobacco has also been linked to the development of malignancies of the aerodigestive tract. Tobacco smoke may predispose to the development of lung cancer by triggering oncogenic genetic mutations, particularly of the *p53* gene. Reduction of smoking, or ideally cessation, reduces the risk of lung cancer, with the extent of risk reduction depending on the duration of abstinence.

Patients may be asymptomatic, and treatment often entails surgical resection, radiation or chemotherapy, or a combination of treatments depending on cell type.

Hypersensitivity Pneumonitis (Extrinsic Allergic Alveolitis)

A variety of molds, including *Aspergillus* and thermophilic actinomycetes, may be present on tobacco plants, which then are inhaled by workers harvesting the crop or, theoretically, by smokers inducing hypersensitivity reactions. If exposure is long-standing, pulmonary fibrosis may develop.

MARIJUANA

The pyrolysis products of cannabis are similar to those of cigarettes and exert the same effects on the airway epithelium, increasing the possibility of lung cancer. Marijuana smoke has deleterious effects on respiration, depositing three times more tar than cigarette smoke (because the marijuana cigarettes are not filtered and because inhalation tends to be significantly deeper and is associated with prolonged breath-holding) and causing a fivefold higher carboxyhemoglobin level in the blood than cigarettes. Marijuana smoke increases oxidative stress within the lung and impairs alveolar macrophage function. Cases of squamous cell carcinoma of the oropharynx in heavy marijuana smokers also have been reported.

Obstructive Lung Disease

Although heavy regular marijuana smoking is not associated with accelerated decline in FEV1, as is tobacco smoking, marijuana smokers may suffer some of the same complications as do those who smoke tobacco, including chronic bronchitis and bullous emphysema.

Pathogen-Associated Complications

Pulmonary aspergillosis associated with smoking marijuana is reported among immunocompromised patients. This association may become more important as increasing numbers of immunocompromised patients turn to medicinal uses of marijuana.

COCAINE

Cocaine has local anesthetic effects but also crosses the blood–brain barrier and stimulates the CNS where it can increase respiratory rate. It causes fewer tracheobronchial mucosal abnormalities than either smoked tobacco or marijuana, but it may augment the injury induced by those smoked drugs. Cocaine is a highly potent bronchoconstrictor when inhaled. Through its effect on vasculature, cocaine smoking causes vasoconstriction and permeability changes and reduction in diffusion capacity similar to that of smoking tobacco. Cocaine also causes alveolar hemorrhage and noncardiogenic pulmonary edema. Symptoms commonly associated with cocaine use, particularly use of crack cocaine, include cough productive of carbonaceous sputum, pleuritic chest pain, wheezing, dyspnea, and hemoptysis.

Cocaine's effect on the immune system impairs the function of natural killer cells, B and T lymphocytes and alveolar macrophages. After in vivo inhalation or injection of cocaine, neutrophils are activated and have enhanced production of IL-8, which has been implicated in a number of inflammatory lung disorders, including acute lung injury.

Combining cocaine with various depressants such as heroin or morphine ("speedballing") has led to overdose deaths. "Freebasing" is the practice of using volatile solvents to convert cocaine from a salt to a base and to remove adulterants. This potentially incendiary chemical process can lead to extensive cutaneous and inhalational burns.

Barotrauma

Barotrauma is common with crack cocaine inhalation and is associated with prolonged and forceful deep inhalation, Valsalva maneuver, or "shotgunning" (forceful exhalation of crack smoke into another individual's respiratory tract).

Upper Airway Complications

Upper airway complications associated with inhaled cocaine include burns, mucosal irritation or inflammation, nasal septal perforation, sinusitis, epiglottitis, upper airway obstruction, and a vasculitis resembling Wegener granulomatosis.

Bronchitis

Both acute and chronic bronchitis may develop from mucosal irritation, as described earlier. Often, there is concomitant tobacco use, which contributes in large measure to airway obstruction.

Airway Burns

Anesthetic properties of cocaine make the oropharynx and tracheobronchial tree susceptible to thermal inhalational injuries. Thermal injuries of the upper airway can cause airway obstruction and those of the lower airway may lead to airway or tracheal stenosis.

Bronchospasm

Cocaine inhalation may precipitate life-threatening exacerbations of asthma. Cocaine use is associated with severe bronchospasm and inhaled corticosteroid noncompliance.

Hemoptysis

Hemoptysis may result from mucosal irritation or ulceration anywhere within the respiratory tract (as in rhinitis, sinusitis, and bronchitis), from pulmonary infarct, or from diffuse alveolar hemorrhage.

Diffuse Pulmonary Hemorrhage

Autopsy studies show high rates of acute and chronic pulmonary hemorrhage (40%–58%). Diffuse alveolar hemorrhage may be a life-threatening complication.

Pulmonary Edema

Intravenous cocaine causes cardiogenic edema due to arrhythmia, coronary vasospasm–induced myocardial ischemia or infarction, or acute heart failure related to abruptly increased afterload. Noncardiogenic pulmonary edema can also occur with cocaine use.

Pulmonary Vascular Disease and Infarction

There are case reports of cocaine-induced massive pulmonary artery vasoconstriction and, rarely, pulmonary infarction. Vasoconstriction, platelet aggregation, vascular damage, and induction of endothelin-1 release may contribute to this. Pulmonary hypertension may develop over time as a result of interstitial lung disease caused by debris deposited in the lung.

Eosinophilic Hypersensitivity Pneumonitis ("Crack Lung")

A mild Loeffler syndrome has been reported, with transient migratory pulmonary infiltrates and eosinophilia. A more severe reaction may occur 1 to 48 hours after heavy cocaine smoking. This consists of chest pain, cough with hemoptysis, dyspnea, bronchospasm, pruritus, fever, diffuse alveolar infiltrates without effusions, and pulmonary and systemic eosinophilia. Recurrent episodes may occur with continued cocaine inhalation. It is unclear whether this syndrome is specific to cocaine or to impurities present in the inhaled drug.

Bronchiolitis Obliterans-Organizing Pneumonia

A rare complication of cocaine inhalation, bronchiolitis obliterans-organizing pneumonia presents with sub-acute manifestations, including dyspnea, cough, constitutional symptoms, and patchy—usually peripheral—infiltrates. It is diagnosed reliably by open lung biopsy and treated with steroids.

Panlobular Emphysema

Bullous pulmonary emphysema may develop with chronic cocaine use and may be potentiated by tobacco inhalation.

Interstitial Pulmonary Fibrosis

Pulmonary fibrosis may occur as a result of intensive or chronic use of cocaine, either inhaled or injected. Silica or talc is usually found histopathologically. Occasionally, the degree of fibrosis is extensive and leads to pulmonary hypertension.

AMPHETAMINES AND OTHER STIMULANTS

Amphetamines were used in the early part of the last century to treat respiratory illness. They have sympathomimetic effects and can induce some bronchodilation and vasoconstriction. Amphetamines have adverse effects on the immune system which may affect the delayed hypersensitivity response to microbial pathogens.

Metabolic Acidosis and Respiratory Alkalosis

Extreme agitation and hyperthermia may result in rhabdomyolysis and severe metabolic acidosis, with an associated increased respiratory drive. A direct central effect also may increase respiratory drive.

Barotrauma

Pneumomediastinum, subcutaneous emphysema, and retropharyngeal emphysema have been reported with the use of inhaled MDMA.

Respiratory Depression

CNS and respiratory depression may be seen, particularly in overdose. Patients are at increased risk of aspiration from a depressed mental status or from seizures.

Pulmonary Edema

Amphetamines may cause cardiogenic and noncardiogenic pulmonary edema, as well as myocardial infarction or acute cardiomyopathy. Users can also develop pulmonary edema through a neurogenic mechanism or because of aspiration.

Pulmonary Hypertension

Appetite suppressants, such as fenfluramine and its derivatives, may be causal or may hasten the development of pulmonary hypertension. The drug increases circulating levels of serotonin and results in vasoconstriction of the pulmonary vasculature which may lead to proliferation of pulmonary vascular smooth muscle. Intravenous injection and chronic inhalation of methylphenidate has also been reported to cause pulmonary hypertension.

OPIOIDS

Opioids bind to specific receptors, with distribution to the CNS and the cardiovascular, immune, and respiratory systems. Opioid receptors in the respiratory tract are found mostly within the alveolar walls but also are associated with tracheal and bronchial smooth muscle.

Opioid binding to μ_2 receptors in the CNS causes a reduction in responsiveness to carbon dioxide and depresses the pontine and medullary centers that regulate respiratory automaticity and cough. Consequently, breathing becomes irregular and apnea may develop. This effect is dose related.

Opioids can induce histamine release from mast cells, which may lead to pulmonary vein constriction, increased pulmonary capillary permeability and pulmonary edema, and bronchoconstriction. Opioids have significant effects on the immune system, which may account for the reported association with infections.

Although morphine often is used for the relief of dyspnea, opioids also can exert adverse effects on the lung, acutely and with chronic abuse. Acutely, particularly with inhalational use, opioids may induce bronchospasm, bronchitis, and hypersensitivity pneumonitis. Respiratory depression and failure, pulmonary edema, respiratory infections, chronic bronchitis, septic pulmonary emboli, pulmonary hypertension, and talc-related complications are associated with chronic (particularly intravenous) opioid abuse. Pulmonary edema probably is the most common complication of overdose, while respiratory arrest is the most serious.

Bronchospasm

It has long been recognized that asthma exacerbations may be precipitated by heroin use. Opioids can induce bronchospasm in histamine-sensitive asthmatics, but it is unclear whether histamine-insensitive asthmatics are also prone to opioid-induced bronchoconstriction.

Pulmonary Edema

Opioid overdose, particularly with heroin, is a common cause of pulmonary edema in patients younger than 40 years, and it accounts for many drug-related deaths. It is believed to be dose-related rather than an idiosyncratic reaction.

Several mechanisms of opioid-induced noncardiogenic pulmonary edema have been offered. Whether it is a direct toxic effect on the alveolar capillary membrane, an effect on the CNS that induces a vast neurogenic efferent response, a hypersensitivity reaction, or an acute hypoxic effect, the outcome is increased alveolar capillary permeability and fluid extravasation.

Clinically, this complication manifests as dyspnea and somnolence, usually within minutes, depending on the route of administration. Affected individuals become obtunded and cyanotic and develop hypoxemia and hypercapnia.

Treatment is supportive and may include noninvasive or invasive mechanical ventilation, positive end-expiratory pressure, oxygen, and judicious use of diuretics. It is estimated that as many as 50% to 75% of patients with pulmonary edema develop a superimposed pneumonia.

ALCOHOL

Alcohol ingestion may cause acute intoxication accompanied by respiratory depression and complications such as atelectasis, hypoxemia, respiratory acidosis, aspiration, adult respiratory distress syndrome (ARDS), and respiratory failure. Alcohol ingestion also may cause worsening of underlying respiratory conditions such as sleep apnea. Pneumonia caused by atypical pathogen (e.g., *Klebsiella*) occurs with greater frequency among individuals who abuse alcohol chronically.

Acute Metabolic Acidosis and Respiratory Alkalosis

Respiratory alkalosis can occur in compensation for alcoholic ketoacidosis or ingestion of other alcohols (such as methanol) that cause anion gap acidosis.

Chronic Respiratory Alkalosis

Among patients with cirrhosis, chronic respiratory alkalosis is common, even in the absence of metabolic acidosis.

Asthma

Patients with preexisting asthma, particularly those who are histamine sensitive, may experience worsening of asthma symptoms after consumption of alcohol. Acetaldehyde, generated from ethanol metabolism, leads to mast cell or basophil degranulation and the ensuing release of histamine and other mediators of inflammation induce asthma.

Pulmonary Restriction from Ascites

Massive ascites, with or without hydrothorax, may impede diaphragmatic and pulmonary excursion, leading to rapid shallow breathing, dyspnea, atelectasis, and even hypoxemia.

Hepatic Hydrothorax

Cirrhosis with ascites may lead to the formation of pleural effusion, usually on the right side. If refractory to diuretics and other medical therapy, pleurodesis or transjugular intrahepatic portosystemic shunts (TIPS) may need to be performed.

Hepatopulmonary Syndrome

This syndrome, found in 8% to 15% of patients with cirrhosis, consists of a triad of liver dysfunction, intrapulmonary or other vascular dilatations, and arterial hypoxemia. Arteriovenous shunts are thought to arise from circulating estrogen-like substances, as well as from elevated nitric oxide production in the lung. Symptomatic improvement has been reported when TIPS are performed.

Portal Pulmonary Hypertension

Approximately 2% of patients with cirrhosis develop pulmonary arterial hypertension. The pathogenesis of this complication is not clear, but it probably is mediated by both mechanical and humoral factors. The physical signs of right-sided heart failure from pulmonary hypertension may be missed in cirrhotic patients, who already may have peripheral edema. Vasodilator therapy may be used and, if not contraindicated, liver transplantation has been reported to alleviate portal pulmonary hypertension. This condition may also develop as a consequence of TIPS.

Adult Respiratory Distress Syndrome

Epithelial lining fluid from the lungs of heavy alcohol users is depleted of glutathione, which is important in mitigating the oxidative stress that plays a role in the pathogenesis of ARDS. Chronic heavy alcohol use increases the severity of dysfunction of organs other than the lung in patients with septic shock.

SEDATIVE HYPNOTICS

Sedative-hypnotic drugs may exert significant respiratory depressant effects when abused or when mixed with alcohol and opiates.

Overdose

Benzodiazepine overdose most commonly occurs as part of a polysubstance overdose. Clinically, sedation may progress to coma, with progressive alveolar hypoventilation and respiratory acidosis. Hypotension may follow, with accompanying respiratory arrest (more typically in barbiturate overdose). Most deaths occur as a result of ARDS.

Treatment is supportive and usually entails decontamination, supplemental oxygen, airway protection, and mechanical ventilation as necessary. In benzodiazepine overdose, flumazenil should be used with caution as it is short-acting, its ability to reverse the respiratory depressant effects is controversial, and it can induce seizures. In barbiturate overdose, elimination can be enhanced with alkaline diuresis.

In GHB overdose, recovery is rapid, with full return to baseline within several hours. Recovery from benzodiazepine and barbiturate overdose is longer in duration, but the prognosis is excellent with supportive care alone.

Withdrawal Syndromes

Generally occurring 2 to 5 days after the last dose of the drug, tachypnea is the most common respiratory manifestation of withdrawal from benzodiazepines. To eliminate excess carbon dioxide and as a result of anxiety, the individual experiencing withdrawal hyperventilates. Because seizures are so common in barbiturate withdrawal, airway protection and management are the primary respiratory issues.

Sleep

Benzodiazepines can worsen sleep disorders by decreasing the tone of the upper airway muscles and reducing the ventilatory response to carbon dioxide, leading to worse nocturnal hypoxia and pulmonary hypertension.

VOLATILE SUBSTANCES

When sniffed or vigorously inhaled within a hermetic container ("huffed"), inhalants are readily absorbed in the lungs. Pulmonary complications include severe respiratory depression, barotraumas, persistent cough, and suffocation.

Methemoglobinemia

Butyl and isobutyl nitrites may cause methemoglobinemia, which manifests as cyanosis with normal partial pressure of oxygen. Intravenous methylene blue may be administered for treatment.

Metabolic Acidosis and Respiratory Alkalosis

Metabolic acidosis may occur, with compensatory respiratory alkalosis, resulting from distal renal tubular acidosis or from wide anion gap acidosis.

Tracheobronchitis

Nitrates and other inhalants may be directly irritating to airway mucosa and cause chronic cough.

Asphyxiation

Users of inhalants may develop asphyxiation from plastic bag suffocation or from respiratory depression.

NITROUS OXIDE

Nitrous oxide may bind to the opioid receptors. Pulmonary complications include pneumomediastinum, respiratory depression, and hypoxemia because of displacement of oxygen, leading to asphyxia.

ANABOLIC STEROIDS

Anabolic steroids induce a prothrombotic state and may cause pulmonary embolism, strokes, and complications such as atelectasis, pneumonia, and aspiration.

76

Summary Author: Agnes Kwasnicka
John C.M. Brust

Neurologic Disorders Related to Alcohol and Other Drug Use

As it is not unusual for individuals to use more than one substance, neurological signs and symptoms associated with drug and alcohol use must be interpreted cautiously, taking into account that they could represent intoxication by one agent with simultaneous withdrawal from another.

TRAUMA

The effects of trauma can be masked by coexisting intoxication or other neurologic disturbance. People with alcohol dependence are at particular risk of misdiagnosis. Intracranial hemorrhage must always be considered in a patient who drinks alcohol and who has an altered sensorium, and spinal cord injury must be considered in one who is unable to walk.

INFECTION

Parenteral users of any drug are subject to an array of local and systemic infections involving the central and peripheral nervous systems. Endocarditis, bacterial or fungal, leads to meningitis, cerebral infarction, diffuse vasculitis, abscess (intraparenchymal, subdural, or epidural, including the spinal cord), or subarachnoid hemorrhage from rupture of a septic ("mycotic") aneurysm. Infectious hepatitis can cause encephalopathy or, because of deranged clotting, hemorrhagic stroke. Vertebral osteomyelitis can cause radiculopathy or spinal cord compression. Tetanus is more common after subcutaneous injection of heroin, and botulism can occur at injection sites and in the nasal sinuses of cocaine users.

Those with alcohol dependence are prone to develop bacterial or tuberculous meningitis as a result of their immunosuppressed state. Parenteral drug users are at risk for AIDS and for infection with T-cell lymphotrophic retrovirus type I or type II, with consequent myelopathy. HIV-seronegative heroin-addicted patients are at risk for central nervous system (CNS) infection, including agents such as *Candida* or *Mucor*.

SEIZURES

Seizures can be a feature of either drug toxicity (as with psychostimulants) or withdrawal (as with sedatives or ethanol). In contrast to seizures associated with amphetamine-like psychostimulants, cocaine-induced seizures often occur without other symptoms and signs of intoxication. Seizures occurring many hours after use of cocaine might be related to the proconvulsant properties of the cocaine metabolite, benzoylecgonine. Single grand mal seizures are most common; focal seizures suggest another cause. Status epilepticus tends to be refractory to treatment. New-onset seizures most often follow intravenous administration of cocaine or smoking of "crack"; the reason probably is the higher dose and more rapid delivery to the brain these practices permit.

Except possibly in newborns exposed in utero, seizures are not a feature of opiate withdrawal. Unlike heroin or morphine, meperidine (Demerol) readily causes myoclonus and seizures through the proconvulsant properties of its metabolite, normeperidine. Seizures often follow parenteral use of the mixed agonist-antagonist opiate pentazocine (Talwin) when it is combined with the antihistamine tripelennamine ("Ts and blues").

At high doses (i.e., 1 mg/kg or more), phencyclidine causes seizures and myoclonus along with other signs of severe overdose, including coma with extensor posturing yet open staring eyes, marked hyperthermia, myoglobinuria, respiratory depression, and hypertension progressing to hypotension. Seizures can also occur with very high doses of hallucinogens, acute intoxication with inhalants, and severe anticholinergic poisoning.

In patients with alcohol dependence, seizures can be the result of alcohol-related disorders such as head injury, CNS infection, or stroke. Alcohol can trigger seizures in subjects with preexisting epilepsy, usually after a day or a weekend of heavy drinking.

The term "alcohol-related seizures" refers to seizures in the absence of epilepsy or other predisposing factors. Such seizures most often are a withdrawal phenomenon, occurring within 48 hours of the last drink in persons who have used excessive amounts of alcohol chronically or in habitual binge drinkers. The minimal duration of drinking is uncertain, but the risk is dose-related. Such seizures usually are single or occur in a brief cluster and are grand mal without focality. Other symptoms of early withdrawal may or may not be present, and a patient with alcohol withdrawal seizures may go on to develop *delirium tremens* (DTs), but seizures rarely are observed after DTs is present.

Alcohol blocks glutamate neurotransmission, and up-regulation of N-methyl-D-aspartate receptors theoretically could not only contribute to withdrawal symptoms but also set the stage for excitotoxicity and permanent neuronal damage. Consistent with such a view is evidence that the risk of seizures increases with repeated ethanol detoxification.

Brain CT or MRI is indicated if seizures are of new onset, and lumbar puncture should be performed if meningitis or subarachnoid hemorrhage is suspected. In patients with alcohol-related seizures, the EEG usually is normal.

Given early enough, intravenous lorazepam decreases the likelihood of recurrent alcohol seizures, but by the time a patient is seen, it is often too late for effective anticonvulsant pharmacotherapy as alcohol-related seizures usually occur singly or in brief clusters. In treatment of status epilepticus during alcohol withdrawal, benzodiazepines and phenobarbital have the advantage (compared with phenytoin) of cross-tolerance with ethanol and, thus, efficacy in treating other withdrawal symptoms, including progression to DTs. Long-term anticonvulsant medication generally is not indicated.

As with alcohol, seizures in people with barbiturate dependence occur most often as a withdrawal phenomenon. The risk of seizures and delirium are dependent on the prewithdrawal dose the patient had become tolerant to.

Seizures are a potential symptom of benzodiazepine withdrawal, but a paradoxical toxic reaction featuring agitation, hallucinations and, in some cases, seizures, has also been described. Seizures can occur during withdrawal from the notorious "date rape drug" γ-hydroxybutyric acid (GHB).

STROKE

Stroke stemming from parenteral drug abuse can be as a result of associated predisposing systemic complications (e.g., hepatitis, endocarditis, AIDS, heroin nephropathy). Taken parenterally or, in a few cases, sniffed, heroin has caused ischemic stroke in the absence of intermediary conditions or other evident risk factors. In some cases, angiographic changes and laboratory abnormalities were consistent with cerebral vasculitis or hypersensitivity reaction, but systemic hypotension after overdose and embolization of injected foreign material are also possible. Heroin myelopathy may be vascular in origin. Acute paraparesis, sensory loss, and urinary retention most often occur shortly after injection and sometimes after a period of abstinence.

Users of amphetamine-like drugs (especially methamphetamine) are subject to intracerebral hemorrhage, often associated with acute hypertension and fever or related to vasculitis. Amphetamine-induced vasculitis, which more often causes ischemic stroke, appears to be of more than one type, resembling either polyarteritis nodosa or small-vessel hypersensitivity angiitis.

Methylenedioxymethamphetamine (MDMA, "Ecstasy") has been associated with hypertensive crisis, severe hyperthermia, and both ischemic and hemorrhagic stroke.

Stroke in cocaine or "crack" users may be secondary to drug-induced cardiac arrhythmia, myocardial infarction, or cardiomyopathy, but in many cases, no risk factors are evident. The rates of ischemic and hemorrhagic strokes are about equal. A plausible mechanism for hemorrhagic stroke is surges of systemic hypertension. Ischemic strokes may be the result of direct cerebral vasoconstriction induced by the drug. A contributing factor may be cocaine's effects on platelets and clotting factors and the ability of cocaine to accelerate atherosclerosis.

Phencyclidine causes acute systemic hypertension, which, like the drug's mental effects, can last hours or days. Cerebral infarction, intracerebral and subarachnoid hemorrhage, and hypertensive encephalopathy have followed use of phencyclidine.

As with coronary artery disease, epidemiologic studies suggest that low to moderate doses of ethanol decrease ischemic stroke risk, whereas higher amounts increase it. Possible contributors to the increased risk of occlusive stroke in heavy drinkers include alcohol-related cardiac disease, alcohol-induced hypertension, increased platelet aggregation, acceleration of the clotting cascade, decreased fibrinolysis, direct cerebral vasoconstriction, hemoconcentration, and hyperhomocystinemia secondary to folate deficiency. Protection against ischemic stroke may be related to decreased low-density lipoproteins and increased high-density lipoproteins, increased prostacyclin, decreased platelet aggregation, and decreased fibrinogen levels.

Tobacco is a major risk factor for ischemic and hemorrhagic stroke. This risk decreases but does not disappear with cessation of smoking. Possible mechanisms of tobacco's role in stroke include acceleration of atherosclerosis, reductions in oxygen-carrying capacity because of carbon monoxide in tobacco smoke, nicotine-induced endothelial damage, acute elevations of blood pressure and acceleration of chronic hypertension, elevated blood fibrinogen levels, elevated hemoglobin, increased platelet reactivity, and inhibition of prostacyclin formation.

Strokes have been reported in young athletes using anabolic steroids as they potentiate platelet aggregation, alter fibrinogen, stimulate erythropoietin, and increase systolic blood pressure.

ALTERED MENTATION

Excessive alcohol users are at high risk of lasting cognitive impairment through multiple mechanisms including neurotoxicity and nutritional deficiency.

Wernicke-Korsakoff disease is caused by thiamine deficiency, which can develop within a few weeks of inadequate intake. In the acute syndrome, mental symptoms evolve over days or weeks to a "global confusional state," with varying degrees of lethargy, inattentiveness, abulia, and impaired memory. Usually also present are abnormal eye movements (nystagmus and abduction or horizontal gaze paresis progressing to complete ophthalmoplegia) and ataxic gait (both cerebellar and vestibular), progressing to inability to stand unaided. Without treatment, there is a progression to coma and death. With early treatment (intravenous thiamine and multivitamins), recovery begins within hours or days and can be complete, but if treatment is delayed, the mental symptoms evolve into Korsakoff syndrome, an irreversible disorder in which the predominant abnormality is impaired memory, with inability to store or retrieve recent information, varying degrees of retrograde amnesia, and, especially acutely, a tendency to confabulate. Residual nystagmus and gait ataxia also may be present.

A rare but often fatal disease associated with alcoholism, Marchiafava-Bignami disease consists of demyelinating lesions in the corpus callosum and progressive neurologic symptoms. Mental symptoms predominate, with depression, mania, paranoia, and dementia. Seizures are common, and hemiparesis, aphasia, dyskinesia, and ataxia are variably present.

"Alcoholic dementia" refers to progressive mental decline in people with alcohol dependence without apparent cause. Many with alcohol dependence have mental impairment more gradual in onset and more "global" than would be expected with Korsakoff syndrome. Enlarged cerebral ventricles and sulci often are seen on CT or MRI, may correlate with cognitive decline, and improve with abstinence.

Neuropathologic studies of humans with alcohol dependence without evidence of nutritional deficiency describe neuronal loss in selective regions of the brain, especially the superior frontal association cortex. Difficulty planning, problem solving, and abstracting, as well as disinhibition and lack of insight are features of frontal lobe damage.

Alcohol's effects on cognition follow a J-shaped curve similar to its effects on ischemic cerebrovascular disease; that is, the detrimental effects of alcohol on cognition are dose-related. Mild-to-moderate alcohol intake, compared with abstinence, *reduces* the risk of developing dementia, but ten or more drinks daily cause serious cognitive impairment.

People who use illicit drugs are at risk for altered mentation by indirect mechanisms, including head trauma, infection (especially AIDS), malnutrition, and concomitant alcohol abuse. It is less clear that the drugs themselves cause lasting cognitive or behavioral change as predrug mental status usually is uncertain. Experience with methadone maintenance treatment shows that the great majority of such patients have normal mental function.

Claims of permanent depression in psychostimulant users are unproven. Although lasting cognitive impairment is described in heavy cocaine users, that drug does not directly damage nerve terminals. Widespread microvascular lesions might contribute to the cognitive dysfunction.

Although the existence of an "antimotivational syndrome" in cannabis users has not been confirmed, rigorous neurologic assessment has revealed persistent, if subtle, cognitive impairment in heavy users. Marijuana use during childhood or adolescence has been implicated as a risk factor for schizophrenia.

Among inhalants, the substance most clearly associated with CNS damage is toluene, which is found in many solvents, paints, and glues. White matter lesions can result in dementia, often accompanied by pyramidal, cerebellar, and oculomotor signs. Sniffers of gasoline containing tetraethyl lead have developed lead encephalopathy.

MUSCLE, NERVE, AND SPINAL CORD

Acute rhabdomyolysis with myoglobinuria and renal failure has followed use of heroin, methamphetamine, cocaine, or phencyclidine. In people with alcohol dependence, myopathy may consist of asymptomatic elevation of serum creatine kinase, progressive proximal weakness resembling polymyositis, or acute rhabdomyolysis with myoglobinuria. The cause is toxic, not nutritional.

Sensorimotor polyneuropathy is common in people with alcohol dependence. Paresthesias usually begin in the feet and, with progression, may be accompanied by sensory loss and weakness affecting the four limbs, with severe burning pain in the feet. Autonomic symptoms and signs sometimes appear, caused by both nutritional deficiency and alcohol neurotoxicity. The primary damage is axonal, and so electrodiagnostic studies usually show only mildly reduced nerve conduction velocities, a nonspecific finding. Abstinence and nutritional replenishment are likely to be followed by clinical improvement, although mild distal sensory loss (especially vibratory sensation) can be persistent.

People with alcoholism are subject to pressure palsies from sleeping soundly in unusual positions. Radial nerve palsy with wrist drop and peroneal nerve palsy with foot drop are most common.

Guillain-Barré polyneuropathy and brachial and lumbosacral plexopathy, probably immune-mediated, are described in heroin users.

"Glue-sniffers' neuropathy" is a severe sensorimotor polyneuropathy that affects users of products containing n-hexane. Quadriplegia can evolve over a few weeks, with incomplete improvement after abstinence.

Nitrous oxide oxidizes cobalamin, and sniffers of nitrous oxide develop a myeloneuropathy that is clinically indistinguishable from combined systems disease. The earliest symptoms usually are paresthesias in the feet and unsteady gait secondary to impaired proprioception.

OTHER COMPLICATIONS

Inhaling the vapor of heroin heated on metal foil ("chasing the dragon") has been associated with cerebral and cerebellar spongiform leukoencephalopathy, but the nature of the toxicity is unknown.

Impaired vision with optic atrophy is common in individuals with alcohol dependence. Although it is likely the result of a nutritional deficiency, toxicity of alcohol itself and cyanide in tobacco smoke are other potential causes.

Cerebellar degeneration can occur in nutritionally deficient people with alcoholism in the absence of Wernicke-Korsakoff syndrome presenting as gait and sometimes leg ataxia, usually without ataxia of the arms or dysarthria. With abstinence and nutritional replenishment, improvement is likely, albeit usually incomplete.

Chronic cocaine users can develop dystonia or chorea that outlasts drug use by days or weeks, and cocaine can precipitate symptoms in patients with Tourette syndrome.

CHAPTER

77

Summary Author: Agnes Kwasnicka
Carol A. Sulis

HIV, TB, and Other Infectious Diseases Related to Alcohol and Other Drug Use

Acute infection accounts for 60% of hospital admissions among injection drug users (referred to as IDUs in this chapter) in the United States each year and complicates a substantial proportion of hospital admissions among others who use drugs. Cellulitis, cutaneous abscesses, endocarditis, hepatitis, pneumonia, and tuberculosis have been common problems for people who use drugs. Acquired immunodeficiency syndrome (AIDS) has been recognized as a risk for decades, whereas infection with type II human T-cell lymphotropic virus (HTLV-II) is a relative newcomer.

HOST DEFENSES

Cell-mediated deficiencies may result from effects on T-lymphocyte function caused by infection with human immunodeficiency virus (HIV), tuberculosis, and other intracellular pathogens. Smokers have defective mucociliary function and are predisposed to the development of sinopulmonary infection with *Streptococcus pneumonia* or *Klebsiella pneumonia*.

Repeated, nonspecific stimulation of the immune system can lead to polyclonal elevation of immunoglobulin, which can cause diagnostic confusion in caring for the patient who develops autoantibodies such as rheumatoid factor or who has a biologic false-positive test for syphilis or hepatitis C.

SKIN AND SOFT-TISSUE INFECTIONS

Skin and soft-tissue infections are common among IDUs and often are the reason for hospital admission. The type of infection (cellulitis, abscess, or ulcer), its location and severity, and causative organisms usually are related to the duration and site of injection and local epidemiology. *Staphylococcus aureus* and groups A, C, F, and G β-hemolytic streptococci are the organisms most often seen.

Beginning in 1999, there has been a dramatic increase in the incidence of methicillin-resistant *S. aureus* (MRSA) infection. Risk factors for acquisition include use of alcohol, methamphetamine, and injection drugs. The mainstay of therapy is incision and drainage of the wound, judicious use of appropriate antibiotics, and meticulous hygiene.

IDUs who mix their drugs with saliva or who lick their needles before injecting are particularly prone to the development of polymicrobial infections with viridans streptococci, *Haemophilus* spp., *Eikenella corrodens*, and oral anaerobes. Repeated injection of nonsterile, potentially vasoactive opiates and both inhalation and injection of cocaine can cause ischemic tissue necrosis, rendering the damaged areas susceptible to superinfection. Large necrotic ulcers with extensive loss of tissue are extremely common among IDUs.

The diagnosis of cellulitis is straightforward, but these patients often delay seeking medical care while they attempt to self-medicate with antibiotics or lotions and may develop extensive cellulitis, necrotizing fasciitis, or overwhelming sepsis.

Whereas diagnosis of superficial cutaneous abscess may be straightforward, the presentation of deeper abscesses can be quite subtle, and diagnosis often requires radiologic imaging. A deeper abscess may surround blood vessels (especially in the neck and groin), causing local bland or suppurative thrombophlebitis, or be hidden deep in the mediastinum or epidural space. Deep neck abscess can cause internal jugular vein thrombosis, vocal cord paralysis, airway obstruction, or massive hemorrhage after eroding into the carotid artery.

In IDUs, necrotizing fasciitis, an infection of the deep fascial structures, can be caused by *S. pyogenes* (group A *β*-hemolytic streptococci) or a mixture of aerobic and anaerobic pathogens and most commonly originates at a soft-tissue injection site. The most important diagnostic clue is the presence of pain or hemodynamic instability out of proportion to the physical findings, which may be quite trivial. Classic findings of high fever, crepitus, and progressive edema occur late in the course. Prompt surgical and radiologic evaluations for evidence of fasciitis are crucial for diagnosis. Treatment with antibiotics and urgent surgical exploration with débridement are required.

The clinician should carefully evaluate lesions located in the vicinity of blood vessels (especially in the groin), because a mycotic aneurysm can masquerade as an abscess and should not be blindly incised due to the potential for massive hemorrhage.

An increasing incidence of infection in large skeletal muscles has been recognized. Such infections usually are caused by *S. aureus*. Pyomyositis is characterized by the presence of a suppurative collection without myonecrosis, often without prior trauma or local drug injection at the site. Patients may have fever, pain, and swelling in the involved muscle, but often there is little evidence of local inflammation.

GINGIVITIS

Acute necrotizing ulcerative gingivitis (ANUG; trench mouth, Vincent angina) is characterized by severe pain, gingival necrosis, bleeding, fever, malaise, and fetid breath. Development of ANUG appears to be associated with smoking, stress, immunosuppression, and poor oral hygiene. Treatment may include use of antiseptic mouth wash, systemic antibiotics, or debridement.

Extensive tooth decay ("meth mouth") is common among people who chronically use methamphetamine and is thought to be due to a combination of bruxism, decreased saliva production, and poor dental hygiene.

ENDOCARDITIS

Epidemiology and Pathogenesis

Infective endocarditis (IE) is the most common cardiac complication of injection drug use. While IE generally occurs in previously damaged valves, endocarditis that occurs in structurally normal valves is more likely to occur in an IDU. The resulting lesion, called a *vegetation*, is composed of layers of platelets and fibrin covering clumps of relatively sequestered microorganisms. The sustained bacteremia that characterizes IE occurs when microorganisms are released as the vegetation fragments.

In the IDU, IE most often is caused by *S. aureus* (>50%), of which variable proportions are methicillin-resistant; streptococci (13%), enterococci (7%), and fungi, particularly nonalbicans *Candida* species (5%), are much less commonly involved.

Both IDUs and people with alcoholism have a higher proportion of IE caused by Gram-negative bacilli such as *Pseudomonas aeruginosa*, *P. cepacia*, and *S. marcescens*, although their relative prevalence has significant regional variation. Underlying alcoholism is identified as a risk factor in 40% of episodes of pneumococcal endocarditis, and concurrent meningitis is present in 70% of this subgroup of patients.

Clinical Presentation

Clinical features usually include

- Fever, night sweats, anorexia, arthralgias, myalgias (especially in the low back and upper thighs), and weight loss
- Cardiac abnormalities—*murmur, conduction delay, congestive heart failure, and valvular dysfunction*
- Complications from emboli or from metastatic seeding—*meningitis, brain abscess, osteomyelitis, or splenic abscess*
- Immune complex mediated phenomena—*arthritis, glomerulonephritis, aseptic meningitis, Osler nodes, Roth's spots, splinter hemorrhages, and other manifestations of vasculitis*

The presence of IE cannot be predicted in a febrile IDU on the basis of signs and symptoms alone. Unexplained fever should prompt evaluation for endocarditis.

The most reliable clues are the presence of embolic phenomenon and visualization of vegetations on echocardiography, especially involving a previously normal tricuspid valve. These patients will have pulmonary symptoms, including cough and pleuritic chest pain from septic pulmonary emboli. Radiographs might show pulmonary infiltrate or effusion and septic emboli, which appear as rounded infiltrates ("cannon balls") early in the course, and may cavitate or be complicated by empyema. Murmurs and congestive heart failure usually are absent in these patients. In contrast, IDUs with left-sided endocarditis have murmur, congestive heart failure, and stigmata of systemic embolization.

Mycotic aneurysms complicate IE in 15% of patients. Most are asymptomatic and resolve with treatment.

Diagnosis

Patients should have two or three blood cultures drawn before empiric antibiotics are started. Diagnosis is established by demonstrating characteristic findings on echocardiography in a patient with multiple positive blood cultures, but a negative transesophageal echocardiogram does not exclude the diagnosis. The probability that endocarditis is present is estimated by using major and minor criteria, as shown in Table 77.1.

TABLE 77.1 Criteria for the Diagnosis of Infective Endocarditis (Modified Duke University Criteria)

Definite diagnosis

- Pathologic criteria: histopathology/microbiology of vegetation, embolized vegetation, and intracardiac abscess grow organisms or show active endocarditis; or
- Clinical criteria:
  a. Two major criteria; or
  b. One major plus three minor criteria; or
  c. Five minor criteria

Possible diagnosis: one major plus one minor criteria or three minor criteria

No endocarditis: no pathology at surgery or autopsy, clinical resolution with ≤4 d antibiotic therapy, firm alternative diagnosis.

Major criteria
- Blood culture
  a. Two separate blood cultures positive for viridans streptococcus, *S. bovis*, HACEK (*Haemophilus, Actinobacillus, Cardiobacterium, Eikenella,* and *Kingella*) or *S. aureus*, or community-acquired enterococcus in the absence of a primary focus
  b. Positive blood cultures >12 h apart
  c. Positive blood cultures 3/3 or majority of ≥4 that are ≥1 h apart
  d. Positive blood culture for *Coxiella bumetti* or antibody >1:800
- Endocardial involvement
- Echocardiogram positive for endocarditis: oscillating intracardiac mass on a valve or supporting structure, in the path of a regurgitant jet stream, or on implanted material in the absence of alternative anatomic explanation, valve ring abscess, or new dehiscence of prosthetic valve. (TEE recommended in patients with prosthetic valve or paravalvular abscess.)
- New valvular regurgitant murmur

Minor criteria
- Predisposing heart condition or intravenous drug user
- Fever ≥38°C
- Systemic or pulmonary emboli, mycotic aneurysm, intracranial hemorrhage, conjunctival hemorrhage, Janeway lesions
- Immunologic phenomena: glomerulonephritis, Roth's spots, Osler node, rheumatoid factor
- Microbiologic/serologic findings consistent with but not definitive for endocarditis

Adapted from Li JS, Sexton DJ, Mick N, et al. Proposed modifications to the Duke Criteria for the diagnosis of infective endocarditis. *Clin Infect Dis* 2000;30:633–638.

Treatment

Vancomycin should be considered in areas with a high prevalence of methicillin-resistant *S. aureus* or penicillin-resistant pneumococcus; otherwise, empiric therapy with an antistaphylococcal antibiotic is appropriate. Other antibiotic choices will depend on local epidemiology and ultimately final culture and sensitivity results of blood culture.

The duration of therapy should be a minimum of 4 weeks of intravenous antibiotics, though shorter courses can be effective in IDUs with uncomplicated tricuspid valve endocarditis. An active IDU should not be discharged with an intravascular access device.

Once effective antimicrobial therapy has been initiated, blood cultures should be obtained daily, until sterile. If initial blood cultures remain negative, the possibility of culture-negative endocarditis, an undrained focus of infection such as splenic abscess, or an alternative diagnosis should be explored.

Surgical intervention should be considered when sequelae of endocarditis progress despite appropriate antibiotic management. These include

- Congestive heart failure refractory to medical therapy
- Multiple clinically relevant emboli
- Infection caused by fungi or resistant organisms
- Extension of myocardial abscess
- Inability to sterilize blood cultures
- Infection or dehiscence of a prosthetic valve

Outcome and Prevention

The outcome of an episode of IE is based on age of the patient, virulence of the organism, site of the infection, presence of complications, and the presence of comorbid conditions such as HIV infection. Left-sided endocarditis and infection with Gram-negative bacilli or fungi are associated with a worse prognosis. Heart failure remains the leading cause of death.

Patients remain at a substantially increased risk of reinfection especially if they continue injection drug use. As a result, patients should follow American Heart Association Guidelines and be given prophylactic antibiotics when undergoing certain invasive procedures.

NONCARDIAC VASCULAR INFECTIONS

Epidemiology and Pathogenesis

Vascular complication	Pathogenesis
Endothelial injury and thrombus formation	Injury to blood vessels during injection drug use and vasospasm from cocaine use
Septic thrombophlebitis	Bacterial seeding of the thrombus
Hematoma superinfection	Adjacent to the traumatized or ischemic blood vessel
Arteriovenous fistula	Direct injury or from extension of local infection

During episodes of bacterial endocarditis, a mycotic aneurysm can result when emboli to the vasa vasorum cause a mushroom-shaped swelling at arterial bifurcations. Mycotic aneurysms complicate 15% of cases of IE, usually are silent, but may become symptomatic in 3% to 5% of patients months or years after completion of appropriate therapy.

For most noncardiac endovascular lesions, the predominant pathogen is *S. aureus*; however, Gram-negative bacilli (especially *P. aeruginosa*) are reported with increased frequency in IDUs.

Clinical Presentation

Mycotic aneurysm in:	Symptoms	Clinical findings	Complication
Neck or groin	Painful, tender, enlarging, pulsatile mass	Overlying bruit or thrill various constitutional symptoms Ischemia of a distal extremity or signs of nerve compression	Extension of infection into surrounding soft tissue with abscess formation
Brain	Unremitting headache, visual disturbances, or cranial nerve palsy		Massive hemorrhage from aneurysmal rupture complicates 2%–4% of cases of left-sided endocarditis
Large vessel			Thrombosis of larger vessels with pulmonary embolization or distal ischemia

Patients with endovascular infection may have sustained bacteremia and signs of clinical sepsis. Management of septic thrombophlebitis is controversial but generally includes treatment with both intravenous antibiotics and short-term anticoagulation.

Diagnosis
Early diagnosis before rupture occurs and a high index of suspicion is essential. Arteriographic confirmation remains the standard diagnostic test.

Treatment
Empiric antibiotics guided by local epidemiology can be given after blood cultures have been obtained, later modified on the basis of culture and sensitivity results, and usually are continued for 4 to 6 weeks. Surgical excision is indicated for enlarging mycotic aneurysm, intrathoracic, intra-abdominal, and peripheral mycotic aneurysms and cerebral mycotic aneurysms if enlarging or bleeding.

RESPIRATORY INFECTIONS

Epidemiology and Pathogenesis
Factors that may contribute to the increased risk of respiratory infection in this population include

- Cigarette smoke disrupts mucociliary function and macrophage activation.
- Alteration in the level of consciousness accompanied by depressed gag reflex compromises airway protection and permits aspiration of oropharyngeal flora.
- Alcoholism is associated with oropharyngeal colonization with enteric Gram-negative bacilli and abnormal phagocyte function.
- Injection drug use is associated with bronchospasm, pulmonary edema, and the development of various types of foreign-body granuloma.
- Increased risk of exposure to certain pathogens because of lifestyle (e.g., homelessness or incarceration).
- Increased prevalence of HIV infection.

Pneumonia
Pneumonia is present in up to one third of IDUs evaluated for fever. Septic pulmonary emboli associated with right-sided endocarditis or septic thrombophlebitis and tuberculosis infection are common.

Most pulmonary infections are community-acquired episodes of pneumonia, caused by common respiratory pathogens, but IDUs have an increased incidence of pneumonia caused by *Haemophilus influenzae*, *S. aureus*, and *P. aeruginosa*, especially those coinfected with HIV. Though *Pneumocystis (carinii) jiroveci* is the major pulmonary pathogen in patients with AIDS, pneumonia caused by *Mycobacterium tuberculosis*, *M. avium-intracellulare*, cytomegalovirus, and common bacterial and viral pathogens occurs with increased frequency in this group. Lung abscesses can complicate aspiration pneumonia, necrotizing bacterial pneumonia, or septic emboli. Left-sided pulmonic effusion may be a clue to an underlying splenic abscess or bacterial or tuberculous pleuritis.

Tuberculosis

In the United States, 4% to 6% of the population have latent tuberculosis infection. People who use drugs, especially people with alcoholism and IDUs, have an increased incidence of reactivation for reasons that are unknown. Difficulties in controlling outbreaks are sometimes compounded by homelessness and noncompliance with medical therapy. Infection transmission by the aerosolization of acid-fast bacilli is increased with cough-inducing activities such as smoking cigarettes, crack cocaine, and marijuana. As most people who use drugs are at increased risk of tuberculosis infection, they should have routine tuberculin skin testing.

The classic symptoms of pulmonary tuberculosis include cough with purulent, blood-tinged sputum, and increasing malaise, with the development of night sweats and weight loss as the disease progresses. Diagnosis is made by culturing *M. tuberculosis* from expectorated sputum or by nucleic acid amplification tests. Tuberculin skin tests generally turn positive 4 to 6 weeks after primary infection but can be negative in up to 25% of patients at the time of diagnosis.

Extrapulmonary tuberculosis occurs in one sixth of normal adults and up to 60% to 80% of patients with HIV. Diagnosis generally requires biopsy. Complications include empyema, meningitis, and vertebral osteomyelitis.

Because of the long delay to obtain culture and sensitivity results, treatment usually is initiated before a definitive diagnosis has been established. Treatment should follow American Thoracic Society Guidelines. IDUs are at increased risk of multidrug-resistant tuberculosis. Directly observed therapy is strongly encouraged when nonadherence is anticipated and often is preferred for patients with risk factors, such as homelessness or addictive disorders.

Rifampin can reduce methadone levels, and patients often require adjustment of their maintenance dose. IDUs with underlying hepatitis or who use hepatotoxins such as alcohol have an increased risk of developing hepatitis when using isoniazid, rifampin, or pyrazinamide.

HEPATIC AND GASTROINTESTINAL INFECTIONS

Viral hepatitis often leads to hepatic cirrhosis. Infection is the leading cause of death in patients with cirrhosis. Gram-negative enteric bacilli such as *Escherichia coli*, *K. pneumoniae*, and encapsulated respiratory pathogens such as *S. pneumonia* are the most frequent but severe infections with many other organisms have been described.

Spontaneous bacterial peritonitis is a common and potentially fatal infectious complication in patients with cirrhosis and ascites. Diagnostic paracentesis should be performed in patients with ascites who have fever. Because Gram-negative enteric bacilli and *S. pneumonia* are the most common cause of infection in these patients, a second-generation cephalosporin or a combination of fluoroquinolone plus clindamycin or metronidazole are common starting regimens.

BONE AND JOINT INFECTIONS

Osteomyelitis

Most microorganisms can infect bone but *S. aureus* (60%), *S. epidermidis* (30%), streptococci, Gram-negative bacilli, anaerobes, mycobacteria, and fungi (10%) are most common. Infection can occur by hematogenous seeding (frequently involving the spine because of the vascularity of the vertebrae), by introduction after surgery or trauma, or spread from a contiguous focus.

Patients with osteomyelitis complain of focal pain and tenderness. Fever is present in two thirds of patients; erythema, warmth, and swelling are variably present. In vertebral osteomyelitis, associated symptoms result when inflammation extends beyond the spine. Spinal tuberculosis (Pott disease) is relatively indolent.

Diagnosis of osteomyelitis is made by biopsy and culture of bone. Computed tomography scan and magnetic resonance imaging are helpful in determining the extent of involvement but blood cultures often are negative.

Antibiotics alone may be sufficient therapy to cure acute osteomyelitis and should be chosen based on the isolated pathogen. Surgical debridement generally is required for cure when the infection has been present for longer than 6 weeks.

Septic Arthritis

Septic arthritis occurs when bacteria seed joints previously damaged by trauma, instrumentation, osteoarthritis, or chronic inflammatory conditions. Infection with *S. aureus* is most common, but arthrocentesis with culture and microscopic examination of joint fluid are required for diagnosis.

Two particular syndromes are more common among IDUs than in the normal population and involve fibrocartilaginous joints, which are most susceptible to hematogenous seeding.

1. *Septic arthritis of the sternoclavicular joint caused by P. aeruginosa*—symptoms (fever, tenderness and swelling over the joint, and decreased range of motion of the ipsilateral shoulder) may be present for several months before the patient seeks evaluation
2. *Septic arthritis of the sacroiliac joint or symphysis pubis*—symptoms include fever and various combinations of hip, groin, thigh, or lower abdominal pain that is exacerbated by walking

Treatment may require exploratory arthrotomy, with surgical debridement of infected material followed by prolonged antibiotic therapy directed at isolated organisms.

NERVOUS SYSTEM INFECTIONS

Manifestations of central nervous system infections are easily missed if symptoms are mistakenly attributed to intoxication or withdrawal. Delirium, acute confusional states, encephalopathy, or coma may accompany overdose, intoxication, infection, or a large number of noninfectious etiologies. Clinical features should guide diagnostic strategies, with management based on results of lumbar puncture and neuroradiologic imaging.

Endocarditis can cause meningitis (aseptic or purulent), brain abscess from septic emboli, or hemorrhage from rupture of a mycotic aneurysm. Bacteremia during IE can cause vertebral osteomyelitis, which, in turn, can be complicated by epidural abscess, with evidence of cord compression.

Brain abscess and subdural empyema in the absence of endocarditis usually are caused by extension from a contiguous focus in the mastoid, ear, or paranasal sinuses, seeding of a preexisting subdural hematoma during an episode of transient bacteremia, or direct inoculation of the subdural space after a traumatic wound. A variety of pyogenic bacteria and atypical organisms (including *Nocardia*, *Aspergillus* spp., *Cryptococcus*, mucormycosis, tuberculosis, and *Toxoplasma gondii)*, especially in those with HIV, have been implicated.

A patient with brain abscess may have nonspecific symptoms such as headache or personality change. An abscess can attain enormous size before diagnosis. Management includes antibiotics and drainage, if indicated. In most cases, patients with HIV who have ring-enhancing mass lesions in the brain and appropriate clinical presentation are treated empirically for toxoplasmosis. Meningovascular syphilis has been reported in a number of patients with HIV, despite presumably effective therapy for primary syphilis infection, and it should be considered in young people who present with a new stroke.

Contamination of skin ulcers with spores of *Clostridium* spp. can cause neurologic symptoms from elaboration of neurotoxins. Wound botulism is caused by contamination of injection sites or skin ulcers with *Clostridium botulinum* that release botulinum toxin. Over the past 15 years, there has been a dramatic increase in reported cases of botulism among IDUs who injected black tar heroin, the dark, gummy substance derived from crude preparations of opium that may be contaminated by spore-containing adulterants such as dirt. Treatment with trivalent or type-specific antitoxin can limit disease progression. Botulism has been reported in a patient with colonization of the paranasal sinuses after intranasal cocaine use.

Wounds contaminated by dirt, feces, or saliva provide an appropriate anaerobic milieu for infection with *C. tetani*. Since 1995, fewer than 50 cases of tetanus per year have been reported, but 15% to 18% of these were in IDUs who lacked a history of an acute injury but did inject black tar heroin and presented with infected subcutaneous injection sites. The toxin causes devastating tetany in an otherwise conscious patient. Management should include antibiotics, aggressive wound debridement, tetanus immune globulin, and supportive care. For prevention, all patients should be immunized with tetanus toxoid every 10 years after a primary series (or immediately after a high-risk wound if >5 years has elapsed since the last booster).

EYE INFECTIONS

IDUs have an increased incidence of bacterial and fungal endophthalmitis as a complication of IE. Many investigators have reported *C. albicans* endophthalmitis as part of a syndrome of disseminated candidiasis in IDUs who injected "brown heroin," presumably related to fungal contamination of the lemon juice used to dissolve the drug.

Symptoms of endophthalmitis are similar to the symptoms in people who do not use drugs. Aggressive evaluation and management are required to salvage vision.

Cytomegalovirus retinitis is the most common serious intraocular complication of AIDS and generally occurs after reactivation of latent infection in patients with CD4 cell counts of <50, especially those not receiving antiretroviral therapy.

HUMAN IMMUNODEFICIENCY VIRUS AND ACQUIRED IMMUNODEFICIENCY SYNDROME

Epidemiology and Pathogenesis

Among US adults with known risk factors who were diagnosed with HIV between 2001 and 2005, 33% reported injection drug use and another 17% reported sex with an IDU. Among children diagnosed with HIV infection between 2001 and 2005, >90% of the cases involved transmission from an infected mother. Risk factors for these mothers included injection drug use in 38% and unprotected sex with an IDU in 16%. For both men and women, the estimated number of new cases of HIV related to injection drug use has fallen slightly each year for the past several years, perhaps because of emphasis on prevention strategies.

HIV testing can be postponed during acute mental health and addiction exacerbations but should be done, with appropriate communication of results, implications, and treatment options, as soon as patients are prepared to hear the results of testing even if other health problems (including addictions) are not entirely resolved.

Classification

Stages of HIV infection range from asymptomatic (latent) through early symptomatic infection (B symptoms) to AIDS. Classification follows CDC criteria and stratifies disease according to the CD4 cell count and the presence of various other criteria.

Primary HIV infection causes symptoms in 50% to 90% of cases, which occur 2 to 4 weeks after exposure. Symptoms may include fever, adenopathy, pharyngitis, rash, myalgias, arthralgias, diarrhea, headache, nausea and vomiting, hepatosplenomegaly, thrush, mucocutaneous ulcers, meningoencephalitis, peripheral neuropathy, cranial nerve palsy, Guillain-Barré syndrome, radiculopathy, cognitive impairment, and psychosis.

Diagnosis

Primary HIV infection should be considered in any patient with a history of potential exposure and compatible symptoms. Early on the patient may have no physical findings except for persistent generalized lymphadenopathy.

The diagnosis is best established by demonstrating the presence of p24 antigen, quantitative HIV RNA, or qualitative HIV RNA in association with negative or indeterminate HIV serology. Seroconversion generally occurs at 6 to 12 weeks. By 6 months after transmission, 95% of patients have developed positive HIV serology and stabilization of viral load, with levels correlating with prognosis.

Treatment

Guidelines and algorithms are available to assist practitioners in navigating the complexity of HIV treatment and outlining appropriate laboratory monitoring and screening. Additional guidelines provide disease-specific recommendations for the use of primary or secondary prophylactic antibiotics for the prevention of the most common, serious opportunistic infections. It is strongly recommended that care be comanaged with an expert in HIV treatment.

Patient education and involvement in therapeutic decisions are especially critical for effective HIV treatment. Antiretroviral regimens are complex, have major side effects, and carry serious potential consequences from the development of viral resistance associated with nonadherence to the drug regimen or suboptimal levels of antiretroviral agents.

Past and current high-risk behaviors and exposures that may have resulted in HIV infection should be reviewed and mitigation plans designed to prevent further transmission. Behaviors such as high-risk sexual activity or injection drug use not only increase the risk of HIV transmission to others but also can expose the HIV-infected patient to opportunistic pathogens such as herpes simplex virus, cytomegalovirus, *Cryptosporidium*, human papillomavirus (HPV), human herpes virus type 8, and hepatitis viruses.

Continuing addictive behavior should prompt the offer of referral to addiction treatment services; a history of addictive disorder warrants review of relapse-prevention efforts.

Once the decision has been made to initiate treatment, the goals should be maximal and durable suppression of viral load, restoration or preservation of immunologic function, improvement in the quality of life, and reduction of HIV-related morbidity and mortality. Efficacy of therapy and rate of progression of disease are evaluated by monitoring CD4 counts and viral load.

Drug-drug or drug-food interactions can profoundly affect the absorption and efficacy of certain medications. For example, methadone levels can be significantly decreased when given with certain protease inhibitors (ritonavir, nelfinavir, or lopinavir) and nonnucleoside reverse transcriptase inhibitors (nevirapine or efavirenz) and often require an increase in methadone maintenance dosage. Conversely, use of maintenance methadone can significantly decrease the level of some nucleoside reverse transcriptase inhibitors (stavudine or didanosine), requiring an increase in antiretroviral dosage. In contrast, limited data suggest that buprenorphine needs no dosage adjustment and is less likely to be associated with adverse events when given with HAART regimens that include efavirenz.

Prevention

Prevention messages should encourage sexual abstinence or the practice of the correct and consistent use of latex condoms. Patients should be encouraged to avoid sexual practices that might result in oral exposure to feces (e.g., oral-anal contact) to reduce the risk of intestinal infections. Patients who inject drugs should be encouraged to stop using injection drugs and to enter and complete addiction treatment. If the patient continues to inject drugs, the importance of using a sterile syringe for every injection and the avoidance of sharing any injection-related drug paraphernalia with another person should be emphasized. Such patients should be encouraged to use a needle-exchange program or to safely discard syringes after one use. In areas where needle exchange is illegal, IDUs should be taught to clean their injection equipment with household bleach before use.

SEXUALLY TRANSMITTED DISEASES

Though the prevalence of sexually transmitted diseases is higher in people who use drugs, the presentation, diagnosis, and management of most sexually transmitted diseases (STDs) are not profoundly influenced by drug use. One exception is that the diagnosis and treatment of syphilis in IDUs may be confounded by an increased prevalence of biologic false-positive nontreponemal screening tests such as venereal disease research laboratory or rapid plasma reagin tests for syphilis.

Recent studies suggest that an increasing number of persons, especially men who have sex with men, are participating in high-risk sexual behaviors (often while intoxicated) that place them at risk of acquiring STDs. Related studies have shown that patients who report heavy drug or alcohol use are most likely to report high-risk sexual behavior and to have HIV infection or syphilis.

Pregnant women who use drugs should be screened according to standard protocols and aggressively treated to minimize disastrous maternal or fetal outcomes. Because of the synergistic effect of cigarette smoke in the development of HPV-associated cancers, patients with diagnosed HPV should be strongly encouraged to consider smoking cessation.

Type-one human T-cell lymphotropic virus (HTLV-I) infection is present in widely scattered populations throughout the world and is the etiologic agent in adult T-cell leukemia/lymphoma and HTLV-associated myelopathy. HTLV-II has been reported in IDUs and their sexual contacts, appears to be endemic in IDUs in the United States, and has not been definitively linked to a specific disorder. Both retroviruses appear to be transmitted by sexual intercourse, administration of blood products, and mother-to-child transmission. No effective therapy exists, and prevention of exposure is the only known method of limiting spread.

CHAPTER 78

Summary Author: Agnes Kwasnicka
Sanford Auerbach

Sleep Disorders Related to Alcohol and Other Drug Use

Given the influence of alcohol and other drugs on sleep, sleep problems are likely to be more prevalent in persons with addictive disorders than in the general population.

OVERVIEW OF SLEEP

Lack of adequate sleep is associated with inattentiveness, performance failure, anxiety and excitability, difficulty with concentration and memory, chronic fatigue, aches, stiffness, uneasiness, and withdrawal. "Sleep need" is the amount of sleep required for optimal function during wakeful periods. It may vary from one individual to the next but is generally in the range of 3 to 10 hours.

The nocturnal polysomnogram (PSG) is the standard method of determining the presence and stage of sleep by measuring electroencephalographic (EEG), electromyographic, and electro-oculographic activity.

The multiple sleep latency test is a standard and accepted measure of daytime sleepiness and employs polysomnography while a patient is allowed to take naps on five separate occasions throughout a day.

Sleep need often is translated into the concept of "sleep drive." Thus, relative sleep deprivation leads to increased sleep drive, whereas napping lends itself to a relative decrease in sleep drive. Contrary to popular belief, total sleep over a 24-hour period shows little change as an individual transitions from young adulthood into old age.

Sleep Architecture

Sleep is a dynamic process, featuring fluctuations in brain wave activity, muscle tone, eye movement, and autonomic activity. It consists of two discrete states: rapid eye movement (REM) and non–rapid eye movement (NREM) sleep. Each can be defined in physiologic terms by using the elements of the PSG.

Non–Rapid Eye Movement Historically, NREM sleep has been subdivided into four stages, which are numbered one through four. Stages 3 and 4 usually are consolidated and referred to as *slow wave sleep* (SWS) or *delta sleep*. In brief, each stage is characterized by progressively slower EEG background, lower muscle tone, and decreasing eye movements. More recently, the nomenclature has been changed and NREM sleep is considered as N1, N2, and N3 (formerly SWS).

Rapid Eye Movement REM sleep, sometimes referred to as *paradoxical sleep*, is characterized by lowest state of muscle tone over a 24-hour period (relative muscle atonia) on the background of a relatively active EEG. REM sleep can be subdivided into tonic and phasic components, where REMs and brief muscle twitches occur in the phasic components. It is noteworthy that these components of REM sleep are not rigidly synchronized as is seen in some normal individuals with sleep paralysis as a benign condition, in which the individual is transiently "paralyzed" as he or she awakens from sleep. REM sleep is associated with the well-formed dream and sometimes nightmares.

Sleep Rhythms

The components of sleep occur in a clear rhythm with the "light" stages of NREM (N1,N2) seen first. They are followed by a transition to SWS or N3, followed by lighter stages of NREM again, and then REM sleep. Typically, there are three to four NREM-REM cycles, each lasting 90 to 120 minutes. As the night progresses, the relative amount of time spent in REM increases and the amount of time in SWS decreases.

Sleep-wake rhythms follow a circadian or approximately 24-hour biologic pattern that is tightly synchronized with circadian variations in core body temperature. Falling core body temperature is associated with sleep onset, whereas a rise in temperature makes one susceptible to waking. A rise in body temperature occurs in the early morning hours, usually peaking at about 3 AM, when a secondary arousal time occurs and the individual is susceptible to wakening from any physical or emotional factor (e.g., anxiety, pain, the need to urinate). The most powerful factor influencing the periodicity of the sleep-wake rhythm has proved to be exogenous light that exerts its influence through retinohypothalamic input to the suprachiasmatic nucleus, our endogenous pacemaker.

UNDERSTANDING SLEEP DISORDERS

For a comprehensive listing of specific disorders and their descriptions, the reader is referred to *The International Classification of Sleep Disorders, revised (ICSD-2, 2005)*.

Drive/Sleep Need

As noted previously, sleep drive is based on sleep need, which, in turn, assumes that sleep need is based on otherwise efficient sleep. Identification of an individual's sleep need is the first step in understanding sleep complaints. Careful questioning of the patient is required to account for total sleep time, including both nocturnal sleep and daytime naps. Sleep need will vary with age, season, mood changes, medication/drug use, and other medical conditions.

Timing

In adults, the sleep-wake circadian rhythm often advances with age toward an early bedtime and early rise time (the lark). For a variety of social and biologic reasons, there is a tendency for the adolescent to become delayed and the older adult to become advanced. In addition, the circadian rhythm of the older adult appears to be more fragile and susceptible to disruption, as might be seen in shift workers or patients plagued by the nocturnal arousal of chronic pain.

It is unclear how much of this change is due to biologic changes in the endogenous oscillator that governs the rhythms and how much is the result of changes in exogenous factors such as light exposure, lifestyle changes, and physical activity. The rhythm can be manipulated by well-timed bright light exposure and the use of exogenous melatonin.

Intrinsic Sleep Disorders

Periodic Limb Movements of Sleep Periodic limb movements of sleep (PLMS) (also referred to as *periodic leg movement, nocturnal myoclonus, periodic movements of sleep,* or *leg jerks*) are characterized by episodes of repetitive, stereotyped limb movements during sleep. Movements consist of extension of the big toe, in combination with partial flexing of the ankle, knee, and hip. The arms also may be involved. The movements often are associated with a brief arousal, usually too brief to be considered an awakening. Clinically, the patient may complain of nonrestorative sleep. The amplitude of the movements does not always correlate with the impact on sleep quality. Even when the patient reports sound sleep, he or she may thrash about, while the bed partner reports kicking or even bicycling movements.

Although PLMS can occur in any stage of NREM, they are most common in stage 2 and usually disappear in REM. Although PLMS can be seen in otherwise young, healthy individuals, they may be associated with obstructive sleep apnea (OSA) or with the use of antidepressants. Similarly, withdrawal from certain drugs (including anticonvulsants, benzodiazepines, barbiturates, and other hypnotics) may contribute to the development of PLMS.

Restless Legs Syndrome It has been estimated that restless legs syndrome (RLS) is present in 5% to 15% of the general population. The usual presentation is an urge to move the limbs (usually bilateral, often more prominent in the legs than in the arms) accompanied by uncomfortable sensations. Symptoms tend to be worse when the individual is relaxing and especially at the transition between wakefulness and sleep. They follow a diurnal pattern, becoming more severe late in the day, and tend to improve with movement. Some patients develop myoclonus or sudden jerking movements. It is not uncommon to find an overlap with PLMS.

The pathophysiology of RLS is unknown. Disorders of iron metabolism within the central nervous system and dopaminergic function have been considered. Many medical problems have been found to aggravate the symptoms. Of particular note in addiction medicine is the observation that RLS may be aggravated or triggered by the use of several medications, including antidepressants, lithium carbonate, neuroleptics, and caffeine.

Medications for treatment of RLS include the dopaminergic drugs such as carbidopa/levodopa or dopaminergic agonists such as ropinirole and pramipexole. Success has also been demonstrated with anticonvulsants (especially gabapentin), the opioids, and the benzodiazepine receptor agonists (especially clonazepam). Some patients report that they began to use opioids on a regular basis when they received them for an unrelated disorder and realized that they were able to sleep for the first time in years.

Obstructive Sleep Apnea The prevalence of OSA in the general male population has been estimated to be 0.4% to 5.9%, with the incidence in men outnumbering that in women. Common risk factors include obesity, smoking, alcohol consumption, stroke, and age. It is characterized by repetitive episodes of sleep-related upper airway obstructions, which usually are associated with oxygen desaturation and snoring as a result of upper airway muscles relaxation. The role of upper airway muscle relaxation in the pathophysiology also means that certain medications, such as benzodiazepines or alcohol, may aggravate the severity of the OSA.

The sleep disruption may or may not be apparent to the patient because brief physiologic arousals may not be recalled. Daytime somnolence or an irresistible urge to doze if allowed to sit in a comfortable chair or when confronted with the monotony of highway driving often is the prime complain. Similarly, presenting complaints may be related to difficulties in memory or concentration that reflect suppression of REM sleep. SWS also can be suppressed and may be associated with complaints similar to those associated with fibrositis or fibromyalgia.

There are several cardiopulmonary consequences associated with OSA. Significant oxygen desaturation can lead to arrhythmias, systemic and pulmonary arterial hypertension, and polycythemia.

The severity of OSA can be measured in three dimensions: snoring, sleep disruption, and cardiopulmonary consequences. Upper airway resistance syndrome, a related condition where symptoms may be attributed to events that do not meet the formal criteria for the definition of apneas or hypopneas, may be associated with sleep disruption or frequent EEG alpha arousals.

Central Sleep Apnea Central sleep apnea (CSA) is a disorder characterized by recurrent episodes of apnea during sleep resulting from temporary loss of ventilatory effort. CSA may be associated with desaturations and arousals, as encountered in OSA. Although CSA is much less frequently encountered when compared with OSA, it does pose a particular potential problem in addiction medicine. A pattern of sleep-related irregular respirations has been referred to as ataxic breathing or Biot respirations and has been associated with chronic opioid therapy and the risk seems to be related to the morphine dose equivalents.

Extrinsic Factors

Exercise has long been recognized as a factor promoting sound sleep. Regular exercise, especially in the late afternoon or early evening, is conducive to sleep initiation, either through release of certain endogenous substances or subsequent cooling 5 to 6 hours later, which reinforces circadian factors.

Aging has been associated with increased susceptibility to external stimuli, such as room temperature and light, which may cause arousal. The effect of evening meals is variable. Foods containing tryptophan may promote sleep but heavy bedtime snacks can be disruptive to sleep. Older adults appear to be more susceptible to the contribution of medication and changes in metabolism to sleep disruption.

Medical and Psychiatric Factors

Medical conditions can contribute directly to specific sleep disorders such as OSA or RLS or lead to problems with the wake-sleep transition. Nocturia, headache, gastrointestinal illnesses, cardiopulmonary disease, menopause, and chronic pain can all contribute to waking through the night, including the most vulnerable time in the circadian cycle (i.e., 3–5 AM).

Two specific sleep-related psychiatric disorders have been formally defined. Alcohol-dependent insomnia occurs in nonalcoholics who use alcohol as a hypnotic for sleep onset for >30 days and who may not otherwise meet criteria for alcohol dependence. Substance-induced sleep disorder, with subtypes based on the substance used, is described in the *DSM-IV*.

Sleep disruption is not uncommon in persons with a comorbid psychiatric syndrome. Insomnia is the prominent feature of depression, although hypersomnia may be seen especially when the depression is a component of a bipolar disorder. Similarly, during manic episodes, one may see periods of sleeplessness, with an apparent reduction in sleep need.

Prolonged sleep latency, sleep fragmentation, early morning arousals, decreased sleep efficiency, and daytime fatigue and somnolence have been well documented in depression. PSG features associated with depression include decrease in the amount of SWS, a reduction in REM latency, increased duration of the first REM period, and an increase in REM density.

Insomnia

Insomnia may be transient or chronic, primary, or secondary. Primary insomnia, which is fairly uncommon, is considered to be independent of other sleep disturbances or the other factors cited previously.

In recent years, there seems to have been a paradigm shift in the approach to insomnia from categorizing it as a symptom to looking at it as a comorbid disorder. Thus, the emphasis in management should not only be directed toward the underlying disorder.

ALCOHOL AND SLEEP

Effect of Alcohol on Sleep in the Individual Without Alcohol Dependence

The hypnotic properties of alcohol are summarized in Table 78.1. Alcohol probably is the sleep-promoting agent that is most widely used by the general public. Despite this wide use, it must be remembered that alcohol can be mildly stimulating.

The effects of alcohol on the sleep architecture of the individual without alcohol dependence should be considered in terms of both direct effects and immediate withdrawal. As predicted by the hypnotic effect, sleep latency is shortened and there is an increase in the amount of NREM sleep that occurs at the expense of REM sleep, which is suppressed during the acute phase. As the effects of the alcohol dissipate, there is a rebound effect, in which sleep becomes lighter and more easily disrupted. REM increases, with an associated increase in dreams and nightmares. There is an increase in sympathetic arousals, with tachycardia and sweating. As alcohol consumption continues, the hypnotic effects may diminish, but the late sleep disruption persists. Ultimately, the net effect is a feeling of fatigue during the individual's waking hours.

It would seem that the hypnotic effects of alcohol should be related to direct effects of alcohol on the central nervous system. Even after alcohol is no longer detectable, both sleepiness and delayed sleep latency can

TABLE 78.1 **Summary of Effects of Alcohol on Sleep Architecture**	
Individual without alcohol dependence	Rebound of REM sleep
Initial half of sleep period	Persistent decreased SWS
Shortened sleep latency	Alcohol recovery
Decreased REM sleep	Early (initial weeks)
Decreased SWS	Increased sleep latency
Second half of sleep period	Increased fragmentation
Shallow disrupted sleep	Decreased total sleep time
Increased REM sleep with increased	Increased REM density (exaggerated in
dream (nightmare recall)	depression)
Sympathetic arousal	Persistence of decreased SWS
Individual with alcohol dependence	Chronic
Increased sleep latency	Persistence of sleep fragmentation
Decreased sleep efficiency	Persistence of decreased SWS
Decreased total sleep time	Recovery relapse
Decreased REM sleep	Increased total sleep time
Decreased SWS	Decreased sleep fragmentation
Alcohol withdrawal	Increased SWS
Severe insomnia	
Severe sleep fragmentation.	

REM, rapid eye movement; SWS, slow wave sleep.

be observed. Although it is customary to advise patients with sleep difficulties to avoid late evening alcohol, there is evidence that even alcohol consumed 6 hours before sleep onset may disrupt sleep in the last half of the night.

Effect of Alcohol on Sleep in the Individual with Alcohol Dependence

It is not uncommon for persons with alcohol dependence to report some combination of insomnia, hypersomnia, circadian rhythm disorders, or parasomnias (abnormal sleep-related behaviors). Various objective measures have demonstrated increased sleep latencies, decreased sleep efficiencies, and decreased total sleep, with reductions in both REM and SWS in these patients. As the dependence continues, patients often report that they no longer are able to initiate sleep without a drink and the usual rhythms of sleep become quite disrupted.

Dream Content in Alcoholism Individuals with alcohol dependence suffer from nightly nightmares more often than controls. The use of alcohol to suppress nightmares needs to be considered in the management of other disorders associated with nightmares, such as posttraumatic stress disorder. In fact, some patients may have initiated their substance abuse out of a desire to suppress nightmares.

Alcohol, Sleep, and Other Cardiopulmonary Functions Alcohol consumption before sleep by patients with chronic obstructive pulmonary disease can worsen nocturnal hypoxemia during sleep and increase ventricular ectopic activity.

Sleep in Alcohol Withdrawal The alcohol withdrawal syndrome frequently is marked by severe insomnia and sleep fragmentation. There is reduction of SWS during this period and rebound of REM sleep; in fact, sleep during withdrawal may consist simply of fragments of REM sleep.

Nightmares and vivid dreams are not uncommon features of alcohol withdrawal and may be related to increased REM sleep. It has been speculated that it is the early and abundant REM, with its associated dream content or hallucinations, and the accompanying sympathetic discharge that may account for much of the clinical picture of the *delirium tremens*.

Sleep During Alcohol Recovery In the alcohol-dependent patient, sleep is not immediately recovered with abstinence; in fact, it may require months or even years. In the first 2 to 3 weeks of recovery, increased sleep latency may be seen, accompanied by increased sleep fragmentation and reduced total sleep time. There may be a decrease in SWS and an increase in REM density. The effects on REM may be exaggerated in patients with secondary depression. The elevated percentage of total sleep time spent in REM sleep and thus reduction in the amount of SWS can persist for months or years. It has been demonstrated that the presence of subjective sleep disruption increases the likelihood that the recovering individual will relapse to alcohol use.

Several investigators have attempted to identify the sleep measures that are the most important in predicting relapse. Studies suggested that measures of REM sleep were critical in predicting outcome. In fact, the emergence of markers of REM pressure, as defined by a shortened REM latency, increased REM density, and increased amount of time in REM sleep as a percentage of total sleep, is among the most robust predictors of continued recovery at the 3-month mark.

SPECIFIC SLEEP DISORDERS ASSOCIATED WITH ALCOHOLISM

Alcohol- and Sleep-Related Breathing Disorders

Patients with alcohol dependence appear to be at increased risk of developing OSA, especially if they snore. Alcohol has been shown to increase the frequency and duration of obstructive events in patients with established OSA. Furthermore, alcohol-induced reduction in muscle tone of the upper airway and changes in airflow resistance are sufficient to cause OSA in those who consume moderate to high doses of alcohol in the evening, even if they do not otherwise have OSA. Moreover, the depressant effects of alcohol can decrease the likelihood of arousal from an obstructive event, thus prolonging the duration of each respiratory event. The relationship of alcohol to the development of OSA varies across populations with other factors, such as age, the presence of snoring, and perhaps gender, playing a role in the development of OSA.

In patients with established severe OSA, it has been noted that consumption of two or more alcoholic drinks per day is associated with a fivefold increase in fatigue-related motor vehicle crashes when compared with those who consumed little or no alcohol.

Alcohol and PLMS

The risk of PLMS may be increased by alcohol consumption. The potential increase in fatigue and daytime somnolence associated with PLMS should be considered in the management of these patients.

OTHER DRUGS AND SLEEP

Stimulants

Stimulants suppress sleep by prolonging sleep latency and reducing total sleep time. They have a specific inhibitory effect on REM sleep. Presumably, this effect is attributable to the dopaminergic stimulation of the arousal system, although serotonergic systems also may be involved. When used episodically, these agents contribute to periods of sleeplessness that can last for days, but they usually are followed by a rebound hypersomnia. Tolerance to this effect can develop with continued use.

After a period of persistent, chronic use, withdrawal of stimulants often leads to initial insomnia, which may persist. The sleep abnormalities encountered include a decrease in sleep efficiency, with increased periods of nocturnal wakefulness, increased amounts of REM sleep with a shortened REM latency, and increased stage 1 NREM sleep.

Opioids

The primary effect on sleep of acute administration of opioids to normal subjects or abstinent users is to shorten sleep latency and reduce total sleep time, sleep efficiency, REM sleep, and SWS. Chronic use, however, usually leads to tolerance to some of these effects. Even the longer-acting opioids, such as methadone, contribute to insomnia, with disruption of sleep architecture and increased arousals accompanying chronic administration. The pathophysiology of this effect is not clear, but evidence suggests that the REM-inhibiting properties can be attributed to inhibition of acetylcholine receptors in the pontine reticular formation or to direct agonist effects at specific μ receptors.

Opioids play a role in the treatment and management of RLS and PLMS, although the mechanism of this benefit is not well understood. The risk of becoming dependent on opioids must be weighed against the sleep benefits. Opioids play an obvious role in the management of sleep disorders secondary to pain syndromes.

Little has been written about the characteristics of sleep during withdrawal from opioids, but clinical experience suggests that insomnia often is cited as a troublesome feature of withdrawal.

Nicotine

Smokers experience an increase in sleep latency and an increase in arousals, with resulting poorer sleep maintenance. A possible biphasic response is that low doses promote sleep and higher doses disrupt sleep. Unlike most of the other agents discussed in this chapter, nicotine can increase rather than decrease REM.

Withdrawal from nicotine is associated with sleep disruption and increased daytime sleepiness. The effect of nicotine patches on sleep disruption remains unclear. Some researchers speculate that tobacco and the irritation it causes to the upper airway may contribute to OSA.

Caffeine

The half-life of caffeine ranges from 3 to 7 hours, with effects persisting for as long as 8 to 14 hours. As with other drugs, there is considerable variability in individual responses to caffeine, explaining why some can sleep soundly despite heavy consumption.

Caffeine often is used in combination with alcohol and together they can lead to even further aggravation of insomnia. Although alcohol has hypnotic properties, its half-life is much shorter than that of caffeine and its major effects disappear within a few hours. At that point, the rebound effect of alcohol withdrawal and the persistent stimulatory effect of caffeine jointly contribute to further sleep disruption.

Withdrawal from caffeine occurs within 18 to 24 hours and common complaints include headache, fatigue, irritability, sleepiness, and flulike symptoms.

Benzodiazepines

Benzodiazepines represent an interesting group of medications because they often are used in the management of sleep disorders, in addition to being potential drugs of abuse.

The primary effect of benzodiazepines is to reduce sleep latency, increase total sleep time, and reduce nocturnal arousals. There is minimal effect on REM sleep but acute and chronic use leads to decreases in the amount of SWS. Recent reviews suggest that the development of tolerance to the hypnotic effects of benzodiazepines is variable and that drug effects may persist for extended periods of time.

Marijuana

The hypnotic properties of cannabis, whether direct or by impacting pain, anxiety, and other chronic difficulties, may be of particular concern in addiction medicine. In a study of chronic marijuana users, abstinence from THC increased ratings of anxiety/depression/irritability and decreased the reported quantity and quality of sleep; factors that may contribute to continued use.

Some of the hypnotic effect has been attributed to the ability of cannabinoids to modulate spontaneous neuronal activity and evoke inhibition of the locus coeruleus neuradrenergic neurons. Another major constituent of marijuana, cannabidiol, may actually induce alertness through its impact on dopaminergic release and activation of neurons in the hypothalamus and dorsal raphe nucleus.

Few studies that have looked specifically at the impact of marijuana on sleep architecture. It seems that the acute administration leads to a decrease in REM sleep and an increase in SWS. With the long-term administration (>7 days), some tolerance probably develops to the SWS effects, but not to the REM sleep effects.

CLINICAL APPROACHES TO SLEEP DISORDERS

The clinical approach to patients with co-occurring sleep and addictive disorders poses certain problems. In addition to dealing with specific sleep disorders, it is necessary to address the effect of the substance of abuse on sleep, the effect of withdrawal, and any comorbid psychiatric problems such as depression. The clinical picture may be further complicated because some of the medications used in the treatment of specific sleep disorders have a potential for abuse. Therefore, a systematic approach is critical.

1. Obtain a careful history of the amount of sleep obtained in a 24-hour period.
2. Address the issue of timing and determine the patient's probable circadian rhythm. A sleep diary can be helpful.
3. Consider the potential for medical or psychiatric issues that can interfere with sleep. Review medications, exercise, nicotine, alcohol, and other drug use, symptoms of anxiety, depression, nightmares, and posttraumatic stress.
4. Inquire about possible features of intrinsic sleep disorders.
5. Inquire about the sleep environment. Is the sleep area conducive to the relaxation required to allow the wake-to-sleep transition?

Occasionally, additional diagnostic studies are required. A PSG should be considered if OSA, narcolepsy, or parasomnia is suspected.

Any strategy to address the sleep problem needs to take the addictive disorder into consideration, including careful selection of medications. RLS and PLMS can be treated with medications that are not subject to abuse. OSA usually is treated with continuous positive airway pressure devices. Special attention then can be directed to issues of sleep hygiene. In working with a patient with mood disorders for whom addiction is an issue, it is wise to consider the sedating antidepressants or the more active agents used to treat other anxiety-related disorders, such as the selective serotonin reuptake inhibitors.

CHAPTER 79

Summary Author: Agnes Kwasnicka
Linda C. Degutis • David A. Fiellin • Gail D'Onofrio

Traumatic Injuries Related to Alcohol and Other Drug Use

Alcohol and other drugs (AODs) use contributes to a substantial proportion of injury events. These people suffer more frequent and severe complications than other injured patients. This chapter provides data on the effectiveness of screening instruments for injured patients in emergency department and inpatient settings.

EPIDEMIOLOGY OF ALCOHOL AND OTHER DRUG-RELATED INJURY

Overall Risks

Nearly 50% of major trauma cases and 22% of minor trauma cases have been found to be alcohol-related. Data from the 1989 National Health and Nutrition Epidemiologic Survey show that persons who consumed five or more drinks per occasion were twice as likely to die of injuries as nondrinkers and that consuming nine or more drinks on one occasion increased the risk of injury-related death more than threefold.

Alcohol and Motor Vehicle Fatalities

According to the National Highway Traffic Safety Administration, 41% of motor vehicle fatalities were alcohol-related in 2006, and 11% of people who were injured were in an alcohol-related crash. More than 50% of those who are arrested for driving under the influence (DUI) have alcohol problems, and many require medical care for injuries related to MVCs. In fact, an arrest for DUI is an independent indicator of risk of death in a future MVC in all age groups. Nearly half of the approximately 35,000 fatal MVCs in the United States each year are related to alcohol use.

Alcohol and Non-Motor Vehicle–Related Injuries

Alcohol is involved in 42% of pedestrian fatalities, 60% of fatal burns (often related to cigarette smoking), and an unknown percentage of work-related injuries and drownings. Studies of boating fatalities show that 60% of the victims tested positive for alcohol, and 30% had blood alcohol concentrations (BACs) >100 mg%.

Persons older than 30 years who sustained violence-related injuries were more likely to have a positive alcohol breath test, to report drinking before the event, and to report a significant history of alcohol-related problems as compared with persons who experienced other types of injuries.

In adolescents, alcohol use is associated with MVC-related injuries (including 38% of drivers), attempted suicide, and assault.

Relationship Between Alcohol, Other Drugs, and Injury

Alcohol is an important risk factor for fire and burn injuries associated with cigarette smoking. In one study, nearly half of those who died in fires had BACs above 0.10. Work-related injuries, including injuries requiring hospitalization, were found to be more likely in persons who had an average daily intake of five drinks, compared to abstainers, and in those who used psychoactive drugs. Finally, onset of alcohol use at ages younger than 21 years was associated with experiencing an alcohol-related injury.

Alcohol, Other Drugs, and Trauma Patients Admitted to the Hospital

In one study of substance use disorders in trauma patients, 54% had a lifetime history of a substance use disorder, 24% had a current diagnosis of alcohol dependence, and 18% had a current diagnosis of dependence on other drugs. Alcohol is frequently implicated in fatal and nonfatal falls.

In a study of the role of alcohol in bicycle injuries, persons who died were more likely to have had positive BACs (30% vs. 16%) than were those who were injured but did not die.

Cocaine Use and Injuries

The role of cocaine use in injuries or fatalities has been studied less frequently than that of alcohol but has been associated with MVCs (especially when combined with alcohol), homicide, and risk-taking behavior.

An evaluation of 14,842 fatal injuries, including overdose, homicides, suicides, MVCs, and falls, found evidence of cocaine in 27%.

Drugs and Motor Vehicle Injury

A study of drug use with and without concomitant alcohol use among injured drivers found that 14 (6.6%) of 211 injured drivers tested positive for drugs (amphetamines, barbiturates, benzodiazepines, cocaine, cannabis, and opiates) alone, while 12 (5.7%) of 211 tested positive for alcohol and drugs in combination.

EFFECTIVE SCREENING IN INJURED PATIENTS

Screening for Alcohol Problems in the Emergency Department

Screening and intervention when needed may take place at almost any time during the emergency department visit, after admission if necessary. Depending upon the particular situation, intervention may range from a brief conversation to a referral to specialized treatment.

Studies of screening instruments for alcohol problems in emergency department and trauma settings have focused primarily on the recognition of the most harmful spectrum of alcohol consumption, including alcohol abuse and dependence, and so provide little empirical evidence to guide screening for at-risk drinking. Evidence supports the use of brief, formal screening questionnaires such as the CAGE, TWEAK, or AUDIT in preference to clinical recognition or laboratory analyses such as the BAC or SAT. For patients who met the criteria for alcohol dependence

- Two positive responses on the CAGE had a sensitivity of 76% to 87% and a specificity of 84% to 90%.
- A score of 3 on the TWEAK had a sensitivity of 84% to 89% and a specificity of 81% to 86%.
- A score of 8 on the AUDIT had a sensitivity of 83% to 91% and a specificity of 81% to 90%.

Although other instruments are being studied, the wealth of information on the use of the CAGE plus quantity and frequency questions from the AUDIT make these the preferred screening methods at this time.

When planning screening programs it is important to keep in mind that the operating characteristics of screening instruments for alcohol problems in emergency settings have been shown to vary with ethnicity, gender, and nature of the alcohol problem.

There are no comparable screening instruments for drug abuse and dependence other than alcohol. One attempt to identify problems is to add an additional question to the CAGE to ask about specific drugs. Asking about specific classes of drugs may yield a better history.

INTERVENTIONS WITH INJURED PATIENTS

When an alcohol or other drug-related injury occurs, the negative consequences of the injury can create what has been described as a "teachable moment"—a unique opportunity to motivate patients to change their behavior or to encourage them to seek further treatment.

Brief interventions can reduce not only alcohol use but also the incidence of alcohol-related injuries. Brief interventions involve counseling sessions that require 5 to 45 minutes. Such interventions often incorporate the six elements proposed by Miller and Sanchez, which are summarized by the mnemonic FRAMES: **F**eedback, **R**esponsibility, **A**dvice, **M**enu of strategies, **E**mpathy, and **S**elf-efficacy.

Results from studies of the efficacy of brief interventions for alcohol problems in emergency departments and inpatient trauma centers have been mixed. Cohort studies without control groups demonstrated a significant benefit of brief intervention, with reduction of alcohol and drug use at 3- to 12-month follow-up. One study with a quasi-experimental comparison group also demonstrated significant reduction in alcohol use in the group receiving brief intervention, and at-risk drinkers appeared to benefit more than did dependent drinkers. In randomized controlled studies, results have been varied. Whether these mixed results are due to methodologic challenges such as extensive assessments, or enrollment of patients with lower levels of drinking, remains to be answered. In terms of admitted trauma patients, there are also disparate results.

In January 2006, the American College of Surgeons Committee on Trauma passed a resolution mandating that screening and brief intervention services be included as an essential component of Level I Trauma Center verification. Moreover, recent reports underscore that education in the use of formal alcohol and drug screening questionnaires is lacking in emergency medicine residency programs but that residents who are exposed to a structured skills-based educational program do improve their knowledge and performance in screening and brief intervention with patients who have alcohol problems.

TABLE 79.1   **Screening for Alcohol Problems in Injured Patients**

Ask the NIAAA quantity and frequency questions:
1. On average, how many days per week do you drink alcohol?
2. On a typical day when you drink, how many drinks do you have?
3. What is the maximum number of drinks you had on any given occasion during the past month?

Use the CAGE (In the past 12 mo...):
C: Have you ever felt you should *C*ut down on your drinking?
A: Have people *A*nnoyed you by criticizing your drinking?
G: Have you ever felt bad or *G*uilty about your drinking?
E: Have you ever had a drink first thing in the morning to "steady your nerves" or get rid of a hangover ("*E*ye opener")?

The screen is positive if
A positive response on one or more questions from the CAGE and/or at-risk consumption is identified.
At-risk consumption
Men: >14 drinks/wk or >4 drinks per occasion
Women: >7 drinks/wk or >3 drinks per occasion
Both genders older than 65 y:
>7 drinks/wk or >3 drinks per occasion

Then assess for
• Medical problems: blackouts, depression, hypertension, injury, abdominal pain, liver dysfunction, sleep disorders
• Laboratory tests: liver function tests, macrocytic anemia
• Behavioral problems
• Alcohol dependence

Intervene
If the patient is an "at-risk drinker"
• Advise the patient of his or her risk.
• Set drinking goals.
• Provide referral to primary care.

If the patient is an alcohol-dependent drinker
• Assess the acute risk of intoxication or withdrawal.
Negotiate a referral for detoxification, to Alcoholics Anonymous, and to primary care.

Reprinted from National Institute on Alcohol Abuse and Alcoholism. *The physician's guide to helping patients with alcohol problems* (NIH Publication No. 95-3769). Rockville, MD: National Institute on Alcohol Abuse and Alcoholism, 1995.

INCORPORATING SCREENING AND BRIEF INTERVENTION INTO PRACTICE

In most settings where injured patients are treated, such as emergency departments and trauma centers, time is short and competing priorities make screening and brief intervention a challenge. Therefore, screens that are short and simple and that can be administered by a variety of providers have a greater chance of being used.

One screen for alcohol problems that can be adapted to the emergency department and trauma center setting and which has been recommended by the National Institute of Alcohol Abuse and Alcoholism (NIAAA) includes three quantity and frequency questions (to elicit information as to whether the patient exceeds the guidelines for moderate drinking), as well as the CAGE questionnaire (which is better at identifying alcohol dependence). Because the CAGE originally was designed for lifetime prevalence, it is helpful, though less well validated, to modify it by specifying "in the past 12 months" (Table 79.1).

Brief interventions may include advice only or incorporate some motivational enhancement techniques. Some suggested interventions

- At-risk drinker or patient who has sustained an alcohol-related injury but is not alcohol-dependent—set goals within safe limits, refer to primary care physician
- Patient with nondependent drug use—negotiate abstinence or harm reduction
- Patient who is dependent on drugs or alcohol or clinician is uncertain as to where a patient fits on the continuum of alcohol and drug problems—seek further assessment or referral to a specialized treatment program.

Brief intervention for injured patients may include the following components but should be tailored to each institution's or community's needs.

1. Raise the subject
2. Give feedback
3. Compare to norms
4. Make a connection (between cause of visit and substance use)
5. Assess readiness to change
6. Develop discrepancy
7. Elicit a response
8. Negotiate a goal
9. Give advice
10. Summarize and provide agreement form and primary care follow-up

CHAPTER 80

Summary Author: Christopher A. Cavacuiti
Alan Ona Malabanan

Endocrine and Reproductive Disorders Related to Alcohol and Other Drug Use

The impact of substance use on the endocrine system is very complex. Drugs of abuse affect multiple hormone systems, and these systems have a wide range of actions. When one adds to this inherent complexity the effects on the endocrine system of gender, mental status, and mental illness, the heterogeneity of illicit drugs, the prevalence of polydrug use, the addition of adulterants, the endocrine effects of drug withdrawal, and differences between the effects of acute and chronic substance use, it becomes clear that the study of the endocrine effects of alcohol and other drugs is very difficult. Generalizing many of these effects to clinical practice is even more difficult. Because of this complexity, this chapter focuses only on the most clearly established and clinically relevant endocrine effects. These effects are given in Table 80.1.

DISORDERS RELATED TO ALCOHOL

Hypoglycemia

Alcohol causes hypoglycemia by producing malnutrition (thereby reducing the body's production of glucose); alcohol also impairs the body's endocrine response to hypoglycemia. While hypoglycemia is not a common consequence of alcohol abuse, it is one of the most serious. It can lead to neurologic damage, coma, seizures, or even death.

Hyperglycemia

The impact of alcohol on glycemic control varies both in terms of acute versus chronic consumption and low versus high amounts of alcohol. Some studies have found an association between low to moderate alcohol use and improved insulin sensitivity and a decreased risk of diabetes mellitus in men. Others found no effect.

Chronic heavy use of alcohol can lead to alcoholic pancreatitis, which in turn can lead to pancreatic exocrine and endocrine insufficiency. When diabetes mellitus results from pancreatic insufficiency, it is an indication that >90% of the pancreatic beta cells, which produce insulin, and the alpha cells, which produce glucagon, are destroyed. The secondary diabetes mellitus that results from alcoholic pancreatitis often leads to extremely labile blood sugars that are typically very difficult to control.

Acute ethanol consumption has also been shown to increase peripheral insulin resistance, which can make type 2 diabetes more difficult to control.

Reproductive Consequences

The reproductive effects of alcohol use are gender-specific. In men, alcohol use is known to raise prolactin and lower testosterone. The consequences of this include sexual dysfunction, gynecomastia, and hypogonadism, particularly in men with alcoholic cirrhosis.

In women, the effects of alcohol use depend on menopausal status and hormone therapy use. In premenopausal women and postmenopausal women on estrogen, acute alcohol consumption leads to an increase in

TABLE 80.1	Endocrine Syndromes Associated with Alcohol and Other Drug Use

Alcohol
- Diabetes insipidus
- Gynecomastia
- Hyperadrenalism
- Hyperglycemia
- Hypoglycemia
- Hyperlipidemia
- Hyperprolactinemia (possibly)
- Hypogonadism/infertility
- Hypertension
- Osteoporosis

Amphetamines
- Hyperadrenalism
- Hypertension
- Weight loss

Anabolic steroids
- Gynecomastia
- Hyperlipidemia
- Hypogonadism/infertility
- Hypertension
- Hyperthyroidism (possibly)
- Virilization

Barbiturates
- Hypoadrenalism (possibly)
- Hypothyroidism (possibly)
- Osteoporosis

Benzodiazepines
- Hypoadrenalism (possibly)
- Hypoglycemia (possibly)
- Syndrome of inappropriate antidiuretic hormone (possibly)

Caffeine
- Hyperglycemia
- Hyperlipidemia (possibly)

- Hypertension
- Osteoporosis (possibly)

Cocaine
- Hyperglycemia
- Hyperprolactinemia
- Hypertension
- Weight loss

Inhalants
- Hypogonadism/infertility
- Hypothyroidism (possibly)
- Osteoporosis (possibly)

Lysergic acid
- None known

Marijuana
- Gynecomastia (possibly)
- Hypoadrenalism
- Hypoglycemia (possibly)
- Hypogonadism/infertility (possibly)

Opioids
- Hyperprolactinemia
- Hypogonadism/infertility
- Osteoporosis

Phencyclidine
- None known

Tobacco/cigarette smoking
- Hyperlipidemia
- Hypogonadism/infertility
- Hypertension
- Hyperthyroidism
- Hypothyroidism (possibly)
- Osteoporosis
- Syndrome of Inappropriate antidiuretic hormone

estradiol levels through reduced metabolism of estradiol. This increase in estrogen level may explain why alcohol use is associated with menstrual irregularities, an increased risk of breast cancer, and a delay in menopause. Pregnant women with a high alcohol intake have a higher incidence of miscarriages, placental abruption, preterm deliveries, and stillbirths than do controls.

Bone Health Consequences

Chronic alcoholism is associated with decreased bone mass and an increased risk of skeletal fractures. In contrast, low to moderate alcohol consumption may actually lead to increased bone mineral density and a decreased risk of fractures. Heavy alcohol use is associated with osteonecrosis of bone. Alcohol may be responsible for up to one third of cases of femoral head osteonecrosis.

Other Endocrinologic Consequences

Alcohol use increases triglyceride synthesis, leading to hypertriglyceridemia and hepatic steatosis. Moderate alcohol increases the high-density lipoprotein (HDL) fraction of cholesterol, which may be associated with reduced cardiovascular morbidity and mortality.

DISORDERS RELATED TO TOBACCO

Tobacco smoke contains myriad chemical compounds, most notably nicotine, tar, thiocyanate, 2,3-hydroxypyridine and carbon monoxide, which may have multiple endocrine effects.

Thyroid Disease

Cigarette smoking is a risk factor for Graves disease. There is conflicting evidence in terms of smoking and hypothyroidism.

Insulin Resistance and Dyslipidemia

Cigarette smoking, as well as nicotine gum use, is associated with an increase in insulin resistance and an increased risk of developing diabetes mellitus. Mild decreases in HDL cholesterol and mild elevations in triglycerides are associated with cigarette smoking, though these changes may be due to components of cigarette smoke other than nicotine.

Reproductive Function

In women, cigarette smoking is associated with decreases in estrogen levels and early menopause. In men, cigarette smoking is associated with quantitative and qualitative decrements in sperm.

Bone Health

Cigarette smoking decreases intestinal calcium absorption, affects vitamin D levels, and disrupts a number of hormones involved in calcium regulation. Smoking is associated with decreased bone mineral density and increased bone loss and is an independent risk factor for osteoporotic fracture and femoral head osteonecrosis.

Other Endocrinologic Effects

Cigarette smoke stimulates antidiuretic hormone from the pituitary and catecholamines from the adrenal medulla. In addition, smoking is associated with noradrenergic stimulation, which can lead to hypertension.

DISORDERS RELATED TO OTHER DRUGS

Marijuana

There is conflicting evidence regarding the effect of marijuana smoking on plasma levels of male and female reproductive hormones. Heavy marijuana use is associated with hypoadrenalism, suppression of cortisol, and reduced growth hormone levels.

Opiates

The endocrine effects of acute administration of opiates occur primarily in the hypothalamus and pituitary. Gonadotropins (follicle-stimulating hormone [FSH] and luteinizing hormone [LH]) are suppressed by inhibition of gonadotropin-releasing hormone (GnRH) secretion. Prolactin secretion is stimulated, while adrenocorticotropic hormone (ACTH) and cortisol secretions are suppressed. Chronic administration of opiates can produce partial tolerance to many of the endocrine effects.

In many (though not all) studies, use of opioids (including methadone and heroin) has been associated with a decline in serum testosterone levels and diminished sperm motility. The variability in findings may be due in part to the different opioids studies, the variability of doses, the presence of other drugs, and the possible effect of malnutrition on the reproductive system.

Studies suggest that >50% of women on methadone maintenance will have hypothalamic and pituitary dysfunction that can lead to oligoovulation and menstrual irregularities.

There is evidence showing a decrease in bone density with opiate use in both men and women.

Cocaine

Cocaine acts primarily by increasing catecholamines (*norepinephrine* and *dopamine*) at the synaptic junctions. These catecholamines act as counterregulatory hormones that antagonize insulin. They stimulate glucose production and inhibit glucose clearance. This can lead to hyperglycemia as well as diabetic ketoacidosis.

Dopamine inhibits the secretion of prolactin. Acute cocaine increases dopamine levels and results in suppressed prolactin secretion. With chronic cocaine use and with cocaine withdrawal, dopamine levels often become depleted and hyperprolactinemia results.

Amphetamines

Well-described acute endocrine effects of amphetamine administration include increased corticosteroid release and increased growth hormone release.

Caffeine

Caffeine is one of the world's most widely used drugs. The many forms in which it is delivered and prepared have confounded its study. Caffeine is a neuroendocrine stimulant with action mediated by central adenosine receptor antagonism. Caffeine ingestion leads to the release of epinephrine and norepinephrine, which can increase blood pressure.

Caffeine's impact on glucose metabolism remains confusing. On the one hand, acute caffeine ingestion has been shown to decrease insulin sensitivity. On the other, chronic coffee consumption is associated with a decreased risk of type 2 diabetes.

Caffeine's impact on bone mass is equally confusing. Caffeine is associated with increased urinary calcium excretion, decreased serum free estradiol and serum insulin-like growth factor I levels. All three of these actions can lead to reductions in bone mass and increased fracture risk. However, not all studies have found an association between caffeine and fractures and some have actually found that caffeinated tea can protect against hip fractures.

Benzodiazepines

Benzodiazepines act by stimulating γ-aminobutyric-acidergic (GABAergic) neurons, which usually are inhibitory in function. Benzodiazepines appear to suppress basal serum levels of cortisol and also suppress the body's cortisol and ACTH response. There is evidence to suggest that this effect is even greater in elderly patients than in young.

Inhalants

Occupational exposure to inhalants is associated with infertility, increased risk of spontaneous abortion, and a variety of birth defects. It is not known if these actions are due to endocrine dysfunction. To date, no specific endocrine consequences of inhalant use have been described.

Anabolic Steroids

The adverse endocrine consequences are a direct result of androgenic effects and suppression of the hypothalamic-pituitary-gonadal axis. These effects include testicular atrophy; decreases in testosterone, LH, and FSH; increases in estrone; and suppression of spermatogenesis in men. Gynecomastia can result from aromatization of the androgens to estrogen. In women, there can be menstrual disturbances, deepening of voice, and development of acne and male-pattern body hair.

Summary Author: Christopher A. Cavacuiti
Martha J. Wunsch • Michael F. Weaver

Alcohol and Other Drug Use During Pregnancy: Management of the Mother and Child

Some women are able to stop using alcohol and other drugs when they learn they are pregnant, but many others others may have difficulty stopping due to the severity of addiction or withdrawal. The prevalence of substance use during pregnancy is substantial. Ten percent of pregnant women drink alcohol, with 4% reporting heavy drinking. The prevalence of illicit drug use varies by drug type during pregnancy, with 8.5% to 15% reporting marijuana use, around 2% using opioids, and 1.1% to 9.5% using cocaine.

APPROACH TO THE PREGNANT WOMAN

Those who provide health care to substance-using pregnant women (SUPW) should be sensitive to the fact that the use of alcohol or illicit drugs is much more stigmatized in pregnancy, so these patients may minimize or deny their drug use, its harmful effects, and the need to seek help. In many cases, a woman may have abused alcohol or drugs during a previous pregnancy, experiencing negative consequences such as stigmatization and loss of custody of other children.

Screening

Perinatal substance use and addiction affect women of all races and socioeconomic levels. Though a number of questionnaires have been validated to detect alcohol use, few instruments have been validated for detection of illicit drug use during pregnancy (see Chapter 18, "Screening and Brief Intervention for Pregnant Women"). Certain factors in a patient's history should raise the index of suspicion in terms of substance use during pregnancy:

- Family history (children of alcoholics have a threefold to fourfold increase in risk of developing alcoholism themselves)
- Frequent encounters with law enforcement agencies
- Substance use, abuse, or addiction by the current "significant other"
- A past history of substance abuse or addiction in the SUPW
- A history of medical conditions associated with substance use (hepatitis C, endocarditis, etc.)

The combination of screening questions and urine toxicology has been shown to be more effective for detection of perinatal addiction than use of either one alone.

Common Substances

Tobacco Forty percent of women who smoke and become pregnant quit during pregnancy. Nicotine replacement helps reduce the amount smoked during pregnancy, which improves birth outcomes, and nicotine replacement therapy does not produce fetal complications.

Alcohol and Sedative Hypnotics More than 60% of women who use alcohol and become pregnant quit during pregnancy. Increased use, abuse, and addiction, progressing to severe withdrawal from alcohol or sedative hypnotics carries a significant mortality risk, so early recognition and treatment are essential. The normal physiologic changes that accompany pregnancy can make it difficult to recognize early withdrawal. Table 81.1 displays similarities and differences between sedative-hypnotic withdrawal syndrome and pregnancy.

Stimulants Stimulant use is associated with a number of perinatal complications including preterm labor, premature rupture of membranes, placental abruption, and intrauterine growth restriction (IUGR). Discontinuation of stimulants does not cause significant physiologic sequelae. Stimulants do not need to be tapered or replaced with a cross-tolerant drug. In cases of extreme withdrawal induced agitation, low doses of a benzodiazepine may be used if necessary.

Opioids Infections such as endocarditis, recurrent cellulitis, or thrombophlebitis should raise suspicion for injection drug use. Opioid withdrawal syndrome during pregnancy can lead to fetal distress and premature labor. Premature labor may occur in 29% to 41% of pregnant women abusing opioids (rates for other illicit drugs are considerably lower; cocaine users, for example, have around a 6% rate of premature labor). Methadone is frequently used to treat acute withdrawal symptoms from opioids, including other shorter acting prescription opioids. Naloxone should not be given to a pregnant woman except as a last resort in life-threatening opioid overdose. Withdrawal precipitated by an opioid antagonist can result in spontaneous abortion, premature labor, or stillbirth.

Office Care of the Substance-Using Pregnant Woman

Support involvement of the patient's significant others in the treatment of the pregnant addicted woman. With the consent of the woman, involvement of family members who comprehend and accept the need for treatment may be helpful. Pregnant women with substance use disorders often require treatment of other psychiatric diagnoses. Thus care should include screening for depression and other mental health diagnoses. Blood-borne disease and sexually transmitted disease (STD) testing is usually part of routine prenatal care in most women, but it is particularly important in SUPW as these infections are more common in this population. Evaluation of the need for psychosocial support system (and referral to appropriate community services) is essential.

Screening for domestic violence should be routine in this population. Up to 8% of pregnant women are victims of physical abuse, but 34% of SUPW report physical abuse.

Labor and Delivery

The pain and emotional stress of labor (and the similarity of labor symptoms to those of withdrawal) make this a high risk period for relapse. Education of SUPW that labor and delivery can be a "trigger" for substance use can aid in planning coping strategies and help prevent relapse after the birth.

Patients addicted to drugs are subject to pain in the same manner as any other patient. The pregnant addicted woman benefits from appropriate treatment for pain. Pain medication should not be withheld based on a history of addiction.

TABLE 81.1 Pregnancy and Sedative-Hypnotic Withdrawal

Signs and symptoms common to both sedative-hypnotic withdrawal and pregnancy	Signs and symptoms of sedative-hypnotic withdrawal not common to pregnancy
Restlessness	Impaired memory
Insomnia	Distractibility
Nausea and vomiting	Agitation
Hypertension	Tremor
Tachycardia	Fever
Tachypnea	Diaphoresis
Seizures	Hallucinations

MATERNAL ADDICTION TREATMENT

In most cases of addiction, simple admonitions to stop using are insufficient. Therefore, most SUPW need to be referred for comprehensive and intense treatment. While a wide variety of treatment programs exist, very few have been specifically studied in SUPW. Studies show that for SUPW/new mother-specific addiction treatment programs to be successful, they must provide childcare. Unfortunately, very addiction treatment programs do so.

Opioid Maintenance Treatment

Medical withdrawal of the pregnant opioid-dependent woman is not recommended because of high rates of relapse to illicit prescription opioid and heroin use and the increased risk to the fetus of intrauterine death. Methadone maintenance treatment (MMT) in pregnancy has been shown to reduce illicit opioid use, improve maternal psychosocial function, and lead to better birth outcomes. MMT is therefore the treatment of choice for opioid-dependent pregnant women.

Maternal methadone dose does not correlate with neonatal abstinence symptoms, so maternal benefits of methadone are not offset by harm to the newborn. It is not unusual for the methadone dose requirement to increase during the third trimester of pregnancy. This is due to larger plasma volume, decreased plasma protein binding, increased tissue binding, increased methadone metabolism, and increased methadone clearance in the mother. Splitting the total daily methadone requirement into two doses, given in the morning and evening, is preferred if possible.

Sublingual buprenorphine, a partial agonist prescribed for the treatment of opioid addiction, is not yet approved in the United States for use in pregnancy but has been used successfully in other countries for opioid maintenance in pregnant women.

Other Pharmacotherapy

Disulfiram (Antabuse) is a known teratogen and is contraindicated during pregnancy. The effects of acamprosate (Campral) and naltrexone (Revia) have not been studied in pregnancy. Women taking any of these medications for alcohol dependence should stop the medication if they are planning to become pregnant.

EVALUATION OF THE SUBSTANCE-EXPOSED NEWBORN

Physical examination of the newborn, maternal social and legal history, and maternal addiction history may lead the clinician to request laboratory screening for substances in mother and/or child. When indicated, infant urine, meconium, and cord blood may be tested for legal and illegal drugs of abuse. A request for infant body fluid testing must be accompanied by informed consent.

The advantage of testing neonatal urine is ease of collection; however, many drugs are cleared rapidly in the urine, and therefore urine testing only provides information about fetal exposure shortly before delivery. The theoretical advantage of meconium testing is that it is produced from 14 weeks of gestation onward and thus allows for evaluation of a much longer window of prenatal exposure (essentially from 14 weeks to delivery). However, comparison studies have shown little advantage for analysis of meconium compared with analysis of maternal urine and first infant voided urine). Testing of cord blood is also feasible. However, it only provides data about exposure around the time of birth and is less often available.

Health care practitioners must be familiar with legislation in their community dictating legal duty to report positive results to Child Protective Services.

Confirmed or suspected history of addiction in the mother should lead to infant screening for hepatitis B or C, human immunodeficiency virus (HIV), or other STDs.

NEONATAL INTOXICATION AND ABSTINENCE SYNDROMES

In SUPW using psychoactive substances, *polysubstance* abuse is the norm rather than the exception. Because of this, determination of specific perinatal effects of individual drugs may be difficult. The substance-exposed newborn may have any or all of the symptoms described below (Table 81.2).

Neonates with intrauterine drug exposure should be followed up in the hospital for at least 72 to 96 hours after birth to monitor for signs of a neonatal intoxication or signs of neonatal abstinence syndrome (NAS). If >7 days has elapsed between the last maternal use and delivery, the incidence of NAS is low.

Initial Treatment

Initial treatment of NAS should be primarily supportive, as pharmacotherapy may prolong hospitalization and subject the neonate to exposure to medications that may not be indicated. Supportive measures include reducing

TABLE 81.2	**Signs of Neonatal Intoxication and Abstinence**

- Poor weight gain
- Instability in heart rate, respiratory rate, and temperature
- Hyperactivity
- Irritability
- Hypertonia or hypotonia
- Difficulty sucking or excessive sucking
- Sleep disturbance
- High-pitched cries
- Feeding difficulties

ambient light and noise exposure, quieting the infant with swaddling, frequent small feedings, and intravenous replacement of fluids and electrolytes (if required). Indications for pharmacotherapy include seizures; diarrhea or vomiting resulting in dehydration or excessive weight loss; inability to sleep; or significant autonomic instability with bradycardia or tachycardia, apnea or tachypnea, or temperature instability not due to infection.

The differential diagnosis for NAS includes sepsis, hypoglycemia, perinatal anoxia, intracranial bleed, and hyperthyroidism.

Opioids
Neonatal opioid withdrawal syndrome occurs in 60% to 80% of infants with intrauterine exposure to heroin or prescription opioids, including methadone and buprenorphine. The most commonly used and comprehensive assessment is Finnegan Neonatal Abstinence Score.

Other Drugs
There is no specific alcohol/sedative-hypnotic scoring scale, in part because of the predominance of polysubstance exposures. Exposure to alcohol and/or sedative hypnotics commonly occurs in tandem with other substances, with tobacco being the most commonly co-occurring substance. Phenobarbital is the agent of choice for severe sedative-hypnotic withdrawal syndrome.

FETAL EFFECTS OF PSYCHOACTIVE SUBSTANCE USE IN PREGNANCY

In the human, it is difficult to attribute causation to exposure when there are confounding variables such as malnutrition and concurrent use of other substances. Alcohol and tobacco, alone and in combination with other substances, are known to have the most potential to cause teratogenicity in the human, but psychoactive substance use in pregnancy, whether illicit or medicinal, always involves some degree of risk of teratogenicity to the developing embryo or fetus.

Alcohol

Fetal Alcohol Syndrome The classic phenotype and diagnosis of fetal alcohol syndrome (FAS) includes the following:

1. *Evidence of growth retardation (prenatal and/or postnatal)*: Height and or weight equal to or less than the 10th percentile, corrected for racial norms
2. *Evidence of deficient brain growth and/or abnormal morphogenesis*, including one or more of the following: structural brain anomalies or head circumference equal to or less than the 10th percentile (microcephaly)
3. *Evidence of a characteristic pattern of minor facial anomalies*, including two or more of the following: short palpebral fissures (equal to or less than the 10th percentile), thin vermillion border of the upper lip, smooth philtrum

Fetal Alcohol Spectrum Disorders The umbrella term *fetal alcohol spectrum disorder* expands the classification of prenatally alcohol-exposed individuals to include the following:

1. FAS with and without confirmed maternal alcohol exposure.
2. Partial FAS (displays some but not all of the FAS phenotypic features or displays milder versions of these characteristics).

3. Alcohol-related birth defects: These include a number of alcohol-related organ anomalies not listed in the strict FAS definition. Commonly involved organs include the heart, skeleton, kidneys, eyes, and ears.
4. Alcohol-related neurodevelopmental disorder: This is the name given to the impaired neurodevelopment that can occur from fetal alcohol exposure. It is characterized by marked impairment of complex developmental tasks, higher-level receptive and expressive language deficits, and disordered behavior. It often co-occurs with FAS and other fetal alcohol spectrum disorders (FASDs).

In the United States, it is estimated that between 0.5 and 2 per 1,000 live births meet diagnostic criteria for FAS. FASD is more common, and up to 1% of live births may be affected.

Sedative-Hypnotic Medications

Barbiturates In one study, the relative risk of major congenital malformations in anticonvulsant-exposed offspring (which include barbiturates such as phenobarbital) was 4.2. Features of anticonvulsant embryopathy include increased major malformations, growth retardation, and hypoplasia of the midface and fingers.

Benzodiazepines The use of benzodiazepines during pregnancy has been associated with various degrees of teratogenic effects, particularly cleft lip and palate.

Opioids

A review of the animal and human literature provides no evidence that prescribed and illicit use of opioids are in themselves teratogenic. The most common ill effect of opioid abuse and addiction in pregnancy is IUGR. IUGR is not felt to be due directly to the opioids per se. Rather, it is thought to be a result of lifestyle consequences of opioid addiction (such as poor maternal nutrition and recurrent intoxication and withdrawal secondary to fluctuating opioid levels). The offspring of women prescribed opioids for the treatment of pain, with steady-state levels of opioid medications, have no increase in pregnancy complications and deliver infants of normal weight and length.

Stimulants

Cocaine The effects of cocaine are thought to be through direct neurotoxicity by causing vascular damage. Multiple studies over the last decade have identified neurologic, developmental and behavioral deficiencies in the infant, toddler, and young child exposed prenatally to cocaine.

Methamphetamine Effects of prenatal exposure include neurobehavioral alterations and IUGR.

Tobacco Cigarette use exposes the fetus to wide variety of toxic substances including carbon monoxide, nicotine, tar, cyanide, and lead. An inverse relationship exists between birth weight and the number of cigarettes smoked per day. A meta-analysis of >60 studies concluded that nearly one third of sudden infant death syndrome (SIDS) deaths may be prevented with cessation of smoking in pregnancy.

Cannabis

Studies of effects on neurodevelopment and growth have produced conflicting results. Additionally, the concurrent use of alcohol and tobacco in pregnancy confounds understanding of the teratogenicity of cannabis.

BREAST-FEEDING

Women actively engaged in addiction treatment should be encouraged to breast-feed as long as urine drug screens are negative and the mother is negative for HIV. Women prescribed opioid agonists for treatment with either methadone or buprenorphine should be encouraged to breast-feed if they are in stable recovery. While small amounts of methadone and buprenorphine may be present in breast milk, concentrations are not enough to cause harm to the infant and may actually reduce NAS severity.

Negligible amounts of methadone are excreted in human milk, and the American Academy of Pediatrics lists methadone as a medication compatible with breast-feeding. Breast-feeding should also be encouraged in mothers prescribed buprenorphine.

The substance-exposed nursing infant will often display signs similar to those with prenatal exposure (see Table 81.2 above).

LEGAL ISSUES

Many states require hospitals to report pregnant women suspected of heavy alcohol or other drug use to local public health authorities or the criminal justice system when they present for delivery, whether they have or have not sought treatment. This reporting may cause SUPW to be even more wary of acknowledging that they are abusing or addicted to drugs or medications. For this reason, it is very important for a physician who recognizes perinatal addiction to address this with the patient in a compassionate, nonjudgmental manner.

POSTPARTUM CARE

A number of studies have documented a strong association between parental active addiction and child maltreatment. Helping an addicted parent obtain effective treatment is the most important intervention for the child exposed to substances, both prenatally and during his or her childhood. Effective treatment and intervention is cost-effective in the short and long term and becomes the first and most effective prevention intervention for children.

Many SUPW also suffer from a lack of family and social support, depression and other psychiatric problems, inadequate housing or homelessness, exposure to violence, and financial difficulties. These challenges may pose as much risk to successful child rearing as the diagnosis of addiction.

Summary Author: Christopher A. Cavacuiti
Daniel P. Alford

Surgical Interventions in the Alcohol- or Drug-Using Patient

There are a number of reasons why it is important to consider alcohol and drug issues within the surgical setting:

- Many of the complications of active substance use require surgical management (common examples include traumatic injuries, infections of the skin and soft tissues, infective endocarditis, and certain cancers).
- Due to the health consequences of addiction, alcohol and drug abuse is a risk factor for perioperative complications.
- There is growing evidence that surgical teams with procedures to identify and appropriately manage patients with alcohol drug abuse have better outcomes.

PERIOPERATIVE CARE OF THE ALCOHOL-DEPENDENT PATIENT

Unhealthy alcohol use is common especially in patients seeking medical and surgical care. The prevalence of alcohol use disorders is as high as 40% in emergency room and various surgical inpatient settings and up to 50% in patients with trauma.

Preoperative Evaluation

Physicians often fail to identify alcohol use disorders in surgical patients. In one study, only 16% of people with alcoholism were identified in the perioperative setting. In screening for alcoholism, it is important to remember that patients with unhealthy alcohol use are often asymptomatic and often minimize consumption. Adults undergoing preoperative evaluation should be screened using validated questionnaires such as the CAGE questionnaire. The CAGE mnemonic refers the following questions.

- Have you ever felt you should *C*ut down on your drinking?
- Have people *A*nnoyed you by criticizing your drinking?
- Have you ever felt bad or *G*uilty about drinking?
- Have you ever taken a drink first thing in the morning (*E*ye opener) to steady your nerves or get rid of a hangover?

The Alcohol Use Disorder Identification Test (AUDIT) questionnaire is longer but detects a fuller spectrum of unhealthy alcohol use.

Any patients who screen positive for alcohol-related problems should be further evaluated in terms of risk for withdrawal. Risk factors associated with severe and prolonged alcohol withdrawal include amount and duration of alcohol use, prior withdrawal episodes, recurrent detoxifications, older age, and comorbid diseases. The incidence of alcohol withdrawal in hospitalized patients is as high as 8% and is two to five times higher in hospitalized trauma and surgical patients.

Any patients who screen positive for alcohol-related problems should also be evaluated for evidence of alcohol-related medical complications (particularly liver, pancreatic, nervous system, and cardiac disease). Heavy alcohol use is associated with a number of cognitive problems (such as Korsakoff syndrome, hepatic and

Wernicke encephalopathy). These neurologic conditions can worsen during the perioperative period and may be confused with other postoperative neurologic complications. Therefore, preoperative baseline mental status and cognition should be assessed and documented. Anemia is common in patients with alcohol dependence as well as decreased platelet count.

Management of Alcohol Withdrawal

One of the most common complications of hospitalized alcohol-dependent patients is withdrawal. The spectrum of alcohol withdrawal ranges from minor symptoms of autonomic hyperactivity including diaphoresis, tachycardia, systolic hypertension to tremor, insomnia, hallucinations, nausea, vomiting, psychomotor agitation, anxiety, and grand mal seizures to life-threatening delirium tremens. Recognizing withdrawal risk and treating early withdrawal can often prevent the complications of severe withdrawal.

Benzodiazepines are the drugs of choice for both the prevention and management of alcohol withdrawal. This subject is covered in detail in Chapter 42, Management of Alcohol Intoxication and Withdrawal.

Alcohol Use and Surgical Risk

Heavy alcohol use (even in the absence of clinical liver disease and even in the absence of alcohol dependence per se) is an independent risk factor for postoperative complications. Patients with chronic alcohol problems have longer intensive care unit stays, more postoperative septicemia, and pneumonia requiring mechanical ventilation as well as increased overall mortality. Abstinence before surgery has been shown to decrease postoperative morbidity.

Alcoholic Liver Disease

Unhealthy alcohol use can lead to liver disease of varying severity. More severe liver disease carries higher surgical risk and requires more special considerations.

Alcoholic Fatty Liver   Alcoholic fatty liver (hepatic steatosis) is the mildest form of alcohol-related liver disease. It occurs in 90% of heavy drinkers and is often asymptomatic and reversible. Common findings include right upper quadrant pain, nausea, and a mild elevation in liver transaminases with preserved liver function. While patients with fatty liver seem to tolerate surgery well, it is prudent to delay elective surgery whenever possible until reduced alcohol consumption (or abstinence) is achieved and signs and symptoms have resolved.

Alcoholic Hepatitis   Alcoholic hepatitis is a serious inflammatory disease of the liver, which occurs in up to 40% of heavy drinkers. These patients often present extremely ill with nausea, vomiting, anorexia, abdominal pain, fever, and jaundice. Elevated transaminases and prolonged coagulation studies are common. Surgical risk is very high in this group. It is recommended that elective surgery be delayed until clinical and laboratory parameters normalize, sometimes taking up to 12 weeks.

Alcoholic Cirrhosis   Cirrhosis occurs in 15% to 20% of heavy drinkers and refers to the irreversible necrosis, nodular regeneration, and fibrosis of the liver as a result of multiple episodes of hepatitis. Surgery in patients with cirrhosis is high risk. These patients are at increased risk for uncontrolled bleeding, poor wound healing, infections, and delirium. Cirrhosis can be subdivided into various levels of hepatic decompensation. Two of the most commonly used classification schemes are the *Pugh Classification* and the *Model for End-Stage Liver Disease (MELD)* score. Both schemes are effective predictors of surgical risk.

Preoperative Considerations in Patients with Cirrhosis   Preoperative abstinence should be the goal before all elective procedures. Vitamin K deficiency is common in these patients, and therefore coagulopathy management should start with the administration of vitamin K. Electrolytes should be monitored closely. Perioperative hemodynamic monitoring is often needed because these patients may have large fluid shifts, especially during abdominal surgeries. Ascites should be optimally managed preoperatively with sodium restriction and appropriate diuretic therapy. Thrombocytopenia should be identified and treated. Aggressive preoperative treatment of hepatic encephalopathy using lactulose and dietary protein restriction is recommended. Patients with known gastroesophageal varices should be monitored closely for gastrointestinal bleeding and should be considered for β-blocker prophylaxis preoperatively. Nutritional status should be optimized with multivitamins, thiamine, folate, and nutritional supplementation preoperatively. Cirrhotic patients may develop hepatopulmonary syndrome. Therefore, continuous monitoring oxygen saturation should be part of postoperative care.

PERIOPERATIVE CARE OF THE OPIOID-DEPENDENT PATIENT

Opioid-dependent persons are at high risk for medical complications, which often require surgical intervention. In injection opioids users, infections of the skin, soft tissue, bones, and joints are common and often require surgical drainage and debridement. These patients are also at risk for infectious endocarditis and may require surgery for valve replacement. Hepatitis B and C infections are common in intravenous drug users and are the leading causes of liver transplantation.

Preoperative Evaluation
Patients with a history of active injection drug use should be evaluated for a history of endocarditis and the need for antibiotic prophylaxis. These patients should also be evaluated for HIV/AIDS and active hepatitis B and C. Hospitalized patients with active opioid dependence are at risk for acute opioid withdrawal.

Management of Opioid Withdrawal
It is important for providers of perioperative care to be able to recognize and manage acute opioid withdrawal, which is likely in hospitalized opioid-dependent surgical patients. One approach to treating opioid withdrawal in the hospital setting involves treating the physiologic manifestations of acute withdrawal (including the hyper-adrenergic signs and symptoms, insomnia, nausea, vomiting, diarrhea, and muscles aches) with clonidine, benzodiazepines, dicyclomine, and nonsteroidal anti-inflammatory drugs. A much more effective method employs a long-acting opioid agonist such as methadone. There are a variety of protocols for titrating methadone on an inpatient basis. These protocols are beyond the scope of this chapter. After acute withdrawal is controlled, discussions regarding daily dose taper versus continued daily dose until the day of discharge (as well as postoperative addiction treatment aftercare and referral) should be discussed.

Management of Patients on Opioid Agonist Treatment
Approximately 350,000 patients are maintained on opioid agonist therapy (OAT) in the United States, using methadone or buprenorphine. Such patients should be maintained on their usual maintenance dose during the perioperative period. The correct maintenance dose should be determined by calling the patient's treatment program, prescriber, or pharmacy. When opioid agonist treated patients are being discharged, it is important to discuss the discharge plan with the addiction treatment program's clinical staff. This is important so that special arrangements can be made for "medical" take-home doses of methadone or buprenorphine in clinically appropriate cases (i.e., for clinically stable patients with impaired postoperative ambulation).

Management of Acute Pain in Patients on Opioid Agonist Therapy
Acute postoperative pain management in patients maintained on long-acting OAT can be challenging. The daily methadone or buprenorphine dose a patient receives is not adequate analgesia for acute pain. The lack of analgesia occurs because of the patient's high tolerance to opioids and the pharmacodynamics of methadone and buprenorphine. All methadone- and buprenorphine-maintained patients have a high tolerance to other opioids (cross-tolerance). As a result, OAT patients often require higher and more frequent doses of opioid analgesics to adequately treat acute pain. The appropriate treatment of acute pain in these patients includes uninterrupted OAT to address the patient's baseline opioid requirement and aggressive pain management. Clinical experience supports consideration of patient-controlled analgesia use in patients on OAT; increased patient control over analgesia minimizes patient anxiety over pain management. Mixed agonist/antagonist opioid analgesics such as pentazocine (Talwin) and butorphanol (Stadol) must be avoided due to their ability to precipitate acute opioid withdrawal in these patients.

PERIOPERATIVE CARE OF THE BENZODIAZEPINE-DEPENDENT PATIENT

Benzodiazepines, which are commonly prescribed to treat anxiety, panic attacks, and insomnia, have a high abuse potential. Patients who abuse benzodiazepines often are addicted to multiple drugs. Some studies have found up to 15% of heroin users and 40% of alcoholics also abuse benzodiazepines. The withdrawal syndrome ranges from severe anxiety, insomnia, autonomic hyperactivity (including tachycardia and hypertension), to seizures, delirium and even death. Patients with physical dependence to prescribed benzodiazepines should be maintained on their usual dose during the perioperative period. Patients dependent on illicit benzodiazepines should be maintained on an equivalent dose of long-acting benzodiazepine (e.g., diazepam, chlordiazepoxide) during the perioperative period.

PERIOPERATIVE CARE OF THE NICOTINE-DEPENDENT PATIENT

Nicotine-dependent patients (particularly those with preexisting cardiovascular disease and chronic obstructive pulmonary disease [COPD]) are at risk for a variety of surgical complications. Providers of preoperative care should encourage smoking cessation. Pharmacotherapy, including nicotine replacement, bupropion, and varenicline, consistently increases abstinence rates and should be considered preoperatively. Nicotine replacement therapy also should be offered postoperatively to patients at risk for nicotine withdrawal.

PERIOPERATIVE CARE OF THE STIMULANT-DEPENDENT PATIENT

Intravenous stimulant use may result in all the complications attributable to injection drug use such as endocarditis, pulmonary hypertension, hepatitis B and C, and HIV/AIDS. Stimulants use is associated with a variety of cardiopulmonary conditions, including pulmonary edema, dilated cardiomyopathy, left ventricular hypertrophy, arrhythmias, and myocardial infarction. Therefore, it is critically important to identify stimulant use during preoperative assessment and to evaluate carefully for clinical evidence of cardiopulmonary disease.

ORGAN TRANSPLANTATION IN PATIENTS WITH ADDICTIONS

Hepatitis B and C infections from injection drug use and alcoholic liver disease are the most common causes of end-stage liver disease requiring liver transplantation in the United States. In the past, patients with a history of addictive disorder have been kept off of transplantation lists because of fears of posttransplant noncompliance, with subsequent loss of graft, but also because of moralistic arguments that the patients had "self-inflicted" diseases. While some studies have found that former alcohol- and drug-using transplant patients have high relapse rates, high graft loss, and poor survival, other studies have not found this to be the case. Because organ transplantation in patients with addiction disorders is unusually complex, some medical centers have added addiction specialists to the transplant team.

CONCLUSIONS

Perioperative morbidity associated with acute abstinence syndromes can be prevented with proper preoperative treatment. It is therefore essential that surgical providers identify addiction disorders and ensure that they are effectively managed during the perioperative period. Because of the high prevalence of polydrug abuse, patients who acknowledge an addiction to one substance should be carefully screened regarding their use of other substances. If possible, elective surgery should be postponed to allow time for complete detoxification. Management of patients with addiction disorders going for surgery often requires consultation with addiction and pain specialists. All patients with active addiction should be encouraged to engage in addiction treatment postoperatively.

CHAPTER

83

Summary Author: Ashok Krishnamurthy
R. Jeffrey Goldsmith • Richard K. Ries • Christine Youdelis-Flores

Substance-Induced Mental Disorders

PREVALENCE OF SUBSTANCE-INDUCED PSYCHIATRIC DISORDERS

Prevalence of Substance-Induced Mood and Anxiety Disorders

Prevalence rates of substance-induced psychiatric disorders vary considerably depending on the study subjects (treatment-seeking populations vs. epidemiologic surveys) and the research diagnostic criteria used to define the disorders.

It can be very difficult to differentiate between substance-induced and independent depressive disorders and the diagnosis may change if the patient is followed over time.

Several studies have reported high rates of anxiety symptoms among alcoholics in withdrawal, with 80% of alcohol-dependent male subjects experiencing repeated panic attacks during alcohol withdrawal.

Prevalence of Substance-Induced Psychotic Disorders

The prevalence of substance-induced disorders varies across studies undertaken, from 53% reporting transient cocaine-induced psychosis in one study to 13% that had psychotic symptoms and 23% experiencing clinically significant psychotic symptoms in the past year in another.

In studies conducted in Japan, chronic intravenous methamphetamine use is associated with increased rates of prolonged psychosis persisting for several months to over 2 years after abstinence that closely resembles paranoid schizophrenia.

Substance-Associated Suicidal Behavior

For many individuals with substance dependence, one of their biggest fears is that the dysphoria and hopelessness that frequently accompany their substance use (and substance use withdrawal) will never improve. Patients can be reassured, however, that existing evidence suggests that substance-induced depression tends to improve far more quickly than many other forms of depression. Although substance-induced depression tends to dissipate rapidly, it can be as dangerous as major depressive disorder in terms of the risk of suicide and self-injurious behavior. When completed suicides are investigated, the rate of comorbidity is high.

Among schizophrenics, however, it was found in one study that it was the severity of the depression, not the substance abuse, that explained suicidal behavior.

SPECIFIC SUBSTANCES: SUBSTANCE-INDUCED SYMPTOMS

Caffeine

Caffeine is the most commonly used addictive substance.

The effects of **caffeine** include the induction of anxiety with consumption of "large amounts"; however, the range of **caffeine** doses that can induce anxiety is considerable. **Caffeine** can increase the frequency of panic attacks in those individuals who are physiologically predisposed to them.

Nicotine

Nicotine is the deadliest psychoactive drug and the third most popular in the United States, with about 25% of the adult population smoking cigarettes, about 5% using smokeless tobacco, and about 5% smoking pipes and cigars.

Nicotine-dependent patients experience more depression than nonusers and that some use nicotine to regulate mood.

Alcohol

Although light consumption of alcohol is associated with a slight euphoria or "buzz," *moderate to heavy consumption may be associated with depression, suicidal feelings, or violent behavior in some individuals.*

In those who are physiologically dependent, one usually sees a hyperadrenergic state that is characterized by

- Agitation
- Anxiety
- Tremor
- Malaise
- Hyperreflexia
- Mild tachycardia
- Increasing blood pressure
- Sweating, insomnia
- Nausea or vomiting
- Perceptual distortions

A few chronic heavy drinkers experience hallucinations, delusions, and anxiety during acute withdrawal, and some have grand mal seizures.

Sedatives

Sedatives are able to induce depression, anxiety, and even a psychotic-like state with prolonged use and dependence.

Withdrawal symptoms include mood instability with anxiety or depression, sleep disturbance, autonomic hyperactivity, tremor, nausea or vomiting, transient hallucinations or illusions, and grand mal seizures.

A protracted withdrawal syndrome has been reported to include anxiety, depression, paresthesias, perceptual distortions, muscle pain and twitching, tinnitus, dizziness, headache, derealization and depersonalization, and impaired concentration.

These symptoms can last for weeks, and some (such as anxiety, depression, tinnitus, and paresthesias) have been reported for a year or more after withdrawal.

Cocaine and Amphetamines

Individuals occasionally become paranoid and even delusional after prolonged heavy use of cocaine or amphetamine.

Unlike other psychotic states, the patient experiencing a paranoid state induced by cocaine has intact abstract reasoning and linear thinking, whereas the delusions, if analyzed, are poorly developed delusions of a nonbizarre nature.

If abstinence is maintained for several weeks, many stimulant addicts report a dysphoric state that is prominently marked by anhedonia and/or anxiety, but which does not meet the symptom severity criteria to qualify as a *DSM-IV* disorder.

This anhedonic state can persist for weeks.

Metamphetamine

Studies in Japan report that chronic and heavy methamphetamine users, particularly those who use intravenously, have an increased rate of psychosis and depression lasting several months or more that closely resembles paranoid schizophrenia.

Methylenedioxyamphetamine (MDMA)

Chronic MDMA users may develop more severe longer term problems such as dysphoric states and cognitive impairments in memory, concentration, and executive functioning, which are thought to be due to serotonergic neurotoxicity.

Opiates

If opiates are used for a long period, moderate to severe depression is common.

In withdrawal, some opiate addicts are acutely anxious and agitated, whereas others report depression and anhedonia. Anxiety, depression, and sleep disturbance, in a milder form, can persist for weeks as a protracted withdrawal syndrome.

Hallucinogens

Tetrahydrocannabinol, lysergic acid diethylamide (LSD), mescaline, and dimethyltryptamine produce visual distortions and frank hallucinations.

All hallucinogens are associated with drug-induced panic reactions that feature panic, paranoia, and even delusional states in addition to the hallucinations.

A cannabis withdrawal syndrome is described that is generally mild and consists of anxiety, irritability, physical tension, depressed mood, decreased appetite, restlessness, and craving.

Recent literature has emerged that early use of cannabis is a risk factor for the development of psychotic symptoms later in life.

A few hallucinogen users experience chronic reactions, involving

1. Prolonged psychotic reactions
2. Depression, which can be life threatening
3. Flashbacks
4. Exacerbations of preexisting psychiatric illnesses

PCP

PCP is known for its dissociative and delusional properties. It also is associated with violent behavior and amnesia of the intoxication.

Users who once exhibit an acute psychotic state with PCP are more likely to develop another with repeated use.

Differential Diagnosis and Treatment

Diagnosing and treating a substance-induced mental disorder is very much dependent on the attitude and training of the clinician.

1. Is he or she attuned to the prevalence of alcohol and drug use? Without this awareness, there is less inclination to search for the problem.
2. Does the clinician think that it is relevant to the current problem to take the time to elicit an alcohol and drug use history?
3. Has the clinician received adequate training to counteract the therapeutic nihilism acquired during medical school and residency training?
4. Is he or she adversely affected by the distortions and denial that are exhibited by many alcoholics and drug addicts?
5. Does the clinician routinely seek corroboration of an alcohol and drug use history from family or friends of the patient?
6. Will the clinician order a drug screen?

   A. Making the diagnosis of a substance use disorder is the first step in the differential diagnosis and treatment of a substance-related problem.
   B. In the second step, the substance-induced symptoms must be differentiated from the symptoms of major psychiatric disorders.
   C. Finally, the substance-induced disorders must be differentiated from the dual disorders: substance abuse or dependence combined with a comorbid, nonsubstance Axis I disorder.

The *DSM-IV* contains five criteria for substance-induced mood disorders:

1. A prominent and persistent disturbance in mood predominates, characterized by (a) a depressed mood or markedly diminished interest or pleasure in activities; or (b) an elevated, expansive, or irritable mood.
2. There is evidence from the history, physical examination, or laboratory findings that the symptoms developed during or within a month after substance intoxication or withdrawal, or medication use are etiologically related to the mood disturbance.
3. The disturbance is not better explained by a mood disorder.
4. The disturbance did not occur exclusively during a delirium.
5. The symptoms cause clinically significant distress or impairment.

In making the diagnosis of substance use disorder, it is helpful to order a drug screen. Even if the results come back hours after the clinical decision is made, they can be used to confirm the presence of a substance despite the patient's denial.

Such a screen also can clarify the history in some future episode. Sometimes, addicts report part of their history, but not all. For example, it may be useful to know that a depressed patient used both alcohol and cocaine.

Although either substance can induce symptoms of anxiety (or depression), a slightly different treatment plan may be necessary for a patient dependent on both.

Mood Disorders

Establishing whether there is a relationship between the use of psychoactive substances and the symptoms prominent at the moment is a crucial step.

Chronic use of alcohol, sedatives, and opiates can cause depressed mood, as can withdrawal from stimulants and sedatives.

Exploring the mood during periods of sustained abstinence from all depressant drugs is critical.

Anxiety Disorders

For the substance-induced anxiety disorders, the criteria are almost identical to substance-induced mood disorders. However, the first is different: prominent anxiety, panic attacks, obsessions, or compulsions predominate.

CHAPTER **84**

Summary Author: Ashok Krishnamurthy
Edward V. Nunes • Roger D. Weiss

Co-Occurring Addiction and Affective Disorders

OVERVIEW

Significance

Depressive disorders, major depression, and dysthymia are among the most common psychiatric disorders in the general population. Estimates from community surveys show that >10% of the general population has experienced a depressive disorder at some point in their lifetime.

Major depression is the most common co-occurring psychiatric disorder encountered among patients presenting for treatment for substance use disorders, with lifetime prevalence rates ranging from 15% to 50% across samples studied from various treatment settings.

Among drug- and alcohol-dependent patients, *major depression has been associated with worse outcome, including worse substance use outcome, worse psychiatric symptoms, and increased suicide risk.*

Clinical trials suggest that treatment of depression among substance-dependent patients with medication or behavioral therapy can improve outcome.

Bipolar disorder is less common than major depression among samples of patients seeking treatment for substance use disorders in routine outpatient settings. However, *the strength of association between bipolar disorders and substance use disorders is larger than for depressive disorders*, with the presence of a bipolar disorder *increasing the likelihood of a substance use disorder by a factor of 4 or more.*

Hence, among patients with bipolar disorder, the prevalence of substance use disorders is 40% or more.

Distinguishing Substance-Related Mood Symptoms from Mood Disorders

Mood symptoms (e.g., sadness, apathy, irritability, pessimism, hopelessness, fatigue, anxiety, insomnia, euphoria, hyperactivity) *are extremely common among patients with drug or alcohol use problems* (Table 84.1)

Often such symptoms are components of substance intoxication or withdrawal and will resolve with abstinence; in that case, the indicated treatment is aggressive treatment of the substance problem.

At other times, the mood symptoms are components of an independent mood disorder that needs to be treated in addition to treating the substance problems.

Abstinence or Initiation of Substance Abuse Treatment Improves Depression Initiation of treatment for the substance use problem and efforts to achieve abstinence should always be a first step in the treatment of patients with co-occurring mood and substance use disorders.

Some Cases of Depression Will Persist Despite Abstinence or Substance Abuse Treatment Despite abstinence or reductions in substance use, some cases of depression will persist.

Evidence suggests that a careful clinical history can distinguish mood disorders that are independent of substance use and will persist in abstinence from those that will resolve with abstinence.

Importance of the Clinical History The history should examine the course of mood symptoms in relation to substance use over the patient's lifetime, *looking particularly for onset of a mood disorder syndrome prior to the onset of substance problems*, or the *persistence or emergence of a mood disorder during abstinent periods over the lifetime.*

TABLE 84.1	Similarities and Differences between *DSM-IV* Intoxication or Withdrawal Symptoms and Symptoms of *DSM-IV* Mood Disorders		
	Intoxication or withdrawal symptoms that resemble major depression or dysthymia	Intoxication or withdrawal symptoms that resemble mania or hypomania	Intoxication or withdrawal symptoms that are distinct from symptoms of mood disorder
Alcohol or sedatives	Intoxication: mood lability	Intoxication: inappropriate sexual or aggressive behavior, mood lability, impaired judgment, impaired functioning, impaired attention	Intoxication: slurred speech, incoordination, unsteady gait, nystagmus, impaired memory, stupor, coma
	Withdrawal: anxiety, insomnia	Withdrawal: insomnia, agitation, auditory hallucinations	Withdrawal: autonomic hyperactivity (e.g., sweating, increased pulse, blood pressure, temperature), tremor, nausea/vomiting, visual or tactile hallucinations, seizures, delirium
Cocaine or amphetamines	Intoxication: anxiety, anger, psychomotor agitation or retardation, weight loss	Intoxication: euphoria, increased sociability, hypervigilance, anger, impaired judgment, impaired functioning, agitation, auditory hallucinations, paranoia	Intoxication: stereotyped behaviors, vital sign abnormalities, pupillary dilation, sweating or chills, nausea/vomiting, respiratory depression, cardiac symptoms (chest pain, arrhythmias), confusion, coma, dyskinesia, dystonia, seizures, visual or tactile hallucinations or illusions
	Withdrawal: dysphoria, fatigue, insomnia or hypersomnia, increased appetite, psychomotor agitation or retardation	Withdrawal: insomnia, agitation	Withdrawal: vivid unpleasant dreams
Cannabis	Intoxication: social withdrawal, anxiety, increased appetite	Intoxication: euphoria, impaired judgment	Intoxication: impaired coordination, conjunctival injection, tachycardia
	Withdrawal: depressed mood, irritability, anxiety, insomnia, decreased appetite, restlessness	Withdrawal: irritability, anger, increased aggression, insomnia	Withdrawal: strange dreams, headache, shakiness, sweating, stomach upset, nausea

(Continued)

TABLE 84.1	Similarities and Differences between *DSM-IV* Intoxication or Withdrawal Symptoms and Symptoms of *DSM-IV* Mood Disorders (*Continued*)		
	Intoxication or withdrawal symptoms that resemble major depression or dysthymia	Intoxication or withdrawal symptoms that resemble mania or hypomania	Intoxication or withdrawal symptoms that are distinct from symptoms of mood disorder
Opioids	Intoxication: apathy, dysphoria, psychomotor retardation	Intoxication: euphoria, agitation, impaired judgment or social functioning	Intoxication: pupillary constriction, slurred speech, drowsiness, respiratory depression, stupor, coma (pupillary dilation and other signs of anoxia)
	Withdrawal: dysphoria (irritability, anxiety), insomnia, fatigue	Withdrawal: irritability, insomnia	Withdrawal: nausea, vomiting, muscle aches, lacrimation, rhinorrhea, pupillary dilation, piloerection, sweating, diarrhea, yawning, fever
Hallucinogens	Intoxication: anxiety, depression, paranoia	Intoxication: euphoria, paranoia, impaired judgment or functioning	Intoxication: ideas of reference, fear of losing one's mind, perceptual changes (depersonalization, derealization, hallucinations, synesthesia), pupillary dilation, tachycardia, sweating, palpitations, tremors, blurred vision, incoordination
PCP	Intoxication:	Intoxication: belligerence, impulsiveness, agitation, impaired judgment or functioning	Intoxication: nystagmus, tachycardia, hypertension, decreased responsiveness to pain, unsteady gait, slurred speech, muscular rigidity, seizures, coma, hyperacusis
Nicotine	Withdrawal: dysphoria, insomnia, irritability, anxiety, difficulty concentrating, restlessness, increased appetite, weight gain	Withdrawal: irritability, impaired concentration, restlessness, insomnia	Withdrawal: bradycardia

Note: The table lists *DSM-IV* symptoms for intoxication or withdrawal from each of the main substance classes and shows where there is overlap with similar symptoms of *DSM-IV* depressive syndromes (major depression, dysthymia) in column 2 or bipolar syndromes (mania, hypomania) in column 3. Column 4 lists intoxication and withdrawal symptoms that are not consistent with mood disorder symptoms and would be helpful to distinguish substance effects from mood disorders.

PREVALENCE AND PROGNOSTIC EFFECTS OF CO-OCCURRING MOOD AND SUBSTANCE USE DISORDERS

General Population

Odds ratios are at least 2.0 for most combinations of disorders, showing that the presence of alcohol or drug dependence at least doubles the odds of a mood disorder, or other disorder, being present.

For bipolar disorder, the odds ratios are substantially larger than for major depression or dysthymia. Again, when depressive symptoms are present, it is very important to search the history carefully for past episodes of mania or hypomania, as *bipolar illness has a particularly strong association with substance use disorders* and it has specific treatment implications that differ from those for unipolar depression. *When evaluating a patient with bipolar illness, it is especially important to inquire about substance use problems, as they are likely to be present and to complicate the clinical course.*

Common anxiety disorders (social phobia, panic disorder with or without agoraphobia, and posttraumatic stress disorders) have substantial associations with substance use disorders of at least the same magnitude as major depression or dysthymia.

Their cardinal symptoms (fear of social interactions, spontaneous panic attacks and fear of public places, and reexperiencing symptoms triggered by reminders of traumatic events) are distinctive and not attributable to substance toxicity or withdrawal.

When a substance-dependent patient presents with depression, the history should include a detailed inquiry for each of these anxiety disorders. Their presence can be very useful in ruling out substance intoxication or withdrawal as the sole source of mood symptoms.

In a patient with chronic substance abuse, it is often difficult to establish in the history whether depressive symptoms are independent of substance use, as so many of those symptoms may be toxic or withdrawal effects of substances.

However, the presence of one of these anxiety disorders strongly suggests the presence of an independent disorder, warranting specific treatment.

Attention deficit hyperactivity disorder (ADHD) has strong associations with alcohol and drug dependence as well, with odds ratios of 2.8 and 7.9, respectively.

It is also strongly associated with major depression (odds ratio 2.7), dysthymia (odds ratio 7.5), and bipolar disorder (odds ratio 7.4).

Thus, in any patient with a substance use disorder and a mood disorder, a careful history for ADHD should be taken and direct treatment of ADHD considered if detected alongside treatment of the mood and substance use problems.

The differential diagnosis between early-onset bipolar disorder and ADHD is difficult and a matter of controversy owing to the substantial similarities between the clinical presentations of these disorders in childhood.

Substance Use Disorder Treatment Populations

Lifetime prevalence rates of major depression ranges from 20% to 50%, with rates of current major depression in the 10% to 20% range, substantially exceeding rates found in the general population.

Bipolar disorder is relatively uncommon in these samples, consistent with its low prevalence rate in the general population.

Thus, clinicians seeing patients in these typical addiction treatment settings should expect to see high rates on co-occurring depression and should remain alert for cases of bipolar disorder.

Depression symptom scales such as the Beck or Hamilton can be useful as screening tools, but these need to be followed up with a careful clinical history, establishing presence or absence of depressive disorder.

History of a depressive disorder is important information, as it indicates increased risk for depression in the future, *but it is current major depression that is most clearly associated with worse outcome among substance-dependent patients and should be attended to in the treatment plan*: chronic low-grade depression, and depression that persists after initiation of treatment for the substance problem also warrants clinical attention.

Psychiatric and Primary Care Populations

Among patients presenting in psychiatric and primary care treatment settings for treatment of depression, the prevalence of substance use disorders depends upon the setting and associated severity of the mood disorder.

Among psychiatric inpatients, a more severely ill group, substance use disorders are common among both patients with major depression and bipolar disorder.

Among patients in treatment for bipolar disorder, substance use disorders are common, with rates of current substance use disorders of 30% or more.

The co-occurrence of mood and substance use disorders may be especially common among patients with serious co-occurring medical disorders such as HIV.

The majority of individuals with substance use disorders, depression, and other common mental disorders do not present at specialty treatment settings such as substance abuse treatment programs or even psychiatric clinics.

Instead, they often present at the offices of primary care physicians, where substance abuse and depression are likely to go undetected and may be associated with over- or underutilization of services and poor outcome.

Patients may be unaware of these problems or may avoid discussing them with health care providers because of the considerable stigma attached to the idea of having such a problem or of seeking treatment at an addiction program or a psychiatrist's office.

DIFFERENTIAL DIAGNOSIS

Etiological Relationships between Mood and Substance Use Disorders

All mood symptoms are not caused by toxic and withdrawal effects of substances nor is all substance abuse caused by underlying psychopathology (as in "self-medication").

One must be cautious in formulating causal mechanisms between co-occurring disorders.

For any given patient, it may be difficult to prove which of several causal mechanisms may be operating. (See Table 84.2.)

TABLE 84.2	Summary of Possible Etiological Relationships between Co-Occurring Affective Symptoms/Syndromes and Substance Use Disorders	
Relationship	**Mechanism**	**Clinical presentation and implications**
Substance abuse causes affective symptoms.	Substance intoxication, withdrawal, or biologic effects of chronic substance use	Substance use disorder is chronologically primary; mood symptoms resolve with abstinence or reduced substance use; treatment focuses on substance abuse.
Substance abuse causes affective syndrome, which then takes on a life of its own.	Stress and loss (e.g., relationships, jobs) engendered by substance abuse promote depression; biologic effects of chronic substance exposure trigger a vulnerability to affective disorder.	Affective syndrome is chronologically secondary but persists after abstinence; treat both affective and substance use disorders.
Affective syndrome causes substance abuse.	Self-medication (taking substances to relieve symptoms of affective disorder—e.g., low mood, low energy, poor sleep in depression; lack of sleep, excessive energy in mania or hypomania)	Affective syndrome is chronologically primary or emerges during abstinence, preceding relapse; pure self-medication—where self-medication is the only mechanism operating, and treatment can focus exclusively on the affective disorder—is relatively rare.
Substance abuse is part of a pattern of increased activity and impulsivity in mania or hypomania.	Impulsivity, seeking out new experiences	Substance abuse is chronologically secondary, beginning during episodes of mania or hypomania, and resolves with return to euthymia or depression; treatment can focus on bipolar disorder, but as with pure self-medication, this may be relatively rare.

(Continued)

TABLE 84.2   Summary of Possible Etiological Relationships between Co-Occurring Affective Symptoms/Syndromes and Substance Use Disorders (*Continued*)

Relationship	Mechanism	Clinical presentation and implications
Affective syndrome causes substance abuse, which then takes on a life of its own.	Exposure to substances during an episode of affective disorder triggers a vulnerability to substance dependence.	Substance abuse is chronologically secondary but persists after mood disorder is treated; treat both disorders.
Independent disorders	Both affective and substance use disorders are common in the general population and will co-occur by chance.	Any chronological pattern; each disorder persists during remissions of the other; treat both disorders.
Affective and substance use disorders stem from common underlying risk factors.	Common genetic factors, stress, trauma	Any chronological pattern; both disorders need to be treated; reduction of stress may help both.
Affective symptoms and substance use become related over time.	Moods become a conditioned cue triggering substance abuse.	Substance use disorder may be chronologically primary, but moods (e.g., sadness, anger) trigger episodes of substance use or cravings; management of unpleasant moods becomes important part of therapy.
Co-occurrence worsens prognosis.	Presence of multiple disorders interferes with coping or treatment seeking.	Any chronologic pattern; each disorder needs specific treatment.
Affective symptoms/syndrome may prompt treatment seeking for substance problems.	Affective symptoms (sad mood, trouble sleeping, functional impairment) engender motivation.	Any chronological pattern; focus on treatment of substance use, but affective disorder may need to be treated if it persists.

DSM-IV Independent and Substance-Induced Mood Disorders

Independent Mood Disorder   Also referred to in the literature as "primary," *DSM-IV* defines an independent mood disorder as *one that precedes the onset of substance abuse or persists during significant periods of abstinence* (1 month or more is suggested as the minimum).

The historical data needed to establish these criteria (ages at onset, presence of periods of abstinence, and mood syndromes occurring during abstinent periods) can be determined with good reliability from a clinical history.

Substance-Induced Mood Disorder   Substance-induced mood disorder was established to recognize the phenomenon of co-occurring mood syndromes *that cannot be established as chronologically independent of substance use, yet the mood symptoms seem to exceed what would be expected from mere intoxication or withdrawal effects from the substance(s) the patient is taking.*

Usual Effects of Substances

DSM-IV clearly specifies that the symptoms of either an independent or a substance-induced mood disorder must exceed the expected effects of intoxication or withdrawal from the substances the patient is taking, leaving this as the default category when substances are involved. These are the predominant symptoms expected when using the substances on their own.

Diagnostic Methods and Predictive Validity of *DSM-IV* Approach

The PRISM is a semistructured interview that was designed *specifically to evaluate mood and other co-occurring psychiatric disorders in the setting of substance use disorders.*

PRISM provides more specific criteria for substance-induced mood disorder and its distinction from an independent mood disorder on the one hand or usual effects of substances on the other.

To make a diagnosis of substance-induced mood disorder, PRISM requires full criteria for a mood disorder (e.g., major depression, or dysthymia) to be met *and that each symptom contributing to the diagnosis (e.g., insomnia, loss of appetite, low energy) exceeds the expected effects of the substances that the patients are taking.*

Thus, PRISM establishes criteria for substance-induced mood disorder that are more specific and stringent than those required by the letter of *DSM-IV.*

Diagnosing Bipolar Disorder in the Setting of Substance Abuse

Intoxication with cocaine or other stimulants may resemble mania in regard to grandiosity, hyperactivity, talkativeness, impulsivity, insomnia, and paranoia.

The impulsivity of alcohol or sedative intoxication may sometimes also resemble that of mania.

However, *full-blown mania must last for at least a week*, during which the symptoms should be persistent, whereas symptoms of intoxication are usually intermittent. Further, the marked impairment or psychosis required for mania is usually well in excess of what would be produced by intoxication. For example, cocaine intoxication may produce paranoia that lasts for a few hours and resolves during the crash period, whereas the psychosis characteristic of mania, often either paranoid or grandiose, is persistent.

Hence, in establishing a diagnosis of mania, persistence of symptoms over time and severity of impairment are key markers as well as occurrence of the symptoms during clear periods of abstinence.

Frank mania is distinctive, despite ongoing substance use.

Hypomania, which involves the same core symptoms as mania but may be briefer (at least 4 days) and with less impairment in functioning, may be more difficult to distinguish from substance intoxication or withdrawal effects.

The same may be true of cyclothymia, which may be difficult to distinguish from alternating periods of intoxication and withdrawal, mimicking hypomanic and depressive symptoms, respectively.

Rapid cycling bipolar disorder is diagnosed when there have been at least four mood episodes over the past 12 months, punctuated either by periods of remission or by switches in polarity.

Twenty percent of cases of bipolar disorder are rapid cycling—the pattern is associated with greater impairment and poorer response to treatment.

Some evidence suggests that the rapid cycling subtype is associated with increased prevalence of substance use disorders.

It is important to establish in the history that hypomanic or manic syndromes have persisted over days or weeks before switching to depression as well as seeking to establish occurrence of the symptoms during periods of abstinence.

Substance intoxication is likely to exacerbate the disinhibition and poor judgment associated with mania and is associated with poor medication adherence—this promotes relapse. *Thus, patients who present to emergency departments or other acute psychiatric settings with worsening mania are likely to also have substance abuse in the clinical picture.*

However, for most patients with bipolar disorder, particularly those who have had the disorder for an extended period of time, the clinical course predominantly consists of depression, with occasional episodes of mania or hypomania. *Thus, in a depressed patient with substance abuse, it is important to carefully review the past history for episodes of mania or hypomania that would indicate that the diagnosis is bipolar disorder.*

In patients with chronic substance abuse, in whom it is difficult to establish the presence of independent mood symptoms, *clear-cut episodes of mania or hypomania, because they are distinctive from the usual effects of substances,* are valuable in establishing that an independent mood disorder is indeed present and is in need of treatment.

MANAGEMENT OF CO-OCCURRING MOOD AND SUBSTANCE USE DISORDERS

Depressive Disorders

Antidepressant Medication

Effect on Outcome of Depression Antidepressant medication has been the most thoroughly studied treatment modality for co-occurring mood disorders with numerous placebo controlled trials in the literature.

Two meta-analyses reached similar conclusions that antidepressant medication is more effective than placebo in improving outcome among alcohol-dependent patients with depressive disorders, with the evidence less clear among cocaine- or opioid-dependent patients.

Effects of Antidepressant Medication on Substance Use Outcome Treatment of a co-occurring depression with antidepressant medication is helpful in reducing substance abuse when the depression improves, but it is not a stand-alone treatment and cannot be expected to resolve substance problems by itself; concurrent treatment for the substance use disorder (counseling or medication) is also indicated.

Placebo Response Low placebo response rate was the strongest moderator of medication effect, accounting for approximately 70% of the variance in effect sizes across studies.

Studies with low placebo response rates (in the 20%–30% range) showed large medication versus placebo differences.

In contrast, about half the studies had high placebo response rates in the 40% to 60% range.

High placebo response is a well-known effect in studies of treatment of depression.

In the studies of antidepressant treatment of depressed substance abusers, placebo response is particularly meaningful, as it suggests *some patients respond to the background treatment they receive*, which in most of these trials involved some form of treatment for the substance use disorder.

This is part of what underlies our recommendation that *treatment of the substance use disorder is a first priority in the management of patients with co-occurring depression and substance abuse.*

Treatment of the substance use disorder may, in many cases, result in improvement in both substance abuse and depression.

Antidepressant Response in Alcohol-Dependent Versus Cocaine- or Opioid-Dependent Samples There is greater evidence for efficacy of antidepressant medications among depressed alcoholics than among drug-dependent patients.

Among studies of the treatment of depression among cocaine- or opioid-dependent patients, there was more heterogeneity of effect across the studies, meaning that there were some studies demonstrating benefits of antidepressants among depressed cocaine- or opioid-dependent patients and other studies showing little or no effect.

The treatment of depressed cocaine-dependent patients has been studied least.

Diagnosis of Depression During a Period of Initial Abstinence An effort should be made to help patients initiate abstinence and observe the response of the depression during early abstinence, prior to initiating antidepressant medication.

Depression that persists during an initial period of abstinence would be consistent with what *DSM-IV* would call an independent major depression.

Another clinical implication stems from the high level of severity of depression in the inpatient samples and suggests that the greater the severity of the depression, the more consideration should be given to treatment with antidepressant medication from the outset.

For example, a patient with a clear history of independent major depression with suicide attempts, who presents with suicidal ideation, should be considered for initiation of antidepressant medication without delay.

Class of Antidepressant Medication SSRIs have the advantage of being generally well tolerated, with less potential for sedation or other adverse effects.

TCAs generate a number of concerns including risks of sedation, overdose, and seizures.

Recommend SSRIs as the first-line treatment and move to a non-SSRI antidepressant, such as **venlafaxine**, **duloxetine**, **mirtazapine**, or **bupropion**, if the SSRI trial fails.

The exception might be a patient with early-onset substance use and prominent externalizing symptoms or antisocial personality features for whom the data suggest caution in the use of SSRIs.

Concurrent Psychosocial Intervention These interventions generally have components that focus on managing mood symptoms and thus may have inherent antidepressant effects. Also, the focus of the interventions on substance use disorders may result in reduced substance use, which in turn improves mood.

It is very important that the initiation of treatment for the substance use disorder is the first step with any patient with co-occurring substance use disorder and depression.

Behavioral Treatments for Depression and Substance Abuse
There are fewer controlled studies of psychosocial treatments for depression, compared to control treatments, among substance-dependent patients with depression.

Several studies that have suggested addition of cognitive-behavioral therapy (CBT) for depression to smoking cessation treatment improved smoking outcome among patients with histories of major depression or greater severity of depression symptoms.

A controlled trial among cocaine-dependent patients found that voucher incentives plus the CRA was superior to a control group that received only voucher incentives, in terms of not only improving cocaine use outcome but also reducing depressive symptoms.

In summary, these studies, while in some cases small and preliminary, *support the effectiveness of behavioral therapies among depressed, substance-dependent patients.*

Medication Treatments for Substance Use Disorders Depressive symptoms decrease substantially during the first 1 to 2 weeks of **methadone** maintenance treatment for opioid dependence, and about half of major depressive syndromes in patients presenting for **methadone** maintenance can be expected to resolve during those initial weeks of treatment.

Naltrexone and **disulfiram** were both shown to be safe and effective among alcohol-dependent patients with co-occurring psychiatric disorders, including major depression.

The treatment effect is likely attributable to reduction in substance use, which in turn reduces substance-induced depressive symptoms, which reduces patient stress and anxiety, leading to an improvement in functioning.

Adolescents and Treatment of Co-Occurring Depression and Substance Abuse Effective intervention early in the course of these disorders has the potential to improve functioning during adolescence and prevent progression to chronic mood and substance use problems during adulthood.

Treatment research on mood and substance use disorders in adolescents lags behind research in adults in part owing to the greater difficulties conducting research in adolescents.

Late Life and Treatment of Co-Occurring Depression and Substance Abuse The pattern of substances abused may differ, with more alcohol and prescription drugs problems among the elderly, again, often undiagnosed and untreated.

Importantly, identification and effective treatment of depression (either with pharmacotherapy or behavioral therapy) may improve sleep, pain tolerance, and general functioning and in that instance could be expected to reduce the need for other prescription medications.

Alcohol intake at treatment outset does not interfere with the treatment of depression and that depression and drinking outcome tend to be correlated.

Suicidal Behavior and Co-Occurring Depression/Substance Abuse Depression and substance abuse are both important risk factors for suicide, and thus, the potential for suicide needs to be carefully assessed in any patient presenting with this combination of disorders.

Recent evidence suggests that both *DSM-IV* independent and substance-induced depression are associated with increased suicidal thinking and behavior among drug- and alcohol-dependent patients.

Other common risk factors for suicide are

- Family history of suicide
- History of trauma
- History of irritability or violence
- Current support systems
- Physical illness

A general consensus, based on recent data, is that the benefits of antidepressant treatment (in terms of improved symptoms) outweigh the risks, *although exacerbations of suicidal thinking or behavior may occur,* and patients should *be informed and closely monitored.*

Interventions at the Level of Service Delivery and Primary Care Most patients with depression, substance use problems, or both present not to specialty clinics or practitioners but rather to primary care physicians and settings such as emergency rooms or primary care clinics.

Depression and the Treatment of Nicotine Dependence The prevalence of nicotine dependence is increased among patients with mood disorders and is very high among patients with substance use disorders.

In regard to clinical recommendations, available evidence suggests that patients in treatment for substance use disorders are interested in attempting to quit smoking and that treatment with nicotine patch and counseling is modestly effective.

Depressed patients, with or without concurrent substance use disorders, should be assessed for smoking, encouraged to make a quit attempt, and assisted in the quit attempt with pharmacotherapy and counseling.

Patients should be carefully monitored for the emergence of depression, or worsening of depression symptoms, during quit attempts and particularly if the quit attempt is successful.

Summary of Treatment Recommendations for Co-Occurring Depression and Substance Use Disorder

1. Treat the substance use disorder
2. Evaluate the mood symptoms

All patients presenting for treatment of substance use disorders should receive a brief screening for depression. Patients who screen positive should receive a thorough psychiatric evaluation, according to the *DSM-IV*.
The diagnostic evaluation should also carefully probe for evidence of bipolar disorder.
The diagnostic evaluation should also assess the severity of depression, including suicide risk, as this will influence the urgency with which treatment of depression is initiated.

3. Treat the depressive disorder
Recommend SSRI antidepressants as the first line of treatment: good tolerability, evidence of efficacy
Practitioners should monitor closely for lack of effect or clinical worsening and be prepared to switch away from an SSRI to an antidepressant with a different mechanism of action.

Bipolar Disorder

Pharmacological Treatments

Overview of Medication Treatment for Bipolar Illness *Pharmacologic treatment is the mainstay of the treatment of bipolar disorder.*

Substance abuse often accompanies acute mania or hypomania, and brief hospitalization can be invaluable in the beginning to bring this under control as well, establishing initial abstinence and evaluating the extent to which manic symptoms are reflective of substance intoxication.

Substance abuse is more likely to occur in manic or hypomanic episodes than in depressive phases of bipolar illness.

There is little evidence regarding the use of medications for targeted treatment of substance use disorders among patients with bipolar illness.

However, as a general principle, if a medication is indicated (e.g., **methadone** or **buprenorphine** for opioid dependence, or **naltrexone** for alcohol dependence), it should be initiated with careful monitoring.

In most cases of bipolar disorder, *depression is the predominant mood disturbance*, with mania or hypomania occurring less frequently.

Medication Treatments for Co-Occurring Bipolar and Substance Use Disorders Appropriate pharmacological treatment of a carefully diagnosed co-occurring *DSM-IV*–independent mood disorder improves outcome of both mood and substance use symptoms.

Studies support the efficacy of mood stabilizers both for improving mood and reducing substance use, and one study looked at and found that mood and substance use improvement were correlated.

Medications for Substance Dependence New onset hypomania has been observed in an opioid-dependent patient after detoxification and induction onto naltrexone.

This suggests that clinicians should carefully monitor patients with co-occurring bipolar and alcohol use disorders for side effects or clinical worsening when using naltrexone.

Behavioral Treatments

Behavioral Treatment Approaches to Bipolar Disorder The goals of behavioral and psychosocial treatment for bipolar disorder include

1. Maintaining a treatment alliance and continuity of care
2. Securing adherence to medication treatment
3. Coping with symptoms and addressing stressors/other circumstances that lead to symptomatic exacerbations

Bipolar disorder generally runs a chronic, if waxing and waning, course, and maintaining continuity of care is an essential challenge.

Poor adherence to medications is a frequent cause of relapse and poor outcome in bipolar disorder.

Several specific behavioral/psychosocial treatments for bipolar disorder have been developed and have shown evidence of efficacy, including psychoeducation, CBT, interpersonal social rhythm therapy, and family focused therapy.

Behavioral Treatment Approaches to Co-Occurring Bipolar and Substance Use Disorders Integrated group therapy (IGT) is the first group-based behavioral approach developed specifically for patients with both bipolar disorder and substance use disorders and has been shown to be effective in reducing substance use.

IGT is a manually guided group treatment designed to serve as an adjunct to pharmacotherapy for bipolar disorder.

Founded on cognitive-behavioral principles and focused on relapse prevention, IGT incorporates aspects of the earlier reviewed behavioral treatments for bipolar disorder while addressing the unique interrelationships between bipolar disorder and substance use disorders.

The core principles of IGT include similar patterns of thought and behavior promote relapse to both mood episodes and substance use disorders.

As IGT is designed as an adjunctive treatment, it can be incorporated into a range of practice settings including either substance abuse treatment programs or psychiatric clinics serving bipolar patients or office-based practice.

Summary of Treatment Recommendations for Co-Occurring Bipolar Disorder and Substance Use Disorders
Evidence on behavioral or services interventions suggests the importance of approaching the treatment of combined bipolar and substance use disorders simultaneously in an integrated fashion.

The available evidence on use of mood stabilizers and neuroleptic medications among patients with combined bipolar and substance use disorders suggests these medications are effective in improving both bipolar symptoms and substance use outcome.

When the diagnostic assessment suggests a bipolar spectrum disorder (e.g., cyclothymia or subthreshold bipolar disorder), the differential diagnosis between an independent bipolar disorder and a substance-induced mood disorder may be less clear.

This differential is more difficult if the mood swings are less severe, of shorter duration, and consonant with intoxication or withdrawal symptoms of the substances the patient is abusing.

In this instance, aggressive treatment of the substance use disorder, combined with careful monitoring of the mood symptoms, may be warranted.

Summary Author: Ashok Krishnamurthy
Angela E. Waldrop • Karen J. Hartwell • Kathleen T. Brady

Co-Occurring Addiction and Anxiety Disorders

PREVALENCE

General Population

A number of epidemiologic studies conducted in the United States over the past 20 years have concluded that anxiety disorders and substance use disorders (SUDs) co-occur more commonly than would be expected by chance alone.

Addiction and Psychiatric Treatment Populations

Because the relationship between anxiety and SUDs is fraught with symptom overlap and diagnostic difficulties, estimates of co-occurring disorders in treatment settings are variable and dependent on diagnostic techniques used and specific disorder being assessed.

Primary Care Population

Recognition of anxiety is poor with only 23% of anxiety patients recognized within primary care as compared to 56% of depression cases.

SUDs are also common in primary care settings with estimates that 15% to 20% of men and 5% to 10% of women seen in primary care clinics have problem drinking or an alcohol use disorder (AUD). The prevalence of primary care practice patients with lifetime use of illicit drugs of more than five times was 20%, which is higher than national average.

Prescription drug misuse and abuse are also common problems in primary care settings.

Substances of abuse have profound effects on neurotransmitter systems involved in the pathophysiology of anxiety disorders and, with chronic use, may unmask a vulnerability or lead to organic changes that manifest as an anxiety disorder.

The best way to differentiate substance-induced, transient symptoms of anxiety from anxiety disorders that warrant treatment is through observation of symptoms during a period of abstinence.

Long half-life drugs (e.g., some benzodiazepines, **methadone**) may require several weeks of abstinence for withdrawal symptoms to subside, but shorter acting substances (e.g., alcohol, cocaine, short half-life benzodiazepines) require shorter periods of abstinence to make valid diagnoses.

A family history of anxiety disorder, the onset of anxiety symptoms before the onset of SUD, and sustained anxiety symptoms during lengthy periods of abstinence all suggest an independent anxiety disorder.

GENERAL TREATMENT CONSIDERATIONS

Among psychosocial treatments, cognitive-behavioral therapies are among the most effective for both anxiety disorders and SUDs.

In cases where the relationship of psychiatric symptoms and substance use is unclear, the risk/benefit ratio of using medications must be carefully considered.

Despite their effectiveness in immediate relief of panic and other anxiety symptoms, *benzodiazepine use is generally avoided in substance-using populations because of their abuse potential.*

Benzodiazepines may be considered as adjunctive medication during the early treatment phase when activation or latency of onset of the antidepressants is an issue.

If a benzodiazepine is prescribed to a patient with a co-occurring SUD, close monitoring for relapse and limited amounts of medication should be given.

As a rule, *benzodiazepines should be avoided in patients with a current SUD and used with caution in those with a history of substance use.*

If necessary, a benzodiazepine with a low abuse potential such as **oxazepam** and **chlordiazepoxide** may be considered.

ALCOHOL AND ANXIETY

The short-term relief of anxiety from alcohol use in combination with long-term anxiety induction from chronic drinking and withdrawal can initiate a feed-forward cycle of increasing anxiety symptoms and alcohol consumption.

Generalized Anxiety Disorder (GAD)

In adolescents, the presence of GAD is associated with a more rapid progression from age of first drink to alcohol dependence.

GAD follows a chronic course with low rates of remission and frequent relapses/recurrences. Comorbid SUD decreases the likelihood of recovery from GAD and increases the risk of exacerbation.

Differential Diagnosis GAD symptoms have considerable overlap with acute intoxication from stimulants and withdrawal from alcohol, opiates, sedative, and hypnotic drugs.

The *DSM-IV* diagnostic criteria of GAD require a 6-month duration of symptoms not directly related to the physiologic effects of a substance; however, many substance abusers will have difficulty maintaining abstinence for 6 months, so earlier diagnosis could be important to successful recovery. Careful history taking can establish the timing of GAD relative to the SUD.

Treatment There is little evidence-based research to direct treatment decisions for individuals with GAD and comorbid SUDs.

Benzodiazepines should be used with caution in this population and *never as a first-line agent.*

Psychosocial treatments are efficacious in the treatment of GAD. Cognitive-behavioral therapy (CBT) has been most often used in combination with SUD treatment with goals of managing anxious states without medications.

Social Anxiety Disorder (SAD)

Approximately 20% of individuals with SAD also suffer from an AUD.

Differential Diagnosis Symptoms of social anxiety typically precede the onset of SUDs.

Treatment Current treatment recommendations for SAD include selective serotonin reuptake inhibitors (SSRIs) or β-blockers in combination with integrated psychosocial treatment.

There are few studies examining the treatment options in comorbid populations.

Obsessive Compulsive Disorder (OCD)

The association of OCD and AUDs is less robust than for other anxiety disorders.

Differential Diagnosis Craving in SUDs has been compared to the intrusive recurrent thoughts that drive behavior in OCD, but thoughts and compulsions in individuals with SUDs are restricted to alcohol and drug use and easily distinguished from OCD.

Treatment There are no controlled studies of pharmacologic treatment of co-occurring OCD and SUDs.

First-line medications for OCD are **clomipramine, fluoxetine, fluvoxamine, paroxetine,** and **sertraline**. In individuals with SUDs, SSRIs are preferable to **clomipramine** because of more favorable side effect profiles.

Panic Disorder

Drug dependence was the most strongly associated SUD, although the lifetime risk of alcohol dependence was also elevated.

In a recent review of the literature, *the risk of panic disorder in the presence of AUDs was two to four times higher than in the absence of AUD.*

Differential Diagnosis Individuals with panic attacks may use alcohol to decrease panic symptoms and consequently develop an AUD.

Panic attacks early in recovery that decrease in frequency may respond to support and reassurance. However, if the panic attacks continue or increase over several weeks of abstinence, the diagnosis of panic disorder should be made.

Without treatment, the risk of relapse to alcohol use is increased.

Treatment The SSRIs **fluoxetine**, **sertraline**, **paroxetine**, and **fluvoxamine** have each demonstrated effectiveness in clinical trials and are the best choice for individuals with co-occurring panic disorder and SUD.

NICOTINE AND ANXIETY DISORDERS

The 12-month prevalence rate of nicotine dependence was 13% in the general population and 25% among individuals with anxiety disorders.

The risk of anxiety disorder among individuals with nicotine dependence *was more than twice that of any other psychiatric disorder.*

Conversely, the prevalence rates of nicotine dependence were also increased in individuals with anxiety disorders (panic disorder 40%, SAD 27%, and GAD 33%).

Differential Diagnosis

The anxiety and arousal associated with nicotine withdrawal can be distinguished from independent anxiety disorders by the time course.

Prospective research suggests that nicotine withdrawal symptoms typically return to baseline within 10 days and anxiety decreases within 4 weeks of quitting among smokers without comorbid psychiatric disorders.

Panic Disorders

Daily smoking is associated with an increased risk for the first occurrence of a panic attack or panic disorder and the risk is higher in active smokers than in past smokers.

Early smoking increases the risk for the development of panic disorder, and the initiation of smoking may precede the onset of panic disorder by many years (median 12 years).

Individuals with panic disorder who smoke regularly report more severe anxiety symptoms and social impairment as compared to nonsmokers.

SAD

Few studies have investigated the relationship between SAD and smoking.

GAD

Higher rates of smoking have been observed among individuals with GAD.

OCD

The prevalence of smoking is lower in individuals with OCD compared with other anxiety disorders.

Nicotine administration decreases some forms of compulsive behavior in both human and animal studies and obsessive thoughts can be reduced by transdermal nicotine in humans.

Treatment

Given the high prevalence rates of anxiety disorders among smokers, treatments aimed at the specific needs of this population need to be developed; however, there is little empiric evidence to guide treatment at present.

OPIATES AND ANXIETY DISORDERS

Among individuals with opiate use disorders (OUDs), lifetime prevalence of any anxiety disorder was 36.3% with a much higher rate in opioid dependence (61%) than opioid abuse.

Across studies, lifetime rates of SAD in individuals with OUDs have been reported between 3% and 39%.

The lifetime prevalence of panic disorder with agoraphobia, 5%, was lower compared with panic disorder without agoraphobia, 14%, in individuals with OUDs.

Differential Diagnosis

Few studies have investigated diagnostic issues at the interface of OUDs and anxiety disorders.

Treatment

No evidence-based literature exists to guide treatment of co-occurring anxiety and opioid use disorders; however, general treatment principles apply.

A comprehensive treatment plan is necessary to address the opioid use, anxiety, other comorbid SUDs, and chronic pain if present.

MARIJUANA AND ANXIETY DISORDERS

Marijuana is the most frequently used illicit drug in the United States.

The relationship between marijuana and anxiety remains unclear. Some studies suggest that marijuana use increases the long-term risk of anxiety; others find that marijuana use results in acute anxiety symptoms during intoxication only, and anxiety symptoms can develop as part of marijuana withdrawal.

Studies suggest that the use of marijuana as a coping strategy may serve to enhance anxiety through an avoidance-anxiety cycle and users who report coping motives for their use also use marijuana more often.

STIMULANTS AND ANXIETY DISORDERS

There is relatively little research on co-occurring anxiety disorders and cocaine, methamphetamine, and amphetamine use.

These agents stimulate noradrenergic systems and acute intoxication is often associated with anxiety.

Because of these anxiogenic effects, it has been postulated that individuals who are vulnerable to anxiety may be less likely to abuse or become dependent on this class of drugs.

Prevalence

Thirty-nine percent of individuals with amphetamine use disorders and thirty-one percent of those with cocaine use disorders reported lifetime anxiety disorders.

Of individuals with anxiety disorders, 4.8% reported lifetime amphetamine use disorder and 5.4% reported lifetime cocaine use disorder.

Studies of treatment-seeking individuals indicate that anxiety disorders are relatively less common in cocaine-dependent treatment-seeking patients as compared with alcohol- and other drug-dependent individuals.

Diagnosis

Cocaine has been reported to precipitate panic attacks in patients without previous panic disorder.

Stimulant withdrawal symptoms may also include low levels of anxiety in the first few days of abstinence, so a period of abstinence before diagnosing an anxiety disorder in stimulant abusers is recommended.

Treatment

There is a paucity of research focused on the treatment of co-occurring stimulant use and anxiety disorders.

Repeated cocaine administration is associated with neuronal sensitization leading to increased limbic excitability—thus, it has been hypothesized that this is the mechanism of cocaine-induced panic.

Panic disorder in patients with comorbid psychostimulant use may be linked to a sensitization mechanism and may respond particularly well to anticonvulsant medications. This hypothesis warrants further investigation.

There are a number of psychosocial treatments with demonstrated efficacy in the treatment of stimulant dependence including contingency management and CBT. Individuals with co-occurring disorders should be engaged in evidence-based psychosocial treatment for their stimulant use.

CHAPTER 86

Summary Author: Ashok Krishnamurthy
Douglas Ziedonis • Aurelia N. Bizamcer • Marc L. Steinberg • Stephen A. Wyatt
David A. Smelson • Adrienne D. Vaiana

Co-Occurring Addiction and Psychotic Disorders

PREVALENCE OF CO-OCCURRING ADDICTION AND PSYCHOSIS

General Population

Although addiction is common amongst patients with psychotic disorders in psychiatric treatment settings, schizophrenia has a low prevalence rate of about 1% in the general population.

Because of the low frequency of schizophrenia in the general population, large community-based epidemiologic surveys of substance abuse often exclude these disorders from their reports.

Forty-seven percent of persons with schizophrenia have a lifetime experience of substance use disorders, including thirty-four percent who have an alcohol use disorder and twenty-eight percent who have a drug use disorder, including sixteen percent abusing cocaine. Of note, about 70% and 90% of patients with schizophrenia are nicotine dependent and that nicotine is not routinely included in reported rates of substance use, making the actual numbers even higher.

Addiction Treatment Populations

Among patients in addiction treatment settings, a range of severity of psychotic symptoms can occur for vulnerable individuals with many substances—including alcohol, cocaine, amphetamine, club drugs, and marijuana.

For example, evidence suggests that chronic amphetamine use can result in long-term neurobiologic changes, which may persist even after prolonged abstinence and present as a protracted psychosis that is phenomenologically similar to schizophrenia.

Psychiatric Treatment Populations

Cannabis is increasingly linked to an earlier onset of schizophrenia and increased severity of positive symptoms among schizophrenic patients.

Some data suggest that the use of drugs or alcohol can lead to the earlier onset of schizophrenia in an already vulnerable individual.

The addition of drugs of abuse often increases and exacerbates psychotic symptoms in psychiatric patients. In this population, ingestion of even relatively small amounts of drug over a short period can result in

- An exacerbation of psychiatric problems
- Loss of housing
- Use of emergency department services
- Increased vulnerability to exploitation (sexual, physical, or other) within the social environment

Substance use has also been linked to emergence of medication resistance in populations of patients with schizophrenia.

Primary Care or Other Health Care Settings

Drug-induced exacerbation of psychotic disorders and transient substance-induced psychotic symptoms are not uncommon in the emergency room setting; however, these cases are far less common in general primary care practices.

DIFFERENTIAL DIAGNOSIS (TABLES 86.1 AND 86.2)

The type and duration of psychotic symptoms are important in making a differential diagnosis.

In clinical practice, patients are often seen with a mix of symptoms that may not fit neatly into a diagnostic category such as schizophrenia or manic depression.

Schizoaffective disorder is diagnosed when symptoms of a psychotic disorder and a mood disorder (depression, mania, or mixed states) occur during separate time periods.

In contrast to major depression with psychotic features, schizoaffective disorder features a period of psychotic symptoms in the absence of mood disorder symptoms.

For many reasons, differentiating schizophrenia from a substance-induced psychotic disorder is not an easy task, especially if the physician does not know whether the patient has a history of serious mental illness.

Medication side effects can be mistaken for negative symptoms, and negative symptoms can be mistaken for depression.

Substance abusers also may be poorly compliant in taking their medications, so that a presenting psychotic relapse may be the result of noncompliance.

MANAGEMENT OF CO-OCCURRING PSYCHOSIS AND SUBSTANCE ABUSE

Acute/Subacute

At the time of the patient's initial presentation for treatment, the clinician should have four primary goals: patient safety, staff safety, elicitation of the patient's history, and formulation of initial impressions that will lead to a set of treatment recommendations.

The most appropriate setting for the evaluation of an acutely psychotic patient is a hospital emergency department, although some psychiatric triage settings also are appropriate.

Patient safety should be addressed by providing a setting in which external stimuli are minimized to ensure the physical safety of the patient and staff members and to provide a modicum of dignity while the workup is under way.

Physical restraints are used less frequently in mental health settings, and there is an increased use of a quiet room to reduce a patient's level of anxiety and agitated psychotic symptoms.

"Medications to control agitation," examples of which include, but are not limited to, benzodiazepines and antipsychotic medications, may be warranted but should be given only after the primary assessment has taken place, because sedation may be a side effect.

Included in the primary assessment is the gathering of history from anyone with information about the patient before his or her arrival at the hospital.

TABLE 86.1	**Medical Conditions That Present with Psychotic Symptoms**

- *Neurologic conditions*: neoplasms, stroke, epilepsy, auditory nerve injury, deafness, migraine, central nervous system infection
- *Endocrine conditions*: hyperthyroid or hypothyroid, parathyroid, or hypoadrenocorticism
- *Metabolic conditions*: hypoxia, hypercarbia, hypoglycemia
- *Fluid or electrolyte imbalances*
- *Hepatic or renal failure*
- *Autoimmune disorders* with central nervous system involvement (systemic lupus erythematosus)
- *Delirium*
- *Dementia*: Alzheimer disease, vascular, HIV related, Parkinson disease, Huntington disease, head trauma, and the like
- *Neoplasm*: lung

TABLE 86.2	**Substances That Cause Psychotic Symptoms**

During Intoxication

- Sedatives (alcohol, benzodiazepines, barbiturates)
- Stimulants (amphetamine, cocaine)
- Designer drugs ("Ecstasy" and the like)
- Marijuana/THC
- Hallucinogens (LSD, ketamine, psilocybin, and the like)
- Opioids
- Phencyclidines

During Withdrawal

- Sedatives (alcohol, benzodiazepines, barbiturates)
- Anesthetics and analgesics
- Anticholinergic agents
- Anticonvulsants
- Antihistamines
- Antihypertensives
- Antimicrobial medications
- Antiparkinson medications
- Cardiovascular medications
- Chemotherapeutic agents
- Corticosteroids
- Gastrointestinal medications
- Muscle relaxants
- Nonsteroidal anti-inflammatory drugs
- Various over-the-counter medications
- Toxins (anticholinesterase, organophosphate insecticides, nerve gases, carbon monoxide, volatile substances such as fuel or paint)

Initial laboratory information should include complete blood count, electrolytes, liver enzymes, glucose, blood urea nitrogen, calcium, blood alcohol, and urine analysis with toxicology screen.

CT scanning of the acutely psychotic patient's head always should be considered; however, CT scanning is of little help in differentiating between schizophrenia and drug-induced psychosis.

Pharmacological Treatments Medications that best treat schizophrenia include traditional and atypical antipsychotics and, in some cases, long-acting injectable depot antipsychotics.

Pharmacotherapy of the acute psychosis induced by substances should be treated symptomatically and managed with short-acting antipsychotic medication, and side effects from these medications should be closely monitored, especially acute dystonias and oversedation.

Management of Drug-Specific Psychotic Symptoms

Alcohol and Psychosis The most obvious psychotic symptoms associated with alcohol use generally occur in the withdrawal stage.

Auditory and visual hallucinations encountered in alcoholic hallucinosis occur in a clear sensorium (the absence of delirium) to differentiate from alcohol withdrawal delirium, which can also present with visual hallucinations and acute agitation.

The auditory hallucinations most often are of the threatening or command type. In this condition, individuals can be in an extremely agitated and paranoid state as a result of the hallucinations and physical discomfort they are experiencing.

The most typical time for emergence of symptoms is within 2 days of abstinence.

Some evidence suggests that individuals with symptoms that are prolonged for weeks or months may have a predisposition to a psychotic illness.

Withdrawal has been associated with the development of extrapyramidal symptoms, including dystonia, akathisia, choreoathetosis, and parkinsonism.

Cannabis and Psychosis   Some evidence suggests that certain users seek the more psychotomimetic effects achieved through chronic high-dose use of marijuana. At doses >0.2 mg/kg, the potential for development of psychotic-like symptoms increases dramatically.

At this level of use, symptoms include

1. Suspiciousness
2. Memory impairment
3. Confusion
4. Depersonalization
5. Apprehension
6. Hallucinations
7. Derealization

There is some evidence that chronic use of cannabis is related to the onset of a primary psychotic disorder.

First-time use, large amounts, and route of ingestion (oral more so than smoked) may be factors in the higher incidence of cannabis-related psychosis.

Cannabis use often is associated with a more affective type of psychosis.

Typically, the psychosis associated with cannabis is acute and of short duration. However, there are case reports of chronic psychosis attributed to cannabis.

Frequently, the evaluating clinician must decide whether chronic schizophrenia is secondary to the past use of cannabis.

Cocaine and Psychosis   Transient paranoia is a common feature of chronic cocaine intoxication.

Psychotic symptoms associated with cocaine use are almost exclusively seen in the intoxication phase.

There is epidemiologic evidence that men have a greater propensity toward psychosis than women and that Whites are affected more frequently than nonwhites.

High-dose use of cocaine over time is strongly associated with the onset of psychotic symptoms.

Sensitization occurs with chronic administration of cocaine and amphetamines.

Onset of psychotic symptoms has been associated *with reduction in individual doses* and the *desire for treatment.*

Most frequently reported psychotic symptoms are paranoid delusions and hallucinations.

Auditory hallucinations are the most common, often associated with paranoid delusions. Visual hallucinations are the next most common, followed by tactile hallucinations.

Evidence suggests that the character of the psychotic symptoms experienced is associated with the setting in which drugs are ingested.

Observation by studies shows an orderly progression in the effects of cocaine intoxication.

Euphoria to dysphoria and finally to psychosis.

This progression is related to dose, chronicity, and genetic and experiential predisposition.

Amphetamines and Psychosis   Amphetamine psychosis has been described as a three-stage illness:

First stage: increased curiosity and repetitive examining, searching, and sorting behaviors
Second stage: first stage behaviors followed by increased paranoia
Final stage: Paranoia leads to ideas of reference, persecutory delusions, and hallucinations, which are marked by a fearful, panic-stricken, agitated, overactive state.

Amphetamine-induced psychosis develops over time in association with large amounts of the drug, delivered by any route of administration.

The strongest correlation has been seen in those individuals who use large amounts by intravenous injection.

A common presentation of the psychotic, amphetamine-intoxicated patient involves paranoia, delusional thinking, and hypersexuality. The hallucinatory symptoms may include visual, auditory, olfactory, or tactile sensations.

Treatment should be initiated by providing a safe, secure place for the patient and should reduce external environmental stimuli.

Physical restraints should be avoided or used in a time-limited fashion (to prevent dehydration rhabdomyolysis).

Caution should be noted for amphetamines lowering the seizure threshold, inducing hyperpyrexia, and stimulating cardiovascular compromise.

Clinical experience suggests that amphetamine psychosis can last for 3 to 6 months in extreme cases of high-dose use. There is little evidence to suggest that these drugs cause schizophrenia.

Hallucinogens and Psychosis

The primary model for hallucinogens is LSD, an indole-type drug with structural similarities to serotonin.

LSD crosses the blood–brain barrier readily and has a potent affinity for the 5-HT2A receptor.

The *most common hallucinations are visual*; the least common, auditory.

The occurrence of synesthesia—the blending of the senses—is uncommon but not unknown.

There often is a loss of the concept of time.

Paranoia and aggression can be profound, but the more frequent experience is that of euphoria and security.

The setting can have an effect on the experience, and much has been written on proper preparation for the "trip."

"Talking down" the patient is the most common way to ease his or her anxiety around the psychotic features of LSD and related drugs.

The persistently agitated patient may be treated pharmacologically with a benzodiazepine. If neuroleptics are used, **haloperidol**, 1 to 5 mg, or an equivalent dose of high-potency antipsychotic medication may be appropriate.

No clear evidence exists that LSD causes a prolonged psychotic-like illness.

Although there is no hallucinogen-induced schizoaffective disorder in DSM IV TR, the symptoms of LSD-induced psychosis also often include affective symptoms.

Phencyclidine, Ketamine, and Psychosis

Evidence suggests that, in the case of PCP, the psychotic-like state can last for prolonged periods beyond the period of intoxication.

Ketamine, at potency 10 to 50 times lower than PCP, has been shown to produce far fewer of these psychotic-like episodes and was released for use as an anesthetic. Children do not appear to develop the associated psychotic-like symptoms.

PCP and **ketamine** can be smoked, ingested, snorted, or injected intravenously. The drugs are rapidly absorbed and excreted in the urine. The intoxicating effects last for approximately 4 to 6 hours. The recovery period is highly variable.

The behavioral effects of these drugs appear to be mediated by their effect on the excitatory amino acid NMDA subtype of glutamate receptor.

The clinical appearance is

1. Altered sensory perception, with bizarre content
2. Impoverished thought and speech
3. Impaired attention, disrupted memory
4. Disrupted thought processes in healthy individuals
5. There also may be protracted psychosis.

There is considerable symptom variation, depending on dose.

Treatment of the acutely disturbing effects of PCP-like drugs can be achieved with benzodiazepines in doses equivalent to **diazepam** 10 mg and greater, titrated until the patient is satisfactorily sedated.

Neuroleptics also can be considered for treatment of the psychotic symptoms. Most typically, a high-potency neuroleptic such as **haloperidol** (1–5 mg) is used.

MDMA ("Ecstasy") and Psychosis

Hallucinations associated with use generally are mild.

The mechanism is unclear, but, as with a serotonin syndrome, it may be that MDMA can have a direct effect on the thermoregulatory mechanisms that are potentiated by the context of the drug use.

Long-term users can suffer serotonin neural injury associated with psychiatric presentation of panic attacks, anxiety, depression, flashbacks, psychosis, and memory disturbances.

Cases of paranoid psychosis indistinguishable from schizophrenia have been associated with chronic use.

Management of Psychotic Disorder

The first step in medication management is to consider the best approach to treating the patient's schizophrenia or chronic psychosis.

Improving medication compliance in an outpatient setting can be enhanced by

- Reducing positive and negative symptoms
- Providing psychoeducation and social skills training in medication management
- Using motivational enhancement techniques to improve compliance
- Switching the route of administration of the medication from oral dosing to a long-acting injected antipsychotic medication

Second-generation antipsychotic medications have the added benefit of decreasing extrapyramidal side effects, reducing negative symptoms, and improving cognition when compared with traditional antipsychotics.

Complications of Substances with Antipsychotic Medications

Most of the substances of abuse interact with psychiatric medications by reducing their effectiveness, but some can alter blood levels of medications and increase side effects.

Smoking is known to decrease blood levels of **haloperidol**, **fluphenazine** and **thiothixene**, **olanzapine**, and **clozapine** by increasing the metabolism of these medications and other medications and substances such as caffeine.

Abstinence from smoking increases blood levels of neuroleptic medications.

Because of the altered metabolism of medications, *smokers often need double the dose of traditional neuroleptic medications that is given to nonsmokers.*

Additional Medication Decisions

After clinicians have chosen a primary medication treatment option that stabilizes the psychotic symptoms, they can consider the use of additional medication, as necessary, to manage comorbid depression, comorbid substance abuse, or another psychiatric problem.

Psychosocial Treatment

Individuals with substance-induced psychosis will benefit from medications as well as a supportive treatment team and environment.

Psychosocial treatment requires an awareness of the perceived "self-medication" aspects of why individuals with schizophrenia believe they continue to use substances.

Some individuals with schizophrenia report that using substances helps them cope with symptoms of their schizophrenia; some report using substances for pleasure; to alleviate boredom; to relieve feelings of anxiety, sadness, or distress; and to share the excitement of "getting high" with friends who also are using.

Another self-medication theory suggests that individuals with schizophrenia use substances to help ameliorate the distressing side effects of the medications used to treat their schizophrenia.

The term *neuroleptic dysphoria* is used to describe the unpleasant feelings elicited by treatment with conventional antipsychotic medications, including irritability, fatigue, listlessness, and lack of interest or ambition.

Some studies suggest that individuals with schizophrenia may smoke to help improve their attention and concentration. Despite the self-medicating experience of some smokers with schizophrenia, tobacco use is associated with more positive symptoms of schizophrenia and more hospitalizations.

LONGER TERM MANAGEMENT

Patients who continue to display an affective or psychotic disorder despite a significant period of abstinence may require formal treatment of that disorder.

Long-term psychotherapy should consider a dual recovery therapy approach that integrates the best of mental health and addiction psychotherapy.

Psychosocial Treatment

Three specific psychosocial treatments that appear fundamental to dual diagnosis treatment are

1. MET
2. Relapse prevention
3. Twelve-Step facilitation

In most cases, treatment of this dual diagnosis subtype is best suited to the mental health setting, provided that mental health staff members receive adequate training in substance abuse and dual diagnosis treatment strategies.

Clinicians should have skills and knowledge in integrating mental health and addiction treatment approaches, with special emphasis on MET, relapse prevention, and Twelve-Step facilitation for addiction, as well as social skills training and behavioral therapies for psychiatric disorders.

Prochaska et al. defined motivation in relation to a five-stage scale: precontemplation, contemplation, preparation, action, and maintenance.

Individuals enter treatment at various stages, and therefore, interventions need to be tailored accordingly.

Interventions that address individual stages of change have an impact not only on rates of substance use but also on the severity of psychotic symptoms and on the need for antipsychotics.

Certain conditions can work to accelerate a patient's motivation to change through use of external motivators, a realization that led to the development of the community reinforcement approach.

Because external motivation often is lacking among dually diagnosed patients, the community reinforcement approach searches out a range of possible motivators—disability income, probation, family, and so forth—and uses those motivators to engage, support, and monitor patients in treatment.

Recovery

Recovery is a journey of healing and transformation enabling a person with a mental health and/or substance abuse problem to live a meaningful life in the community of his or her choice while striving to achieve his or her full potential.

Unfortunately, stigmatization of people with mental health disorders, including substance abuse, has persisted throughout history and can impact recovery. Stigma is manifested by bias, distrust, stereotyping, fear, embarrassment, anger, or avoidance; can be found throughout our society; and can even include people with mental illness and the professionals and health care systems who serve them.

Addressing Tobacco Addiction in Recovery

Nicotine cessation therapy has received less clinical attention and often has gone untreated, despite the fact that *nicotine is the substance most commonly abused by schizophrenics*. The development of treatment guidelines can correct this oversight and lead to the inclusion of tobacco dependence as a component in clinical treatment plans.

Although few studies have examined the treatment of tobacco dependence in smokers with schizophrenia, specialized smoking cessation programs appear to benefit this population.

CHAPTER 87

Summary Author: Ashok Krishnamurthy
Frances R. Levin • John J. Mariani • Maria A. Sullivan

Co-Occurring Addiction and Attention Deficit/Hyperactivity Disorder

ETIOLOGY OF ADHD

Evidence of a genetic basis for the pathophysiology of ADHD derives from family, twin, and adoption studies, as well as molecular genetics research.

Neuroanatomic explanations for ADHD have also been proposed. For example, neuroimaging studies of ADHD patients have demonstrated reduced volume of the prefrontal cortex.

Structural imaging studies of ADHD patients have revealed several common findings: smaller volumes in frontal cortex, cerebellum, and subcortical structures.

Certain environmental risks have also been associated with ADHD: maternal smoking during pregnancy, low birth weight, low social class, maternal respiratory viral infection, moderate to severe physical illness in the mother during pregnancy, maternal alcohol exposure, febrile seizures, and moderate brain injury.

The finding that traumatic brain injury results in symptoms of ADHD has been documented by a large number of studies.

EPIDEMIOLOGY OF ADHD AND SUDs (SUBSTANCE USE DISORDERS)

ADHD is the most common behavioral disorder of childhood, affecting 8% to 18% of children and adolescents worldwide.

Given that up to 60% of children with ADHD continue to have symptoms into late adolescence and adulthood, *it was estimated that the rates for adult ADHD in the general population would be from 1% to 5%.*

Clinical experience suggests that many patients do not meet full criteria in adulthood but do continue to have significant impairment as a result of persistent ADHD symptoms.

Individuals with ADHD also have a greater likelihood of nicotine dependence. Adults with ADHD have higher rates of nicotine dependence than the general population.

THE IMPACT OF HAVING ADHD ALONE AND WITH SUDs

ADHD has substantial morbidity in and of itself.

Children with ADHD who were followed into adulthood were more likely

- To have completed less schooling
- To hold occupations with less professional or social status
- To suffer from poor self-esteem
- To have social skill deficits
- To have antisocial personality disorder

Persistent ADHD symptoms appear to place these individuals at great risk for antisocial personality disorder and substance abuse.

Adult ADHD conservatively costs the United States >$31 billion per year in work- and health-related costs for patients and their families.

An individual's response to addiction treatment is adversely affected by comorbid ADHD.

Progression of substance may occur with ADHD; for example, adults with ADHD were more likely to transition from an alcohol use disorder to a drug use disorder and to continue to abuse substances than were similar patients without ADHD.

POSSIBLE REASONS FOR LINKAGE OF ADHD AND SUD

There is considerable evidence that individuals diagnosed with childhood ADHD who also have conduct disorder as children are more likely to develop problems related to substance use.

A critical risk factor for having an ongoing substance abuse in adolescence or adulthood is the persistence of ADHD symptoms.

After regular substance use is established, the presence of ADHD symptoms may increase the likelihood of heavy and impairing use.

A growing preclinical and clinical literature suggests that impulsivity is associated with increased likelihood of developing or having a substance use problem.

Impulsivity, a common feature of ADHD, is associated with the inability to inhibit responses. More broadly, individuals with ADHD are often thought to have difficulties in executive function including difficulties in impulse control, attention, planning, and goal-directed behavior.

Increased impulsivity may facilitate risk-taking behavior, involvement with drug-abusing peers, and poor cognitive skills to weigh the negative consequences of drug experimentation and continued substance use.

Deregulation and overexpression of the dopamine transporter also have been implicated in the pathophysiology of ADHD. The 10-repeat allele of the dopamine transporter gene has been associated with ADHD. Dopamine transporter density is significantly higher in adults with ADHD than in healthy controls.

DIAGNOSIS OF ADHD

ADHD is characterized by inattention, impulsivity, and hyperactivity. Importantly, the current criteria require that some symptoms have caused impairment before the age of seven and that impairment must occur in more than one setting (Table 87.1).

The more settings in which deviant behavior occurs, the more justified one is in saying that the behavior interferes with the child's functioning and therefore warrants a diagnosis.

A child who appears distracted and inattentive in only one setting (such as at school) but can listen well and pay attention in other settings may have a learning disability rather than ADHD.

Individuals can meet full criteria for ADHD in three ways:

1. ADHD, inattentive type
2. ADHD, hyperactive/ impulsive type
3. ADHD, combined type

Use of Neuropsychologic Testing to Confirm ADHD Diagnosis

Given the high comorbidity of ADHD with other psychiatric disorders, what is most needed are computer tests that would distinguish ADHD. Computer testing shows areas of dysfunction that may or may not be consistent with ADHD. Testing may be useful for treatment or educational planning.

Difficulties in Diagnosing Adult ADHD in Substance-Using Populations

Diagnostic ambiguity often arises when one attempts to apply these criteria to individuals who abuse alcohol and other drugs.

Potential Reasons for Underdiagnosis Childhood sources of information may not be available during assessment of the adult patient, particularly a substance-abusing patient.

If the patient or family cannot recall symptoms before age seven but does remember substantial impairment related to ADHD symptoms in elementary school, it is reasonable to make the late-onset ADHD-NOS (Not otherwise Specified) diagnosis. This designation is for disorders with prominent symptoms of inattention or hyperactivity-impulsivity that do not meet the formal criteria for ADHD. However, it is important to inquire specifically about childhood inattention, hyperactivity, and impulsivity, because not all disruptive behavior during the school years can be attributed to ADHD.

TABLE 87.1	**Criteria for Attention Deficit/Hyperactivity Disorder**

A. Either (1) or (2):

1. Six (or more) of the following symptoms of inattention have persisted for at least 6 mo to a degree that is maladaptive and inconsistent with the developmental level:

   Inattention
   a. Often fails to give close attention to details or makes careless mistakes in schoolwork, work, or other activities
   b. Often has difficulty sustaining attention in task or play activities
   c. Often does not seem to listen when spoken to directly
   d. Often does not follow through on instructions and fails to finish schoolwork, chores, or duties in the workplace (not due to oppositional behavior or failure to understand instructions)
   e. Often has difficulty organizing tasks and activities
   f. Often avoids, dislikes, or is reluctant to engage in tasks that require sustained mental effort (such as schoolwork or homework)
   g. Often loses things necessary for tasks or activities (such as toys, school assignments, pencils, books, or tools)
   h. Often is easily distracted by extraneous stimuli
   i. Often forgetful in daily activities

2. Six (or more) of the following symptoms of hyperactivity-impulsivity have persisted for at least 6 mo to a degree that is maladaptive and inconsistent with the developmental level:

   Hyperactivity
   a. Often fidgets with hands or feet or in seat
   b. Often leaves seat in classroom or in other situations in which remaining in seat is expected
   c. Often runs about or climbs excessively in situations in which it is inappropriate (in adolescents or adults, may be limited to a subjective feeling of restlessness)
   d. Often has difficulty playing or engaging in leisure activities quietly
   e. Often is "on the go" or often acts as if "driven by a motor"
   f. Often talks excessively

   Impulsivity
   a. Often blurts out answers before questions have been completed
   b. Often has difficulty awaiting turn
   c. Often interrupts or intrudes on others (e.g., butts into conversations or games)

B. Some hyperactive-impulsive or inattentive symptoms that caused impairment were present before 7 years of age.

C. Some impairment from the symptoms is present in two or more settings (such as at school [or work] and at home).

D. There must be clear evidence of clinically significant impairment in social, academic, or occupational functioning.

E. The symptoms do not occur exclusively during the course of a pervasive developmental disorder, schizophrenia, or other psychotic disorder and are not better accounted for by another mental disorder (such as mood disorder, anxiety disorder, dissociative disorder, or a personality disorder).

Code based on type:
- Attention Deficit/Hyperactivity Disorder, Combined Type: if Criteria A1 and A2 are met for past 6 mo.
- Attention Deficit/Hyperactivity Disorder, Predominantly Inattentive Type: if Criterion A1 is met but Criterion A2 is not met for the past 6 mo.
- Attention Deficit/Hyperactivity Disorder, Predominantly Hyperactive-Impulsive Type: if Criterion A2 is met but Criterion A1 is not met for the past 6 mo.

Coding note: For individuals (especially adolescents and adults) who have symptoms that no longer meet full criteria, "In Partial Remission" should be specified.

Reprinted from American Psychiatric Association. *Diagnostic and Statistical Manual of Mental Disorders*, 4th ed. (*DSM-IV-TR*). Washington, DC: American Psychiatric Press, 2000, with permission.

Other reasons for lack of proper diagnosis of ADHD are

1. Many persons with both SUDs and adult ADHD were not diagnosed as children and attribute their impatience, restlessness, or procrastination to character traits of being "hotheaded," "easily bored," or "lazy."
2. Many of the consequences of ADHD (such as work failure and poor educational attainment) also are associated with SUD.
3. Patients often develop ways to partially compensate for their ADHD symptoms, so that the symptoms of the disorder may not be obvious to the evaluating clinician.
4. Because questions regarding childhood behaviors—particularly behaviors associated with ADHD—may not be part of the "standard" assessment, it is an easy diagnosis to overlook.
5. The current diagnostic criteria for adult ADHD are problematic and need to be reexamined.

Potential Reasons for Overdiagnosis Overdiagnosis of adult ADHD also can occur if one ignores the functional impairment criterion.

Adults with ADHD have had significant occupational, interpersonal, or psychologic impairment as a result of their impaired ability to start and complete tasks.

It is incumbent on the clinician to ensure that a patient's current symptoms of ADHD are not limited to one setting.

Another way in which the clinician may overdiagnose ADHD is by failing to confirm that a patient shows a continuity of symptoms from childhood into adulthood. Also, a good medical evaluation is important because anemia and thyroid problems may mimic some of the symptoms associated with ADHD.

Some individuals may feign symptoms of ADHD to get special consideration with test taking or obtain stimulant medication. Although these possibilities exist, secondary gain is more likely to occur in adolescent, non–drug-dependent groups. In substance-abusing populations, it has been our clinical experience that substance abusers are more likely to be surprised when a clinician suggests that they may have ADHD.

Other Psychiatric Comorbidity

The last criterion listed in the *DSM-IV* for ADHD emphasizes that ADHD should not be diagnosed if the observed symptoms are better accounted for by another mental disorder. Unfortunately, some clinicians may interpret this to mean that if depression or bipolar illness is present, ADHD should not be diagnosed. In reality, these disorders may coexist.

For example, in one study, prevalence rates of depression were 18.6% in the ADHD group and 7.8% in the non-ADHD group. Similarly, the prevalence rate of bipolar illness was 19.4% in the ADHD group and 3.1% in the non-ADHD group.

Individuals with

1. Major depression may experience symptoms of inattention *but are less likely to have hyperactivity and talkativeness associated with ADHD: If suicidality is present, this is unlikely to be from ADHD alone.*
2. Bipolar illness are more likely to describe discrete periods of *increased restlessness, talkativeness, and hyperactivity,* and the like, whereas those with adult ADHD will be more likely to describe a lifelong constellation of these symptoms to a lesser degree
3. *ADHD typically do not exhibit psychotic symptoms*
4. ADHD adults have first-degree relatives with ADHD

TREATMENT OF CO-OCCURRING ADHD AND SUD

1. Compared with other patients with SUDs, individuals with ADHD may have greater difficulties in processing information and in sitting through group meetings—a common format for addiction treatment.
2. Individuals with ADHD have a tendency to act impulsively; they also may be more likely than those without ADHD to drop out of treatment.

PHARMACOTHERAPEUTIC OPTIONS FOR TREATMENT OF ADHD CO-OCCURRING WITH SUD

Stimulant Medications

Amphetamine analogues and **methylphenidate** are the stimulant medications most commonly used to treat ADHD in children and adults.

Methylphenidate

- Is a piperidine derivative that is structurally related to **amphetamine**
- Mechanism of action: dopamine reuptake blockade in the striatum
- Is safe and effective for the treatment of ADHD in children and adults
- Is available in multiple immediate and sustained-release preparations for delayed absorption

Amphetamine

- Stimulates the cerebral cortex and the reticular activating system primarily by enhancing dopamine release
- Blocks dopamine reuptake
- Is safe and effective for the treatment of ADHD in children and adults

Abuse Potential of Psychostimulants

Despite concerns that prescription stimulant use may lead to increased craving and cocaine or **amphetamine** use, these effects have not been reported in the controlled clinical trials conducted to date.

Although prescription stimulant medications may be diverted for nonmedical use, clinical data suggest that the use of stimulants in a structured therapeutic context can be accomplished safely.

Use and Misuse of Stimulant Medication

Individuals who receive medication for ADHD are twice as likely to be asked to divert their medication than those receiving medications for pain, sleep, or anxiety.

For the 5.4% of undergraduates who had illicitly used prescription stimulants in the past year at one college campus, nearly 60% reported using stimulants to concentrate.

The reasons for use are multifactorial and may or may not be associated with abuse or dependence.

Abuse Liability of Short- and Long-Acting Formulations of Prescription Stimulants in the General Population

Long-acting preparations of stimulant medications were initially developed to reduce the frequency of dosing and provide consistent therapeutic blood levels throughout the day. However, evidence is accumulating that long-acting preparations may have lower abuse potential and may have particular utility for patients with co-occurring SUD.

Sustained-release **methylphenidate** produced fewer subjective effects than immediate-release methylphenidate.

An additional advantage of delayed-release preparations is greater difficult to using via a nonoral route (e.g., injected, intranasally), which should also reduce the potential for misuse and diversion.

Abuse Liability of Prescription Stimulants in Individuals with ADHD with and Without Active Substance Dependence

Even though misuse and diversion of prescription stimulants, particularly long-acting preparations, is not widespread in the general population or substance abusers in treatment, there is reason for concern.

It is crucial that patients who are prescribed stimulants for their ADHD, regardless of whether they are current abusers, past substance abusers, or have no history of abuse, be warned about the risks associated with prescription stimulant use, understand why it is important not to "share" their medication with others, and be given strategies of how to safeguard their medication so that it is not diverted.

Nonstimulant Medications

With the exception of **atomoxetine**, all nonstimulant medications are "off-label" for ADHD and are generally considered second- or third-line treatments.

There are certain instances where nonstimulant medications would be considered first line, such as if a motor tic disorder is present or in the case of cardiovascular disease.

Atomoxetine

- Centrally acting noradrenergic reuptake inhibitor
- Onset of therapeutic effects are more gradual than stimulant medication—takes several weeks to manifest

- Common side effects: sedation, appetite suppression, nausea, vomiting, and headache
- No known abuse potential

Other Nonstimulating Medications

Tricyclic antidepressants, which block the reuptake of norepinephrine, have some efficacy in reducing ADHD symptoms but are considered to be less effective than the stimulant medications.

Monoamine oxidase inhibitors have been shown to have efficacy for ADHD, but the potential for hypertensive crises associated with tyramine-containing foods and medications (both illicit and prescribed) limits their utility, and MAOIs should be considered contraindicated in patients with SUD.

Clonidine, a noradrenergic alpha-2 agonist antihypertensive agent, has been shown to be effective for the treatment of ADHD.

Modafinil, a novel wake-promoting agent that is U.S. Food and Drug Administration approved for narcolepsy and shift work sleep, has recently been reported to improve ADHD symptoms in children and adolescents, and limited evidence suggests that it may be effective for adult ADHD as well. Some data suggest that **modafinil** may have potential as a treatment for cocaine dependence and is deserving of further study in the treatment of co-occurring ADHD and SUD. Although **modafinil** has some stimulant-like properties, it has minimal abuse potential reported and has not been shown to be as effective as traditional stimulant medications, so for the purposes of discussion, it is being grouped with nonstimulant second-line agents.

PHARMACOTHERAPY SELECTION FOR ADHD AND CO-OCCURRING SUD

The most important clinical variable in considering the use of stimulant medication is whether the SUD is active or in remission.

Patients with a remote history of an SUD and a long period of abstinence from substance use likely represent a low-risk group for prescribing stimulant medications.

Patients with ongoing substance use, but not consistent with a diagnosis of abuse or dependence, likely represent an increased risk of misuse and diversion of prescription stimulants; frequent office visits, urine toxicology testing, and monitoring the pattern of substance use are prudent measures.

Patients with an active SUD represent a high-risk group for prescription stimulant treatment of ADHD. For these patients, given the elevated risk of misuse or diversion, nonstimulant medications are likely to be a first-line choice.

Certain precautions are warranted when using stimulants in substance-abusing patients:

- Keeping careful records (number of pills, dates, etc.)
- Seeing the patient on a frequent basis
- Regular urine toxicology screens
- Taking medication on a regular schedule (i.e., no PRN)
- Using long-acting preparations for ADHD in patients with SUD to reduce the potential for misuse although clinical data are lacking to support this approach

NONPHARMACOLOGIC INTERVENTIONS

In the treatment literature for both childhood ADHD and for SUDs, positive outcomes are reported with the use of behavioral approaches. Such approaches include contingency management, cognitive–behavioral interventions, and combined pharmacologic and behavioral interventions.

Whereas positive contingencies have been stressed as an appropriate treatment for adults with SUDs, there have been no contingency management strategies targeted to persons with both adult ADHD and SUD.

Adults, in contrast to children, have a greater potential to understand the effects of ADHD symptoms on their lives and thus may be better able to use cognitive-behavioral approaches. However, such approaches may need to be modified for persons with ADHD and SUD.

Summary Author: Ashok Krishnamurthy
Linda A. Dimeff • Katherine Anne Comtois • Marsha M. Linehan

Co-Occurring Addiction and Borderline Personality Disorder

PREVALENCE OF BORDERLINE PERSONALITY DISORDER TREATMENT AND OUTCOMES FOR BORDERLINE PERSONALITY DISORDER

Borderline personality disorder (BPD) and substance use disorders (SUDs) are both severe, difficult to treat disorders characterized by frequent relapse.

BPD, in particular, is considered by many to be difficult, if not impossible, to treat and is often associated with treatment noncompliance, poor treatment outcomes, premature termination of treatment, clinician burnout, and suicide.

Dialectical behavior therapy (DBT) is an efficacious treatment for BPD as well as SUD.

BPD DEFINED AND REDEFINED

BPD is a severe Axis II personality disorder (PD) characterized by intense and labile negative emotions including

- Shame
- Anger
- Sadness
- Significant interpersonal conflict
- Extreme behavioral dyscontrol: characterized by impulsivity and disinhibition (Table 88.1)

All BPD criterion behaviors are understood as functioning to regulate emotions or are direct consequences of emotion dysregulation.

PREVALENCE OF BPD AND BPD-SUD

Between 0.2% and 1.8% of the general population meet criteria for BPD. Between 8% and 11% of outpatients seeking mental health services and between 14% and 20% of inpatients meet criteria for BPD.

SUDs commonly co-occur with BPD and result in serious and complex behavioral problems.

Prevalence of current SUDs among patients receiving treatment for BPD range from approximately 25%.

The presence of a PD, such as BPD, among individuals with SUD significantly increases the degree and severity of behavioral dyscontrol and resultant problems.

Specifically, individuals with a PD and an SUD have higher rates of alcoholism, depression, and more extensive legal and medical problems than patients without PDs and engage in significantly more high-risk HIV behavior compared to those with SUD only or individuals with a PD but without SUD.

Among the personality disorders, BPD was associated with the most severe psychiatric problems.

TABLE 88.1	*DSM-IV* Criteria for Borderline Personality Disorder

BPD involves a pervasive pattern of instability of interpersonal relationships, self-image and affects, and marked impulsivity, beginning by early adulthood and present in a variety of contexts, as indicated by five or more of the following:

- Frantic efforts to avoid real or imagined abandonment. (Note: Do not include suicidal or self-mutilating behavior.)
- A pattern of unstable and intense interpersonal relationships, characterized by alternating between extremes of idealization and devaluation, identity disturbance, and markedly and persistently unstable self-image or sense of self
- Identity disturbance: markedly and persistently unstable self-image or sense of self
- Impulsivity in at least two areas that are potentially self-damaging such as spending, sex, substance abuse, reckless driving, binge eating. (Note: Do not include suicidal or self-mutilating behavior.)
- Recurrent suicidal behavior, gestures, or threats, or self-mutilating behavior
- Affective instability due to marked reactivity of mood (e.g., intense episodic dysphoria, irritability, or anxiety), usually lasting a few hours and only rarely more than a few days
- Chronic feelings of emptiness
- Inappropriate, intense anger or difficulty in controlling anger such as frequent displays of temper, constant anger, or recurrent physical fights
- Transient, stress-related paranoid ideation or severe dissociative symptoms

Reprinted from American Psychiatric Association. *Diagnostic and statistical manual of mental disorders*, 4th ed. DSM-IV Washington, DC: American Psychiatric Press; 1994:654, with permission.

RISK OF SUICIDE AND NONSUICIDAL SELF-INJURY AMONG BPD

BPD is the only *DSM-IV* diagnosis for which suicide attempts and/or nonsuicidal self-injuries (SASIs) *are a criterion*, and *SASIs are thus considered a "hallmark" of BPD.*

Rates of SASI among individuals diagnosed with BPD range from 69% to 80%.

Patients with BPD and SUD combined may be at higher risk for suicide than BPD patients without SUD or SUD patients without BPD.

BPD AND UTILIZATION OF PSYCHIATRIC AND MEDICAL SERVICES

Several studies of high users of inpatient psychiatric hospitalizations found that 9% to 40% of high users are diagnosed with BPD.

Studies have found that, over their lifetime, 97% of individuals with BPD have received outpatient treatment from an average of 6.1 therapists.

Presenting medical concerns frequently include asthma, diabetes, hepatitis, and ulcers, as well as chronic fatigue syndrome, irritable bowel syndrome, and fibromyalgia.

Prevalence estimates of childhood abuse in the population with BPD range from 67% to 86% for sexual abuse and 71% for physical abuse, compared with rates of 22% to 34% for sexual abuse and 38% for physical abuse in non-BPD populations.

TREATMENT AND OUTCOMES FOR BPD

Two to three years after index assessment, 60% to 70% of patients diagnosed with BPD continued to meet the criteria. An average of 15 years after index assessment, 25% to 44% continued to meet the criteria.

BPD also has been associated with poorer outcomes in the treatment of Axis I disorders, such as major depression, obsessive-compulsive disorder, bulimia, and SUDs.

Despite advances in the treatment of BPD with medications, it is widely assumed that some form of ancillary behavioral treatment of BPD is necessary.

There are few randomized controlled studies of treatments designed specifically for BPD.

DBT IN A NUTSHELL

Though treatment of severe disorders requires the synthesis of many dialectical polarities, that of acceptance and change is the most fundamental.

This simultaneous embrace of change and acceptance is consistent with the philosophical approach found in Twelve-Step programs, captured in the Serenity Prayer (*"God, grant me the serenity to accept the things I cannot change, the courage to change the things I can, and the wisdom to know the difference."*).

The spirit of a dialectical point of view is never to accept a proposition as a final truth or an undisputable fact. Instead, the client and therapist ask,
"What is being left out of our understanding?" or
"What is the synthesis between these two positions?"
DBT is a comprehensive treatment program composed of five essential functions:

1. Improving client motivation to change
2. Enhancing client capabilities
3. Generalizing new behaviors
4. Structuring the environment
5. Enhancing therapist capability and motivation

DIALECTICAL ABSTINENCE IN DBT

"Dialectical abstinence" seeks to maintain an unrelenting insistence on total abstinence while the person is off drugs, then shifts to radical acceptance and nonjudgmental problem solving after a slip, and follows a quick return to the absolute abstinence pole the moment the person stops using.

In DBT, absolute abstinence involves teaching patients specific cognitive self-control strategies that allow them to turn their minds fully and completely to abstinence.

APPLYING PRINCIPLES OF DBT IN MANAGEMENT OF BPD PATIENTS

Principle 1: Do Not Give Lethal Drugs to Lethal People
For those suicidal patients with a history of overdosing on prescription medications, we recommend prescribing nonlethal medications should they be needed. If it is not possible to prescribe a nonlethal, safe medication, then prescribe a limited nonlethal quantity at a time or have the patient arrange with a friend or family member to hold the bulk of the prescription for him or her.

Principle 2: Combine Pharmacotherapy with a Psychosocial Treatment
The rationale for this principle stems from the chronicity and severity of BPD and the absence of data demonstrating that pharmacotherapy is sufficient for BPD patients.

Principle 3: Do Not Reinforce Dysfunctional, Ineffective Behavior
It is not uncommon to inadvertently reinforce dysfunctional behavior, including suicidal behaviors, in the process of attempting to help patients with BPD. In many treatment settings and systems, for example, patients with BPD receive more time, attention, warmth, sympathy, favors, and services (all of which are often highly reinforcing for many BPD patients) when their behavior is most extreme, egregious, and dysfunctional. Though this may be temporarily helpful at reducing the immediate problem behavior and perhaps curative for a small percentage of BPD patients, it is seldom effective in the long run.

Principle 4: Catch the Patient "Being Good" (e.g., Acting Skillfully)
It is also important to reinforce functional, effective behaviors emitted by the patient.

Application of this principle requires paying close attention to the patient's behavior in order to detect *"just noticeable"* improvements to reinforce.

Second, what constitutes a reinforcer is highly individualized.

Principle 5: Validate Valid Behavior
Use of validation was associated with treatment retention.
However, it is important not to validate maladaptive, ineffective (e.g., invalid) behavior.

Behavioral Skills to Help Your Client Not Use Drugs

For most patients with BPD and SUD, drug use and other dysfunctional behaviors function as a means of regulating or escaping negative emotions and tolerating distress (albeit ineffectively). If patients are to succeed in their efforts to get off and stay off drugs, they require a new set of functional behavioral skills to replace their dysfunctional behaviors.

Linehan's *Skills Training Manual for Borderline Personality Disorder* includes a plethora of such skills in four modules:

1. Mindfulness
2. Interpersonal effectiveness
3. Emotion regulation
4. Distress tolerance

DBT Skills for Newly Abstinent Patients

Though most BPD-SUD patients need all skills across all these modules at some time or another in order to successfully maintain their abstinence, distress tolerance skills are particularly important for patients as they get off drugs.

DBT crisis survival strategies, a subcomponent of the DBT distress tolerance skills, are intended to help a person get through an immediate crisis without making matters worse by engaging in dysfunctional behavior, such as using drugs.

Crisis survival strategies are intended as *short-term* strategies to get through a crisis (e.g., an intense urge or craving to use drugs, a very upsetting event); they are not intended to feel better or to solve the problem.

CHAPTER 89

Summary Author: Ashok Krishnamurthy
Joan E. Zweben • Richard K. Ries

Integrating Psychosocial Services with Pharmacotherapies in the Treatment of Co-Occurring Disorders

WORKING WITH COUNSELORS AND PSYCHOTHERAPISTS

Understanding the background and orientation of specific staff can enhance communication and teamwork.

Counselors

Nonlicensed, recovering personnel

- Found in short-term, Minnesota Model, chemical dependency inpatient programs
- In a growing number of co-occurring disorder programs, and in community-based addiction treatment programs
- Also are dominant in therapeutic communities, which have their own conceptual model that integrates Twelve-Step elements to varying degrees.

Noncredentialed counselors vary widely in talent, experience, and skill.

Some have little training, except for occasional in-service training sessions. Others have completed comprehensive credentialing programs and are far more sophisticated than some licensed staff.

Physicians should draw conclusions about the skill level of the counselors with whom they work from *direct observation, not from inferences based on the presence or absence of credentials.*

Licensed Professionals

Unfortunately, graduate schools do not usually integrate thorough training in the assessment and treatment of addiction into their core curricula, even though many of the clinical populations with whom graduates will work are using alcohol and drugs.

Clinical experience alone may tell little about qualifications.

Many therapists have evolved practices with which they have grown comfortable but which bear little relation to those supported by an empirical literature or by the experience of clinicians who are addiction specialists.

In selecting good therapists for referral, *physicians should look for evidence of recent systematic training*, either through conferences or course work. Such evidence increases the likelihood that the therapist will be familiar with sound treatment practices.

Collaboration with Psychotherapists in the Community

Addiction treatment typically is highly structured, with multiple behavioral expectations.

Psychotherapy usually has minimal structure other than the scheduled sessions.

Most outpatient addiction treatment is abstinence-oriented. Though this goal may be difficult to reach, the goal itself normally does not vary. Abstinence usually is viewed as the foundation that must be in place before meaningful progress can be made on other issues.

Psychotherapy has a wider range of goals and less consistent priorities. Some psychotherapists may not understand or endorse the need for abstinence over some form of controlled use.

Addiction treatment often includes breath and urine testing if resources permit, whereas psychotherapists rarely arrange such testing, and many consider it invasive and abhorrent.

Therapists and counselors in addiction treatment are active and directive, whereas psychotherapists in private practice have a variety of styles, which can be more or less compatible with addiction treatment.

USE OF PHARMACOTHERAPIES

In settings wherein physicians see patients only when specific problems emerge, counselors need a screening tool that incorporates warning signals (such as prescriptions for benzodiazepines) that indicate a need for physician review.

Family members or Twelve-Step program participants may criticize the patient or pressure for discontinuation of medication, generating conflict that undermines treatment.

Achieving Adherence

Adherence to treatment recommendations is a key factor in successful treatment outcomes.

Many behavioral strategies yield poor results because time is not taken to identify the real obstacles to compliance.

Sympathetic listening, combined with well-timed doses of information, can improve medication adherence significantly.

Rejecting a recommendation for medication may reflect the "all-or-none" thinking characteristic of the alcohol- or drug-addicted person.

Adherence with medication regimens can be monitored through refill requests as well as through regular inquiry by the counselor.

Communication with other treatment staff is essential when noncompliance is suspected. Discontinuation of psychotropic medication often is a harbinger of relapse to alcohol and drugs, as distressing psychiatric symptoms begin to reemerge. It also can be an indicator that a relapse to drug use already has occurred.

It is important for counselors to identify medication side effects that influence adherence, discuss them with the patient, and facilitate a plan to coordinate with the physician.

Moreover, the physician needs to discuss with the patient and other members of the treatment team the indications for discontinuing medications (if any) and the process by which such discontinuation should occur. The physician needs to educate both patients and nonphysician therapists about the dangers of psychiatric and addiction relapse that attend such a decision.

Office-Based Opioid Therapy

The U.S. Food and Drug Administration (FDA) has determined that medical maintenance treatment can be provided through program-wide exemptions under the current opioid treatment regulations. Stable, socially rehabilitated patients may receive up to a month's supply of take-home medications, and can reduce the frequency of other clinic visits accordingly.

A psychotherapist with expertise in addiction may be able to provide sufficient assistance if the therapist is clear as to what constitutes an appropriate level of intensity and structure, given the patient's condition in the opioid treatment program.

RECOVERY-ORIENTED PSYCHOTHERAPY

Therapy funded by insurance has been limited to relatively brief interventions that are limited in scope. They often permit management of the initial crisis that brings the patient to treatment but little beyond that.

In a recovery-oriented model, the therapist focuses his or her activity according to the tasks faced by the recovering person.

Engagement

For patients who seek psychotherapy without recognizing that their alcohol or drug use is problematic, motivational enhancement strategies have proved beneficial.

Harm reduction approaches are increasingly available in the community and may be effective as engagement strategies, as damage control, or as sufficient intervention for mild-to-moderate problems.

Addressing the Patient's Self-Medication Hypothesis

Patients often have strong beliefs that their substance abuse is a form of self-medication—that they will be overwhelmed with unmanageable feeling states if they discontinue. *They like the rapid change of state that occurs with the use of alcohol and other drugs.*

It is important for the counselor to explore these beliefs and experiences in detail—it is important to validate the patient's belief that the substances appear to help and their effects are generally faster than prescribed medications.

However, it is usually possible to demonstrate that the overall effect of substance use is to

- Increase the number of crises
- Increase hospitalizations
- Increase housing instability
- Decrease adherence to medication regimens
- Decrease in overall quality of life

For the counselor or therapist, the key concept to work with *is the difference between the initial effects of a drug and the ones that unfold over time.*

Patients focus on the initial effects and often do not track those that unfold over time.

Patients should be encouraged, through the use of logs and discussion, to monitor longer time frames in an effort to better identify the negative consequences of their drug use.

Integrating Psychosocial Approaches

Cognitive-behavioral strategies have been well studied and shown to be effective. In such therapy, the therapist focuses on how the patient can become and remain abstinent.

The recovery-oriented therapist does not mechanistically focus on behavior but blends approaches while maintaining a clear perspective about the immediate goals to be achieved.

Collaboration Issues

Many issues of collaboration may arise between the treating physician and the attending counselor.

For example, the importance of urine and breath testing may be underappreciated by a counselor and can weaken patient cooperation by conveying a sense to the patient that it is somehow degrading to comply with testing requirements. In this case, the counselor can be made aware that such testing often functions as a key element in the support structure for outpatient treatment, permitting prompt relapse identification.

Patients should be helped to understand that urine and breath testing serve as a deterrent to impulsive use and make the option of using seem further removed. It also provides documentation of progress.

Ongoing Recovery Issues

The therapist will have some understanding of relapse precipitants in order to be able to detect signs of early relapse. Current pressures to shorten the duration of addiction treatment will place more burdens on psychotherapists to handle these issues.

Sensitivity to later relapse issues and a willingness to restore addiction issues to first priority when relapse threatens is a necessary characteristic of the therapist capable of good work with recovering patients.

CO-OCCURRING DISORDER PATIENTS IN SELF-HELP GROUPS

Participation in self-help groups is a major element in achieving a positive outcome, so it is important for clinicians to facilitate such participation.

Self-help groups are important in two ways:

1. They provide access to a culture that supports the recovery process, from which participants can recreate social networks that are not organized around alcohol and drug use.
2. They provide a process for personal development that has no financial barriers.

Though many different groups exist, *Twelve-Step programs are the largest self-help system in the world.*

Patients with co-occurring addictive and mental disorders may encounter a variety of difficulties in engaging in self-help programs, particularly if they are severely disturbed.

Initially, most patients have some form of "stranger anxiety"—an understandable reluctance to enter an unfamiliar group where many or most participants appear to know one another.

Encouraging patients to go with someone, pairing them with other patients who attend regularly, or encouraging case managers to go with them (at least initially, and perhaps regularly) can reduce some of this awkwardness.

Patients who object or are ambivalent about calling themselves an addict or alcoholic can be assured that AA is for anyone concerned about drinking and that they can introduce themselves by name only or as a guest.

Those who are concerned about "that religious stuff" can be encouraged to attend meetings less dominated by religious overtones, where they can "take what you need and leave the rest."

Despite a well-articulated AA position that medication is quite compatible with recovery, it is common to encounter negative attitudes toward medications on the part of AA participants.

Patients should be given a copy of the AA pamphlet entitled "The AA Member—Medications and Other Drugs: Report From a Group of Physicians in AA" and provided an opportunity to discuss or role-play potentially difficult situations. It also is possible to find meetings that are more receptive to those on medication. Hospital-based meetings are good candidates in this regard.

The best preparation for practitioners is first-hand familiarity with self-help programs through a "field trip" to meetings.

Interns, residents, and new staff can be asked to attend a specified number of meetings, preferably involving groups recommended by staff or others familiar with community offerings.

Those who are not alcoholics or addicts should be advised to select an open meeting and introduce themselves as a student or a guest.

Summary Author: Ashok Krishnamurthy
Michael E. Saladin • Sudie E. Back • Rebecca A. Payne

Posttraumatic Stress Disorder and Substance Use Disorder Comorbidity

The highly comorbid nature of posttraumatic stress disorder (PTSD) and substance use disorders (SUDs) indicates that persons presenting to treatment for either PTSD or SUD should be screened for both disorders to ensure accurate assessment and appropriate treatment.

EPIDEMIOLOGY

The prevalence of comorbid PTSD and SUDs has been examined in various populations, with war veterans being one of the most extensively investigated groups.

Studies from the civilian population indicate that PTSD and SUDs frequently co-occur. Careful examination of the civilian data reveals that men and women differ in the prevalence of comorbid psychiatric illnesses and PTSD.

The most common comorbid diagnoses in women with PTSD are (in order) depression, other anxiety disorders, and alcohol use disorders.

In men (veteran and civilian), the most common comorbidities in those with PTSD are, in order, (a) alcohol use disorders, (b) depression, (c) anxiety disorders, (d) conduct disorder, and (e) drug use disorders.

Finally, distinct populations, including adolescents, young adults, elderly adults, and minorities, have evidenced similar high prevalence rates of comorbid PTSD and SUD.

ETIOLOGIC RELATIONSHIP BETWEEN PTSD AND SUD

Various theories have been proposed to characterize the development of comorbid PTSD and SUD.

One of the most prominent, *the self-medication theory*, postulates that substance use serves to alleviate PTSD symptoms.

The most common competing theory hypothesizes that SUDs precede the development of PTSD, in two ways:

1. *The lifestyle of a substance abuser*—typically considered to be high risk with dangerous environments and behaviors associated with obtaining or using alcohol or drugs, thus increasing the likelihood of experiencing a traumatic event and subsequently developing PTSD.
2. *Increased anxiety and arousal* that accompanies chronic substance use may increase one's biologic vulnerability to develop PTSD after trauma exposure.

NEUROBIOLOGIC FACTORS IN COMORBID PTSD AND SUD

The model for the human stress response, in which the hypothalamic-pituitary-adrenal (HPA) axis plays an integral role, is also thought to be a key component in the biologic development and maintenance of PTSD.

In patients with PTSD, basal cortisol levels are lower, lymphocyte glucocorticoid receptors are upregulated, and there is increased suppression of cortisol after dexamethasone administration.

These findings suggest that glucocorticoid feedback is enhanced in PTSD.

Individuals with SUDs commonly report stress as a trigger for relapse, and studies have shown that exposure to stress results in increased craving and salivary cortisol, suggesting HPA axis activation similar to activation in PTSD.

ASSESSMENT OF PTSD IN SUD

Given the high rates of trauma and PTSD among individuals with SUDs, it is important to screen all SUD patients.

Brief PTSD assessment measures appear to perform as well as longer, more complicated measures.

As a general rule, *PTSD assessment should be conducted after a patient has emerged from acute alcohol or drug intoxication and withdrawal.*

In contrast to other anxiety disorders (e.g., generalized anxiety disorder), less abstinence may be required in order to establish a diagnosis of PTSD among SUD patients because of the unique nature of the diagnostic criteria (i.e., requirement of exposure to a criterion A traumatic event).

Intrusive PTSD symptoms (e.g., recurrent thoughts or images related to the trauma) *are uniquely characteristic of PTSD and are less likely to be mimicked by substance use or withdrawal.*

If there is any diagnostic uncertainty, reassessment of PTSD symptoms as the patient becomes abstinent can provide helpful information.

Interviewer-Rated Assessment of PTSD

The most widely used interviewer-rated PTSD assessment is the *Clinician Administered PTSD Scale* (CAPS).

A checklist of potentially traumatic events is included at the beginning of the interview to assess lifetime trauma exposure. Seventeen items assess the frequency and intensity of diagnostic PTSD symptoms.

In addition, associated features of PTSD (e.g., survivor guilt, homicidality, hopelessness), social and occupational functioning, and global PTSD severity are also rated.

Other commonly used, clinician-applied scales include

1. Structured Clinical Interview for the *Diagnostic and Statistical Manual of Mental Disorders*
2. Potential Stressful Events Interview and the National Women's Study Posttraumatic Stress Disorder Module
3. PTSD Symptom Scale—Interview (PSS-I)
4. Structured Interview for PTSD (SIP)
5. MINI International Neuropsychiatric Interview PTSD Module
6. Composite International Diagnostic Interview (CIDI)

Some popular self-report scales also exist:

1. Impact of Events Scale-Revised
2. Posttraumatic Stress Diagnostic Scale
3. Modified Posttraumatic Stress Disorder Symptom Scale (Self-Report)
4. Mississippi Scale for Combat-Related Posttraumatic Stress Disorder

TREATMENT OF PTSD AND PTSD-SUD COMORBIDITY

There have been very few studies of therapies specifically designed to address PTSD and SUD concurrently.

Current treatments tend to fall into two general classes: psychotherapy and pharmacotherapy or, in rare cases, their combination.

Cognitive-behavioral therapies (CBTs) for PTSD are emphasized here because *they are widely accepted as the most empirically valid treatments for PTSD.*

Additionally, it has been suggested that *the treatment of one disorder in dually diagnosed individuals often yields clinical benefits for the untreated comorbidity.* This being the case, treatment of PTSD in PTSD-SUD comorbid individuals is important because it can be expected to have positive impact on substance use.

Cognitive-Behavioral Therapy for PTSD

Exposure-Based Therapy Exposure therapies are based on conditioning or information-processing theories of fear and anxiety, both of which argue that exposure to fear and anxiety-eliciting situations/stimuli (i.e., physical location where a motor vehicle accident occurred) without traumatic outcome (i.e., motor vehicle accident) results in anxiety abatement.

Cognition-Focused Therapy Two therapies constitute this class: cognitive therapy (CT) and cognitive processing therapy (CPT).

Originally used for depression, CT, as applied to PTSD, is built conceptually around the notion that it is the *meaning* that individuals assign to traumatic events, rather than the traumatic events, which determines duration and intensity of emotion/mood states that ensue.

The goal of CT is to aid individuals in implementing corrective cognitive procedures to identify and challenge inaccurate, irrational thoughts and beliefs and to replace them with ones that are more evidence-based, rational, and beneficial.

The other therapy in this class, CPT, is similar to CT but has a decidedly more emotional focus. Though originally developed to address PTSD resulting from sexual assault, it has been extended to victims of other types of trauma.

The primary feature of this treatment is the CT component that involves identification and challenging of key cognitive distortions. Specific areas of belief that are targeted for challenge relate to themes of safety, trust, power, esteem, and intimacy. The therapy generally concludes with an analysis of beliefs, including changes to dysfunctional thinking, and discussion of future goals. Completion of CPT can be achieved in approximately twelve 60- to 90-minute therapy sessions.

Anxiety Management Therapy As applied to PTSD, the main goal of this therapy is to provide individuals with a sense of mastery over their PTSD symptoms by teaching them a variety of coping skills and then permitting them to practice the skills both inside and outside of treatment sessions.

Effectiveness of Cognitive-Behavioral Therapy for PTSD The treatments appear to benefit a range of populations including those with civilian and combat-related PTSD. Treatment dropout rates tend to be similar across studies, at approximately 20% to 25%.

The bulk of clinical studies point to exposure therapy (in vivo and imaginal combined) as the dominant therapeutic approach for resolving PTSD.

Integrated Cognitive-Behavioral Therapy for PTSD-SUD Comorbidity The majority of patients with PTSD and comorbid SUDs receive treatment for the SUD only.

Subsequent to the successful completion of SUD treatment, patients are often, but not always, referred to PTSD treatment.

Proponents of this treatment model, known as "sequential" treatment, in which the SUD is first treated and then the PTSD is treated, posit that continued substance use during therapy impedes therapeutic efforts to address PTSD and that addressing the trauma increases the risk of relapse.

"Integrated" treatment models, in which both the SUD and PTSD are simultaneously addressed in therapy, have been developed over the past decade: integrated treatments show that alcohol and drug use typically decrease significantly and do not increase with the addition of trauma-focused interventions.

Proponents of integrated treatments assert that PTSD symptoms may, at least in part, drive substance use and that untreated PTSD symptoms place SUD patients at risk of relapse.

A substantial proportion of PTSD-SUD comorbid patients express a preference for integrated treatment.

Seeking Safety (SS) is the most widely known and empirically studied integrated CBT.

SS is

- Involves at least 25 sessions
- Is present-focused
- Is a manualized treatment that provides psychoeducation
- Teaches coping skills
- Helps clients gain more control over their lives
- Was first developed for adult women
- Leads to abatement of substance use, PTSD, psychiatric symptom severity

Pharmacotherapy of PTSD The primary goals of the pharmacologic treatment of PTSD include

- Decreasing PTSD symptoms
- Improving overall functioning
- Improving resilience to future stressors
- Decreasing symptoms of comorbid psychiatric conditions
- Reducing risk of PTSD relapse

Long-term pharmacologic treatment is recommended based on evidence that PTSD is likely to return after discontinuation of shorter treatment.

Two medications, both selective serotonin reuptake inhibitors (SSRIs), are currently FDA-approved for the treatment of PTSD: **sertraline (Zoloft)** and **paroxetine (Paxil)**.

These are considered the first-line pharmacotherapeutic treatment options for PTSD based on their demonstrated efficacy in treating PTSD and other comorbid conditions and their relative safety in overdose.

SSRIs have been shown to diminish all three symptom clusters of PTSD and improve overall quality of life, particularly among civilian PTSD patients.

Findings from other studies examining the use of mood stabilizers and anticonvulsants fail to show clear benefit in the treatment of PTSD.

Encouraging evidence exists that antipsychotic medications, in particular **risperidone**, may be beneficial as an augmentation medication to partial responders of SSRIs.

Benzodiazepines are contraindicated as a monotherapy or preventive strategy based on preliminary findings that their use was associated with increased risk of PTSD relative to placebo.

Medications that reduce central nervous system activity (e.g., **clonidine, prazosin**) may be helpful in decreasing nightmares and hyperarousal symptoms, which do not respond particularly well to SSRIs.

Research on the pharmacologic prevention of PTSD is limited and methodologically problematic. Consequently, there are no medications that effectively prevent/curtail the development of PTSD.

There are preliminary data indicating that propranolol administration immediately after trauma cue exposure in individuals with PTSD dampens emotional reactivity during subsequent trauma cue exposure.

Pharmacotherapy of PTSD-SUD Comorbidity

Most studies suggest that patients with PTSD and comorbid SUDs respond as well to standard PTSD pharmacotherapies as compared to patients without comorbid SUDs.

Several studies have examined the use of SSRIs, the pharmacologic treatment of choice for PTSD, among patients with comorbid SUDs. All of these studies have evaluated **sertraline**.

All have shown significant reductions in all three PTSD symptom clusters, and the studied substance use parameters (e.g., number of drinking days, number of drinks per day).

CHAPTER **91**

Summary Author: Ashok Krishnamurthy
Lisa J. Merlo • Amanda M. Stone • Mark S. Gold

Co-Occurring Addiction and Eating Disorders

Eating disorders can be described as an unhealthy relationship with food.

The eating disorders comprise a category of psychologic illnesses characterized by disturbed eating patterns and dysfunctional attitudes related to food, feeding, and body shape.

ANOREXIA NERVOSA (TABLE 91.1)

Anorexia nervosa (AN) may be the most widely recognized eating disorder, though it is not well understood by the general public; individuals with AN are characterized by extremely low body weight for their age and height, making their disorder difficult to conceal. Akin to addiction patients, they are often adamant in their denial of the disorder.

Just as an individual with alcohol abuse/dependence may boast about high tolerance, individuals with AN rarely have insight into their problem and frequently note significant weight loss as an achievement, despite the medical concerns associated with their condition.

Rates of completed suicide in this population range from 0.9% to 6.3%.

Other symptoms include
1. Amenorrhea (or delay of menarche) in females
2. Severe disturbance in body image
3. Fear of gaining weight

Associated physical symptoms:
1. Constipation
2. Cold intolerance
3. Lethargy
4. Lanugo (fine body hair that develops along the midsection and appendages)
5. Bradycardia
6. Hypotension
7. Cardiac arrhythmias
8. Mitral valve prolapse
9. Metabolic alkalosis or acidosis
10. Hypokalemia
11. Hypoglycemia
12. Leukopenia
13. Anemia
14. Carotenemia
15. Acrocyanosis
16. Thrombocytopenia
17. Peripheral neuropathy
18. Hypothermia
19. Dehydration
20. Hair loss
21. Dry skin

TABLE 91.1	*DSM-IV* Criteria for AN

Individuals display each of the following symptoms:

A. Failure to maintain at least 85% of expected body weight based on gender, age, and height
B. Significant fear of weight gain or being fat, despite underweight status
C. Distorted perceptions of body shape and/or weight, overemphasis of body shape or weight on self-concept, or failure to admit the severity of current underweight status
D. Amenorrhea (i.e., absence of menstruation for at least three cycles in a row) or delayed menarche

Subtypes

A. Restricting type: characterized by restriction of food intake without accompanying binge-eating or purging behaviors
B. Binge-eating/purging type: characterized by regular binge-eating and/or purging behaviors within the context of a current anorectic episode

Adapted from the American Psychiatric Association. *Diagnostic and Statistical Manual of Mental Disorders,* 4th ed. [Text revision]. Washington DC: American Psychiatric Association, 2000:589.

BULIMIA NERVOSA (TABLE 91.2)

Bulimia nervosa (BN) differs from AN in that markedly low body weight is not a required symptom, *but presence of binge eating and compensation for that bingeing are necessary for the diagnosis.*

Compensatory actions involve purging by self-induced vomiting in approximately 90% of BN cases but can also include misuse of laxatives, diuretics and/or enemas, excessive exercise, or periods of fasting.

Because of frequency of vomiting, it is common for dental enamel to show significant erosion.

Other significant medical complications associated with BN include

- Fluid and electrolyte abnormalities
- Cardiac arrhythmias
- Parotid enlargement
- Submandibular adenopathy
- Menstrual irregularity

TABLE 91.2	*DSM-IV* Criteria for BN

Individuals display each of the following symptoms:

A. Regular binge-eating episodes characterized by
   (1) Eating an abnormally large amount of food within a short time period (e.g., within 2 h) and
   (2) Experiencing a subjective lack of control over one's ability to stop or limit eating during the binge episode
B. Participation in compensatory behaviors to prevent weight gain (e.g., vomiting; use of laxatives, diuretics, enemas; excessive exercising; fasting)
C. On average, symptoms are present at least two times per week for 3 mo.
D. Body shape/weight has excessive impact on one's overall self-evaluation.
E. Symptoms are not present exclusively during an episode of AN.

Subtypes

A. Purging type: characterized by regular purging behaviors (e.g., vomiting or misusing laxatives, diuretics; enemas)
B. Nonpurging type: characterized by participation in only nonpurging compensatory behaviors (e.g., fasting or excessive exercise)

Adapted from the American Psychiatric Association. *Diagnostic and Statistical Manual of Mental Disorders,* 4th ed. [Text revision]. Washington DC: American Psychiatric Association, 2000:594.

- Constipation
- Reproductive problems

BINGE-EATING DISORDER (TABLE 91.3)

Though it is similar to BN in that regular binge eating occurs, the key distinction is that *individuals with binge-eating disorder (BED) do not engage in compensatory behavior for their overeating.* Approximately 20% of individuals with BED are overweight, and approximately 70% are obese.

BED is currently listed in the *DSM-IV* under the category of Eating Disorder, Not Otherwise Specified. It is being considered for possible inclusion as a separate disorder in the *DSM-V*.

Though not currently included in the *DSM-IV*, obesity represents another serious condition related to a disturbance in eating. Generally, a diagnosis of obesity is made on the basis of an individual's body mass index (BMI) score.

PREVALENCE

General Population

In general, the prevalence of eating disorders is higher in urban environments. Though AN occurs relatively equally among areas of diverse urbanization levels, BN appears to be much more common in cities than in rural areas.

As with addiction disorders, heritability appears to be an important factor in the development of eating disorders, with genes accounting for 58% to 71% of the variance for AN and 30% to 83% of the variance for BN.

Unlike addiction disorders, it is commonly accepted that *the prevalence of eating disorders is much higher in females*, with the incidence of eating disorders in males being approximately one-tenth that of females.

However, it is likely that eating disorders have been underdiagnosed among boys and men.

Symptom onset rarely occurs past the age of 40 years, and point prevalence rates are much higher during adolescence and early adulthood.

The prevalence of subclinical AN among girls of ages 16 to 25 is estimated to be approximately 10%.

Recent studies have determined the lifetime prevalence of AN in females to be between 0.9% and 1.9% and have found the lifetime prevalence of AN in males to be between 0.29% and 0.3%.

With regard to BN, recent research has demonstrated the lifetime prevalence of BN to be much higher than that of AN, at 1.5% to 2.9% in females and approximately 0.5% in males.

TABLE 91.3 *DSM-IV* **Suggested Research Criteria for BED**

Individuals display each of the following symptoms:

A. Regular binge-eating episodes characterized by
   (1) Eating an abnormally large amount of food within a short time period (e.g., within 2 h) and
   (2) Experiencing a subjective lack of control over one's ability to stop or limit eating during the binge episode
B. Binge-eating episodes are associated with at least three of the following:
   (1) Abnormally rapid eating
   (2) Continued eating until one feels uncomfortably full
   (3) Eating large amounts of food despite lack of hunger
   (4) Concealing one's eating owing to embarrassment over eating habits
   (5) Experience of self-disgust, depression, or shame after binge episode
C. Individual experiences marked distress as a result of binge eating.
D. On average, binge episodes occur at least twice per week for 6 mo or more.
E. Individual does not regularly utilize compensatory behaviors to prevent weight gain, and symptoms are not present exclusively during an episode of AN or BN.

Adapted from the American Psychiatric Association. *Diagnostic and Statistical Manual of Mental Disorders,* 4th ed. [Text revision]. Washington DC: American Psychiatric Association, 2000:787.

Recent studies have suggested that BED is the most common eating disorder, with lifetime prevalence rates of 1.9% to 3.5% in females and 0.3% to 2.0% in males. The estimated 12-month and lifetime prevalence of BED greatly exceeds the prevalence of both AN and BN. BED onset typically occurs later than AN or BN and most frequently in the early to mid-20s, though many patients do not present for treatment until their 40s.

Much as the prevalence of substance use exceeds the prevalence of substance abuse or dependence, more individuals display subclinical eating disturbances than a full diagnosable eating disorder.

Addiction Treatment Populations

Drug use, abuse, and dependence can have dramatic and consistent effects on eating.

In addition, certain addiction disorders appear to co-occur with specific diseases of eating. Treating one may exacerbate the other, but ignoring one may cause a new life-threatening disease to emerge.

Among individuals receiving treatment for an addiction disorder, approximately 0.02% to 3.4% also suffer from an eating disorder. It has been estimated that 17% of women with eating disorders have a lifetime history of an addiction disorder.

Specifically, results of several studies demonstrate that binge eating is frequently associated with excessive alcohol consumption. *Up to 57% of men and 28% of women with BED meet criteria for an addiction disorder.*

Animal research has demonstrated that abstaining from alcohol may promote bingeing on sugary foods, whereas restricting sugary food intake may promote excessive alcohol consumption.

Human studies have demonstrated that weight gain frequently occurs after treatment and recovery from addiction disorders.

Dieting and purging are frequently associated with the use of cocaine and other stimulants. AN patients also frequently abuse prescription and over-the-counter medications and may use drugs to suppress their appetite in order to lose weight.

Psychiatric Treatment Populations

Individuals with eating disorders frequently display other psychiatric disorders.

The most common axis I psychiatric comorbidity among individuals with AN is a mood disorder, particularly depression, with approximately *94% of AN patients meeting criteria for a depressive disorder.*

Between 56% and 66% of those with an eating disorder experience one or more anxiety disorders.

Obsessive compulsive disorder is the most common comorbid anxiety disorder, with a prevalence rate between 29.5% and 41% among individuals with AN or BN.

Axis II disorders are extremely common among individuals with eating disorders. Research has demonstrated that approximately 68% of patients meet diagnostic criteria for one or more personality disorders.

Patients with AN most commonly display cluster C (anxious/avoidant) personality disorders, whereas those with BN are more likely to display cluster B (dramatic/erratic) personality disorders.

Individuals with BED are three times more likely to suffer from major depressive disorder than are individuals from the general population.

Obesity is also associated with increased psychiatric conditions, including major depressive disorder and generalized anxiety disorder.

Primary Care or Other Health Care Populations

Within a family practice setting, the prevalence of AN is estimated to be between 4.2% and 6.3%, and the prevalence of BN is estimated to be between 6.3% and 12.2%.

Among female athletes, rates of subclinical eating disorders range from 15% to 32%, and these symptoms also commonly occur among male athletes. Participation in aesthetic sports (e.g., ballet, gymnastics, figure skating) or sports in which "making weight" is required (e.g., wrestling, horse racing) results in increased risk for disordered eating.

DIFFERENTIAL DIAGNOSIS

Research suggests that more than half of individuals with an eating disorder go undiagnosed.

In addition, just as addiction disorder patients are unlikely to self-refer for treatment, eating disorder patients often resist acknowledging their symptoms and impairment or accepting their diagnosis. Moreover, several medical disorders share symptoms with eating disorders, complicating the diagnostic process.

Ideally, all substance-misusing, -abusing, and -dependent patients should be evaluated for comorbid psychiatric disorders and diseases of eating.

All patients would benefit from an analysis of diet, exercise, eating behaviors, and BMI. In particular, patients undergoing treatment for alcohol abuse/dependence should always be evaluated for binge-eating symptoms; those in treatment for stimulant abuse/dependence should always be assessed for purging behaviors and excessive dieting; and patients abusing caffeine or laxatives should always undergo a general eating disorder screening.

In addition, as treatment for the addiction disorder progresses, the patient's weight and BMI should be monitored to track significant gain or loss.

Addiction clinicians may find it helpful to use these questionnaires in their initial evaluation and intermittently throughout treatment. Some example questionnaires are listed below.

Eating Disorders Inventory—Second Edition

The Eating Disorders Inventory—Second Edition (EDI-2) has excellent psychometric properties and *is the most widely used self-report measure of disordered eating and related symptoms of AN and BN.*

Eating Disorder Diagnostic Scale

The Eating Disorder Diagnostic Scale (EDDS) is a 19-item self-report questionnaire that assesses eating disorder symptoms over the previous 3 months. The authors have developed algorithms to determine whether diagnostic criteria are met for AN, BN, and/or BED. The EDDS has demonstrated excellent psychometric properties.

Eating Disorder Examination Questionnaire

The EDE-Q assesses disordered eating behaviors and attitudes over the previous 4 weeks. The EDE-Q contains 36 items which are scored using a 7-point forced choice scale. It has demonstrated good psychometric properties.

Bulimia Test—Revised (BULIT-R)

The BULIT–R is a 36-item self-report measure of BN symptoms. Reliability and validity have been well established, and the BULIT-R has been used with both clinical and nonclinical populations. The BULIT-R is recommended for individuals 16 and older.

Binge Eating Scale (BES)

The BES is a 16-item measure used to assess binge-eating symptoms. The BES has strong psychometric properties and published cutoffs to determine whether an individual displays clinically significant binge-eating symptoms.

Night Eating Symptom Scale (NESS)

The NESS is a self-report instrument that contains 12 items assessing symptoms of night eating syndrome (e.g., percentage of food consumed after supper, frequency of nighttime snacking). The NESS has demonstrated treatment sensitivity, but its psychometric properties have not been reported.

Eating Behaviors Questionnaire

The Eating Behaviors Questionnaire (EBQ) is a 20-item self-report measure that was developed to assess for symptoms of food addiction.

MANAGEMENT

Like addiction treatment, the treatment of eating disorders can be a long and arduous process marked by alternating periods of relapse and recovery.

Motivational interviewing interventions may be useful in helping the patient to recognize the need for treatment and to increase his or her willingness to enter and participate in a treatment program.

Management of an eating disorder typically involves a multidisciplinary team and includes psychosocial, behavioral, and pharmacologic interventions.

Depending on the severity of symptoms and presence of comorbid addiction or psychiatric disorders, treatment may be administered in outpatient, partial hospitalization, inpatient, or residential settings.

Biologic Management

While the establishment of weight gain is a goal, it is important to be certain that an electrolyte, cardiac, or other disease does not kill the patient or compromise the patient's ability to be treated or recover.

Once medical issues are resolved, it is generally recommended that addiction treatment take priority unless the patient is at immediate medical risk owing to malnutrition.

AN

Individuals with AN are generally terrified of gaining weight, so weight gain should be implemented gradually (e.g., 0.5–1.0 lb per week).

The American Dietetic Association recommends nutrition intervention and nutritional counseling by a registered dietician as an integral part of treatment for AN.

Referral to a mental health professional who specializes in eating disorders may also be beneficial for many patients.

Thus far, *no pharmacologic treatments have proved effective in treatment of the primary symptoms of AN.*

However, selective serotonin reuptake inhibitors (SSRIs) may help to decrease associated symptoms such as depression, obsessive-compulsive symptoms, and lack of interoceptive awareness.

BN

As in AN, patients with BN who have a comorbid addiction disorder should be treated first for their addiction.

Once in stable sobriety, biologic management of BN generally involves medication with an SSRI.

Fluoxetine has demonstrated efficacy in reducing the core symptoms of BN acutely, and has been shown to lower treatment dropout rates.

Other medications with demonstrated efficacy:

- **Imipramine**, up to 300 mg per day
- **Desipramine**, up to 300 mg per day
- **Topiramate**, titrated from 25 mg per day up to 250 or 400 mg per day

With any medication, it is recommended that pharmacotherapy be combined with cognitive-behavioral therapy (CBT). Individuals with a comorbid addiction disorder who prefer not to take prescription medication should be referred directly for CBT for BN.

In addition, given the detrimental effects of digestive juices on tooth enamel and oral health, a dental exam is recommended for those with purging-type BN. Physicians should monitor patients with BN to assess for fluid and electrolyte abnormalities, cardiac arrhythmias, gastrointestinal symptoms, and reproductive problems.

BED

There are several options for medication management to assist with BED symptoms.

Several SSRIs (**sertraline**, 50–200 mg per day; **fluvoxamine**, 50–300 mg per day; **fluoxetine**, 20–80 mg per day; and **citalopram**, 20–60 mg per day) have demonstrated efficacy. **Topiramate** (50–600 mg per day) has shown utility in decreasing the number of binge-eating episodes per week, decreasing BMI, and shortening the time to recovery.

Psychologic Management

For AN patients, both family therapy and individual therapy have demonstrated efficacy, though family therapy may be particularly beneficial for younger patients.

CBT has consistently been shown to reduce the risk for relapse and improve outcome. Many of the skills developed during CBT for an addiction disorder can be easily transferred to eating disorder treatment.

Combining pharmacotherapy with CBT generally enhances management of BN. CBT is currently recommended as the first-line treatment for BN. CBT can be administered either individually or in a group setting and is generally included as part of both residential and outpatient treatment programs.

Social Management

Eating disorders occur frequently within close-knit groups, particularly among adolescent females and young adults. Socially valued behaviors (e.g., food restriction) appear to increase with social proximity, whereas nonvalued behaviors (e.g., binge eating, purging) appear to decrease. However, levels of binge eating appear to grow more similar among females as their friendship grows closer.

As a result, large-scale prevention and intervention programs are important and can be effective in managing the incidence and prevalence of AN, BN, and BED.

While normally group therapy may be helpful in supporting AN or BN individuals in treatment and recovery, it may be contraindicated in individuals admitted to treatment involuntarily (and particularly those with AN). In some cases, this may lead to competition among the patients to be the "thinnest" in the group or sharing of maladaptive strategies to continue losing weight.

Among motivated individuals, particularly those who have participated successfully in Alcoholics Anonymous (AA) or Narcotics Anonymous (NA), referral to a Twelve-Step program for eating disorders may be beneficial as well.

Recovery Issues

Comorbid Addiction Disorders Eating disorder symptoms may serve as a coping mechanism for some patients with addiction disorders. *Therefore, it is typically recommended that individuals be treated first for their addiction disorder.*

Moreover, when substance abuse is comorbid with AN, it is generally suggested that treatment occur in a residential treatment facility where both issues can be addressed.

Recovery rates for AN with comorbid substance abuse, especially alcohol abuse, are generally poor; indeed, *suffering from these conditions in combination is a strong predictor of fatal outcome.*

However, studies have shown that those receiving treatment for BN as well as an addiction disorder have treatment outcomes similar to those without a history of substance abuse.

Similarly, individuals who suffer from BED with a comorbid addiction disorder show outcomes similar to those without an addiction disorder.

General Recovery Rates Research has demonstrated recovery rates for eating disorders to be between approximately 40% and 94%, with recovery rates and outcome for BN being more encouraging than those for AN.

BN generally is not fatal, *whereas the mortality rate for those with AN is about 10%.*

Among BED patients, there is some evidence that the disorder will spontaneously remit over time, though other research has suggested a more chronic nature, particularly among patients who are older, who are more obese, and who meet full diagnostic criteria.

Disordered Eating After Addiction Treatment Presence of an eating disorder is associated with increased risk for a relapse to substance use.

Individuals who are attempting to manage their disordered eating symptoms may turn to drugs or alcohol as an alternate coping strategy.

CHAPTER

92

Summary Author: Christopher A. Cavacuiti
Peggy Compton • Rollin M. Gallagher • Issam A. Mardini

The Neurophysiology of Pain and Interfaces with Addiction

INTRODUCTION

As our understanding of pain has evolved, so too have the various systems of pain classification. Unfortunately, there is no single universally accepted system and current classification of pain can often be confusing and contradictory. To name just a few examples, pain may be classified as acute or chronic, physiologic or unphysiologic, nociceptive or neuropathic, central or peripheral, or as belonging to Category I or Category II. In an attempt to resolve some of this confusion, the American Academy of Pain Medicine has recommended updated terminology that is based on the functional origin of the pain. **Category I pain is "eudynia":** pain that occurs as a symptom of an underlying disease process. It incorporates nociception (pain resulting from exposure to noxious stimuli) and is considered physiologic. In contrast, **Category II pain is referred to as "maldynia,"** pain that serves no useful purpose to the organism. Of interest, both scientifically and clinically, is the profound overlap between those neural and opioid systems that regulate pain and those responsible for addiction responses. This chapter provides a review of the pathophysiology of maldynia and of the theoretical and clinical evidence for overlap with addiction responses.

CHRONIC PAIN

In contrast to our presently well-established ability to prevent, minimize, and manage acute pain, the management of chronic pain often presents a daunting challenge in clinical practice. First, the physiology of pain after initial onset becomes much more complex almost immediately—the longer the pain, the more complex the process. Second, with chronic pain, every new episode or change in pain intensity, character, or localization activates cognitive processes and emotions that are influenced by current context and are conditioned by past pain experience. Therefore, theoretically at least, virtually no two pain experiences are ever the same. Clinically, this means that chronic pain management plans must be tailored to suit various clinical settings as well as the unique biopsychosocial and neural needs of the patient.

Pain Anatomy and Physiology

Wall and Melzack's postulation of the gate theory of pain provided the first pathophysiologic model to coherently explain how a variety of factors (setting, mood, past experience) can influence perception of pain. One of the earliest descriptions of the "gating system" occurred when delivering babies for women trained in Lamaze techniques in 1971 to 1973. Women trained with Lamaze breathing and delivering in a secure familiar environment (personalized, informed, longitudinal prenatal care by their doctor in a small hospital in their own community and with a participating family member) would manage childbirth in almost all cases without systemic analgesia and, in many cases, at their preference, without regional blocks. In contrast, mothers in unfamiliar medical setting with no prenatal care experienced severe pain and high anxiety and almost always required systemic opioid analgesics and neural blockade.

The neurobiological basis of Wall and Melzack's functional gating system, now better understood, provides a conceptual framework for understanding the clinical presentation of pain and helps explain the often complementary effects of different types of treatment for pain. Three major "stages" of pain have been proposed involving different neurophysiologic mechanisms depending on the nature and time course of the originating stimulus. The three stages are

Stage 1: Consequences of a brief noxious stimulus
Stage 2: Consequences of a prolonged noxious stimulus leading to tissue damage and peripheral inflammation
Stage 3: Consequences of neurologic damage, including peripheral neuropathies, central pain states, and peripheral and central sensitization

These stages are not mutually exclusive. Their end result is chronic pain perpetuated by one or more of several mechanisms: loss of descending inhibitory controls; chronic inflammation; enhanced excitability of pain neurons; neuro-structural reorganization so that touch, movement, and temperature changes cause the sensation of pain. At any given time, one or a combination of these pathophysiologic mechanisms may be contributing to the experience of maldynia.

Stage 1 Pain

A sufficiently strong noxious stimulus activates nociceptors leading to depolarization of pain afferents (A delta and C fibers), which transmit the pain message from the peripheral tissue centrally to the dorsal horn of the spinal cord. If the signal is strong enough (many nociceptive neurons firing) and/or repetitive enough, second-order neurons depolarize, sending the message rostrally in the spinal cord to the brain. Lateral projections from the thalamus to the somatosensory cortex convey localization and intensity information, resulting in the conscious perception of pain.

Stage 2 Pain

Stage 2 pain occurs when a noxious stimulus is sufficiently intense or prolonged to lead to tissue damage and inflammation. In the absence of tissue damage, most nociceptors are inactive and unresponsive. However, cell damage and death from injury or disease and accompanying inflammation can cause an "awakening" of nociceptors, which may spontaneously discharge (ectopic firing) and become more sensitive to peripheral stimulation. This state is termed *peripheral sensitization*. The sensitization of nociceptors depends on activation of second-messenger systems by the action of inflammatory mediators released in the damaged tissue, such as bradykinin, prostaglandins, serotonin, and histamine. Stage 2 pain is also modulated by various receptors on the surface membrane of sensory axons (including opioid, GABA, bradykinin, histamine, serotonin, and capsaicin).

The consequence of this *peripheral sensitization* is an increase in the depolarization (firing) of primary afferent pain fibers, leading to an increase in the pain signal to the spinal cord and brain. Clinically, this can result in more pain than normal from a noxious stimulus; this is termed *hyperalgesia*. Also, peripheral sensitization can lead pain signals being sent in response to what is normally innocuous stimulation, such as light touch that activates sensitized A β fibers; this is termed *allodynia* (algesia felt in response to an innocuous stimulus).

Along with nociceptor sensitization, stage 2 changes also take place in the central pathways. Under normal circumstances, a variety of inhibitory inputs reduce or eliminate the transmission of pain signals to the brain. The balance of these excitatory and inhibitory processes provides an explanatory basis for gate theory of pain transmission. In stage 2 pain, these normal inhibitory effects are reduced, resulting in more pain signals reaching the brain. In addition, the interneuronal networks in the dorsal horn of the spinal cord transmit nociceptive information not only to neurons that project to the brain but also to spinal motor neurons, which leads to enhanced reflex actions in response to a noxious stimulus, including muscle spasm.

In *central sensitization*, persistent pain input to the central nervous system (CNS) sets off a process of enhancement of responsiveness in the dorsal horn neurons of the spinal cord. Central sensitization is thought to play a significant role in *secondary hyperalgesia* (hyperalgesia in sites away from the site of initial injury) and *allodynia*. The rationale for *preemptive analgesia* (analgesics or neural blocks that are given prior to a painful surgical procedure) is that this is thought to prevent central sensitization.

Stage 3 Pain

Stage 3 pain states are abnormal pain states, often termed as *maldynia* (bad pain), which are generally the consequence of chronic inflammation (e.g., arthritis), damage to peripheral nerves (e.g., neuropathy), damage to the CNS (e.g., thalamic stroke, multiple sclerosis), or changes in the CNS itself (e.g., neuroplasticity, central

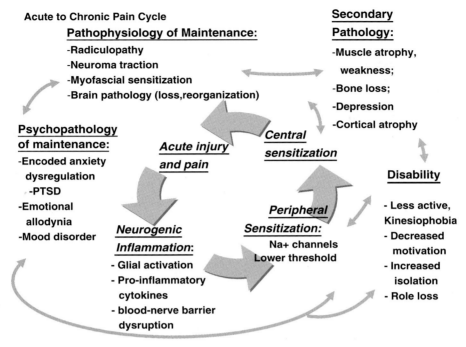

FIGURE 92.1   Acute-to-chronic pain cycle.

sensitization and alteration in modulatory systems, such as complex regional pain syndrome [RSD]). *Maldynia* is characterized by a lack of correlation between the intensity of a peripheral stimulus and the intensity of pain (manifest by exaggerated responses to noxious stimuli) and also by pain that is spontaneous or triggered by innocuous physical or psychologic stimuli. The development of stage 3 pain may also involve genetic, cognitive, and emotional factors that remain to be clarified.

Our growing understanding of the neurophysiology of pain is now beginning to help explain the underlying basis for many forms of chronic pain management. For example, placing laboratory mammals in a challenging novel environment leads to changes in the hippocampal region of the brain that enhance the ability of the CNS to inhibit transmission of pain signals. This finding helps to explain the effectiveness of stimulating, goal-directed activity and exercise in suppressing pain, enabling improvements in functional ability and even reducing the clinical manifestations of central sensitization (e.g., allodynia and hyperpathia). This mechanism is thought to underlie the effectiveness of comprehensive rehabilitation programs for chronic pain. Figure 92.1 illustrates the sequence of biopsychosocial processes involved in the transition from acute injury to maldynia. The complexity of this acute to chronic pain cycle also highlights the need for chronic pain treatment plans to involve a comprehensive approach that identifies the patient's biopsychosocial profile in this pathway and addresses specific pathophysiologic factors that perpetuate pain and pain-related and disease-related impairments and comorbidities.

Pain and Emotions

Emotional states that activate sympathetic arousal, such as anxiety or anger, can increase the level of pain in any episode of acute pain and reactivate or worsen chronic pain. Not surprisingly, chronic pain is more frequent and severe in those with significant mood disorders such as post traumatic stress disorder (PTSD), depression, or anxiety disorders. Moreover, certain personal traits, such as the tendency to catastrophize, also predict worse outcomes. Comorbid substance abuse can also complicate the use of analgesics for pain control.

Historical Notes on Psychosomatic Concepts
A large number of studies over several decades demonstrate a strong association between depressive and anxiety disorders and chronic pain. The same environmental factors that trigger depression (stress, trauma, etc.) also tend to trigger chronic pain. Furthermore, family history of mood disorders is a strong predictor of chronic pain and vice versa.

One interpretation of these aforementioned studies is that central pain states such as fibromyalgia and central mood disorder states such as depression share a genetic and/or biologically mediated vulnerability. It is postulated that individuals with this vulnerability tend to respond to stressful or traumatic events with psychological and/or pain-related symptoms. This interpretation is consistent with several recent studies:

- Persons with fibromyalgia are more likely to develop PTSD in response to the same traumatic event than those without fibromyalgia.
- Women with fibromyalgia (a central pain state) who were primed to experience negative mood prior to stress showed greater subsequent pain elevations than similarly primed women with osteoarthritis (a peripheral pain state).
- Functional polymorphisms in the promoter region of the serotonin transporter gene seem to influence the development of both depression and fibromyalgia.

Pain and Anxiety   Experimental and epidemiologic evidence points to a strong association between anxiety disorders and pain conditions. Anxiety and pain share common neurochemical pathways and can interact in a way that leads to the reorganization of normal perceptual pathways in the brain. The subjective experience of pain is mediated in part by the amygdala, which appears to play a key role in the up-regulation or down-regulation of the emotional response to pain. The hippocampus, a structure with robust connections to the amygdala, is a center for memory formation, storage, and retrieval. This may explain why the same noxious stimulus (e.g., a back strain) can cause far more severe and dramatic anxiety when the pain is experienced during traumatic events associated with high emotional content (like a car accident). Individuals who have suffered very traumatic experiences (such as those with PTSD) have chronic changes in the amygdala, hippocampus, and other areas of the limbic system. This may explain why a disproportionate number of individuals with PTSD experience maldynic pain.

It has also been demonstrated that involvement in goal-oriented, motivating, engrossing activities can help reverse hippocampal sensitization and downregulate the emotional response to pain. In addition, the cortex plays an essential role in the categorization, appraisal, and attenuation of our reactions to pain and other frightening stimuli. Thus, higher cortical connections to the more primitive fight, flight, and reward circuitry of the amygdala, hippocampus, and other areas of the limbic system are what allow us to have a degree of conscious recognition and control over these processes.

CLINICAL INTERFACE BETWEEN PAIN AND ADDICTION

Pain and addiction interface in a variety of clinically significant ways:

- Pain and drug reward share common neuroanatomic and neurochemical substrates.
- The physiologic sequelae of addiction (i.e., tolerance, physical dependence, altered stress response) have clear effects on pain management.
- Drugs of abuse often have analgesic and hyperalgesic properties.
- The disease of addiction brings with it physical symptoms, mood states, behaviors, and social losses that serve to worsen the pain experience.

Physiologic Mechanisms of Addiction

The physiology of addiction often is characterized by two incompletely understood yet related allostatic states: *tolerance* and *withdrawal*. Like pain, addiction is an extremely complex human response, with strong behavioral components that cannot be entirely understood by analyzing its physiology. Addiction is identified by a cluster of aberrant patterns of behavior that, while partially motivated by these physiologic changes, is also evident in much broader domains.

Tolerance   Ongoing use of certain psychoactive drugs results in the development of drug tolerance, which is defined as a reduction in response to a given dose of drug after repeated administration. The *opponent process theory* offers a theoretical explanation for development of tolerance. In order to maintain homeostasis over the course of repeated exposures to a psychoactive stimulus, a counteracting or opposing psychoactive response develops. In other words, in order to maintain a "normal" or homeostatic level of reward system activity, "antireward" systems are recruited to counteract drug effects. These "antireward" systems become stronger with each exposure and are extinguished more slowly than the original response.

Withdrawal As habituation develops, this counteracting "antireward" response eventually becomes the predominate state when the drug is absent. Upon abrupt drug withdrawal, the tolerance-producing processes are revealed. When drug blood level falls below a critical point, the homeostatic changes associated with tolerance predominate and become profoundly nonadaptive. Suddenly unopposed by drug effects, the "antireward" effects become evident as the characteristic *autonomic* and *affective* drug-specific withdrawal symptoms.

Role of Stress Stress-related activation of the hypothalamic-pituitary-adrenal (HPA) axis plays a significant role in reward responses to addictive drugs. Both stress and repeated, chronic administration of glucocorticoids to animals have been shown to enhance their behavioral sensitization to addictive drugs.

Analgesic Effects of Drugs of Abuse

It is important to recognize that many classes of abused drugs have demonstrated analgesic properties. For example, opioids are defined by their direct analgesic effect, and at high doses, alcohol is a potent anesthetic. The sedative hypnotics, particularly benzodiazepines, are used to treat muscle spasm secondary to upper motor neuron damage and are the standard anxiolytic adjuncts for procedural sedation and analgesia. CNS stimulants, such as cocaine and caffeine, produce and potentiate analgesia, and cannabinoids alter pain perception.

General Effects of Addiction on Pain

Studies have demonstrated that addiction can effect the input, modulation and processing of pain signals in a variety of ways. Abused substances tend to be ingested in short-acting formulations and via routes of rapid onset (i.e., inhalation, intravenous) to boost psychoactive effect. This results in frequent and rapid fluctuations in blood levels of the drug. These rapidly alternating states of intoxication and withdrawal can result in activation of the sympathetic nervous system and thereby augment to the pain experience.

In addition to these physiologic effects, the interpersonal conflicts, role adjustments, and social support losses that characterize the social context of addiction can worsen the experience of pain. Further, the chaotic and drug-oriented lifestyle of individuals with an addiction makes it difficult to comply with prescribed pain management regimes.

Unique Effects of Opioid Addiction and Pain

The effects of addictive disease on pain become especially pertinent in the case of individuals addicted to opioid drugs, because the class of drug abused also is the primary pharmacologic tool for the treatment of moderate-to-severe clinical pain. Opioid addiction and opioid analgesia are both dependent upon opioid agonist activity at the μ-opioid receptor.

Pain and Methadone Maintenance Patients There are significant cross-sectional data to indicate that methadone-maintained (MM) patients are more sensitive to pain than are matched normal controls. As early as 1965, Martin and Inglis described significantly lower tolerance for cold pressor (CP)-induced pain in a sample of incarcerated, known narcotic-abusing females, in comparison to matched nonaddict controls. Ho and Dole found that both MM patients and formerly opioid-dependant patients had significantly lower thresholds for CP pain than did matched nonaddict sibling controls. Existing evidence suggests that patients not only receive *no* underlying analgesic effect from daily, high-dose administration of methadone but also present a case for the *antianalgesic* (hyperalgesic) effects of chronic methadone therapy. Early data suggest that patients maintained on the *partial agonist* buprenorphine for the treatment of opioid addiction are less hyperalgesic than those maintained on methadone, a *full agonist*.

Opioid-Induced Hyperalgesia Accumulated evidence indicates that opioid administration not only provides analgesia but concurrently sets into motion certain antianalgesic or hyperalgesic processes, which counteract or oppose the opioid analgesic effects.

Withdrawal Hyperalgesia The phenomenon of hyperalgesia has long been recognized as a fundamental symptom of the opioid withdrawal syndrome in both animals and humans. Opioid administration produces a biphasic response in which analgesia is an early response, followed by the longer-lasting hyperalgesic state.

Opioid-Induced Hyperalgesia and Tolerance The presence of hyperalgesia with ongoing opioid use demands reconsideration of the well-described phenomenon of analgesic tolerance. That which appears to be opioid analgesic tolerance, and therefore increased opioid need, may in fact be caused by a decrease in pain thresholds secondary to opioid-induced hyperalgesia (OIH). Reconceptualizing tolerance as a reflection of OIH raises significant concerns about the utility of chronic opioid therapy.

Mechanisms of Opioid-Induced Hyperalgesia Various physiologic explanations for the development of OIH have been offered. Like the hyperalgesia of neuropathic origin, OIH appears to be partially mediated at the dorsa horn level and can be prevented by NMDA-receptor antagonism and calcium channel blockers. Opioids also enhance descending nerve conduction from the brain to the spinal cord, which can result in an augmented spinal hyperalgesic response. Various spinal neuropeptides, distinct from excitatory amino acid systems, have also been implicated in the development of OIH. Exogenously administered opioids are theorized to bind to opioid receptors located on the astrocytes of the blood–brain barrier, activating these and resulting in the subsequent expression and release of proinflammatory (and pronociceptive) chemokines and cytokines.

Clinical Evidence of Opioid-Induced Hyperalgesia In abdominal surgery patients, postoperative reports of pain severity and/or opioid consumption were significantly higher in those patients receiving high-dose opioids during surgery in comparison to those receiving placebo or low-dose opioids. It is theorized that the increased opioid exposure experienced during surgery produced a hyperalgesic state that resulted in increased pain perception and opioid need in the postoperative period. In a study of patients with chronic nonmalignant low back pain, 30 days of morphine at therapeutic doses not only resulted in analgesic tolerance but also diminished tolerance to CP pain by almost 25% from baseline.

As noted in several recent meta-analyses of the extant clinical trial data, the benefits of opioid therapy for chronic nonmalignant pain beyond 6 to 8 weeks of treatment have yet to be demonstrated. Clinical trials involving the use of chronic opioids often tend to have very high (>50%) rates of dropout. Most commonly, these dropouts are attributed to side effects (nausea, constipation, drowsiness, and dizziness), and to a perceived lack of efficacy, perhaps reflecting OIH.

In addition, patients on opioid therapy for the treatment of chronic nonmalignant pain are often less likely to achieve key outcomes (pain relief, improved quality of life and functionality) than those not on opioid therapy.

Genetic Factors Underlying Pain and Addiction Response

Well-recognized individual differences in pain tolerance and opioid response have long been appreciated at the clinical level, and the genetic factors that underlie these differences are increasingly elucidated. Individuals who are extensive "metabolizers" of opioids (i.e., those with high P450 activity) receive less analgesia and reward from a given opioid dose, theoretically putting them at decreased risk for addiction but increased risk for unrelieved pain.

Genetics of Pain and Addiction

Murine studies demonstrate that strains of mice with poor pain tolerance find opioids to be highly reinforcing, whereas those with good pain tolerance receive little reinforcement from opioids. Furthermore, pain-tolerant murine strains receive robust opioid analgesia and demonstrate increased opioid receptor-binding activity as compared to pain-intolerant strains. Much of the research to explain findings such as these has focused on polymorphisms in the µ-opioid gene receptor (OPRM). One of the most researched is the A118G polymorphism of the OPRM. Human subjects with the variant allele have been shown to require almost twice as high a plasma level of morphine to achieve the analgesic response of those with the nonmutated allele.

Genetics and Opioid-Induced Hyperalgesia

Studies in mice have demonstrated have demonstrated significant differences in OIH among various murine strains. Genetic analyses revealed that differential expression of a gene coding for the nonspecific P-glycoprotein transporter (*Abcb1b* gene) best accounted for strain-related differences in the development of OIH.

CONCLUSIONS

Pain is the most modulated of the sensory modalities. The conscious perception of pain can be modified in complex ways and at a variety of anatomic levels including the nociceptor, the peripheral nerve, the spinal cord neurons and tracts, the thalamus, the hippocampus, or the cortex; modulation typically occurs at one or more of these sites. Psychoactive drugs can profoundly disrupt the complex neuromodulation that controls pain. Through a wide variety of mechanisms, the presence of addictive disease appears to augment the experience of pain. The congruence between the approaches for the treatment of pain and addiction (i.e., cognitive therapy, behavior modification, involvement of family, treatment of concurrent psychiatric disorders, and group support) provides further evidence that these phenomena have similar bases and are not entirely unrelated.

Summary Author: Christopher A. Cavacuiti
Edward C. Covington • Margaret M. Kotz

Psychological Issues in the Management of Pain

This chapter addresses primarily chronic, nonmalignant pain, as its management differs from that of acute, malignant, and recurrent acute pain. Although the focus is on psychologic interventions, it should be recognized that such interventions are most effective when combined with rehabilitation and medications. For many chronic pains psychosocial variables predict onset, chronicity, and outcomes better than do somatic variables.

PSYCHOLOGIC COMPONENTS OF PAIN

Both the onset of pain and its transition from acute to chronic are determined at least as much by psychologic and environmental factors as by medical and disease-related ones.

Disease Onset

The progression from acute to chronic pain has been studied most thoroughly in low back pain, the leading cause of disability in industrialized nations. Studies suggest that job dissatisfaction, low socioeconomic status, physical work stress, and poor performance appraisals are all strong predictors of acute back pain.

Disease Progression

The progression from acute to chronic back pain is associated with a number of occupational, medical, and demographic factors including significant self-rated disability at onset, a protracted initial episode, multiple recurrences, a history of back pain or hospitalization, somatization, depression, catastrophizing, stress, and compensation. Occupational predictors include blue-collar jobs, labor requirements beyond the subjects' capabilities, job dissatisfaction, poor performance ratings, being new at the job, prior spine-related compensation, sickness payments, and disease-related litigation. Social and economic predictors included lack of schooling, language problems, and low income. Patients who apply for and receive workers' compensation benefits seem to fare worse with virtually all interventions than those not so encumbered. Workers must continually prove how sick they are to obtain the care they believe they need. In disputed cases, physicians and attorneys for each side may take polarized and improbable positions.

Litigation is thought to prolong disability, although the issue is controversial. Disability associated with "whiplash" injuries appears much less common in countries with a less developed tort system than the United States, where that complaint accounts for two thirds of all bodily injury claims.

Chronic pain syndrome (CPS) must be distinguished from chronic nonmalignant pain (CNMP). CPS refers to pain that is persistent and *not associated with progressive tissue destruction*. The term *CPS* is used to describe those with *inordinate impairment* and *behavioral abnormalitie*s, and is defined as intractable pain of 6 months' or more duration, accompanied by

- Marked alteration of behavior, with depression or anxiety
- Marked restriction in daily activities
- Excessive use of medication and frequent use of medical services
- No clear relationship to organic disorder
- History of multiple, nonproductive tests, treatments, and surgeries.

Some of the controversy regarding chronic opioid analgesia may be an argument between those who have found opioids useful in treating chronic pain and those who have found them harmful in CPS. Pain patients who have an active addiction disorder are at risk for CPS as well, because they are prone to inordinate disability, symptom exacerbation, and health care utilization. Psychological factors modulate, for better or worse, the intensity with which pain is felt, the associated affective distress, and the extent to which the person is functionally impaired.

Developmental Issues

Adverse childhood experiences (particularly deprivation and trauma) have been implicated as causes and exacerbating factors in various chronic pains.

Researchers speculate that psychologic trauma, in a process akin to kindling, can evoke a hypersensitivity not unlike that seen in neurogenic sensitization in pain, and that this hypersensitivity involves cross-sensitization, so that the individuals are hypersensitive to psychic (loss, humiliation) and physical (injury) trauma, both of which elicit both physical and affective symptoms. The term *polymodal allodynia* has been coined to describe the vulnerability experienced by these patients.

Cognitive Factors in Pain

Cognitive approaches to pain are based on the premise that individuals react not to events per se, but to their understanding of them. Maladaptive cognitions have the quality of being automatic and habitual, so that they rarely are examined for validity. They are accepted by the patient, even when it is obvious to others that they are illogical.

The Meaning of Pain

The aversive quality of pain is modified by its interpretation so that it is more distressing if thought to presage disaster.

Catastrophizing

One example of maladaptive cognition is catastrophic thinking, a trait associated with poor pain tolerance and coping. "Catastrophizing" describes the automatic interpretation of events (including pain) in catastrophic terms.

Helplessness

Cognitive influences on pain include not only beliefs regarding the pain, but also those regarding the person experiencing it. One's sense of personal power and competence modify coping. Those who feel unable to control events in their lives tend to respond passively to them, become depressed, and experience increased disability and pain. Conversely, belief in self-efficacy is a major determinant of successful coping.

Locus of Control

This refers to the perception that events are determined by one's own behavior ("internal loss of control [LOC]"), as opposed to outside forces, such as family members and physicians ("powerful others"), or chance. In several chronic pain studies, those with an internal LOC felt and functioned better and had more successful rehabilitation. In contrast, those with a "chance/external" LOC reported depression and anxiety, felt helpless, and relied on maladaptive coping strategies.

Blame

Blame attribution can be an important modifying factor in recovery from injury. Chronic pain patients who blame others for their pain report greater mood distress and behavioral disturbance, poorer response to past treatments, and lower expectation of future benefits.

Behavioral Contingencies in Pain

Operant conditioning refers to the process in which behaviors increase in frequency when reinforced and decrease when they are not. An immediate small reinforcer may be more powerful than a delayed large one, which is reflected in the human propensity to engage in behaviors that produce immediate small rewards despite substantial delayed adverse consequences. In the case of chronic pain, rest and inactivity often provide the small immediate reward of decreasing pain. However, prolonged inactivity can have substantial long-term consequences (such as physical deconditioning, depression, and loss of identity, friendships, jobs, and recreational activities).

Above and beyond the internal rewards (reduced immediate pain) arising from inactivity and disability, there are also often significant external rewards. Although disability income is often meager, there are nonetheless a number of *secondary gains* to be had by remaining on disability. Disability income is not contingent on one's ability to compete in the work marketplace, or the viability of one's industry in precarious economic times. In addition, access to health care may be contingent on remaining disabled. It also appears that the factors listed above not only reinforce *pain behavior*, but also *pain perception*. Sometimes, it is in the interest of family and friends for an individual to remain disabled; the phenomenon where a third party supports an individual's helplessness and disability is referred to as *tertiary gain*.

Fear and Deconditioning

The profound impairment that results from prolonged inactivity often begins with fear of injury. A vicious cycle begins, in which inordinate fear leads to inactivity, which in turn leads to deconditioning and a state of increased fragility, as loss of strength and range of motion increase susceptibility to further injury. The term *kinesophobia* has been coined to denote an inordinate fear that movement or activity will lead to reinjury.

Distraction

Perceptions, including pain, are amplified when attended to and attenuated by distraction. Patients often respond to chronic pain by retreating into the bedroom, isolating socially, and limiting stimulation in an effort to feel better. These behaviors may so limit competing stimulation that pain becomes all-consuming. ("If life is empty, pain will fill it up.")

Emotional Distress

Depression is common among those with chronic pain and probably reflects a multitude of factors, including pain, loss of gratifying activities, loss of self-esteem/identity, powerlessness, and drug-induced affective changes. *Anxiety* is also common in chronic pain and can both amplify physical symptoms and provide disincentives for recovery. *Anger*, a major cause of suffering in pain patients, has been somewhat neglected in comparison to other mood states. It seems to increase pain-related suffering and interferes with life activities, while it reduces response to treatment. Chronic pain is also often associated with emotional symptoms that do not meet criteria for a psychiatric diagnosis, but nevertheless contribute substantially to overall suffering and require treatment.

AXIS I DISORDERS

Psychiatric conditions are generally more frequent in chronic pain patients than they are in the general population. The four most frequent psychiatric illnesses in pain patients probably are somatoform disorders, anxiety disorders, depression, and substance abuse disorders.

Depression

An extensive literature documents widely varying estimates of the prevalence of depression in CNMP, with figures ranging from 10% to 83%. The wide variance reflects differences in settings, methodology, and criteria as well as the confounding effects introduced by overlap of affective symptoms with those of pain. For example, insomnia from pain and drugs, loss of energy from deconditioning, and guilt from having become a burden all mimic symptoms of mood disorders. In fact, there seems to be a vicious cycle in which pain behavior, isolation, inactivity, helplessness, depression, loss of reinforcers and distractions, and pain are mutually reinforcing. This vicious cycle has a number of elements: (a) mood disturbance can *elicit* pain and vice versa, (b) mood disturbance can *exacerbate* pain and vice versa, and (c) mood disturbance can make pain *treatment-resistant* and vice versa. The greatest fear in depressed patients is, of course, suicide, and in the case of those with CNMP, suicide ideation and behaviors were elevated even after depression was controlled for. Fortunately, depression in CPS is highly responsive (up to 98% in some studies) to nonpharmacologic interventions provided in an interdisciplinary pain rehabilitation program.

Anxiety Disorders

The prevalence of anxiety is elevated in CNMP. The relationship between panic and pain is likely multifactorial, and involves such disparate elements as hypervigilance, hypothalamic pituitary-adrenal (HPA) axis activation, and the elaboration of alpha receptors on injured nociceptors. That severe trauma promotes somatization is an additional explanation. Anxiety not only compounds the suffering in CNMP, it also impedes treatment. Baseline anxiety, as well as depression, predicted poor functional and symptomatic outcome in sciatica.

SOMATOFORM DISORDERS AND PSYCHOGENIC PAIN

Psychogenic pain is a concept whose existence is disputed. The term is widely criticized, in part because pain is defined as an *experience,* and to label an experience psychogenic may be tautologous. Additionally, a number of pains thought to be nonphysiologic have subsequently been explained by neurologic plasticity and sensitization. Even granting the validity of the concept, the diagnosis is fraught with difficulty. Nevertheless, pains of various sorts are prominent in somatization disorder, in which there is no evidence of physical disease, and it is certainly worthwhile, if only to avoid costly and potentially harmful studies and treatments, to distinguish complaints based on "hardware dysfunction" from those resulting from "software bugs." The current term for what was previously called psychogenic pain is *pain disorder associated with psychologic factors.* It is difficult to distinguish conversion symptoms from malingering, because the distinction relies primarily on patient intent and consciousness of the situation, which are not observable.

Addiction

The management of intractable pain can be quite challenging in the presence of comorbid addiction disorder, which tends to magnify complaints, impede diagnosis, and confound interventions. Despite these difficulties, such patients can be treated successfully. The prevalence of addiction disorder in CNMP is disputed, with some researchers even finding a prevalence substantially lower than the population baseline. Such low figures strain credulity for several reasons: (a) many common causes of CNMP are associated with substance use; (b) chronic pain often follows accidents, which are more common in those who are chemically dependent; and (c) the similar neurophysiologic adaptations that occur in pain and addiction suggest these disorders will trigger and reinforce one another. Most of the research in this area has generally reached the conclusion that substance use problems are common in pain patients, and they are also high in health care consumers in general. However, despite the fact that pain and addiction are frequently comorbid, available evidence suggests a high likelihood that most substance use disorders will not be detected in health care facilities.

Diagnosing addiction disorder in those with CNMP poses special challenges. Two of the major diagnostic criteria of DSM-IV-TR, tolerance and physical dependence, are virtually universal in those on chronic opioid therapy and do not distinguish the person with addiction disorder from those not so afflicted. Continued use despite adverse consequences, which is often an obvious clue to addiction to recreational substances, is less obvious in addiction to prescribed drugs. Even when the diagnosis of comorbid pain and addiction is clear, getting patients to accept the diagnosis can be challenging. Patients with pain have often experienced a major blow to self-esteem as they have become nonproductive and burdensome to loved ones, and they may be especially reluctant to accept a stigmatized diagnosis.

Malingering

It is somewhat politically incorrect to discuss malingering in the context of CNMP, and indeed it should be. For decades our failure to understand and appreciate the significance of the neurologic processes that generate and amplify pain that is disproportionate to the peripheral stimulus (if any) has led to default diagnoses of psychogenic pain, malingering or faking. For this, if no other reason, the burden must be on the clinician to demonstrate the presence of conscious, wilful deception before making such a diagnosis. This does not, however, imply that malingering is nonexistent or rare.

IDENTIFYING PSYCHOGENIC COMPONENTS OF PAIN

A number of findings may support a conclusion that pain and disability are not fully explained by medical pathology:

- Patients who choose predominantly affectively charged terms (e.g., agonizing, torturing, unbearable) on the McGill Pain Questionnaire are likely to have substantial psychological components or sequelae of pain.
- Scores higher than 10 on a 0 to 10 Likert pain scale indicate exaggeration (i.e., pain greater than "the worst imaginable") and may reflect a desire to emphasize the severity of suffering present.
- Bizarre locations, multiplicity of pain locations, and pain outside the body may suggest functional components.

ESSENTIAL ELEMENTS OF A CHRONIC PAIN EVALUATION

Functional Impairment

Evaluation should always include an assessment of functional impairment, including such activities as work, household chores, social and recreational activities, and activities of daily living.

Emotional Symptoms

Depression, anxiety, and irritability should be noted, along with such symptoms as crying spells and changes in sleep, energy, interest, libido, humor, concentration, appetite, and weight. Suicidality should be assessed.

Family Response

It is most helpful when family and friends accept the person, validate the pain, provide assistance when necessary, and encourage function. Hostility and challenges to the validity of the pain may increase distress and elicit efforts to "prove" the existence of the illness. On the other hand, inappropriate caretaking can promote regression and should be considered a form of "enabling."

Stresses

Work, family, and entitlement agencies are perhaps the most common stressors mentioned, and the patient may have observed that these issues are related to pain severity.

Litigation/Disability

The presence or absence of disability income may be less relevant than the process of trying to obtain it, which requires continued demonstrations of dysfunction. It is difficult to recover while trying to prove how sick one is.

Collateral Information

Poor recollection, drug-induced confusion, and the desire to portray oneself in a favorable light may combine to produce an unreliable history and highlight the need for clinicians to obtain collateral information whenever possible.

Physical Examination

It is important to note whether findings are consistent internally and with known pathology, while recognizing that our understanding of pathology is incomplete.

Mental Status Examination

Cognitive function should be assessed for dementia or baseline cognitive limitations that create disincentives to rehabilitation. Locus of control should reflect the patient's acceptance of responsibility for recovery.

PSYCHOLOGICAL APPROACHES TO THE TREATMENT OF PAIN

Psychologic interventions should focus on treating psychiatric (including addictive) comorbidity, correcting cognitions, reinforcing healthy behaviors, and reducing such psychophysiologic components as tension and anxiety.

Physical Therapy

In the patient with chronic pain, physical therapy is a critical form of psychotherapy. Deconditioning commonly results from fear and causes such psychologic changes as perceived helplessness. A major consequence of deconditioning is that many activities become difficult or painful, reinforcing the belief that one is handicapped. Physical therapy thus becomes a form of systematic desensitization for patients who are immobilized and deconditioned because of the fear of reinjury. It is a powerful antidote to "learned helplessness" and directly reduces symptoms such as anxiety and depression. Passive modalities should be used with caution because of their potential to teach that improvement is achieved by being a passive recipient of others' ministrations.

Behavior Modification

The management of CNMP has as much to do with behavioral changes as perceptual ones. In physical therapy, praise, rest, and other "rewards" should follow goal completion, rather than "trying." Families can learn that unnecessary coddling promotes invalidism. They must learn to distinguish ignoring pain behavior from ignoring the person, and must be encouraged to provide social reinforcers for healthy behavior. This involves a role change from that of caregiver to companion or friend.

Education

Patients are often bewildered about the significance of their pain. In many cases, patients avoid activities because of an unwarranted fear that they will cause more damage. Therefore, teaching should include the pain pathology, if known, its benign nature, and the difference between hurt and harm, so that patients are not deterred from reconditioning programs that may initially increase pain. Education also should involve families, lest they promote unwarranted regression. Much maladaptive behavior on the part of patients and families can be understood as an inappropriate extension of appropriate *acute* pain management (which is how most *chronic* pain began) into the chronic phase, so that the regression and caretaking that initially protected injured parts and promoted healing come to promote deconditioning, increased pain, and destruction of quality of life.

Cognitive-Behavioral Therapy

Cognitive-behavioral therapy (CBT) is an amalgam of cognitive therapies, relaxation techniques, and behavioral therapy. In this most common psychotherapeutic approach for chronic pain, patients are trained to identify, challenge, and alter automatic inappropriate thinking patterns and self-defeating behavior. CBT approaches generally share the principle that thoughts largely determine emotional reactions. Therapies are time limited, somewhat didactic in structure, with homework assignments. Studies show that CBT leads to improvements in activity, psychological function, pain, and medication use.

Mindfulness

CBT has evolved over the years, and increasingly focuses on such concepts as mindfulness and acceptance. Early versions of CBT focused primarily on reducing pain and other (primarily emotional) symptoms. However, strategies that focus primarily on symptom control can be backfire if they fail. Mindfulness-based CBT focuses less on the end result (reduced pain) and more on the process (inappropriate thinking and self-defeating behavior).

Acceptance

As with mindfulness, newer CBT approaches hold that there can be value in acceptance of pain. As noted by McCracken et al., "Somewhat paradoxically, there may be occasions when helpful change in the quality of a patient's life can only occur when some aspects of the problem are accepted as they are. Change efforts may then be directed away from struggles that keep the person stuck, such as with unwanted thoughts, feelings, or sensations, toward situations that yield overall better results, such as a course of action that is personally meaningful and satisfying." Thus, acceptance of pain, which may initially sound like giving up, actually is about changing the things that can be changed and accepting the things that cannot. Studies suggest that patients who accept the idea that they cannot completely eliminate pain and so choose to have a good quality of life despite it are the ones who feel and function best over time.

Stimulus Reinterpretation

Patients can be taught to identify and reframe inappropriate cognitive responses and catastrophic statements that they make in regard to their pain. For example, "My back is breaking" can be replaced with, "Although it feels as though my back is breaking, it's probably another muscle spasm, and it won't last forever."

Assertiveness Training

Those who are uncomfortable directly expressing their desires and declining requests have an intrinsic incentive for remaining "sick." Pain elicits nurture and is an excuse to avoid unpleasant responsibilities or situations. Patients, especially passive ones, may have concerns that assertive training will encourage them to be demanding or unpleasant. However, by teaching individuals more appropriate ways of saying "no," assertive training often makes these individuals less demanding. As patients set limits on how others treat them, what they are willing to do, and to communicate their needs, the sick role becomes less necessary.

Biofeedback/Relaxation Training

Clinical biofeedback/relaxation training (BFT) achieves symptom control by using electronic feedback to teach patients to regulate such functions as skeletal muscle tension, palmar sweating, gastrointestinal motility, and digital blood flow. It is commonly used to train autonomic responses in complex regional pain syndrome (reflex sympathetic dystrophy) and has also been used for the treatment of tension headache, fibromyalgia, and back pain. There may be a synergistic effect from combining BFT with cognitive therapies.

Family Therapy

It is perplexing that, despite almost universal agreement as to the importance of the family in perpetuating and ameliorating inordinate functional impairment in pain, there is very little literature devoted to the subject of how best to intervene. Family members often find themselves torn between overly solicitous responses which can promote increased pain and decreased function, and rejecting responses that can promote anger and depression. As general principles, the optimal response is one that validates a person's pain, and conveys unconditional affection and acceptance of the person, while at the same time providing strong "social reinforcers" for behaviors that enable patients to abandon their sick role.

Interdisciplinary Pain Rehabilitation Programs

Combined approaches seem more effective than unitary treatments for CNMP. Accordingly, combinations of interventions should be tailored to maximize comfort and function. Typical services in multidisciplinary pain rehabilitation programs include

- Education
- Reconditioning physical therapy
- Medications
- Biofeedback/relaxation training
- Operant conditioning
- Psychotherapy (personal and family)
- Detoxification
- Addiction treatment
- Treatment of psychiatric comorbidity
- TENS
- Interventions such as spinal cord stimulator or nerve blocks

Studies suggest that Interdisciplinary Pain Rehabilitation Program (IPRP) are the most efficacious and cost-effective, evidence-based treatment extant for CNMP.

Addressing Pain/Addiction Comorbidity

Of the psychologic problems that beset the patient with CNMP, perhaps none is more insidious and difficult to manage than addiction. Addiction (to prescribed substances) is more difficult to diagnose in the presence of CNMP, more difficult to enlist patient efforts to combat, and more difficult to treat. Yet treatment is essential, because addiction recovery seems to be a *sine qua non* for pain recovery.

Diagnosis of Pain/Addiction Comorbidity

Often one of the most difficult challenges faced in terms of pain/addiction comorbidity is related to patient willingness to accept the diagnosis. Patients with CNMP have often lost the ability to be the breadwinner, to parent, to function sexually, and even to be a desirable friend or companion. In this context, it is easy to see why individuals who have already lost so much may have difficulty accepting a diagnosis that may stigmatize them yet further. Second, the person who is addicted to recreational substances, even if in considerable denial, is likely to know that substance use is the reason for job loss, legal consequences, marital discord, and the medical consequences of toxic substances. For the person who is addicted to prescribed drugs, on the other hand, virtually all consequences, from reduced libido to poverty, can be attributed to pain rather than the drugs themselves. Finally, the person addicted to medical substances often has the approval of physicians who may perceive the medications as helpful and may lack skills in diagnosing addiction disorders.

Treatment of Pain/Addiction Comorbidity Contentious Terms

Addicting Drugs and Iatrogenic Addiction The term *addicting drugs* should be used in the way that "photosensitizing drugs" is used—that is, it does not affect everyone, but suggesting sunscreen is still a good idea. While some have argued that *iatrogenic addiction* is something of a scientific oxymoron (since it is the individual, not the physician, who is responsible for taking his or her drugs), it is nonetheless true that numerous physicians have been successfully sued for "causing addiction."

As a general rule, patients with a prior/current addiction to recreational substances who go on to develop opioid dependence secondary to CNMP often respond to traditional addiction care in a setting appropriate to the severity of the disease. In contrast, the person with no prior history of addiction who has become addicted in the course of pain treatment (and perhaps the person who has an "iatrogenic relapse," associated with prescription of opioids after a prolonged period of sobriety) seems to respond better if treatment is initiated in a chronic pain treatment program.

The concept of cross-addiction suggests that a patient with any prior addiction is at heightened risk for new addiction, even to unrelated substances. The treatment of pain in patients with comorbid addiction raises the question of whether to use opioids, and, if so, how to protect the person's recovery. It is generally considered unethical to withhold opioid analgesia from persons/patients with an addiction disorder, yet patients should not be given treatments that fail to help or harm them.

Distinctions must be made between acute pain and chronic nonmalignant pain, and between the patient who is actively engaging in substance abuse and the patient in recovery.

Acute Pain

Acute injuries and surgery in persons/patients with an addiction disorder, even with sustained recovery, may require more aggressive analgesia than in patients with no addiction history. Patients should be encouraged to inform the surgeon/anesthesiologist in advance of elective procedures that they are in recovery; will likely require higher than usual doses of analgesics; but wish to preserve their sobriety by avoiding their previous drug of choice, transitioning to long-acting oral agents as soon as possible, and making arrangements for safe use of opioids after discharge.

Chronic Pain

It is reasonable to conclude that chronic opioid analgesic therapy can help some patients with CNMP if managed meticulously. The issue of ensuring that addiction is being adequately treated is often a key to management of the patient with comorbidity. Experts in the addiction/pain have provided recommendations for treating the patient with chronic pain and addiction.

- Wean opioids if pain can be managed with nonopioids, although detoxification alone is ineffective treatment for addiction.
- The risks of treating must be balanced against risks of not treating, because unrelieved pain may promote addiction relapse or use of street drugs.
- Do not withhold opioids from patients with addiction, but integrate them into a plan to relieve pain and treat addictive disease.
- Address the "false promise" that opioids enable one to avoid pain.
- Provide treatment in a pain center if the primary physician is reluctant to prescribe opioids.
- Require a treatment "contract" to establish treatment boundaries.
- Educate patients about tolerance, dependence, withdrawal, and interactions between opioids, other medications, and alcohol.
- Optimize adjunctive medications and nonpharmacologic strategies (e.g., physical conditioning, coping skills, daily time management skills, lifestyle modifications).
- Address psychiatric disorders and risk factors—survivors of childhood trauma may require psychotherapy.
- Involve families in rehabilitation efforts.
- Require drug abuse treatment.
- Slowly titrate opioids to the point of maximum function.
- Monitor analgesic misuse.
- Reevaluate addictive disease if drug seeking persists despite increased dosing in the absence of disease progression.
- Provide multiple dated small prescriptions to those who cannot adhere to instructions.
- Do not replace lost medication.
- Do not expect addiction-controlling doses of methadone to effectively manage pain.
- Expect relapse, especially early in treatment, during stress, or with unrelieved pain. Treat relapse; do not abandon the patient.
- Terminate opioids in the case of selling prescriptions.
- Strict contracts and frequent follow-ups with urine toxicology screening are essential elements to promote and ensure compliance with treatment plans.

Opioid Selection The goal of opioid selection is to optimize analgesia with minimal risk of relapse. This suggests selection of slow-onset, long-acting agents, and avoidance of the fast-in, fast-out products.

Several strategies have been proposed to help opioid users remain in control. It is common to request that patients always bring their pill bottles to visits for pill counts. Some clinicians phone patients to bring in the bottle at random times, the idea being that the unpredictable oversight will help the patient to take the drugs as prescribed. Patients may be required to return used transdermal patches to receive a prescription for new patches, thereby demonstrating that they were not sold, opened, or cut into pieces.

Additional Medications Comorbid psychiatric symptoms are the rule in pain and addiction disorder, and their management should also be conducted with an eye to protecting sobriety. There seems little justification for prescribing benzodiazepines or other controlled substances for anxiety, "muscle spasm," and insomnia, because nonaddicting alternatives abound.

Nonopioid Treatments It has been compellingly demonstrated over the course of several decades that many patients with chronic pain (including those with comorbid pain and addiction) are more comfortable and functional without opioids. CNMP patients who fail to respond to moderate-high dose opioids often have pain reduction with opioid elimination as part of a comprehensive treatment approach.

Physician Protection

The issue of physician self-protection must be raised, because persons/patients with an addiction disorder may seek compensation from physicians who they claim caused their addiction. Risk of litigation and sanctions can be minimized by

- Obtaining written informed consent that notes the risk of addiction
- Meticulously seeking and documenting the presence of prior addiction
- Carefully documenting unambiguous benefit from opioids if these are to continue being prescribed
- Whenever possible, obtaining independent corroboration of benefits and harms from family
- Weaning opioids when benefits are unclear
- Monitoring for development of behaviors suggesting addiction

Other Considerations

Self-Help Groups A number of CNMP self-help groups exist. Their focus is on self-management techniques such as daily relaxation, stretching exercises, and such psychologic tasks as working on goal setting, assertiveness, and avoiding pain behavior.

Chronic Cancer Pain Although not the focus of this chapter, cancer pain warrants mention for several reasons:

- Cancer has become a chronic disease, and thus most of the material in this chapter is relevant to those in prolonged remission.
- Most of the comments of this chapter regarding the importance of treating comorbid depression and anxiety and providing coping skills training can be applied to the cancer patient who is not acutely ill.
- Treatments for malignant pain may cause several forms of CNMP such as chemotherapy-induced neuropathy and radiation cystitis.

Acute Recurrent Pain Special difficulties arise in the treatment of patients with conditions such as inflammatory bowel disease, chronic pancreatitis, sickle cell disease, and other illnesses in which there is recurrent, severe, nociceptive pain and a substantial prevalence of addiction disorders. The literature concerning the long-term treatment of pain in these conditions, with the exception of sickle cell disease, is quite sparse. In the case of sickle cell disease, there is a consensus that proper care of acute pain requires rapid and aggressive titration of opioids, typically those with which the patient reports prior success.

CONCLUSIONS

Physicians and patients confronted with the challenges of treating patients who are suffering from intractable pain may experience therapeutic nihilism. In the context of CNMP, hopelessness is seldom helpful. Instead, care providers need to communicate to patients that they can "recover" even when medical interventions have been exhausted. When a patient demonstrates the characteristics of inordinate suffering, medical involvement, disability, or drug use, it is unlikely that solutions will be found external to the patient, whether through pharmacology or technology. Rather, the solution likely will come from the patient's inner resources. It is the physician's task to help that patient find, strengthen, and trust in those resources.

Summary Author: Christopher A. Cavacuiti
James A.D. Otis • Michael Perloff

Nonopioid Treatments in the Management of Pain

Medications can provide effective pain management in most patients. Choosing the appropriate medication requires that the pain state being treated is correctly diagnosed and classified as somatic, visceral, or neuropathic. Nonsteroidal anti-inflammatory drugs (NSAIDs) and opioids are the principal medications for somatic pain, whereas adjuvant medications such as antidepressants, antiepileptics, anesthetics, and adrenergic agents are useful for neuropathic pain.

NONOPIOID ANALGESICS

Nonsteroidal Anti-inflammatory Drugs

NSAIDs, which are the most widely used analgesics, are indicated for somatic pain of mild to moderate intensity. They are most useful in bone and joint pain but can be used in conjunction with opioids for all forms of pain. Bone and joint pains are very responsive to NSAIDs, but neuropathic pain usually is not. The mechanism of action for NSAIDs is thought to be related to the inhibition of cyclooxygenase activity (COX), which in turn inhibits prostaglandin production. Prostaglandins sensitize peripheral nerve endings to noxious stimuli and are the key to the inflammatory cascade. Patients have variable responses to the different classes of NSAIDs: some do not respond at all to one class but have excellent results with a different class.

Significant interactions between NSAIDs and other medications are common. The most important of these involve the potentiation of renal and hepatic toxicity of coadministered drugs and the changes NSAIDs can produce in anticonvulsant levels. Dramatic and dangerous increases in serum levels of lithium, widely used in psychiatric therapy, can result from coadministered NSAIDs resulting from decreased renal clearance.

Adjuvant Analgesics

Medications that have a primary indication other than analgesia, but which have analgesic properties under certain conditions, are termed *adjuvant analgesics*. Most of these medications enhance the body's own pain-modulating mechanisms or the effectiveness of other analgesics.

Antidepressants The tricyclic antidepressants (TCAs) have been used for many years for the management of neuropathic pain. Their analgesic effect appears to be independent of their antidepressant actions. Their mode of action is thought to be that they enhance the body's own pain-modulating pathways and enhance the opioid effect at opioid receptors. Their onset of action is slow, requiring several weeks for the full drug effect to be achieved. The greatest analgesic effect is seen with the older, tertiary amine antidepressants, such as amitriptyline, imipramine, and doxepin. Secondary amine tricyclics, such as desipramine and nortriptyline, are not always as effective, but they generally have less sedation and anticholinergic side effects.

One of the most common side effects of TCAs is sedation. In many cases, this can be avoided by starting at a low dose and instructing the patient to take the medication 10 to 12 hours before rising, rather than at bedtime.

While somewhat less effective than TCAs, duloxetine and venlafaxine may be the preferred drugs for the treatment of depression with comorbid pain syndromes. While low-dose TCAs are often effective for pain, these doses are not particularly effective for depression. At higher doses needed to treat depression, TCAs tend to have significant anticholinergic effects, α blockade (sometimes leading to falls), and QTc prolongation.

Anticonvulsants Carbamazepine, phenytoin, gabapentin, and several other anticonvulsant/antiepileptic drugs (AEDs) have efficacy in neuropathic pain. It is suspected that AEDs may reduce pain by reducing neuronal excitability and local neuronal discharges. While carbamazepine remains first-line therapy standard of care, phenytoin has also been used for the management of a variety of neuropathic pain syndromes, including trigeminal neuralgia and postherpetic neuralgia. Valproic acid has been used for the management of lancinating pain, with mixed results, and for pain of diabetic neuropathy. There are no large studies demonstrating long-term effectiveness. Several newer AEDs, released in the last 10 to 15 years, have been found to be useful in treating neuropathic pain. Gabapentin is well established and multiple studies have demonstrated efficacy in both lancinating and continuous dysesthetic pain. The newest AED with efficacy in neuropathic pain is pregabalin, which has a profile very similar to that of gabapentin. Lamotrigine has showed modest efficacy in treatment of diabetic and HIV neuropathy. However, because of required slow titration of medication to avoid dermatologic side effects and reduced efficacy compared with gabapentin and pregabalin, lamotrigine appears a poor choice for neuropathic pain therapy.

Oral Anesthetics The efficacy and adverse effects of oral anesthetics such as mexiletine are similar to those of other drugs used in neuropathic pain (sedation, dizziness), but the acute onset of these adverse effects is an advantage to the local anesthetics. A recent meta-analysis of oral and intravenous local anesthetics validates their efficacy and safety in acute settings.

α-*Agonists* The α_2-adrenergic agonists have been studied in a variety of pain syndromes. The mechanisms of action are presumed to be an enhancement of endogenous pain-modulating systems and, in the case of sympathetically maintained pain, sympatholysis. Clonidine can be administered epidurally, intrathecally, orally, or transdermally. The major limiting factors in the use of clonidine are hypotension and sedation.

Topical Agents

Topical agents are useful for several types of continuous pain. In general, they are most effective in pain states that have a predominantly peripheral cause. These include painful neuropathies, herpetic and postherpetic neuralgia, and painful arthropathies. Capsaicin, a naturally occurring pepper extract, has been found to have weak to moderate efficacy for neuropathic and musculoskeletal pain. Pain relief does not occur for several days. On initial application, many patients complain of markedly worsened pain and burning. Lidocaine patch use has become popular as a treatment for neuropathic pain. Diclofenac, as a transdermal patch or gel, is the most commonly prescribed topical NSAID and is particularly useful for inflammatory pain. Other topical products with evidence of efficacy include 2% amitriptyline, 1% ketamine, and the combination of these two medications. Eutectic mixture of local anesthetics (EMLA) is a 1:1 mixture of prilocaine and lidocaine, which can penetrate the skin and produce local anesthesia. EMLA has been particularly helpful in postherpetic neuralgia and may help reduce the initial pain and burning that occurs with Capsaicin if EMLA is applied first.

Muscle Relaxants

Several different classes of medications have muscle relaxant properties. Spasmolytic agents such as baclofen, tizanidine, and benzodiazepines are useful for conditions that produce flexor and extensor spasms because of neural injury, as well as chronic muscle spasm. Several other agents also produce muscle relaxation without clear spasmolytic action; these include cyclobenzaprine, carisoprodol, methocarbamol, and chlorzoxazone. While there is evidence to support the short-term use of cyclobenzaprine, there are no controlled studies demonstrating clear efficacy for carisoprodol, methocarbamol, and chlorzoxazone as analgesic agents. Furthermore, they have the potential for abuse and should therefore be avoided.

INTERVENTIONAL PROCEDURES

Interventional procedures include infusions and local blocks with anesthetic agents, administration of epidural steroids, implantable drug delivery systems, and implantable neural stimulators. Anesthetic procedures have been a mainstay of pain management. Although there are many effective procedures for acute pain, evidence of efficacy for chronic pain procedures is somewhat more limited.

Anesthetic Infusions

Intravenous administration of local anesthetics such as lidocaine is sometimes useful in the diagnosis and treatment of neuropathic pain syndromes and for certain forms of vascular headache. The usual method is to infuse lidocaine at a rate of 5 mg/kg of body weight over 30 minutes in a monitored setting. The patient usually experiences relief of paresthesias and lancinating pain within 1 hour of the infusion; this relief can persist for several days.

Trigger Point Injections

Local injection of anesthetic into tender areas in muscle, referred to as trigger points, can provide temporary relief in acute and chronic soft-tissue pain. The main indication for these injections is myofascial pain. Considerable controversy exists as to which agents should be injected and how often.

Local Neural Blockade

Neural blockade is used principally for the relief of acute pain and for diagnostic purposes. Sequential blocks of individual nerves or spinal levels can help to pinpoint sites of pain generation, but they do not identify the specific disease state that may be producing the pain. Unlike neural blocks, which are reversible, neurolytic blocks (using agents such as phenol and absolute alcohol) destroy peripheral myelin causing an irreversible conduction **block.** Neurolytic blocks are reserved for the most intractable cases and for patients with a limited life expectancy. The risk of developing a deafferentation pain syndrome is high and increases over time.

Spinal Steroid Injections and Facet Injections

Local steroid injections into either the epidural space or the facet joints have been used in the treatment of mechanical neck and back pain. Although the indications remain controversial, epidural steroids are used in the management of acute or recurrent pain resulting from root irritation with clinical evidence of radicular dysfunction and in nonoperative spinal stenosis. Facet blocks are useful in patients with neck or back pain with a mechanical component but without radicular signs, presumably arising in the spinal column. There is persisting disagreement regarding the long-term benefit of steroid epidural injections. Some studies see moderate benefit and others find no change in the natural course of the disease with reference to functional impairment, need for surgery, or long-term pain relief. Lumbar facet injections do appear to give short- and long-term pain benefit.

Sympathetic Blockade

Sympathetic blockade may reduce pain involving the sympathetic nervous system and the viscera. Sympathetically maintained nociceptive input from the upper extremities, head, and neck can be blocked by infiltrating the stellate ganglion. Cardiac and thoracic visceral pain can be blocked by infiltrating the thoracic sympathetic paravertebral ganglia. The upper abdominal viscera are innervated by the celiac ganglion, whereas the urogenital viscera are supplied by the superior hypogastric plexus and the ganglion impar. Deep visceral pain can be relieved by blocking the appropriate location. The lumbar sympathetic ganglia are involved in mediating pain in the lower extremities.

Spinal Cord Stimulation

Generally, it is agreed that spinal cord stimulation (SCS) is effective in treating pain of neuropathic origin, particularly sympathetically mediated pain, visceral pain, and ischemic pain. It appears that SCS has no efficacy in acute pain or pain of nociceptive origin. SCS implantation is expensive and labor intensive. Because it usually requires surgical intervention, it should be reserved for patients who have failed more conservative therapies.

PHYSICAL MEDICINE AND REHABILITATIVE THERAPIES

A comprehensive approach to pain management incorporates the use of various physical modalities and rehabilitative therapies. Physical modalities include the therapeutic application of heat, cold, traction, transcutaneous electrical stimulation, acupuncture, and massage.

Heat

Application of heat to muscles or joints can provide analgesia, decrease muscle spasm, and increase flexibility. It also is very useful in decreasing acute pain in soft-tissue injuries and joint inflammation. Evidence suggests that pain relief is greater when heat is combined with exercise.

Cold

The application of cold has a local analgesic effect and reduces inflammatory responses and muscle spasm. There is some evidence that cold may produce pain relief faster than heat and may be more effective in acute pain.

Transcutaneous Electrical Nerve Stimulation

Transcutaneous electrical nerve stimulation (TENS) has been used for a variety of chronic pain conditions. It has demonstrated effectiveness in joint pain and acute pain, but little utility in back pain.

Massage

Massage is one of the oldest and most widely used techniques for decreasing acute and chronic pain. Many different massage techniques are used. The utility of massage seems to be greatest for short-term pain relief after acute injuries. No studies demonstrate that the benefits of massage in chronic low back or neck pain are any greater than those to be derived from rest and reeducation.

Exercise

Pain patients often develop decreased muscle strength, reduced range of motion, and general deconditioning, as well as other functional limitations. Exercise therapy can help overcome those deficits and also reduce pain. In addition to prescribed exercise, simple *aerobic exercises* such as walking and swimming should be part of chronic pain management. Both active and passive *Range of motion exercises* (ROM) can be useful in reducing pain in soft-tissue and joint injuries. It is important to begin with passive ROM and advance to active ROM so as not to overstretch injured tissues, which can decrease tensile strength. Muscle conditioning *exercises* are useful in increasing strength, endurance, and function. Such exercises are divided into isometric and dynamic forms. *Isometric exercise* involves muscle contraction without joint movement; it is used to increase muscle tone and strength in preparation for more vigorous exercise. *Dynamic exercise* is more vigorous and involves the repetitive contraction and relaxation of muscle groups with joint movement. It is the final step in strengthening muscle groups and involves gradually increasing resistance. Patients become discouraged if they focus on pain reduction, because initially exercise may increase pain. Therefore, setting specific functional goals rather than focusing on pain reduction is a key part of exercise therapy.

Acupuncture

In classical Chinese acupuncture, the practitioner attempts to restore energy (Qi) flow by applying treatment at points distributed along specific channels or meridians. Needling is the most common method of applying acupuncture, but heat, pressure, and electrical stimulation also have been used. Acupuncture produces an increase in endorphin release and modulates the firing of high-threshold, small-diameter nerve fibers. The Western approach to acupuncture is based on modulating these elements of pain transmission. Based on the evidence from several controlled studies, acupuncture appears to be effective in controlling the pain of osteoarthritis and fibromyalgia.

There is less evidence to support the effectiveness of acupuncture for neuropathic pain. Verum acupuncture (established points and meridians) and sham acupuncture (avoiding points and meridians) appear to have similar rates of efficacy.

Botulinum Toxin

When pain is directly linked to dystonia or muscle spasm, botulinum toxin (Botox A) has good efficacy and has become a standard treatment for focal dystonias over the past several years. In some cases, electromyographic (EMG) guidance is used to identify hyperactive muscles to be targeted in dystonia. It is not clear whether EMG-guided botox injection is superior to injection at local areas of spasm or tenderness. Effects usually are noticeable within 5 to 10 days after injection and may persist for as long as 3 months, at which point the treatment is repeated.

CHAPTER 95

Summary Author: Christopher A. Cavacuiti
Seddon R. Savage • Ryan Horvath

Opioid Therapy of Pain

Opioids are the most potent analgesic agents clinically available at this time. They have wide efficacy and utility in the treatment of acute and cancer-related pain and may be helpful as a component of the management of chronic nonmalignant pain in some patients. However, opioids may cause euphoria or "reward" in some individuals, which may lead to misuse and, in susceptible individuals, to addiction.

HISTORICAL PERSPECTIVES ON OPIOID USE

Opioids have been used by humans for millennia. There are Sumerian accounts of the use of opioids, the "plant of joy," >5,000 years ago. Theophrastus provides the first written account of the use of opium to relieve pain in 300 BC. In 1805, morphine was purified from opium, but its use did not become widespread until the development of the hypodermic syringe in 1853. By the early 1900s, both the appropriate therapeutic use and misuse of opioids were widespread in North America. In the United States, both the use and misuse of opioids continued to increase until the introduction of the 1970 Federal Controlled Substances Act, which further tightened regulation and required registration of providers. With the enhanced regulation, controlled substance designation, and the understanding of abuse potential of opioids, their use by physicians declined in the latter half of the 20th century. Resurgence in the use of opioids began in the late 20th century as treatment of pain became a higher priority and aggressive marketing of newer opioid formulations emerged.

PREVALENCE AND IMPACT OF PAIN

Pain is one of the most common ailments and is the second leading reason for patients to seek medical care. More than 80 million Americans report serious pain in any given year, and 86% of these have pain on a chronic basis. Pain is also the second leading cause of workplace absenteeism and accounts for an estimated $61.2 billion in lost productivity annually. With the enormous social and economic impact of pain on our society, adequate treatment is paramount.

PREVALENCE OF USE AND MISUSE OF PRESCRIPTION OPIOIDS

The therapeutic use of commonly prescribed opioids has increased dramatically recently, with prescriptions for fentanyl and oxycodone rising by 403% and 227%, respectively, between 1997 and 2002. At the same time, prescription opioid misuse has also risen, with increases of 642% and 347%, respectively, for patients presenting to emergency rooms with harm from fentanyl and oxycodone misuse. Available evidence suggests that misused opioids are often obtained from clinical sources, either directly from prescribers or through diversion of prescribed opioids. It is therefore critical that prescribing clinicians understand and employ clinical strategies to reduce the risk of inappropriate opioid prescribing and diversion.

THE ROLE OF OPIOIDS IN THE TREATMENT OF PAIN

Opioids are essential analgesic agents for the treatment of pain. For the treatment of acute postsurgical or trauma-induced pain, as well as cancer pain, opioid therapy is the gold standard of practice. However, there is less consensus regarding the role of opioids in the treatment of chronic noncancer pain. Although it is clear that opioids are an important component of care for some patients with chronic pain, not all patients benefit from opioids, and some are even made worse. Some of the challenges of using opioids to treat chronic pain patients include prescription drug abuse, addiction, adverse effects, tolerance, and drug interactions. More study is needed to understand what subpopulations of patients with chronic pain benefit from opioid therapy and what therapeutic variables are associated with success.

SPECIAL ISSUES IN THE USE OF OPIOIDS

Like other medications that are scheduled as controlled substances, opioids deserve special consideration for unintended consequences related to their capacity to provide reward and to produce dependence in some individuals. Specific issues include the potential for physical dependence, tolerance, reward, addiction and misuse or diversion for a variety of purposes. Each of these issues is considered separately here.

Physical Dependence

Using the term *addiction* to describe physical dependence is inaccurate. Physical dependence, as defined by a joint consensus statement of several pain and addictions professional organizations, is a state of adaptation that is manifested by a drug class–specific withdrawal syndrome that can be produced by abrupt cessation, rapid dose reduction, decreasing blood level of the drug, and/or administration of an antagonist. Such dependence is an expected occurrence in all patients (with and without addictive disease) after 2 to 10 days of continuous administration of an opioid. In an acute pain setting, dependence generally is not clinically significant, because individuals tend to taper opioids naturally owing to gradual reduction in pain as the acute problem.

Common symptoms of opioid withdrawal include autonomic signs and symptoms, such as diarrhea, piloerection, sweating, mydriasis, and mild increases in blood pressure and pulse, as well as signs of central nervous system arousal such as irritability, anxiety, and sleeplessness. Craving for the medication is expected in the course of withdrawal, and pain (most often experienced as abdominal cramping, deep bone pain, or myalgias) is common.

Tolerance

Tolerance is indicated by the need for increasing doses of a medication to achieve the initial effects of the drug. Tolerance may occur both to a drug's analgesic effects and to its unwanted side effects, such as respiratory depression, sedation, or nausea. Many characteristics of opioid tolerance remain poorly understood. Most investigators agree that absolute tolerance to the analgesic effects of opioids does not occur. That is, opioids may be used over a prolonged period of time in the face of increasing dose requirements and yet continue to provide relief of pain. However, in the context of chronic pain not associated with life-threatening illness, such dose escalation may become impractical owing to cost, side effects, or simply unrelenting requirements for dose escalation. In some cases, increasing pain in the absence of progressive pathology may be due not to opioid tolerance but to the related phenomenon of *opioid-induced hyperalgesia*. In some cases, gradual reduction or elimination of opioids appears to improve pain. There is increasing consensus that very high dose requirements in persons with chronic nonmalignant pain may signal the evolving failure of opioid therapy. It has been suggested on an empirical basis that about 180 mg morphine equivalents per day be considered a point of likely diminishing returns. In one study of 801 primary care patients with chronic pain, quality of life was generally best for patients on between 20 and 40 mg of opioid per day compared with those on no opioids or on high-dose therapy.

Reward

Opioids produce reward in many, though not all, individuals. Some persons, in fact, experience dysphoria or no mood changes in association with opioid use. A clear understanding of the potential issues that may modulate reward experiences when opioids are used for analgesia may be helpful to optimize clinical management strategies, particularly in persons at risk for substance misuse.

Mechanisms of Reward Opioids produce reward by binding to GABAergic interneurons that normally inhibit dopamine production in the limbic reward system. The resulting increase in dopamine and cascade of secondary effects produce feelings of reward or euphoria. Reward may or may not occur in different individuals along with analgesia when opioids are used for pain and is not itself harmful.

Factors Affecting Reward

Rate of Increase Reward increases when the rate of rise in drug blood levels increases: the faster the onset, the better the rush or high. For this reason, smoking or intravenous use of opioids (which have the fastest onset of action) will produce more reward than intramuscular and subcutaneous administration (which has an intermediate onset of action). Oral use of opioids (which has the slowest onset of action) produces the least reward. Similarly, opioids with an inherently slower time to peak effect (such as methadone or levorphanol) produce weaker reward effects than opioids with relatively rapid onset.

Peak Blood Level Attained The higher the opioid blood level relative to the individual's tolerance for the drug, the greater the reward. A dose of an opioid given intravenously achieves a higher peak blood level than the same dose administered by the oral route, with subcutaneous and intramuscular again intermediate.

Receptor Effects μ-Opioid agonists are more likely to cause reward than κ-opioid agonists.

Interference of Pain with Reward Some research suggests that people feel less euphoria if they are in pain when given opioids.

Addiction

In the context of pain treatment with opioids, addiction must be defined through the observation of a constellation of maladaptive behaviors rather than by observation of pharmacologic phenomena such as dependence, tolerance, and dose escalation. Addiction in the context of opioid therapy for pain is characterized by the presence of a combination of observations suggesting adverse consequences due to use of the drugs, loss of control over drug use, and preoccupation with obtaining opioids despite the presence of adequate analgesia. Table 95.1 outlines some of the challenges practitioners face when using current *DSM-IV* criteria to diagnose opioid addiction in pain patients. Existing studies have shown tremendous discrepancies in terms of the risk of developing addiction to opioids in the course of opioid therapy for pain. The prevalence of identified misuse of opioids by patients ranges widely in different studies, between 1% and 38%. These discrepancies can be explained in part by the challenges of diagnosing addiction in the context of chronic pain, as well as by variations in methodology, operative definitions, and quality.

The etiology of addiction in the context of pain treatment likely involves an interplay of biogenetic vulnerability, drug reward effects, and other host and environmental factors including the presence of pain, of stress, and of the psychosocial context of use. The lifetime prevalence of any form of substance dependence (addiction),

TABLE 95.1	**Limitations of Current *DSM-IV* Criteria for Identifying Addiction in Pain Patients**
DSM-IV substance dependence criteria (Reason not specific for addiction)	**Challenges in using criteria to diagnose addiction in opioid analgesia**
Tolerance	Expected with prolonged analgesic use
Physical dependence/withdrawal	Expected with prolonged regular analgesic use
Used in greater amounts or longer than intended	Emergence of pain may demand increased dose or prolonged use.
Unsuccessful attempts to cut down or discontinue	Emergence of pain may deter dose taper or cessation.
Much time spent pursuing or recovering from use	Difficulty finding pain treatment may drive time spent pursuing analgesics. Time spent recovering from overuse is suggestive of addiction.
Important activities reduced or given up	Valid criteria—activity engagement expected to increase not decline with pain treatment
Continued use despite knowledge of persistent physical or psychologic harm	Valid criteria—no harm anticipated from analgesic opioid use for pain

TABLE 95.2	Definition and Indicators of Addiction in Pain Patients

Addiction

American Society of Addiction Medicine, American Pain Society, American Academy of Pain Medicine

A primary, chronic, neurobiologic disease with genetic, psychosocial, and environmental factors influencing its development and manifestations characterized by behaviors that include one or more of the following:

ASAM-APS-AAPM Behavioral criteria	Examples of specific behaviors in opioid therapy for pain
Impaired control over use, compulsive use	Frequent loss/theft reported, calls for early renewals, withdrawal noted at appointments
Continued use despite harm due to use	Declining function, intoxication, persistent oversedation
Preoccupation with use, craving	Nonopioid interventions ignored, opioids only intervention considered, recurrent requests for opioid increase/complaints of increasing pain in absence of disease progression despite titration[a]

[a]May reflect tolerance or hyperalgesia.

ASAM, American Society of Addiction Medicine; APS, American Pain Society; AAPM, American Academy of Pain Medicine.

exclusive of tobacco, is estimated at 3% to 16% of the general population. Therefore, it is not unreasonable to expect that somewhere between 3% to 16% of patients given opioids for pain are at higher risk for the development of addiction. It is appropriate to use special care in implementing opioid therapy in patients who have personal or family histories of alcoholism or other addictions. Opioids should not generally be withheld out of fear of addiction when they are indicated for the relief of pain, but the structure of care may be adapted to reduce risks. Table 95.2 provides some examples and indicators of addictive behaviors that may be seen in pain patients. When addiction is identified in the course of opioid therapy for pain, it is important to address it aggressively, so that the pain is effectively controlled and to prevent the debilitating sequelae of addiction.

Differential Diagnosis of Opioid Misuse

Patients misuse opioids for a variety of reasons with a wide range of implications (Table 95.3). It is important to distinguish clinically between different causes of opioid misuse in order to address each case appropriately. Some patients exhibit distress and engage in behaviors aimed at obtaining more medication because their pain treatment is inadequate. The term *pseudoaddiction* has emerged in the pain literature to describe the inaccurate interpretation of these behaviors in patients who have severe pain that is undermedicated or whose pain otherwise has not been effectively treated. Pseudoaddictive behavior can be distinguished from addiction by the fact that when adequate analgesia is achieved, the patient who is seeking pain relief demonstrates improved function, uses the medications as prescribed, and does not use drugs in a manner that persistently causes sedation or euphoria.

TABLE 95.3	Differential Diagnosis Misuse of Analgesic Opioids

Misunderstanding of instructions
Self-medication of
- Mood/stress
- Sleep
- Disturbing memories
- Undertreated pain
- Other

Elective use for reward or euphoria
Compulsive use due to addiction
Diversion for profit

CLINICAL MANAGEMENT VARIABLES IN THE USE OF OPIOIDS

A number of variables must be considered in planning opioid therapy for pain; these include drug selection, dose titration and scheduling, and management of side effects. It also is clinically important to understand how to appropriately change drugs or withdraw medications when indicated.

Drug Selection

Pure μ agonists, including medications such as morphine, oxycodone, hydromorphone, and fentanyl, have no ceiling analgesic effect and may be titrated as needed to achieve analgesia. Tolerance to side effects generally occurs more rapidly than tolerance to analgesia, though monitoring for respiratory depression is important, especially in opioid-naive individuals, as doses are increased or specific opioids are changed. *Meperidine's* usefulness in pain treatment is limited by its short half-life and because, with high dose use, a neurotoxic metabolite—normeperidine—may accumulate, causing irritability, tremors and, potentially, seizures. *Methadone* differs from other μ agonists in several ways. It has a long and unpredictable elimination half-life (5–130 hours) that necessitates especially careful titration. Methadone has been associated with prolonged QT intervals and cardiac arrhythmias at higher doses. Its dextro-isomer has *N*-methyl-D-aspartate (NMDA) receptor antagonist activity, and it has been suggested that this may result in less tolerance than that occurs with other μ opioids and in greater efficacy in treating neuropathic pain. Incomplete cross-tolerance between methadone and other μ opioid agonists requires the use of a much lower than equianalgesic dose of methadone in the patient who is transitioning from other μ agonists.

Agonist-antagonist—or κ agonist—opioids, including pentazocine, nalbuphine, and butorphanol, have predominantly κ agonist effects while antagonizing the μ receptor. Agonist-antagonist drugs are widely regarded as having less potential for abuse and addiction than the pure opioid agonists, though addiction to these medications has been observed. Their clinical usefulness as analgesics is limited by a number of factors. The agonist-antagonist drugs exhibit a ceiling effect in terms of analgesia. Their use sometimes is associated with dysphoric reactions. Because of their μ antagonist activity, they may reverse analgesia and precipitate withdrawal in individuals who are physically dependent on μ agonists.

Partial μ agonists, including buprenorphine and tramadol, provide analgesia via μ opioid receptors but have relatively low intrinsic efficacy (i.e., they bind μ opioid receptors with high affinity but produce reduced receptor activation compared to full μ agonists). As with the agonist-antagonist/κ agonist drugs described above, partial agonists are thought to possess less potential for abuse and addiction than the pure opioid agonists, though addiction to these medications has been observed. While tramadol is licensed for use as an analgesic in the United States, buprenorphine's use for analgesia is an off-label use.

Routes of Administration

Opioids may be administered orally, rectally, transmucosally, intravenously, subcutaneously, transdermally, and intraspinally. The oral, enteral, transmucosal or transdermal routes generally are preferred when feasible because they are less invasive than many other routes and usually provide satisfactory analgesia, even when high doses are required. Parenteral routes increase both speed of onset and peak blood levels obtained, which not only may be favorable in terms of analgesia but also may increase reward.

Dose Titration and Scheduling

Measuring Efficacy The serial use of a pain scale, such as a numerical 0 to 10 rating scale or a visual faces scale indicating variable levels of distress before treatment and at regular intervals during treatment, is helpful in assessing pain and its response to treatment. It is often helpful to inquire about worst pain, best pain, and typical levels, as well as to document function and quality of life. When assessing a patient on opioids, the "6 A's" can be a useful mnemonic for remembering important elements of a chronic pain history. The "6 A's" are: **A**dherence, **A**nalgesia, **A**buse/**A**ddiction, **A**dverse Effects, **A**berrant behavior, **A**ctivities of Daily Living.

Dose Requirements and Scheduling Considerations Several factors must be considered in determining the dose and interval of administration that will provide effective analgesia in a given patient for a given problem. The pharmacologic characteristics of each drug (onset, relative potency, and duration of analgesic, etc.) as well as the marked variability among patients in intrinsic responsiveness to opioids must be appreciated and accommodated.

Long- Versus Short-Acting Medications and Scheduled Versus As-Needed When patients have persistent pain on an around-the clock basis, longer-acting medications may offer several advantages. They provide relatively stable drug blood levels and, therefore, more consistent analgesia than frequent doses of short-acting medications. Fewer peaks and valleys may result in fewer side effects, including less reward. It is important to be aware that most controlled-release opioids can be altered to become immediate-release drugs through chewing, crushing, snorting, or extracting and injecting. There are several issues that should be considered regarding the use of short-acting opioids, particularly in prescribing for individuals with, or at risk for, substance misuse. First, pairing the perception of pain with the administration of a rewarding, and therefore potentially reinforcing, drug can theoretically reinforce the perception of pain and lead to increased use of the drug and increasing distress. Second, the frequent use of short-acting medications several times a day is thought to result in "on-off effects" as blood levels peak and trough, resulting in alternating analgesia and incipient withdrawal. In the chronic noncancer pain setting, when long-acting opioids are used for continuous baseline pain, some clinicians prefer that patients manage the daily ups and downs of pain with activity pacing and use of nonopioid interventions (heat, ice, stretch, relaxation, etc.) to prevent or address mild exacerbations, rather than using frequent doses of prn short-acting opioid medications.

Enhancing Compliance and Control of Medication Use Strategies include (a) giving specific times for drug administration (i.e., 7 a.m., 3 p.m., 11 p.m. rather than "TID"), (b) having a "trusted other" (such as a visiting nurse, partner, or friend) dispense the medications and do pill/dosage counts, and (c) daily or other short-interval dispensing.

Management of Opioid Side Effects

Opioid side effects can be considered in two groups: side effects of acute and long-term opioid use.

Acute Use Side Effects Respiratory depression is a potentially fatal side effect of opioid administration and is a persistent concern throughout treatment when doses are increased, opioids are changed, or other medications are added. Significant sedation most often is a precursor to respiratory depression and may signal a need to hold medication and adjust the dose. Special care also should be exercised in titrating opioids with long half-lives, such as methadone or levorphanol, because delayed respiratory depression may occur. An opioid antagonist such as naloxone should be used only in emergency situations owing to the risk of inducing acute abstinence syndrome. Other common physical side effects of opioid use include constipation, nausea and vomiting, urinary retention, pruritus, and myoclonus. Persistent physical side effects may be managed through pharmacologic treatments, such as antiemetics for nausea or antihistamines for pruritus. Constipation in particular is a common and persistent side effect of opioid use that may not resolve without treatment. When long-term and/or high-dose use of opioids is anticipated, introduction of constipation treatment on a preemptive basis is recommended. Central nervous system (CNS) side effects of opioids may include sedation, cognitive dysfunction, and affective changes.

Long-Term Use Side Effects Side effects of long-term opioid use include persisting risk of respiratory depression and constipation (as discussed earlier) as well as the potential for hyperalgesia, hormonal imbalance, and immunomodulation. Androgen/estrogen deficiency and osteoporosis have been described in patients receiving long-term opioids. Given the current debate concerning the long-term risk of hormone replacement, sex hormone supplementation is controversial. Numerous studies both in animals and humans have suggested that opioids have immunosuppressive effects. More research is needed to elaborate the clinical significance of this finding.

Changing Opioids Transition from one opioid or form of opioid to another may be indicated in a number of circumstances (e.g., when unrelenting tolerance occurs to a specific opioid with loss of analgesic efficacy, when a patient on chronic oral opioids becomes NPO, or when significant side effects occur and persist). Opioid rotation often results in improved analgesia, sometimes on a significantly lower equivalent dose of the new opioid. When changing from one opioid to another, it is important to understand how to calculate equianalgesic doses of medications and how to modify doses appropriately.

Management of Withdrawal In the acute pain setting, most patients gradually taper their medications without incident as pain gradually improves. However, particularly in the setting of chronic pain and long-term opioid use, tapering sometimes is impeded by withdrawal or craving that occurs during troughs in blood levels. The goal when tapering an individual who is physically dependent on medications is to provide stable but decreasing blood levels of opioid so as to prevent precipitous troughs. Some patients may benefit from having their medications dispensed daily or dose by dose while tapering in order to assist in controlling use as the dose is decreasing.

CLINICAL PAIN MANAGEMENT

Acute Pain

Individuals with addictive disease often experience particularly high levels of anxiety in association with the stress of trauma, illness, or surgery, because they fear that their pain will not be adequately managed; this, in turn, can exacerbate how they experience and react to pain.

Address the Addiction Disorder An open and nonjudgmental approach to the discussion of substance use concerns may help to facilitate information exchange with patients regarding their use. When addiction is understood as a medical disorder, it becomes easier to address it in the same manner as any other medical condition, with respectful, but matter-of-fact, concern. Addiction treatment should be offered when addiction is detected in the course of pain treatment. Many clinicians and individuals in recovery believe that exposure to opioids, sedative hypnotics, or anesthetics may lead to relapse. However, the distress of inadequately treated physical pain may pose an even greater risk of relapse. Effective pain treatment, coupled with an active addiction recovery program, is the best support for continued recovery during periods of acute stress, including periods of pain.

Prevent or Treat Withdrawal It is permissible, under the U.S. Controlled Substances Act, for a treating physician to provide opioids to prevent withdrawal in opioid dependent inpatients who are hospitalized for a diagnosis other than addiction. Though opioids for pain treatment can be continued after discharge, opioids cannot be provided for treatment of addiction after discharge, except from a licensed addiction treatment program (methadone treatment) or from a certified buprenorphine provider.

Include the Patient in Clinical Decision Making It is often helpful to include the individual in pain in the decision-making process regarding medication choices, dosing, and scheduling. This provides the patient with a sense of control and allays anxiety as to whether pain will be adequately treated.

Provide Effective Pain Relief In the acute pain setting, analgesics should be provided in an effective and timely manner. Without adequate control of acute pain, it is unlikely that the patient will be able to engage in addiction treatment. Undertreatment of pain also may create craving for pain-relieving medications as well as anxiety, frustration, anger, and other feelings that tend to feed addiction. Most patients will naturally taper their medications as the cause of acute pain resolves. Some patients with addiction disorders benefit from the negotiation of a structured tapering of medications on a scheduled basis.

Accommodate Preexisting Opioid Dependence

Patients Receiving Chronic Methadone For Pain or Addiction Individuals who are physically dependent on opioids that are prescribed for pain or for addiction or who are dependent on street opioids must have their baseline opioid requirements met in addition to receiving additional opioids required for acute pain treatment. Most often, a patient receiving methadone treatment of addiction should be continued on his or her baseline methadone dose as an inpatient and provided a different opioid for acute pain, rather than being entirely switched to an alternative opioid or having the methadone increased for pain.

Buprenorphine-Maintained Patients Understanding of the analgesic properties of buprenorphine is still in evolution. Buprenorphine binds avidly to opioid receptors and thus tends to block the action of other analgesic opioids provided for pain. Thus, it is difficult, though not impossible, to obtain analgesia by adding another opioid. When acute pain is predicted, such as after elective surgery, in persons on buprenorphine, it is often advisable to discontinue buprenorphine a few days before surgery. Carefully dosed methadone can be added if needed if significant withdrawal symptoms or craving emerge.

If acute pain occurs unexpectedly, such as after an accident or with an acute illness, in a patient on buprenorphine and opioids are required to relieve pain, μ opioids can usually be aggressively titrated to higher doses to overcome the buprenorphine blockade, but close supervision of the patient is critical to safety. Alternatively, if a patient is on a low maintenance dose of buprenorphine (such as 2–8 mg per day), sometimes the daily dose of buprenorphine can be increased and given at 6-hour intervals to control pain.

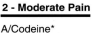

WHO Step Ladder
Cancer Pain Treatment*
*Modified by author for
treatment in addiction*

3- Severe Pain

Morphine
Hydromorphone
Methadone
Levorphanol
Fentanyl
Oxycodone
Continue:
- ASA
- Acetaminophen
- NSAID
Co-analgesics as needed:
- For neuropathic pain
- For other symptoms
Procedures as needed

2 - Moderate Pain

A/Codeine*
A/Hydrocodone*
A/Oxycodone*
Tramadol
Co-analgesics as needed:
- For neuropathic pain
- For other symptoms

*Consider low dose long-acting pure
mu opioid as alternative, with added
ASA, NSAID or acetaminophen*

1 - Mild Pain

ASA
Acetaminophen
NSAIDs
Co-analgesics as needed:
- For neuropathic pain
- For other symptoms

Address addiction recovery   Address addiction recovery   Address addiction recovery

FIGURE 95.1   WHO step ladder for cancer pain treatment.

Document the Pain Treatment Plan It is important to be clear in communicating the treatment plan to all staff involved in caring for the patient. Stigma and misunderstanding regarding addiction disorders are widespread among health care personnel, and these may lead to inadequate pain management when the primary treating clinician is not available and the plan is not clearly documented.

When Pain Persists Beyond Apparent Healing Particularly in the patient with an addiction disorder, continuing complaints of pain may lead to concern that the patient is reflecting behaviors of addiction or relapse to addiction. However, it is important to methodically consider other possible explanations before concluding that this is the case. First, the patient may have an undetected physical problem, related either to the original painful problem or to a separate process. Second, the patient may be physically dependent on analgesic medications and may be experiencing pain related to withdrawal as the medication is discontinued. A third reason that a patient may continue to seek to continue opioids when the underlying pain condition has resolved is that the medications may be ameliorating nonpain symptoms, such as sleep disturbance, intrusive memories, anxiety, or depression. If taper is not possible because of persistent craving or if relapsing use occurs, initiation of opioid agonist therapy for the underlying addiction may be appropriate. Occasional persons may feign pain in order to divert medications for sale, for personal use, or to share with a family member or friend whose therapeutic needs have not been met. It is appropriate to discontinue opioids if an individual is noted to be diverting medications.

Cancer-Related Pain Cancer may occur somewhat more frequently in individuals with addiction disorders than in the general population, probably because of pathologic effects of many substances of abuse, including tobacco and alcohol. Opioids never should be withheld when they are needed for effective pain relief because of concerns regarding the development or perpetuation of addiction. It may, however, be appropriate to have tighter boundaries for patients at high risk for opioid dependence. Such boundaries might include daily dispensing or dispensing by a "trusted other" (such as a visiting nurse, family member, or friend). The "therapeutic ladder" developed by the World Health Organization (WHO) is an accepted model for the treatment of pain in cancer patients, including those with addiction disorders (Fig. 95.1).

Chronic NonCancer-Related Pain Active addiction disorders often have sequelae similar to those of chronic pain. Therefore, when chronic pain and addiction co-occur, they may reinforce one another (Fig. 95.2), and it is important to address each of these conditions. In persons with substance use disorders, the safe and effective long-term use of opioids is challenging and demands a careful balancing of potential risks and benefits, tailored to those individuals.

Universal Precautions in Opioid Therapy for Chronic Pain

Some experts suggest that when opioids are required as a component of chronic pain treatment, a set of universal precautions be used in managing all patients. This concept is predicated on the idea that the risk of an individual

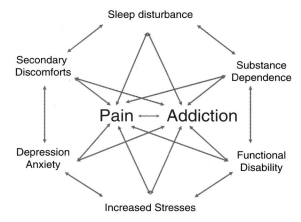

FIGURE 95.2 Synergy of pain and addiction.

patient's misusing opioids cannot be reliably predicted and that the misuse of opioids has potentially seriously negative consequences for both the patient and the prescriber. In addition, application of precautions only to selected patients believed to be at higher risk can result in stigmatizing those patients. For these reasons, it has been suggested that *all* pain patients be assessed in terms of the following:

- A comprehensive pain assessment
- Screen for psychologic and substance use issues.
- Formulate a differential diagnosis of pain.
- Obtain informed consent for treatment.
- Reach and document a clear treatment agreement.
- Set up a trial treatment period with clear goals.
- Assess and periodically reassess of pain level function and salient other issues.
- Document care thoroughly.
- Urine toxicology is increasingly a part of routine supervision of *all* patients on opioid medications.

Risk Assessment There is agreement among most clinical experts and regulatory boards that it is important to screen patients for risk of opioid misuse before initiating long-term opioids in the chronic pain setting. Common screening tools include the *C*utting down, *A*nnoyance by criticism, *G*uilty feeling, and *E*ye-openers (CAGE), and Drug Abuse Screening Test (DAST). In terms of screens specifically aimed at assessing risk of medication misuse in the pain treatment, one promising screen is the Screener and Opioid Assessment for Patients in Pain (SOAPP), which has been validated as a 14- and 20-question screen. Another is the five-question Opioid Risk Tool (ORT) screen.

Adapting the Structure of Opioid Therapy to Match Risks When an increased risk of opioid misuse is perceived, it may be helpful to individualize and tighten the structure of clinical care beyond universal precaution.

Setting of Care Some patients with pain are best managed in a primary care setting; some in a primary care setting with support from specialists; and some by a specialist with specific skills in an area of need, such as a pain specialist, addiction specialist, or psychiatrist. Primary care providers tend to have broader and more longitudinal knowledge of the patient and are in a better position to integrate care of pain with care of other medical issues. Specialists may have particular knowledge and expertise in management of specific aspects of the patient's medical issues and may provide better care when a particular problem such as addiction or psychiatric instability is prominent.

Selection of Treatment The selection of pain treatments, as with that of most medical treatments, is usually based on determination of which are likely to have the most benefit for the patient with the least risk. Clinicians may consider selecting more invasive or expensive treatments earlier in the course of treatment than with a lower-risk patient in whom a trial of opioids would generally be a prerequisite.

Supply of Medications The *amount* of opioid medications available to the patient and the *frequency* with which they are dispensed are two variables that can be controlled. In current practice, it is common for patients to receive a month's supply of analgesic opioids, and some clinicians provide stable patients who have no detected risks with up to a 3-month supply. In persons with addiction disorders or those who tend to overuse medications for other reasons, however, it is often prudent to dispense smaller quantities of medications more frequently, sometimes weekly or even daily.

Supports for Recovery Many persons with recovering addiction disorders who require opioids for pain treatment benefit from active cultivation of their recovery.

Supervision of Care Patients who receive opioid therapy for pain should be seen by their prescribing clinician on a regular basis to monitor pain, functional status, mood, use of medications, and general well-being. Unstable patients or those with more complex problems need to be seen more often. Typical intervals for visits vary between once a week and once every 3 months. Urine drug screens are increasingly routine as part of supervision of all patients using opioids on a long-term basis in order to document use of the prescribed medication and to identify use of illicit or nonprescribed substances. Pill counts are another supervision strategy employed by many physicians to promote adherence to the prescribed medication regimen.

Discontinuation of Opioid Therapy If opioid therapy does not continue to achieve its goals of improved pain, stable or improving function, and enhanced quality of life; if therapy cannot be structured to maintain safety of the patient owing to addictive use; if other concerns such as medications diversion are documented; or if pain resolves, it is sometimes necessary to discontinue opioid treatment. Having a written treatment agreement at the outset of care in order to clarify the conditions under which opioids will be discontinued is enormously helpful when it is necessary to discontinue treatment.

CONCLUSIONS

Opioids have an important role in relieving human suffering. At the same time, it is important to respect their potential to cause harm in vulnerable individuals. In order to use opioids effectively and safely when they are indicated, physicians must understand pharmacologic and clinical issues related to opioids and carefully structure treatment with respect to the particular benefits and risks for individual patients.

96

Summary Author: Christopher A. Cavacuiti
Aaron M. Gilson • Martha A. Maurer

Legal and Regulatory Considerations in Pain Management

Concerns about opioid side effects, adverse events, and abuse, addiction, and diversion have led to restrictions that have at times marginalized their medical use. This is especially true for patients with pain who also have a substance abuse history or use drugs for nontherapeutic purposes. Although treating noncancer pain with opioids continues to be controversial, currently accepted medical practice standards support practitioners assessing patients' pain during the initial evaluation and monitoring their pain and functioning during treatment to determine whether opioids are, and remain, an effective therapeutic option. Such standards often can be found in states' laws, regulations, and guidelines governing drug control and professional practice.

For the purpose of this chapter, a *law* is defined as a rule of conduct with binding legal force adopted by a legislative or other government body. A number of laws have been adopted concerning pain management, with Intractable Pain Treatment Acts (IPTAs) being the most common form of statutory pain policy.

A *regulation* is an official rule issued by an agency. An *agency* is a regulatory body that has been given statutory authority dictate what conduct is or is not acceptable for those regulated by the agency (such as physicians, pharmacists, and nurses). This authority is typically granted by the executive branch of government. Regulations have the force of law.

Guideline, as used here, means an official adopted policy statement that is issued by a government or other regulatory agency, to express its attitude or position on a particular matter. Although guidelines do not have binding legal force, they may outline parameters or standards of conduct for those who are regulated by an agency.

INTERNATIONAL POLICIES

Although the control of diversion and the prevention of illicit drug use typically are perceived as the singular purpose of drug control policy, these policies also have a second and equally important purpose, which is to ensure drug availability; this medicolegal concept is referred to as "Balance." According to international treaty, opioids are necessary for pain relief and must be adequately available for medical purposes.

FEDERAL POLICIES

The U.S. Food and Drug Administration (FDA), according to authority granted to that agency by the federal Food, Drug and Cosmetic Act of 1962, ensures that all drugs, including prescription opioid analgesics, are both safe and effective for human use under medical supervision.

The Controlled Substances Act (CSA) is a federal law that establishes the US drug control system, and is intended to achieve both control and availability of controlled substances by paralleling international treaties. To prevent diversion, the CSA establishes a system of security, record keeping, and monitoring requirements, as well as penalties (both civil and criminal) for violating these requirements. The U.S. Drug Enforcement Administration (DEA) is the agency that administers the Code of Federal Regulations, which is the set of regulations that implements the federal CSA. All persons or business entities that manufacture, order, prescribe, or dispense controlled substances must be registered with the DEA.

CSA Drug Schedules

The CSA classifies controlled substances into five schedules, according to established medical usefulness and relative abuse liability. Each schedule carries a different penalty for unlawful use. Prescription requirements also vary depending on the schedule of medication prescribed. Schedule I contains the drugs that have no accepted medical use and are available only for scientific research (such as marijuana, methaqualone, and heroin). Schedules II through V contain drugs that are FDA-approved for medical use but have an abuse potential, such as opioid analgesics. Medications are placed in a specific schedule based on their abuse potential. Medications considered by the government to have the highest potential for abuse are placed in Schedule II. Schedule V drugs have the lowest abuse potential.

Federal Laws Related to Opioid Prescribing

The DEA monitors all transfers of controlled substances within a "closed distribution system." Prescriptions for Schedule II drugs must be in written form and cannot be refilled, whereas five refills are permitted for drugs in Schedules III and IV. A recent addition to federal regulations permits the issuance of multiple prescriptions for Schedule II drugs, written with "do not fill until" instructions, which can be issued sequentially. Federal law allows oral prescriptions for Schedule II controlled substances in medical emergencies, but these must be followed with a written prescription within a specified period. Federal laws and regulations do not limit, nor have they ever limited, the amount of drug prescribed, the duration for which a drug is prescribed, or the period for which a prescription is valid (although some states do).

The CSA does not permit practitioners to prescribe Schedule II opioids for the purpose of maintenance or detoxification treatment of narcotic addiction. When practitioners have a separate federal registration as an Opioid Treatment Program (OTP), they are allowed to dispense, but not prescribe, narcotic drugs approved for this purpose, such as methadone and buprenorphine, and must comply with federal and state regulations. It is important to note that methadone can be prescribed and dispensed to treat pain, just as one would prescribe any other Schedule II opioid analgesic.

The Drug Addiction Treatment Act of 2000 permits physicians to receive a waiver from these rules, so that they can use specifically approved medications for the treatment of opioid addiction. To date, only sublingual buprenorphine (a Schedule III medication) is approved for this purpose.

STATE POLICIES

Many aspects of medical practice are regulated at the state, not the federal, level. Therefore numerous state laws, regulations, and guidelines can further limit medical practice using controlled substances. State policies may vary considerably from international and federal policies. Many state laws do not recognize the value of controlled medications to the public health, as does the federal law. Furthermore, many restrictive state policy provisions date back 30 years or more and appear to have been based on outdated concepts of addiction and the side effects of opioid analgesics. As a result, state laws, regulations, and guidelines/policy statements may unduly limit prescribing and dispensing of controlled substances, and such requirements or restrictions must be considered when making patient care decisions.

The law provides state health care agencies the authority to license and discipline members of their respective professions, by creating oversight boards, such as medical, pharmacy, and nursing boards. All licensing boards have national organizations: the Federation of State Medical Boards of the United States (FSMB) for medical boards, the National Association of Boards of Pharmacy for pharmacy boards, and the National Council of State Boards of Nursing for nursing boards.

State Prescription Monitoring Programs (PMPs)

Numerous states have laws that establish PMPs. At this writing, 36 states have adopted laws that require using an electronic data transfer system to monitor prescriptions for controlled substances. In the past, PMPs have been limited to medications in Schedule II, but newer programs monitor drugs in other schedules as well. Generally, these programs enable prescribers to quickly determine whether their patients are "multisourcing" (i.e., obtaining controlled substances from multiple providers). Monitoring multiple drug schedules would seem to take the regulatory focus off of Schedule II medications, which research has shown can often motivate practitioners to prescribe lower scheduled medications to avoid being monitored (and has been termed a substitution effect). Current PMPs typically are administered by state health agencies (such as the Pharmacy Board), rather than law enforcement agencies, and the policies that implement the programs often emphasize that this effort to reduce abuse and diversion should not interfere with appropriate patient care. In the past, several states required a government-issued serialized prescription form for controlled substances; however, only Texas still requires an official form for Schedule II medications.

Legislative and Regulatory Definitions of Addiction

Accurately using terminology is central to shaping a balanced policy on drug control, especially in the United States where prescribing opioids to maintain addiction is illegal. Unfortunately, the use and definition of addiction-related terminology remains as much a point of confusion for licensing boards and enforcement authorities as for others in the field. Historically, "addiction" has been synonymous with physical dependence, as indicated by the presence of a withdrawal syndrome. In the past, this has led to numerous patients with chronic pain being admitted to methadone treatment programs primarily or exclusively to obtain analgesia. Fortunately, there has been a growing recognition among licensing boards and enforcement authorities that they must make the distinction between physical dependence and compulsive use despite harm (which is the sine qua non of addiction). The possibility that patients could be admitted to addiction treatment programs only for chronic pain management was minimized when federal regulations governing addiction treatment were modified in 2003. The admission criteria for OTPs now incorporate accepted and updated medical criteria for addiction. However, many states' laws and regulations continue to contain imprecise terminology that could legally label patients who are using opioids to treat their pain as persons with an addictive disease (based on the presence of physical dependence).

Intractable Pain Treatment Acts

Since 1989, a number of state legislatures have adopted IPTAs. Although these policies were designed to reduce physicians' concerns about regulatory scrutiny, they may also unduly restrict physician prescribing and patient access to opioid analgesics. The underlying implication of many IPTAs is that prescribing opioids for chronic pain is outside generally accepted medical practice and should only occur in exceptional circumstances and within the (often narrow) parameters of an IPTA. Further, limiting the use of opioids only to patients for whom other efforts have failed seems to relegate them as a treatment of last resort, even when the patient initially presents with severe pain.

Because many IPTAs have excluded the use of opioids in addiction, such laws also can unintentionally exclude patients with an addictive disease *and* chronic pain from pain management. These provisions appear to conflict with federal policy, which prohibits physicians from prescribing narcotic drugs only for the *purpose* of maintaining narcotic addiction, but does not prohibit prescribing opioids to *persons* who have both pain and an addictive disease.

Model Medical Regulatory Policies to Address the Perceived Threat of Scrutiny

IPTAs were created as a mechanism to protect from regulatory discipline health care professionals who prescribe opioids to treat chronic pain. The perception that practitioners need such protection stemmed from a number of articles reporting physicians' reluctance to prescribe opioid analgesics because of concern about being investigated by a regulatory agency. According to a 1991 survey of American Pain Society's physician members, 40% of members agreed that legal concerns influenced their prescribing of opioids for chronic noncancer pain.

While there have been some improvements since 1991 in terms of physician confidence in using opioids, many physicians continue to be very concerned about the use of opioids—particularly patients with documented drug abuse histories and particularly in the setting of chronic noncancer pain. A 2004 survey of all state medical board members showed that board members continued to be least confident when considering prolonged opioid prescribing to a patient with chronic noncancer pain who also had a documented drug abuse history, with only 21% considering it lawful and acceptable medical practice. Thus, physicians prescribing controlled substances to patients with a prior addiction should be aware that members of their state medical board may subject this practice to heightened scrutiny, and should therefore structure their practice accordingly (e.g., consider appropriate consultation or referral, consider treatment agreements, and thoroughly document rationale for treatment decisions).

In 1998, the FSMB adopted a document entitled "Model Guidelines for the Use of Controlled Substances for the Treatment of Pain" (Model Guidelines) to directly address physicians' concern about regulatory scrutiny and to promote positive state medical board pain policy and greater consistency between the states' policies. The Model Guidelines stated that opioid analgesics may be necessary for the treatment of pain, including pain associated with acute, cancer, and noncancer conditions. If state medical boards adopt this policy, the positive language would communicate to medical professionals that their licensing board recognizes the health benefits of using controlled substances as a part of legitimate medical practice. Another important advantage of the Model Guidelines was that unambiguous definitions of addiction-related terminology were included. Definitions that conformed to accepted clinical and scientific knowledge were provided for *addiction, physical dependence, tolerance*, and *pseudoaddiction*. Finally, the Model Guidelines did not exclude patients with addictive disease from being treated for pain with opioids. In May 2004, the FSMB revised the Model Guidelines, entitled "Model Policy for the Use of Controlled Substances for the Treatment of Pain" (Model Policy). The Model Policy contains substantially the same messages as the 1998 guidelines but also includes language recognizing that physicians' failure to take action to adequately treat pain is a departure from current practice standards and subject to investigation and discipline. At this writing, 32 states have health care regulatory board policies that are based, either in whole or in part, on the Model Guidelines or Model Policy.

CHAPTER

97

Summary Author: Sharon Cirone
Melissa Weddle • Patricia K. Kokotailo

Epidemiology of Adolescent Substance Use

The primary source of information for this chapter is Monitoring the Future, a national survey of drug use that has been administered annually since 1975 and offers a comprehensive view of the factors that influence drug use. In addition to surveying young people about drug use, this survey addresses important factors such as beliefs about the dangers of drugs, and perceived availability.

The 2008 Monitoring the Future surveyed more than 46,000 students from 386 public and private high schools. At-risk and high-risk groups such as out-of-school and homeless youth are not included, perhaps resulting in incidences that are artificially low.

PREVALENCE AND TRENDS

Until 1978, the use of illicit drugs among 12th graders increased steadily from year to year, then decreased until the early 1990s, again climbing through the decade, and more gradually decreasing in the early years of the 21st century (Fig. 97.1).

Alcohol

Trends of alcohol use have overall followed the trends of illicit drug, rising and falling in concert. In 2008, 39% of 8th graders, 62% of 10th graders, and 72% of 12th graders report having tried alcohol. Of greater public health concern is prevalence of episodic heavy drinking or "binge drinking" (defined as five or more drinks in a row at least once during the past 2 weeks).

College students show different trends in alcohol use from those for 12th graders or respondents of the same age not attending college. Daily drinking rates of college students have generally been lower than same-age peers not attending college, but those reporting binge drinking is higher, suggesting a pattern of drinking primarily on weekends, when they tend to drink a lot. Across the adolescent and young adult population, males report binge drinking at higher rates than girls.

Tobacco

Since the survey began in 1975, cigarettes have consistently been the abusable substance most frequently used on a daily basis by high school students. Current smoking (defined as having smoked in the past 30 days) increased from 1991 to 1996, reaching a peak, since then, rates have steadily decreased. In 2008, 7.1% of 8th graders, 14.0% of 10th graders, and 20.4% of 12th graders reported current smoking.

Since 1991, rates of daily smoking have been similar for boys and girls at all grade levels. From 1980 until 1993, college males generally smoked at higher rates than females, but from 1994 through 2007, males and females have smoked at the same rates.

Marijuana

Of the illicit drugs, marijuana use remains the most prevalent. Marijuana use rose sharply during the late 1960s and early 1970s from negligible levels. This rise peaked in the late 1970s and then use gradually decreased

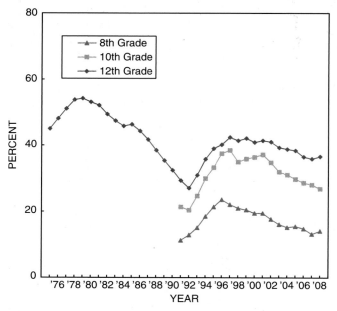

FIGURE 97.1 Illicit drugs. Percentage of students who have used an illicit drug in the past year. (From the Monitoring the Future study, University of Michigan, http:/nmonitoringthefuture.org/data/08data/fig08_1.pdf.)

throughout the 1980s until 1992, when use again rose sharply. Since 2001, there have been significant declines in the annual prevalence rates. In 2008, the annual prevalence rates for marijuana were 11%, 24%, and 32% for grades 8, 10, and 12, respectively. Among older youth, the highest use has been among the young adults not attending college, and lowest use among 12th graders, with college students falling in between.

Amphetamines

Between 1982 and 1992, annual prevalence rates for nonprescription amphetamine use declined considerably. In 2008, 8th, 10th, and 12th graders reported lifetime prevalence use of 4.5%, 6.4%, and 6.8%, respectively.

Methamphetamine

Monitoring the Future has included questions about use of "ice" (crystallized methamphetamine, typically smoked). The use of this drug increased during the 1990s among 12th graders, college students, and young adults. Since 1999, use held steady among 12th graders, and had risen slightly among college students and young adults. More recently, declines have actually been observed. In 2008, 1.2% of 8th graders, 1.5% of 10th graders, and 1.2% of 12th graders reported use of methamphetamine in the preceding year.

Ecstasy

Questions about ecstasy were added to the Monitoring the Future (MTF) secondary school surveys in 1996, because rates of use had increased significantly in 1995. Between 1998 and 2001, use rates increased dramatically in high school students, college students, and young adults. Since 2001, use rates decreased for the next 2 years, and have remained generally stable since 2003. In 2008, 1.7% of 8th graders, 2.9% of 10th graders, and 4.3% of 12th graders reported use of ecstasy in the preceding year.

Cocaine

Crack cocaine (the rock form of cocaine) use rapidly increased during the early 1980s. Thereafter, annual prevalence dropped sharply, where it has remained quite low, likely because of its perception as a dangerous drug. In 2008, 1.8% of 8th graders, 3.0% of 10th graders, and 4.4% of 12th graders reported use of cocaine in the preceding year.

Inhalants

This is the only class of drugs for which use is substantially higher in 8th grade than 10th or 12th grade. Among all high school students, there was a marked increase in inhalant use during the early 1990s, followed by a decrease after 1995. In 2008, 8.9% of 8th graders, 5.9% of 10th graders, and 3.8% of 12th graders report inhalant use in the preceding year.

Heroin

Between 1975 and 1979, the annual prevalence use of heroin among adolescents fell, then remained stable through 1993. Thereafter, the use increased. This upturn was likely related to the decline in perceived risk, as well as the availability of more pure heroin, which allowed use by other means than injection. For 12th graders, college students, and young adults, rates doubled or tripled in 1 to 2 years, remaining at the new higher levels for the rest of the decade. Between 2000 and 2002, use began to decrease. In 2008, 0.9% of 8th graders, 0.8% of 10th graders, and 0.7% of 12th graders reported use of heroin in the preceding year.

Anabolic Steroids

Annual prevalence use for 12th graders was 1.4% in 2007. Rates have been substantially lower among girls than boys.

Prescription Drugs

Overall trends in nonmedical use of opioids, stimulants, and sedative/anxiety medications show increased use since 2000. Young people may perceive prescription drugs as less harmful compared with street drugs and therefore may be more inclined to use them. From a 2005 study, lifetime prevalence use was highest for pain medication (17.7%) followed by sleeping (5.9%), sedative/anxiety (3.5%), and stimulant medications (2.4%). Adolescents identify peers and family members as the primary sources for these drugs.

MORE FREQUENT USE

Experimentation is a normal part of adolescent development, and rare or occasional use of a substance may not constitute problem use for most individuals. Frequency of use provides a more accurate measure of problem use. For marijuana, percentage of 12th graders who reported daily use (used at least 20 of the preceding 30 days) peaked in the late 1970s, dropped steadily until 1992, then increased again through the 1990s. In 2007, 5.1% of high school seniors reported daily marijuana use. Looking at this another way, each classroom would have one or two students who were using marijuana daily.

MULTIPLE DRUG USE

Many adolescents are using more than one substance and modify their drug use patterns over time. Some studies show that adolescent drug use typically begins with alcohol or cigarette use, followed by marijuana use, then by other illicit drugs. There appears to be a change over time of probabilities of progression. More recent generations of youth are substantially less likely to progress from cigarette and alcohol use to marijuana, cocaine, and heroin use. The majority of young substance users are polydrug users.

CORRELATES OF SUBSTANCE USE

Among ethnic/racial subgroups, there are varying associations with substance use. African American 12th graders have consistently lower usage rages than white 12th graders for most drugs. African American students have a lower 30-day prevalence rate of cigarette smoking compared with white students. In the 2007 MTF survey, African American 12th graders were less likely to report heavy drinking (12%) compared with white students (30%) and Hispanic students (23%).

Among white, African-American, and Hispanic 12th graders, whites have the highest rates of use of many drugs, including marijuana, hallucinogens, ecstasy, amphetamines, sedatives, tranquilizers, alcohol, cigarettes, and smokeless tobacco, as well as getting drunk.

Hispanics have the highest usage rates for some of the more dangerous drugs, such as cocaine, heroin, crack, crystal methamphetamine, and inhalants. In 8th grade, Hispanics have the highest rates for not only these drugs but for many of the others as well, such as marijuana and binge drinking.

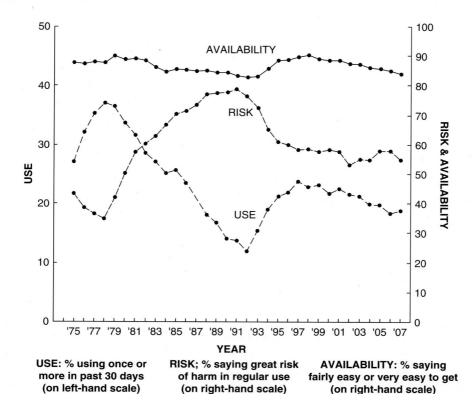

FIGURE 97.2 Marijuana: trends in perceived availability, perceived risk of regular use, and prevalence of use in past 30 days for 12th graders. (From *Monitoring the Future national survey results on drug use, 1975–2007: Volume I, Secondary school students*: http://www.monitoringthefuture.org/pubs/monographs/vol1_2007.pdf.)

Adolescents' Attitudes Toward Alcohol and Other Drugs

An adolescent's perception toward alcohol and other drugs influences his or her decision about whether to use those substances or not. Monitoring the Future includes questions about beliefs and attitudes, specifically about perceived harm of individual drugs and the degree to which the adolescent disapproves of the drug. Overall, the Monitoring the Future data show inverse relationships between the level of drug use and both the perceived risk and disapproval of that drug.

The trends for marijuana use and attitudes strikingly illustrate the relationship between perceived harm and use (Fig. 97.2).

Another drug that demonstrates this relationship is ecstasy. Perceived risk of ecstasy changed little until 2001, when it increased sharply. Accordingly, the use decreased sharply. Amplified media attention to the health consequences of ecstasy have likely contributed to the dramatic decrease in use.

Adolescents perceive a drug's harmfulness to be related to the frequency of use. Twelfth graders attribute a lower level of risk to trying most drugs once or twice (experimental use) than they do to regular use of drugs. For marijuana, only a minority of 12th graders associate great risk with experimenting, compared with over half who see great risk in occasional or regular use. Twelfth graders associate great risk with even experimental use of anabolic steroids, and for any use of ecstasy and heroin, and cocaine.

There are some conspicuous differences in this pattern. One concerning difference is perceived harm of regular cigarette smoking. Among 12th graders, 77% see great risk in smoking a pack or more per day, but only 61% of 8th graders see great risk. Unfortunately, perceived risk is lowest at ages at which smoking initiation is likely to occur.

Another factor in an individual's decision about whether to use a given drug may be the perceived benefits of using that drug. As a new drug becomes available, word may quickly spread about the positive effects, with a delay before information about adverse consequences can be disseminated.

Summary Author: Sharon Cirone
Kenneth W. Griffin • Gilbert J. Botvin

Preventing Substance Abuse Among Children and Adolescents

PREVALENCE RATES AND PROGRESSION OF USE

The onset of substance use typically begins during the adolescent years. Early initiation of substance use is associated with higher levels of use and abuse later in life as well as negative outcomes such as violent and delinquent behavior, poor physical health, and mental health problems. A goal of many prevention initiatives is to prevent early-stage substance use or delay the onset of use.

The prevalence of alcohol, tobacco, and other drug use increases rapidly from early to late adolescence, peaking during the transition to young adulthood. In recent years, prevalence rates of use for most substances have gradually declined among adolescents but remain problematic. The 2007 Monitoring the Future (MTF) study found that among high school seniors, 37% had used one or more illicit drugs in the last year and 48% had done so during their life-time. Though the rates of use for some substances have decreased in recent years, the MTF study also revealed that nonmedical prescription drug abuse and the misuse of over-the-counter medications such as cough syrup to get high are growing problems among adolescents.

Experimentation typically begins with substances that are readily available, such as alcohol, tobacco, and inhalants. Though many individuals discontinue use after experimentation or fail to progress to the use of other substances, some individuals become regular users. A subset eventually develops patterns of use characterized by both psychologic and physiologic dependence. An individual's risk of greater substance use involvement increases at each additional step in the developmental progression. Knowledge of the typical patterns and progression of substance use has important implications for the focus and timing of preventive interventions. The most effective approaches target salient risk and protective factors at the individual, family, and/or community levels and are guided by relevant psychosocial theories regarding the etiology of substance use and abuse.

ETIOLOGY AND IMPLICATIONS FOR PREVENTION

The degree of substance use involvement of any particular teenager is often a function of the negative prodrug social influences in their environment combined with their individual vulnerabilities to these influences.

Developmental Aspects

Substance use is frequently linked to important developmental goals and transitions of adolescence (i.e., separating from parents, gaining acceptance and popularity with peers, developing a sense of autonomy and independence, establishing a personal identity and self-image, seeking fun and adventure, and/or rebelling against authority). Thus, adolescence is a key period for experimentation not only with substances but with a wide range of behaviors and lifestyle patterns.

The Importance of Social Influences

Social influences are the most powerful factors promoting experimentation or initiation of substance use among young people, for example, modeling of substance use behavior by important others (e.g., parents, older siblings, and especially peers) and exposure to positive attitudes and expectations regarding substance use by celebrities and in advertisements.

Risk and Protective Factors

Risk factors occur at the level of the individual, family, school, and community.

Individual Level

1. Cognitive risk factors: knowledge of risks of use, and belief that substance use is "normal"
2. Affect regulation: poor affect regulation may be associated with self-medicating
3. Psychologic characteristics such as poor self-esteem, low assertiveness, and poor behavior control

Family Level

1. Modeling of drug use behavior
2. Positive attitudes regarding use
3. Harsh disciplinary practices
4. Poor parental monitoring
5. Low levels of family bonding
6. High levels of family conflict

School and Community Level

1. Students feeling disengaged from school and/or community
2. Feeling unsafe in their neighborhoods

TYPES OF PREVENTIVE INTERVENTIONS

Primary prevention interventions are designed to reach individuals in the general population before they have developed a specific disorder or disease. Secondary prevention involves screening and early intervention. Tertiary prevention involves preventing the progression of an established disorder to the point of disability.

A more contemporary terminology for prevention was proposed by the Institute of Medicine. In this framework, prevention refers only to interventions that occur prior to the onset of a disorder. Prevention is further divided into three types: universal, selective, and indicated interventions. Universal prevention programs focus on the general population and aim to deter or delay the onset of a condition. Selective prevention programs target selected high-risk groups or subsets of the general population believed to be at high risk owing to membership in a particular group (e.g., pregnant women or children of drug users). Indicated prevention programs are designed for those already engaging in the behavior or those showing early danger signs or engaging in related high-risk behaviors.

School-Based Prevention Approaches

Three types of contemporary approaches to school-based prevention of substance use are as follows:

1. **Social resistance skills**, that is, teaching adolescents how to recognize situations in which they are likely to experience peer pressure to smoke, drink, or use drugs along with ways to avoid or otherwise effectively deal with these high-risk situations.
2. **Normative education** includes content and activities to correct inaccurate perceptions regarding the high prevalence of substance use because adolescents tend to overestimate the prevalence of smoking, drinking, and the use of certain drugs.
3. **Competence enhancement:** Typically involves teaching some combination of the following life skills: general problem-solving and decision-making skills, general cognitive skills for resisting interpersonal or media influences, skills for increasing self-control and self-esteem, adaptive coping strategies for relieving stress and anxiety through the use of cognitive coping skills or behavioral relaxation techniques, general social skills, and general assertive skills.

Effectiveness of School-Based Prevention

Overall, school-based prevention is effective in reducing smoking and other forms of substance use. There is some debate on the long-term effectiveness of school-based prevention in general, though a handful of programs have shown clear evidence of long-term behavioral effects. Effectiveness is increased if the programs are interactive, focus on building skills in drug resistance and general competence skills, are implemented over multiple years, are culturally competent, and are combined with a community component.

Family-Based Prevention Approaches

Family-based drug prevention programs that focus on both parenting skills and family bonding appear to be the most effective in reducing or preventing substance use. An important limitation of family-based prevention is the difficulty in getting parents to participate; families most at risk for drug use are least likely to participate in prevention programs.

Community-Based Prevention Approaches

Community-based drug abuse prevention programs typically have multiple components, including some combination of school-based programs, family or parenting components, mass media campaigns, and public policy components, such as restricting youth access to alcohol and tobacco, and other types of community organization and activities. A limitation of community-based programs is the expense and high degree of coordination needed to implement and evaluate the type of comprehensive program most likely to be effective.

CHAPTER 99

Summary Author: Sharon Cirone
W. Alex Mason • J. David Hawkins

Adolescent Risk and Protective Factors: Psychosocial

Rather than an emphasis on the assessment and treatment of adolescents who are seriously involved in substance abuse, our foremost goal should be to prevent the initiation and progression of substance use in young people before the establishment of substance use disorders.

The physician who cares for children and who knows the risk and protective factors associated with the development of substance use disorders can intervene to avert alcohol and drug problems before they arise.

RISK FACTORS

Individual Factors

Some children appear to be at greater risk for substance abuse by virtue of their family histories, prenatal and birth experience, temperament, and early and persistent displays of behavioral and emotional problems. A family history of alcoholism increases the risk of alcoholism in children by about four times. However, fewer than 30% of the children of alcoholics develop alcoholism.

Perinatal complications (including preterm delivery, low birthweight, and anoxia) and brain damage (from infectious disease, traumatic head injury, or prenatal or postnatal exposure to toxins such as heavy metals, alcohol, tobacco, or cocaine) predispose children to later aggressive behavior, depression and anxiety symptoms, and substance abuse.

Some studies suggest that inherited biologic traits and temperament play a role in substance use behaviors. High physical activity level and negative emotionality are temperament dimensions that predict early drug initiation and substance abuse. Poor self-control and high sensation seeking also increase risk for adolescent substance use and misuse. Attention deficit/hyperactivity disorder, particularly the inattention symptom domain, has been found to predict substance use in late adolescence. A pattern of persistent conduct problems, including aggressive behavior in childhood, is an early behavioral predictor of risk for later substance abuse. There is some evidence that serious and persistent depressive symptoms are linked to adolescent substance involvement, and the co-occurrence of multiple behavioral and emotional problems can exacerbate risk for substance abuse.

Various attitudes, perceptions, and beliefs have been shown to predict greater substance use, including alienation and rebelliousness, positive expectations regarding the effects of alcohol and other drugs, and beliefs that using substances helps one cope with stress or enhances social interactions. Prodrug attitudes tend to precede the initiation of drug use in adolescence and continue to develop as drug involvement progresses.

The younger a child is when he or she first initiates the use of alcohol or other drugs, the greater the frequency of substance use, the greater the probability of extensive and persistent involvement in the use of illicit drugs, and the greater the risk of substance misuse and abuse. Each year that the initiation of alcohol or other drug use is delayed can lead to a 4% to 5% reduction in the likelihood of developing later drug use disorders.

Family Factors

Research shows that risk for substance use increases when parents involve children in their substance-using behavior. Substance use by older siblings increases risk for substance involvement. The influence of sibling substance use on adolescents appears to be stronger than that of parental substance use.

Parents who are permissive or who fail to set clear expectations for their children, who are lax in supervision of their children, and those who are excessively severe and inconsistent in punishing their children increase their children's risk for substance initiation, use, and abuse.

Poor family relationship quality increases risk for substance use and abuse. There is evidence that greater risk may come from parental conflict than from parental absence. High levels of conflict in the parent–child relationship contribute to risk for higher levels of substance use during childhood and adolescence. In contrast, positive family relationships appear to discourage the initiation and progression of substance use.

A twin-family study indicated that low parental monitoring provided opportunities for the expression of genetic predispositions for cigarette smoking among teens, whereas high parental monitoring limited such expression. Parent-child discussions about smoking were associated with decreased risk for cigarette use among teens with nonsmoking parents but not among teens with smoking parents.

School Factors

School experiences appear to contribute to substance nonuse, use, and misuse. School engagement, positive scholastic attitudes, and successful school performance have been shown to reduce risk for the initiation and escalation of alcohol, marijuana, and other drug use. Academic problems have been found to predict early initiation of substance use, levels of use of illegal drugs, and substance misuse.

Peer Factors

Having friends who drink, smoke, or use other drugs is among the strongest predictors of adolescent substance use and misuse. Associating with substance-using peers can exacerbate the effects of risk factors that originate within the family and other domains, synergistically increasing the likelihood of substance initiation, escalation, and abuse.

Interpersonal influences involving the family, school, and peers are particularly important during childhood and adolescence. Whereas parental influences on drug use behaviors tend to be stronger during childhood, peer influences tend to become more important throughout adolescence; still, research indicates that parents continue to play an important role in the lives of their children throughout the teen years and even into early adulthood.

Contextual Factors

Perceived problems with alcohol and drug use in the neighborhood or community predict individual drug use behaviors and drug arrests. Rates of use are higher in communities where alcohol or other drugs are inexpensive and readily available. Changes in laws to be more restrictive on alcohol availability (raising the legal drinking age, raising excise taxes on alcohol, limiting alcohol outlets) have been followed by decreases in alcohol consumption and alcohol-related fatalities.

Broad social norms regarding the acceptability and risk of use of alcohol or other drugs also appear to affect the prevalence of substance use and misuse.

PROTECTIVE FACTORS

There are factors and processes that protect adolescents against substance abuse, even if they have been exposed to multiple risk factors. A general prosocial orientation is a key individual protective characteristic that reduces risk for substance use and abuse. Indicators of this prosocial orientation include bonding to school, religiosity, and an intolerance of deviance.

With respect to alcohol, to delay use until adulthood is protective. Warm and supportive parental involvement, monitoring, consistent discipline, and clear parental expectations against drug use also appear to be protective against substance use and abuse.

Summary Author: Sharon Cirone
Deborah R. Simkin

Neurobiology of Addiction from a Developmental Perspective

What factors lead to early experimentation of tobacco, alcohol, and drugs? Is it genes that make youth more susceptible to use, or environment, or both? To answer this, one must understand the role of genes and environment, that is, epigenetics, on the developing brain.

Prenatal exposure, genetic predisposition, environmental stressors, untreated comorbid disorders, and age of onset of use are factors that may add to the increased risk for using substances of abuse during adolescence and may contribute to a more chronic and severe form of addiction. One must understand risk factors that increase risk and never underestimate the importance of early intervention. No one can understand addiction without understanding when, where, and why risk factors began from a developmental perspective. For these reasons, addiction may be thought of as having pediatric origins. Early intervention can obviously decrease the risk of developing substance abuse. However, missed opportunities to intervene may increase the probability of using substances during adolescence.

PRENATAL EXPOSURE

Though it is unclear whether prenatal exposure to substances of abuse can increase the risk of developing a substance abuse disorder (SUD), studies have shown that prenatal exposure can increase the risk of developing a learning disorder (LD) or comorbid conditions that may increase the risk of abusing drugs and alcohol.

Prenatal Exposure to Nicotine and Marijuana

Prenatal nicotine exposure can increase toddler's negativity, propensity for externalizing disorders, such as attention deficit hyperactivity disorder (ADHD) or conduct disorders. Prenatal cigarette exposure has been associated with lower IQ, poorer auditory functioning, and poorer performance on tests requiring fundamental aspects of visual perceptual performance.

Consistent patterns of cognitive deficits related to prenatal exposure to marijuana have been found, including IQ deficits and inattention, lower verbal reasoning scores, deficits in composite, short-term memory, and lower quantitative scores on testing scales. Those children exposed in utero also displayed more impulsive and more internalizing and externalizing behaviors, executive function difficulty, attention deficit problems, and an increased risk for substance use and psychiatric disorders.

Prenatal Exposure to Alcohol

Research does show a high risk for later alcohol abuse in children exposed to alcohol prenatally; this may be due to their increased impulsivity that could promote increased risk for experimentation during adolescence.

Fetal alcohol syndrome (FAS) is the most common nonhereditary cause of mental retardation. The prevalence varies from 0.5 to 3 per 1,000 live births. Alcohol has become the most teratogenic drug in United States. FAS has shown a sixfold increase between 1979 and 1993.

Children without the facial features commonly associated with FAS are referred to as having alcohol-related neurodevelopmental disorder (ARND). Unfortunately, without the facial features, it becomes more difficult to identify these children, and 60% to 90% escape identification in the normal population. There are four cognitive areas affected by FAS/ARND: learning and memory, visual-spatial processes, executive function, and attention. The percentage of adolescents with FAS in juvenile justice forensic units is three to ten times greater than the accepted worldwide incidence.

Prenatal Exposure to Other Substances of Abuse

Though cocaine can cause developmental delays and LDs, it is clear that findings once thought to be specific to in utero cocaine exposure are more likely to be associated with alcohol, tobacco, and marijuana and the quality of the child's environment. A better home environment was found to reduce many of the effects on lower IQ found at age 4 in cocaine-exposed babies.

Though the number of studies investigating the effect of prenatal caffeine exposure is less, there is little evidence at this time that prenatal caffeine has significant impact on childhood mental and motor development.

PERINATAL AND EARLY LIFE STRESSORS

Certain environmental conditions could cause permanent changes in neural circuitry that, in turn, could confer vulnerability for substance abuse and increase the risk of progression from substance abuse to addiction. Factors such as perinatal and postnatal stress and early life stressful experiences may alter addiction pathology later in life through changes in gene expression. It is crucial to explore the interplay between stressors in the environment and genes (otherwise known as epigenetics) when considering processes that may increase the risk for developing substance abuse. Epigenetics allows us to begin to understand why, for example, stressors such as fetal distress or hypoxia increase the risk for the development of ADHD or LDs, which in turn could lead to an increased risk for substance abuse later in life.

Stress, Drugs, Reward, and the HPA: Antireward System Model

Initially, all drugs of abuse have positive reinforcing effects. During acute use, drugs activate and increase dopamine in the shell of the nucleus accumbens (NAcs), as well as other areas. At the same time, environmental stress and acute drug use can also activate the hypothalamic-pituitary-adrenal (HPA) axis. In the antireward model, it is postulated that environmental stressors and continued drug use can overactivate the HPA axis. This occurs through increases in norepinephrine (NE) in the extended amygdala, which in turn further dysregulates the HPA and increases sensitivity to stress. The increased sensitivity to stress can increase the risk for using substances to relieve this stress. The transition to chronic use of substances to relieve stress exacerbates the dysregulation of the HPA axis, leading to a vicious cycle of worsening sensitivity to stress and substance use.

As these events occur, the individual becomes more sensitive to stress each time drugs are used. At the same time, the individual is more likely to seek out drugs to relieve this stress. All of these changes are referred to as the antireward system. Each time drugs are used, the continued decrease in reward function in the brain reward system relative to the increased recruitment of the brain antireward system moves the brain, from a reversible state where homeostasis could have been reinstated to a more dysregulated state that predisposes to chronic drug use to relieve stress.

The antireward model allows us to understand why, for example, if a person has had chronic stressful experiences, such as childhood sexual abuse and subsequent posttraumatic stress disorder (PTSD) symptomatology, this may cause an alteration of the expression of genes that may dysregulate the HPA axis, which would increase the sensitivity to stress and increase the risk for using substances to relieve this stress. Thus, we can see that chronic stressors, which predate drug use, may set the stage so that the HPA system is less likely to return to normal once drug use and experimentation begins.

Changes in the Brain Reward Circuitry in the Transition to the Addicted State

Certain comorbid conditions may affect the brain reward circuitry, leading to self-medication of these comorbid conditions. Also genes may be inherited that increase the sensitivity to the reinforcing effects of the drugs on the brain reward circuitry.

In general, the shell of the NAc and dopamine are involved in acute drug reinforcement, but the core of the NAc, the basolateral amygdala, and the prefrontal cortex (PFC) are involved in chronic drug use that leads to addiction. Chronic drug use causes intracellular changes, leading to circuitry changes. Changes in the intracellular level have been described as three stages: acute, transition, and end/addiction stage.

Stage 1: Acute Drug Effects After the acute administration of cocaine, dopamine (DA) receptors are stimulated and levels in the NAcs are elevated. At the same time, a cascade of molecular and genetic events occurs to cause dysphoria during early drug withdrawal, thereby decreasing drug reward. Limited exposure to drugs and early changes to the drug reward system will allow the system to return to normal/homeostasis.

Stage 2: Transition to Addiction In chronic repeated administration, long-lasting proteins produced by the DA increase the rewarding effects of drugs, causing an individual to seek out these rewarding effects more often and, when the individual does, more of the drug must be used to give the same rewarding effect (tolerance), and thus a cycle of craving ensues. Chronic use of the drug causes stimulation of the dopamine reward system that is less transient and less flexible to return to homeostasis.

Meanwhile, other protein changes reduce the salience of nondrug motivational stimuli so that normal stimuli such as food are less salient. The PFC becomes hypoactive to previously salient stimuli and the NAcs releases glutamate. These changes move the brain from a transitional stage to the active stage of addiction. Thus, glutamate plays a more important role in drug seeking after chronic drug exposure, versus dopamine playing a role in acute drug use.

End-Stage Addiction With chronic drug use, changes in protein expression move the addiction from temporary and reversible to permanent. Some important brain structures of note in relapse and the end stage addiction are the amygdala, the ventral tegmental area, and the PFC.

Role of Genes The role of genes in transition from drug use to addiction is recognized in a few areas of the brain. As noted above, stressors and initial drug use can turn on genes that can lead to the dysregulation of the HPA axis, in turn leading to a progression in use and abuse.

People born with an increase in dopamine (D2) receptors may be at less risk to develop substance use disorders (SUDs), and those who inherit a decrease in these receptors may beat more risk to progress to addiction.

STUDIES OF INHERITABILITY

Adoption studies of adopted-away children of persons with alcohol dependence have shown increased risk for alcoholism and increased risk for abuse of substances other than alcohol. However, alcohol use by adoptive parents did not increase risk for alcohol abuse in adoptive children.

Adoption studies have shown that genetic susceptibility seemed to be a stronger predictor of risk for substance abuse than exposure to adoptive parents using substances. Both genetic and environmental influences may be correlated to substance initiation, but progression to substance abuse and dependence may be more related to genetic factors alone.

Drug History, Personality, and Comorbidity

Drug History A study of youngsters who began drinking at an early age, 11 to 12 years of age, had a higher probability of meeting the DSM III-R criteria for substance abuse (13.5%) and substance dependence (15.9%) as compared to those who began drinking at age 13 or 14 (13.7% and 9.0%, respectively). Those who drank at age 19 or 20 had rates of 2% and 1%, respectively. One study has noted that a patient with substance abuse was most likely to have started drinking at age 13, when first drunk was at age 15, had his or her first problem associated with drinking at age 18, and first dependence was at age 25 to 40. Death was most likely to occur by age 60. It is important that rapid progression of SUD occurred often with earlier age of onset and frequency, not duration of use. Those individuals with earlier onset had a shorter time span from first exposure to addiction than did adult-onset groups. Adolescent-onset adults had higher lifetime rates of cannabis and hallucinogen use disorders, shorter times between the development of their first and second dependence diagnosis, and higher rates of disruptive behaviors and major depression.

Personality Temperament plays a role in the development of alcohol and drug dependence. Some researchers note that patients with alcohol dependence share common characteristics: early onset of spontaneous alcohol-seeking behavior, diagnosis during adolescence, rapid course of onset, presence of genetic risk factors, deviancy, and greater psychologic vulnerability.

Comorbidity Seldom does any patient with an SUD develop substance dependence without some significant precursors in his or her developmental history, and psychiatric comorbidity may increase the risk or speed of transition from substance abuse to substance dependence.

There are a few psychiatric disorders that are worth mentioning, which, if untreated, will increase the risk for substance abuse perhaps by making the brain neurobiologically more vulnerable to the development of substance abuse.

Mood and Conduct Disorders

Depression may be the primary variable related to SUD in women at any age. Depression in boys may be linked to earlier onset of conduct disorder.

Externalizing disorders in boys are consistently linked to SUDs.

Individuals with adolescent-onset bipolar disorder have an 8.8 times greater risk of developing an SUD than those with childhood-onset bipolar disorder. Though patients may use substances to self-medicate their manic symptoms, it is clear that the use of multiple substances, such as marijuana and alcohol, may, in reality, make the neurobiologic effect even worse.

Anxiety Disorders

The observation of decreased dopamine receptor in patients with social anxiety may help to explain the increased risk of developing substance abuse if social phobia goes untreated.

The predisposition for SUD in young people with a history of chronic childhood physical/sexual abuse, with or without PTSD symptomatology, was discussed earlier.

Attention Deficit Hyperactivity Disorder

It is well recognized that ADHD with conduct disorder has a much greater risk for developing substance abuse than ADHD alone.

Also, if an adolescent has ADHD and is not treated, the risk of developing SUD is two times higher than in those who have ADHD and were treated with stimulants. The explanation for this may lie in the observation that the liability of a drug to cause reinforcing acute euphoric feelings is associated with the instant abuse of that drug, as in the case of cocaine. However, methylphenidate taken orally does not produce this rapid high because it enters the brain barrier more slowly and is less associated with a high that causes a reinforcing effect of the drug. In fact, oral methylphenidate may not induce craving even if it is taken by a subject with cocaine dependence. In rodent studies, consistent methylphenidate treatment (started in adolescence) attenuated cocaine self-administration during adulthood, perhaps through the mechanism of increased D2 receptors in the individuals who had been treated.

Learning Disorders

Academic failure and low commitment to school are other psychobehavioral factors associated with influencing drug use during childhood and adolescence. Beyond early onset of use, poor academic achievement, poor social skills and competence, LDs, and poor self-esteem were found to be related to drug abuse.

Too often, ADHD is assumed to be the reason for school problems, and a comorbid LD goes undetected.

Early detection of LDs is essential to prevent the increased risk for developing substance abuse. However, the timing of the intervention may also be crucial. If these disorders are not detected and intervened upon at the appropriate time in childhood, a window of opportunity may be lost.

Schizophrenia

Adolescent use of marijuana has been associated with earlier onset of schizophrenia in predisposed individuals (i.e., those with family history or a history of prodromal symptoms). Cannabis is also associated with the exacerbation of the positive symptoms of established schizophrenia. New research has revealed an allele variation that may be associated with the onset of schizophrenia in young people who use marijuana.

DEVELOPMENT OF THE ADOLESCENT BRAIN: BIOLOGIC PREDISPOSITIONS

Why do adolescents experiment with risky behaviors? Much of this may be due to the dramatic changes that occur during adolescence. The following is an explanation of these changes.

Immature prefrontal function alone cannot account for adolescent behavior. It has been suggested that perhaps human development researchers should consider adolescence as a period wherein two separate entities are independently working: lack of cognitive control and risk taking. Focusing on these two entities from a neurobiologic level with the consideration of two different trajectories may give more insight to the reasons

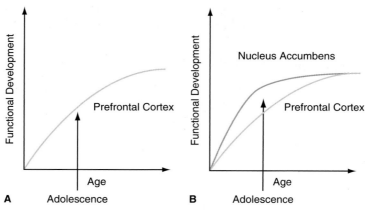

FIGURE 100.1   The traditional explanation of adolescent behavior has been suggested to be due to the protracted development of the PFC (**A**). Our model takes into consideration the development of the PFC together with subcortical limbic regions (e.g., NAcs) that have been implicated in risky choices and actions (**B**).

behind adolescent behavior. Figure 100.1 depicts this model. On the left (A) is the traditional characterization of adolescence as related almost exclusively to the immaturity of the PFC. On the right (B) is a proposed neurobiologic model that illustrates the imbalance of limbic relative to prefrontal control. According to the model, in emotionally salient situations, the limbic system will win over control systems given its maturity relative to the prefrontal control system. Neuroimaging studies corroborate this model and reveal that relative to children and adults, adolescents show exaggerated activation of the accumbens versus prefrontal control regions, which may in turn relate to the increased impulsive and risky behaviors observed during this period of development. Therefore, suboptimal choices win out over rationally considered, goal-directed behavior.

Although adolescents may be more prone to risky choices as a group, individual differences in neural responses to reward predispose some adolescents to take more risks than others, putting them at greater risk for negative outcomes. Impulsivity and risk-taking are associated with immature PFC and increased accumbens activity in some individuals. Knowing that impulsivity plays a major role in risk for developing SUD, these findings provide crucial groundwork by synthesizing the various findings related to risk-taking behavior in adolescence and in understanding individual differences and developmental markers for propensities to engage in negative behavior.

Why Would the Brain be Programmed to Develop this Way?

Evolutionarily speaking, adolescence is the period in which independence skills are acquired to increase success upon separation from the protection of the family. Seeking out same-age peers and fighting with parents, all of which help get the adolescent away from the home territory for mating, are seen in other species, including rodents, nonhuman primates, and some birds. Humans had to engage in high-risk behavior to leave their family and village to find a mate and risk taking at just the same time as hormones drive adolescents to seek out sexual partners. In fact, some have suggested that these risk-taking behaviors may be necessary to sculpt the brain in order to reach the adult pattern necessary for efficient processing. Hence, adolescence is a crucial period of plasticity when brain circuitry and behavior are beginning to be established.

ROLE OF FAMILY AND PEERS DURING KEY DEVELOPMENTAL STAGES

Modeling the use of alcohol or drugs by parents when children are young increases the notion that drugs and alcohol are not harmful substances and this risk factor increases the risk for using as a teen. While parents have a stronger influence in childhood, peers have a stronger influence in adolescence. Peers not only influence initiation of use but also relapse, and adolescents are more likely to seek out risky behaviors especially in the presence of their peers.

CHAPTER **101**

Summary Author: Sharon Cirone
Terri L. Randall • Himanshu P. Upadhyaya

Adolescent Cigarette Smoking

Smoking is the leading cause of preventable death in the United States. Smoking behaviors begin in childhood, with even infrequent, experimental smoking by adolescents leading to symptoms of addiction in a matter of weeks. Once a teen begins smoking regularly, cessation is difficult. Thus, tobacco use among adolescents is an area of considerable public health concern.

EPIDEMIOLOGY

Smoking initiation increases with increasing age and grade. Youth who begin smoking at younger ages are more likely to become dependent and less likely to stop smoking (Table 101.1).

In 2006, young adults aged 18 to 25 had the highest current use of tobacco products (43.9%) according to the National Survey on Drug Use and Health. The study found that the rate of current cigarette use is highest in rural counties. Native American youths use cigarettes and smokeless tobacco at higher rates than other ethnic groups, followed by Caucasians, then Latinos, and then African Americans.

The 2005 results of the Global Youth Tobacco Survey revealed that current tobacco use was highest in the Americas (22.2%) and lowest in the Southeast Asian and Western Pacific regions (12.9% and 11.4%, respectively). Boys were significantly more likely than girls to use tobacco products.

ETIOLOGY

Like many behaviors, the determinants of adolescent smoking are multifactorial. Several individual and environmental risk and protective factors play a role in determining youths' experimentation, initiation, and maintenance of smoking behaviors.

Psychosocial risk factors for smoking include age, race, socioeconomic status, abuse history, and family structure. Being raised in a two-parent family appears to have a protective effect on adolescent smoking. However, a recent study notes that high exposure to deviant peers may nullify the protective effect of being raised in an intact, two-parent family.

Symptoms of depression, anxiety, and attention deficit hyperactivity disorder (ADHD) have all been linked with smoking in youth. Novelty seeking, risk taking, and other problem behaviors such as other drug use, early

TABLE 101.1	Pattern of Tobacco Use among Adolescents	
Monitoring the future results	**1976**	**2006**
Last month use	38%	20% of 12th graders, 9% of 8th graders
Prevalence of daily use	29%	12.2% of 12th graders
Greater than ½ ppd	19%	1.5%–6% of high school students

sexual activity, fighting, low self-esteem, negative self-concept, normative views of smoking, and poor eating habits are associated with youth smoking. Scholastic achievement, a moderate amount of work (<10 hours per week), and involvement in sports and religious activities lessen the risk for youth smoking.

Environmental factors involved in adolescent smoking include parental and peer smoking and influences, media influences, and exposure to secondhand smoke. Increased parental supervision and monitoring is associated with decreased smoking in teens. Compared with parental influences on adolescent smoking, peer factors seem to have a more compelling influence on teen smoking.

School and home smoking bans are associated with decreased rates of youth smoking, perhaps by limiting exposure and perceived approval of cigarette smoking.

There may be gene and environment interactions that lead to smoking. Researchers have explored the connection of the D2 receptor gene, dopamine transporter gene, and the D4 receptor (DRD4) gene to smoking behaviors.

COMORBIDITIES

Smoking is commonly associated with medical and psychiatric comorbidities in children and adolescents. Besides the long-term medical consequences of smoking, such as lung cancer and cardiovascular disease, smoking is also associated with more immediate health problems, including an increased frequency of respiratory symptoms, respiratory infections, a decrease in lung function, an increase in atherosclerotic lesions, and decreases in physical fitness levels.

Psychiatric comorbidities associated with smoking in young people include disruptive behavior disorders such as ADHD and conduct disorder, major depression, anxiety disorders, and other substance use disorders. Youth with a history of mental illness are 50% more likely to increase their smoking over the course of years than those without a history of mental illness.

Youth smoking is associated with increased odds for other substance use disorders. Early-onset smokers are more likely to smoke more heavily, have early onset of drinking alcohol, and have a family history of alcoholism compared with individuals who started smoking at age 17 or older. Early-onset smoking is also associated with increased odds of cannabis and other drug use.

ASSESSMENT

Clinical guidelines recommend that physicians and other health care providers adequately assess children's tobacco use and counsel those who are using tobacco products to quit. Assessment of tobacco use should include queries about the types of tobacco used, patterns of use, severity of use, circumstances of use, context of use, benefits and consequences of use, symptoms of withdrawal, and motivation for cessation.

One of the challenging aspects of working with adolescents is facilitating accurate disclosure of behaviors that are generally not socially acceptable for young people, such as sexual relationships and drug use. Assuring adolescents that their responses will be confidential is one way to decrease the likelihood of underreporting or misreporting of sensitive information. Another way is to ask concrete, specific, open-ended questions, "When was the first time you ever had a cigarette, even one puff? Tell me about the first time you tried smoking." The latter question may provide key information about precipitating and perpetuating factors that maintain cigarette use. Depending on the response, the clinician may follow up by asking, "When did you first smoke a whole cigarette?" or "Do you think you will experiment with cigarettes in the future? If one of your best friends offered you a cigarette would you smoke it?"

After assessing if the adolescent has used or is using any tobacco products, the clinician should ask about frequency of use. Although cigarettes are the most common tobacco product that youth use, it is important to also ask about cigars, cigarillos, bidis (flavored cigarettes from South Asia), water pipes (hookahs), and smokeless tobacco.

It is important for the clinician to ask about children's smoking attitudes and beliefs. Youths' perception of smoking and tobacco harmfulness is inversely proportional to youth smoking prevalence. Providing information to correct misinformation (the majority of people do not smoke; smoking does not make one look more attractive to the opposite sex) is helpful in shaping behaviors.

The clinician should also assess whether the child meets criteria for nicotine dependence. Establishing nicotine dependence in young smokers can be more complicated than in adults because of teen smokers' variable smoking patterns. Keep in mind that youth may develop symptoms of nicotine dependence within days of smoking initiation.

The diagnosis of nicotine dependence is made using clinical judgment, but biochemical markers, such as expired carbon monoxide and cotinine, can aid in assessment and help track success during cessation efforts.

Lastly, the clinician should explore the adolescents' stage of change and motivation to participate in change.

TREATMENT

The Public Health Service published its recommendations that clinicians screen adolescents for tobacco use at every visit and counsel users to quit. It recommended that clinicians use the behavioral counseling model of the 5As (ask about use, advise to quit, assess willingness to make a quit attempt, assist patient in quitting, and arrange follow-up) to guide smoking cessation efforts for all smokers, including adolescents.

Little is known about which pharmacologic treatments are efficacious for smoking cessation in adolescents. To date, nicotine replacement therapies such as the transdermal nicotine patch (TNP) and bupropion SR (Zyban) have been the treatments most explored in adolescent smokers.

Based on the limited data available, behavioral therapy combined with either bupropion SR or TNP should be used as first-line treatment for adolescent smoking cessation. Behavioral interventions such as motivation-enhancement and cognitive-behavioral techniques can be used in individual or group settings. Classroom and school clinic–based treatment programs may be relatively more effective settings compared with interventions based at medical clinics, or delivered via the computer.

PREVENTION

Prevention interventions that target youth include a variety of different tactics including school-based programs, mass media programming, restrictions on advertising and sales to minors, and environmental programs such as clean-air ordinances mandating nonsmoking schools, businesses, and restaurants.

Indoor smoking bans, increased cigarette tax, and antismoking advertising campaigns seem to have made an impact in reducing cigarette smoking among adolescents. School-based prevention programs seem to be less effective.

Summary Author: Sharon Cirone
Sharon Levy • John R. Knight

Screening and Brief Intervention for Adolescents

Substance use is one of the greatest health threats faced by American teenagers. Medical office settings are ideal for early identification of drug and alcohol use by adolescents because they provide a yearly opportunity for a medical professional to interview teenagers in a private and confidential setting. Several professional societies recommend that all adolescents be screened for drug and alcohol use at every primary care visit. Fortunately, easily implemented substance use screens can quickly and reliably determine which teens are at high risk of having a substance use disorder. Teens who are at low risk, who form the majority of any primary care population, can be effectively advised in a primary care setting. Experienced clinicians can follow up a positive screen with a brief assessment to determine the appropriate level of care for teens with more serious substance use disorders and make appropriate referrals. Clinicians who routinely screen all adolescent patients for substance use can have a major impact on the health of their patient population.

SCREENING: OPENING QUESTIONS

Clinicians should begin asking adolescents about substance use and other sensitive questions as soon as the young person is old enough to be interviewed without the parent present. The clinician should review the ground rules of confidentiality while the parent and adolescent are together. Briefly, the clinician should ensure that the details discussed will remain confidential unless the clinician has safety concerns.

The interviewer could ask three straightforward questions: In the past 12 months, did you

1. Drink any alcohol (more than a few sips)?
2. Smoke any marijuana or hashish?
3. Use anything else to get high? ("Anything else" includes illegal drugs, over the counter and prescription drugs, and things that you sniff or "huff".)

Adolescents who report complete abstinence from alcohol and drugs should be given praise and encouragement regarding the good decisions they have made. Any adolescent who reports having used alcohol or drugs should be screened with a developmentally appropriate screening tool.

SCREENING TOOLS

Several tools have been developed to screen patients for high-risk use of alcohol and other drugs, including the AUDIT, POSIT and CRAFFT. In general, these tools fall into two broad categories: written assessments (such as the AUDIT and POSIT) and oral screens (such as the CRAFFT and CAGE).

The CRAFFT screen is a series of six questions developed to screen adolescents for alcohol and other drug use disorders simultaneously. The CRAFFT has been extensively validated with adolescents and is recommended by several professional organizations, including the American Academy of Pediatrics. All adolescents who have used alcohol or another drug should be asked the CRAFFT questions or should be screened with an alternative formal screening tool. Recent research has demonstrated that even experienced adolescent medicine specialists significantly underestimate adolescents' risk level when relying on clinical impressions alone. Adolescents who report abstinence from alcohol and drugs should be asked whether they have ever ridden in a car with a driver who was high or had used alcohol or drugs. After completing the opening questions regarding alcohol and drug use and the follow-up screen, the clinician can determine the appropriate next step.

CRAFFT Questionnaire:

During the past 12 months, have you ever
C Ridden in a **C**ar driven by someone, including yourself, who was high or had been using alcohol or drugs?
R Used alcohol or drugs to **R**elax, feel better about yourself, or fit in?
A Used alcohol or drugs while you are by yourself, **A**lone?
F **F**orgotten things you did while using alcohol or drugs?
F Had your **F**amily or **F**riends tell you that you should cut down on your drinking or drug use?
T Gotten into **T**rouble while you were using alcohol or drugs?

Each "yes" response is scored 1 point. A score of 2 or greater is a positive screen and indicates that the adolescent is at high risk for having an alcohol- or drug-related disorder.

SCREENING AND BRIEF ADVICE: SPECIFIC STRATEGIES

No Use: Praise and Encouragement

Adolescents who have been abstinent from alcohol and drugs and who have never ridden with an intoxicated driver should receive praise and encouragement from their clinician. Adolescents should be encouraged to discuss drug use or ask questions in the future should the need arise. Statements such as, "It sounds as if you have made smart choices by not using drugs or alcohol. If that ever changes I hope you will feel comfortable enough to talk to me about it." aim both to praise the young person's abstinence and leave open the opportunity for open communication in the future.

Car: Contract for life

All adolescents who have ridden with an intoxicated driver should receive risk reduction advice. The "contract for life" is a document developed by Students Against Destructive Decisions (SADD) that asks adolescents to commit to never ride with a driver who has been drinking or using other drugs and also asks parents to promise to provide transportation home without any questions if their child is in need.

CRAFFT 0–1: Brief Advice

Adolescents who report alcohol or other drug use but screen negative (i.e., 0 or 1 on the CRAFFT) are at relatively low risk for meeting criteria for a substance use disorder. These teens should receive brief advice to stop using, such as, "My advice is for you to stop using alcohol or drugs at all, because they pose a serious risk to your health." The clinician should also give specific information related to the health effects of the drug that the teen is using. For example,"Using marijuana during the teen years, when your brain is still developing, greatly increases your risk of developing a serious mental illness, such as schizophrenia or major depression, later in life." The clinician should challenge the patient to a time-limited trial of abstinence (e.g., 3 months) and ask him or her to come for a return visit to discuss how it went.

CRAFFT 2 or Above: Brief Assessment

Adolescents who screen positive (i.e., CRAFFT score of 2 or more) are at high risk of having a substance use disorder and need further assessment. Clinicians who screen adolescents for substance use should be prepared to perform a limited assessment in order to triage referrals for these patients.

BRIEF ASSESSMENT OF ADOLESCENTS WHO ACKNOWLEDGE ALCOHOL OR DRUG USE

Strategies for Interviewing Adolescents and Establishing a Substance Use History

For any patient, a nonjudgmental, empathetic interviewing style that accepts the patient's point of view encourages more information sharing than an interrogative style. The interviewer should use open-ended questions to begin the conversation, with an emphasis on the pattern of drug use over time, including whether drug use has increased in quantity or frequency, whether the teen has made attempts at discontinuing drug use, and why and whether attempts have been successful. Information about the pattern of drug use and associated problems is more important in making a diagnosis of a substance-related disorder than the absolute quantity or frequency. When gathering the information for a substance use history, the clinician should inquire about the pattern of use of not only the identified drug of choice but also other substances of abuse, including alcohol, over-the-counter and prescription medications, and illicit substances.

At times, substance use by an adolescent will present to a clinician as a report by a parent, from a school, or from another adult. In these cases, the clinician should take a careful collateral history. Parents' observations and impressions provide a useful piece of clinical information.

Throughout the interview, cues from the clinician may help the adolescent make connections between drug use and consequences. For example, statements such as "it seems that your grades started to fall at the same time that you started using more marijuana" may help the adolescent associate the two occurrences. A well-conducted

TABLE 102.1	**Stages of Substance Use**
Stage	**Description**
Primary abstinence	No use of alcohol or drugs
Experimentation	The first 1–2 times that a substance is used. At this phase, the adolescent is curious about what it feels like to be intoxicated by a particular substance.
Limited use	Repeated use in social situations, for recreational purposes only, without associated problems.
Problematic use	Use for other than recreational purposes (i.e., to relax or improve mood) or use associated with a single problem (i.e., tension with parents, school suspension)
Abuse	Use that has a negative impact on daily functioning or that is associated with recurrent significant problems (as above) or risks (i.e., driving or babysitting while intoxicated), as defined by DSM-IV-TR[23] criteria below. Patient must meet one or more for a diagnosis of substance abuse: • Failure to fulfill obligations at work, school, or home (e.g., repeated school absences, suspension) • Use in physically hazardous situations (e.g., drinking and driving) • Substance-related legal problems • Continued use despite social or interpersonal problems related to substance
Dependence	Loss of control over a substance, as defined by DSM-IV-TR[23] criteria below. Patient must meet 3 or more criteria for a diagnosis of substance dependence. • Tolerance • Withdrawal • Substance taken in larger amounts or for longer period than intended • Persistent desire or unsuccessful efforts to cut down/control use • Great deal of time spent obtaining, using, or recovering from effects of substance • Important activities given up or reduced because of use • Continued use despite physical/psychologic harm from substance

American Psychiatric Association. Diagnostic and Statistical Manual of Mental Disorders, 4th Edition. Washington DC: American Psychiatric Association; 2000.

history has therapeutic value as it encourages the adolescent to consider the consequences of drug use that she or he has already experienced.

Physical Exam

Adolescents who have a positive screen for high-risk substance use should have a physical exam to look for signs of acute intoxication or chronic drug use. Signs of chronic drug use are rare in teens but should be both discussed with the adolescent and recorded in the chart if present.

Laboratory Testing

Laboratory testing may be useful in some situations, but testing is a complex procedure that yields limited information that must be interpreted within the context of history and physical exam. A positive drug test may serve to open an honest conversation, but does not confirm a substance use disorder. A single negative test does not prove that an adolescent has not used drugs.

SUBSTANCE USE SPECTRUM

The goal of brief assessment is to triage adolescents who screen positive for high-risk substance use to the appropriate level of intervention. Based on the information from the clinical interview, the clinician can conceptualize the adolescents' substance use on a spectrum that varies from primary abstinence to substance dependence. As with other developmental phenomena, the amount of time spent in any given phase of the spectrum depends on the specific substance and the adolescent's individual characteristics; however, most adolescents will pass through the stages in the identical order (Table 102.1).

Adolescents who have had problems related to drug use but do not have a substance use disorder may benefit from a brief intervention and follow-up, either by the primary care clinician or by an allied mental health worker such as a social worker or psychologist.

If assessment suggests a serious substance use disorder, the adolescent should be referred to a mental health or addiction specialist for a full evaluation and treatment recommendations. Clinicians should consider involving parents whenever possible as adolescents are unlikely to follow through with a referral on their own. In many instances parents will already be aware of drug use (though they may underestimate the extent), and the adolescent may be willing to include parents in treatment planning. Even if parents are not aware, the clinician should ask permission to get them involved. An adolescent who reveals significant drug use may be looking for help and support.

CHAPTER 103

Summary Author: Sharon Cirone
Ken C. Winters • Tamara Fahnhorst • Andria Botzet • Randy Stinchfield

Assessing Adolescent Substance Use

THE COMPREHENSIVE ASSESSMENT

When screening suggests a possible drug use problem, the assessor should conduct a more comprehensive assessment in order to determine details of drug use history, consequences of such use, whether the teenager meets criteria for a substance use disorder (SUD), and what other behavioral and mental co-occurring problems may exist. Finally, the assessor should evaluate the adolescent's problem recognition and readiness for treatment. These questions may help determine the initial treatment goals.

The determination of an SUD requires that the assessor review the criteria for substance abuse and dependence for specific substances. Abuse criteria focus on negative social and personal consequences as a result of repetitive use; dependence criteria address symptoms associated with the continued use of drugs in the face of negative consequences and loss of control over use.

DEVELOPMENTAL CONSIDERATIONS

Identifying Clinical Significance

It can be difficult to determine when adolescent drug use will have short-term and minimal health effects versus when drug use may escalate to negative long-term repercussions. Most often, adolescents use legal drugs (alcohol or tobacco) within a social context. The majority of youth will not progress beyond the use of these "gateway drugs," yet some will progress to use illicit drugs and to develop serious problems.

Applicability of SUD Criteria

The applicability of DSM-IV-TR criteria to adolescent drug use has been met with reservation for several reasons, including the following: the distinction of abuse and dependence criterion as applied to adolescents are not well-supported by research; some criteria have limited utility among adolescents (e.g., an important criterion for dependence, tolerance, has low diagnostic specificity among adolescents given that this symptom can take extended lengths of time to develop); and the meaning of symptoms for adolescents, who are relatively inexperienced with the effects of drugs, may lead to higher rates of false positive endorsements (e.g., "drinking more than intended" may be endorsed more frequently among teenagers because of poor judgment).

Neurobiology

Recent research has indicated that the adolescent brain does not fully develop until early adulthood. In some regions of the brain, particularly the prefrontal cortex region, that are associated with judgment (resisting impulses and other executive functioning), nearly 50% of the neurons are "pruned" and undergoing transformation during adolescence. Because of this immaturity, there is speculation that the developing adolescent brain may be highly vulnerable to the effects of drug use. Therefore, adolescents may be less capable of moderating their alcohol intake as compared to adults.

Other Factors

Other developmental issues are relevant with respect to assessing adolescent drug use. Girls tend to utilize drug use as a coping mechanism for stress, whereas boys tend to use drugs for the pleasurable effects. Also, delays in social and emotional functioning, diminished respect toward authority, and tendencies to be egocentric and to minimize negative consequences may contribute to inaccurate reporting of personal drug use behaviors and to poor motivation to change. All of these issues should be taken into consideration when deciding the questions to pose and the mode of enquiry when assessing adolescents for SUD.

SELF-REPORT: VALIDITY AND ALTERNATIVES

The utilization of self-report is a hallmark of a clinical assessment. Convenience, comprehensiveness, low cost, ease of administration, and the perception that the individual is the most knowledgeable reporter have encouraged the use of this method. The overall validity and reliability, however, of the self-report method for assessing adolescent drug use and related problems is still debated in the literature. The findings are not surprising given the circumstances under which an adolescent assessment may be conducted. Defiance, fear, and apprehension can influence the results of an assessment. In addition, youth may see the assessment as an opportunity to "cry for help" and exaggerate their responses.

The alternatives to self-report include drug testing (urine, hair, saliva, and sweat), direct observation by the assessor for behavioral and psychologic indicators of drug use, and reports by others, such as parents or peers.

CLINICAL CONTENT OF THE ASSESSMENT

Course of SUDs

Understanding the course of adolescent SUDs provides a vital perspective in our understanding of the etiology and prognosis of SUDs. A detailed assessment should include a detailed inquiry into the age of onset and progression of use for specific substances, the types of drugs used, circumstances, frequency and variability of use, and usual times and places of drug use, since initiation until the time of assessment.

The differential diagnosis of adolescent SUDs requires consideration that the symptoms of drug use are not due to premorbid or concurrent problems, such as conduct disorder or family issues. Given the frequent comorbidity of SUDs and other psychiatric disorders, it is important that the assessor comprehensively review, in a timeline fashion, the past and present history of psychiatric symptoms. Such a timeline approach can help the assessor sort out the interrelationship between drug use and comorbid psychopathology.

The course of SUDs while in treatment is also relevant. Documentation about some of the variables that have been found to predict the course of SUDs among adolescents in a drug treatment setting is important. Pretreatment characteristics that are associated with more favorable substance use outcomes include a lower substance use severity level at admission, greater readiness to change, and fewer conduct problems or other co-occurring psychopathology. Factors influencing better outcomes during treatment include a longer length of treatment and family involvement in treatment. Posttreatment predictors of better outcome include participation in aftercare, low levels of peer substance use, ability to use coping skills, and continued commitment to abstain. Of all these factors, the posttreatment predictors accounted for more variance in the teenagers' outcomes at 1 year after treatment than did the pretreatment and during-treatment variables.

Psychosocial Factors

Documentation of the various psychosocial dimensions and consequences that are related to the adolescent's drug use behaviors provides beneficial information regarding the onset and maintenance factors of the drug use and aids in treatment planning.

Dimensions that should be included in the assessment protocol include interpersonal relationships; school, work, social, and psychologic functioning; history of criminal justice involvement and delinquency; recreational activities; and sexual behavior.

Peer factors and family environment should be included in the assessment. Multiple research studies indicate that variables such as peer pressure to use drugs, access to drugs through peers, and normative attitudes toward drugs by peers are prominent factors contributing to the onset and maintenance of drug use. Family influences also encompass several variables, including familial genetic risk, parenting styles and practices, and parental alcohol and drug use or psychopathology. Initiation of alcohol use in mid-adolescence is predominantly influenced by factors such as parental monitoring and father's drinking level, rather than genetic factors. However, after drinking is initiated, it appears that the genetic factors increasingly influence the frequency of alcohol and other drug use, as well as the prevalence of SUDs.

Psychological Benefits

In spite of the detrimental effects incurred when using drugs, many adolescents use drugs because they serve psychological need states. Psychological advantages of adolescent drug use include mood enhancement, stress reduction, and relief from boredom. The clinician should ask the adolescent about perceived benefits of alcohol or drug use during the assessment.

Co-Occurring Mental Health Disorders

The clinician should include a review of psychological symptoms and stressors; previous psychiatric consultations, admissions, and diagnosed disorders; history of suicidal ideation or attempts; and family history of psychopathology and psychiatric disorders.

The most common types of comorbid psychiatric conditions include externalizing disorders and internalizing disorders. The clinician should ask about childhood aggression, rebelliousness, theft, and destructiveness, along with related externalizing diagnoses such as Conduct Disorder and Oppositional Defiant Disorder. Enquiries about attentional and behavioral hyperarousal symptoms, as well as assessments for or diagnoses of ADHD, should be included. A review of symptoms of depression and anxiety should be included. The clinician should ask about internalizing symptoms and disorders such as eating disorders, self harm, and self-esteem issues. Adverse life events including childhood maltreatment (i.e., physical abuse, sexual abuse, neglect) should also be documented along with questions about symptoms and sequelae of abuse.

COMPREHENSIVE ASSESSMENT INSTRUMENTS

Significant advances have occurred since the mid 1980s in the development and evaluation of adolescent drug abuse assessment instruments.

Clinicians and researchers can employ various diagnostic interviews, problem-focused interviews and multiscale questionnaires. These instruments yield information that can definitively assess the nature and severity of the drug involvement, typically assign a substance use disorder diagnosis, and identify the psychosocial factors that may predispose, perpetuate, and maintain the drug involvement.

Diagnostic Interviews

Diagnostic interviews, which focus on DSM-based criteria for SUDs, include both general psychiatric interviews that address all psychiatric disorders and SUD interviews that focus primarily on drug use and related domains of functioning. The majority of the diagnostic interviews are structured; that is, the format directs the interviewer to read verbatim a series of questions in a decision-tree format, and the answers to these questions are restricted to a few predefined alternatives.

The Diagnostic Interview for Children and Adolescents and the Diagnostic Interview Schedule for Children (DISC) are two well-researched psychiatric diagnostic interviews that address SUDs as well as the full range of child and adolescent psychiatric disorders.

Interviews that primarily focus on diagnostic criteria for SUDs include the Adolescent Diagnostic Interview, the Customary Drinking and Drug Use Record, and the Global Ascertainment of Individual Needs.

Problem-Focused Interviews

Problem-focused interviews measure several problem areas and consequences associated with adolescent drug involvement, but do not provide a means to obtain a formal diagnosis of a substance use disorder. These include the Addiction Severity Index (ASI), the Teen Severity Index (T-ASI), and the Comprehensive Adolescent Severity Inventory.

Multiscale Questionnaires

The third group of comprehensive instruments consists of self-administered multi-scale questionnaires. These instruments range considerably in terms of length; some can be administered in <20 minutes, whereas others may take a full hour to administer. As a group, many of them share several characteristics: measures of both drug use problem severity and psychosocial risk factors are provided, strategies are included for detecting response distortion tendencies, the scales are standardized to a clinical sample, and the option of computer administration and scoring are available. Four examples of instruments in this group are the Adolescent Self-Assessment Profile, the Hilson Adolescent Profile, the Juvenile Automated Substance Abuse Evaluation, and the Personal Experience Inventory.

Summary Author: Sharon Cirone
Steven L. Jaffe • Ashraf Attalla • Diana I. Simeonova

Adolescent Treatment and Relapse Prevention

Treatment of adolescent substance use disorders involves a number of issues that are quite different from those seen in adults with substance abuse problems. First, the adolescent's biopsychosocial level of development must be considered. For example, it is normal for young adolescents (age 12–14 years) to be self-centered, experience mood shifts, and have minimal capacity for introspection. This profile makes therapy with early adolescents very different from the treatment of older adolescents. Second, because adolescents still are developing within a family system, family members must be part of the treatment program. Third, adolescents differ from adults in their patterns of substance use, as adolescents are more apt to use multiple drugs and are more likely to use inhalants in early adolescence and club drugs in late adolescence and early adulthood. Fourth, some studies have shown that current comorbidity is more common among adolescents than adults, and integrated treatment of the comorbid condition is especially important in adolescents.

TREATMENT MODALITIES

Significant progress has been made in adolescent treatment and relapse prevention in the past two decades. A number of treatment approaches have been used alone or in various combinations for the treatment of adolescent substance use, abuse, and dependency disorders. The three most commonly employed treatment approaches are family therapy, Twelve-Step–based programs, and therapeutic communities (TCs). Three treatment approaches—multidimensional family therapy (MDFT), functional family therapy, and group cognitive-behavioral therapy—are well-established models for treatment of this population. No single treatment modality has been demonstrated to be clearly superior. All therapies have a significant percentage of failures. Multiple approaches can be integrated in an attempt to improve outcome.

FAMILY THERAPY

Family therapy is the most studied modality in adolescent substance abuse treatment. Family therapy targets specific interpersonal family processes. Some of the goals of the family therapy are to decrease family resistance to treatment, to redefine substance use as a family problem, to reestablish parental influence, to interrupt dysfunctional sequences of family behavior, to assess the interpersonal function of the drug abuse, to implement strategies to change family interpersonal functioning, and to provide assertiveness training to the adolescent.

Multisystemic Therapy

This treatment approach promotes responsible behavior among all family members, and attempts to develop each individual's capacity to manage his or her own problems. Therapists work intensively with each adolescent and family in the home, school, and even neighborhood and peer group. Multisystemic therapy (MST) has demonstrated excellent retention rates and favorable outcomes. Some suggest that integrating MST into juvenile drug court improves substance abuse outcomes.

Multidimensional family therapy (MDFT) has established the most empiric support for efficacy. MDFT is an outpatient family-based treatment that combines substance abuse treatment with multiple system assessments and interventions within the family and the surrounding psychosocial environment.

Brief Strategic Family Therapy

This is a manualized family therapy structural-strategic approach developed for Hispanic families with behavior problem youth.

Functional Family Therapy

Functional family therapy integrates behavioral and cognitive interventions with ecological family relationship strategies.

Behavioral Family Therapy

With this approach, parents reinforce drug-incompatible activities, supervise home urge-control assignments, and employ written specifications of desired behaviors with contingent reinforcers. A recent study showed equal efficacy to cognitive problem-solving therapy.

COGNITIVE-BEHAVIORAL THERAPY

This therapeutic modality combines the learning principles of classical and operant conditioning with approaches to correct cognitive distortions and underlying negative belief systems. Treatment involves teaching the adolescent specific techniques to deal with drugs and alcohol. Specific skills to refuse alcohol and drugs are taught and practiced in role-playing exercises. Because deficits in coping skills for negative feelings and life stresses contribute to continued substance use, more general coping strategies (such as communication skills, problem-solving strategies, anger and mood management, and relaxation training) also are taught and practiced.

Both group and individual CBT interventions are relevant for adolescents with substance use disorders.

TWELVE-STEP APPROACHES

Although Twelve-Step–based treatment is one of the most common treatment models for adolescents, there has been little research into its efficacy. Working the 12 steps is an extremely concrete process that promotes abstinence and does not require abstract thinking.

The following descriptions present the first five steps, modified to make them meaningful for adolescents.

Step 1

Although many adult programs emphasize the concept of "surrendering" and admitting that one is an "addict," these are not useful for adolescents. Rather than surrendering, adolescents envision enhancing power by doing what one needs to do (such as stop using alcohol and drugs) instead of doing what one wants to do (use alcohol and drugs) is emphasized.

Twelve-Step programs accept the concept of addiction as a chronic progressive disorder that renders the "addict" unable to control and moderate his or her drinking or drug use. The only viable alternative is complete abstinence. For many adolescents, it may be helpful to view themselves as "on the way to becoming an addict," if they do not see themselves as already being one.

Step 2

The adolescent workbook approaches this step by recognizing that a child's first Higher Power is the person who raises him or her. For many drug-abusing/addicted adolescents, their parental figures were neglectful or abusive. Mourning the pain and sadness from the disappointments of their childhood higher powers enables them to begin to develop a sense of something positive in the universe that they can turn to for help. The Higher Power concept is not a religious belief, but a spiritual feeling that one can trust something positive (e.g., the group, another person, or nature) to take care of those aspects of one's life that one cannot control. One needs to have trust in the stability of the world and realize one controls one's own behavior, but not what others say or do. For many adolescents, the concrete positive feelings of their relationships to other members become the first Higher Power.

Step 3

The adolescent workbook interprets this step to involve having the adolescents make a decision to commit themselves to working the Steps and having a positive spiritual power. The teenagers are helped to recognize that they turned over their lives to alcohol and drugs. Now they are being asked to turn their lives over to a positive program.

Step 4

The workbook section on inventory taking has the adolescents answer numerous detailed questions covering all aspects of their childhood and present life.

Step 5

In this step, the adolescent verbalizes an inventory to a counselor or a sponsor. It is well recognized that adolescents will return to using alcohol and drugs if they return to contact with their alcohol- or drug-using friends. Twelve-Step programs provide the opportunity of a recovering peer group and mentoring relationships in the form of sponsors.

A recent study of 99 adolescents and Twelve-Step attendance following inpatient treatment demonstrated that Alcoholics Anonymous/Narcotics Anonymous attendance was uniquely associated with improved outcome. The major mechanism identified was that Twelve-Step attendance maintained and enhanced motivation for abstinence.

THERAPEUTIC COMMUNITIES

TCs offer long-term treatment (12–18 months) to adolescents who have multiple severe problems. In the TC approach, the community itself is part of the treatment process. Residents move through stages of increasing responsibility and privileges. Work, education, group activities, seminars, meals, job functions, and formal and informal interactions with peers and staff form the basis of self-development. The presence of staff members who are themselves in recovery and family involvement are important aspects of TCs.

Studies have found that adolescents who stayed in treatment 90 days or more tended to be more involved in self-help activities at the posttreatment follow-up. These adolescents had increased likelihood of attending Twelve-Step meetings and having a Twelve-Step sponsor after leaving treatment.

MOTIVATIONAL TREATMENT

Motivational therapeutic intervention involves helping the adolescent in an empathetic, nonconfrontational manner to move along the stages of change. Brief motivational interventions consisting of one to four sessions have proven effective. Even brief motivational interviews in Emergency Departments for adolescents who have presented with injuries related to alcohol use result in fewer future alcohol-related problems. Longer treatment interventions, workbook-based programs, and group programs are also effective. Motivational interviewing and Twelve-Step facilitation therapy develop motivation in the adolescent to stop using alcohol or other drugs through the adolescent's personal recognition of the negative consequences of such use.

Community Reinforcement Approach and Contingency Management

Community reinforcement approach (CRA) is a treatment approach originally developed for adults, in which the individual's life is rearranged so that abstinence is more rewarding than drinking. Contingency management involves concrete immediate positive rewards for a closely monitored behavior that usually involves vouchers for negative urines, or rewards for engaging in non–drug-using activities.

Pharmacotherapy

The use of medications in adolescent substance abuse treatment is just beginning to be studied. Nicotine replacement therapy for nicotine dependency, disulfiram aversion therapy for alcohol dependency, naltrexone as a blocker of opiates or to decrease cravings for alcohol, and methadone/buprenorphine as substitution therapy for opioid dependence are some of the strategies being tried. Pharmacotherapy of the comorbid disorders (i.e., attention deficit hyperactivity disorder, posttraumatic stress disorder, anxiety, and affective disorders) has been more extensively studied. With adolescents, pharmacologic interventions should always be used with psychosocial treatments.

RELAPSE

The most pressing problem in adolescent substance abuse treatment is the enormous relapse rate regardless of the treatment used. Relapse rates are >60% at 3 to 12 months after treatment completion. Thus, relapse is common and to be expected. With this in mind, it is important not to allow a lapse (return to alcohol or drug use for a few days) to develop into a full relapse (return to use for weeks or months). When counseling an adolescent during a lapse, a nonconfrontational manner that emphasizes learning is critical. The clinician can help the adolescent to identify triggers for use and lapse such as the company of "using" peers. The clinician can help the patient to enhance protective factors by encouraging involvement in aftercare and/or Twelve-Step meetings, seeking out family and peer support for abstinence, and following up with treatment of comorbid disorders.

CHAPTER 105

Summary Author: Sharon Cirone
Marc Fishman

Placement Criteria and Strategies for Adolescent Treatment Matching

Although the fields of adolescent treatment in general and adolescent treatment outcomes research in particular are still in their early stages, recent progress has been considerable. Over the past two decades, much has been learned about the effectiveness and limitations of current adolescent treatment methods and programs. Reviews of the published literature have shown favorable outcomes up to 1 year after treatment and beyond, across various modalities and levels of care. Little is known about the differential effectiveness of various treatment strategies, intensities, and treatment program components.

DEVELOPMENTAL CONSIDERATIONS IN ADOLESCENT PLACEMENT

One of the most important advances in the field of adolescent treatment is the articulation of approaches that are developmentally specific to the adolescent population. These respond to the principle that adolescents must be approached differently from adults because of differences in their levels of emotional, cognitive, physical, social, and moral development. Substance use can prevent a young person from completing the maturational tasks of adolescence, which involve formation of personal relationships, acquisition of social skills, psychologic development, identity formation, individuation, education, employment, and family role responsibilities. Adolescent treatment thus often requires habilitative rather than rehabilitative approaches, emphasizing the acquisition of new capacities rather than the restoration of lost ones.

Among adolescents, there may be special populations to take into consideration. Younger adolescents have a very narrow view of the world, with little capacity to think of future implications of present actions. Some adolescents may adopt a pseudomature ("street-wise") posture, despite their overall immaturity. Adolescents who live in a chaotic family system may have difficulties with normative expectations of behavioral contingency. Adolescents who have various cognitive difficulties may be delayed or impaired in acquiring abstract thinking.

In general, for a given degree of severity or functional impairment, adolescents require greater intensity of treatment than adults. This is reflected in clinical practice by a greater tendency to place adolescents in more intensive levels of care.

THE ASAM PATIENT PLACEMENT CRITERIA

The American Society of Addiction Medicine's (ASAM's) *ASAM Patient Placement Criteria for the Treatment of Substance-Related Disorders, 2nd ed.* revised (*ASAM PPC-2R*; 12) is a clinical guide that has been widely adopted to assist in matching patients to appropriate treatment settings. It contains separate sets of criteria for adolescents and adults. The criteria rest on the concept of enhancing the use of multidimensional assessments in placement decisions by organizing the assessment of the substance-using adolescent into six dimensions and specifying appropriate placements according to gradations of problem severity within each dimension.

Assessment-Based Treatment Matching and Clinical Appropriateness

The ASAM criteria use decision rules to guide placement in specified levels of care, which exist along a continuum. They also attempt to standardize some of the program specifications for each level of care. The principal goal of the ASAM criteria is to facilitate the process of matching patients in need of treatment for substance use disorders (SUDs) with appropriate treatment services and settings to maximize the accessibility, effectiveness, and efficiency of the treatment experience. The reality of limited availability of services is, of course, a major problem, particularly in the treatment of adolescents.

The *ASAM PPC-2R* outlines a full range of treatment services appropriate to the needs of all drug-involved adolescents, whether they are privately insured, publicly insured, underinsured, or uninsured. Although they may not have access to it, many marginalized or homeless adolescents and those in the juvenile justice system may need an even broader continuum of services than those with greater resources. In general, adolescents with fewer supports, less resiliency, and lower levels of baseline functioning may need a higher intensity of services and longer lengths of service at all levels of care than do those with the benefits conferred by economic advantage.

Placement and Treatment Considerations by Assessment Dimension

Dimension 1: Intoxication and Withdrawal Potential Severe physiologic withdrawal and the need for its management are seen less frequently in adolescents than in adults, given typical patterns of use and duration of exposure. Therefore, the provision of detoxification as a stand-alone service is less common and less needed with adolescents versus adults. Services to manage the withdrawal in a setting separate from other treatment services for adolescents with SUD are also clinically undesirable because of the developmental issues involved in the care of adolescents. This phase of treatment frequently requires an initial intensity to establish treatment engagement that will lead to the next steps of recovery.

Dimension 2: Biomedical Conditions and Complications Although the medical sequelae of addiction generally are not as common or as severe in adolescents as in adults, they certainly need to be considered in treatment placement decisions. Some of the acute and subacute medical complications of substance use include seizures caused by stimulant and inhalant intoxication, traumatic injuries associated with any substance intoxication, respiratory depression caused by opioid overdose, acute alcohol poisoning, complications of IVDU such as cellulites and endocarditis, STDs, gastritis caused by alcohol use, and exacerbation of reactive airway disease caused by smoking marijuana. Another notable area of medical complication in adolescents is the exacerbation of chronic illness (such as diabetes, asthma, or sickle cell disease) that results from impaired self-care and poor compliance with indicated medical treatments.

The special needs and medical vulnerabilities of pregnant substance-using teenagers require particular care in selecting treatment services. Overall, the need for contraception and other medical prevention and treatment services related to sexual behaviors in drug-involved adolescents cannot be overemphasized.

Dimension 3: Emotional, Behavioral, and Cognitive Conditions and Complications Drug-involved adolescents typically demonstrate a very high degree of co-occurring psychopathology, which frequently does not remit with abstinence. Many experts estimate that rates of psychiatric comorbidity, or dual diagnosis, are higher in adolescents than in adults. Many issues should be taken into consideration:

1. Previously diagnosed psychiatric illnesses
2. Subsyndromal symptoms such as mood lability or anger issues
3. The nonspecific features of immature or impaired executive functioning including impulsiveness, explosiveness, poor affective self-regulation, or poor strategic planning
4. Cognitive functioning and problems such as borderline intellectual functioning, fetal alcohol effects, assorted attentional deficits, or learning disorders
5. Complications of substance use (such as marijuana-induced amnestic disorder)
6. Behavioral issues
7. Adolescent learning in normal adolescent development as well as in those with the delayed development and immaturity that often accompanies drug use and co-occurring psychiatric disorders.

Dimension 4: Readiness to Change Placement decisions based on Dimension 4 will include consideration of whether the adolescent (and related systems, such as the family) is in the "precontemplation," "contemplation," "preparation," or "action" stage of change.

Motivational interviewing and other motivational enhancement techniques have formed the basis of a variety of intervention models at various levels of care, including early intervention and outpatient treatment.

Dimension 5: Relapse, Continued Use, or Continued Problem Potential

Dimension 5 entails an estimation of the likelihood of resumption or continuation of substance use. Four subdomains have been proposed as issues to take into consideration: (a) historical pattern of use (including amount, frequency, chronicity, and treatment response), (b) pharmacologic response to the effects from particular substances (including positive reinforcement such as pleasure with use and cravings and negative reinforcement such as relief from withdrawal or other negative experiences), (c) response to external stimuli (including reactivity to environmental triggers and acute or chronic stress), and (d) cognitive and behavioral vulnerability and resiliency factors (including traits of impulsivity, passivity, locus of control, and overall coping capacities).

Response to past treatment also may be a way of using individualized treatment effectiveness as a guide to placement.

Dimension 6: Recovery/Living Environment

Dimension 6 aims to assess the ability of the adolescent's home environment to support or impede treatment and recovery. For adolescents, the most important features of the recovery environment generally involve family and peers.

Placement and Treatment Considerations by Levels of Care

The adolescent levels of care in the *ASAM PPC-2R* are similar to the levels of care described and endorsed in other expert consensus documents

Level 0.5 Early Intervention

Early intervention services are designed to explore and address the adolescent's problems or risk factors that appear to be related to early stages of substance use. Their goal is to help the adolescent recognize the potentially harmful consequences of substance use, before such use escalates into substance abuse or dependence. Level 0.5 services may be delivered in a variety of settings, including primary care medical clinics, schools, social service and juvenile justice agencies, and driving under the influence intervention programs. Early intervention services are intended to combine prevention and treatment services for youth. Populations that warrant special attention at Level 0.5 are the children of substance-abusing parents, siblings of substance abusers, and adolescents with other emotional or behavioral problems. Early intervention is not appropriate for adolescents who qualify for a diagnosis of an SUD.

Level I: Outpatient Treatment

Outpatient treatment is by far the most frequently used level of care. It is often the initial level of care for an adolescent with low severity of illness. Level I also may be employed as a "step-down" program for the adolescent who has made progress at a more intensive level of care, for example, after care from a residential program. One of the advantages of outpatient treatment is the possibility of achieving therapeutic goals in the context of the patient's own home environment, where new behaviors can be practiced and solidified in real-life circumstances.

Level II: Intensive Outpatient Treatment/Partial Hospitalization

Intensive outpatient programs (IOPs) generally offer at least 6 hours of structured programming per week, for example, "day programs." Adolescent IOPs generally meet after school or work hours, or on weekends.

Partial hospitalization (Level II.5) programs often have direct access to or close referral relationships with psychiatric and medical services. Partial hospitalization may occur during school hours, and many programs, especially if they are longer term, have access to educational services for their adolescent patients.

Level III: Residential Treatment

Although earlier editions of the ASAM criteria treated all adolescent residential treatment as one broad undifferentiated level of care, the *PPC-2R* divides Level III into three sublevels.

- Level III.1: Clinically managed low-intensity residential treatment: programs typically provided in halfway houses and group homes, offering several hours a week of low-intensity treatment sessions for adolescents who require a longer term structured safe environment to learn recovery skills, relapse prevention, and improved social functioning
- Level III.5: Clinically managed medium-intensity residential treatment: These programs are designed to provide relatively extended subacute treatments with the goal of achieving fundamental personal change for the

adolescent who has significant social and psychologic problems or highly unstable home environments. Such programs are characterized by their reliance on the treatment community as a therapeutic agent of change.
• Level III.7: Medically monitored high-intensity residential/inpatient treatment.

This level is appropriate for adolescents whose problems are so severe that they require medically monitored residential treatment but do not need the full resources of an acute care hospital or medically managed inpatient treatment program (Level IV). Medically monitored services are provided under the supervision of physicians who are specialists in Addiction Medicine. Services typically provided include medical detoxification, titration of a psychopharmacologic regimen, and high-intensity behavior modification.

Level IV: Medically Managed Intensive Inpatient (Hospital) Treatment Delivered in an acute care inpatient setting in which the full resources of a general or psychiatric hospital are available, Level IV treatment tends to be brief, generally consisting of emergency or crisis interventions aimed at stabilization in preparation for transfer to a less intensive level of care for ongoing treatment.

Treatment Dose and Utilization Management

The ASAM criteria emphasize the concept of treatment as a dynamic, longitudinal process rather than a discrete episode of care or particular program enrollment. However, current treatment delivery systems do not generally support the necessary continuum of care.

CONFIDENTIALITY IN DEALING WITH ADOLESCENTS

Confidentiality is an essential component of health care for adolescents. Without some promise of confidentiality at the beginning of an office visit, the adolescent patient is less likely to disclose information about his or her behaviors, particularly concerning sensitive areas such as sexual activity or substance use. Health care professionals must understand the key principles underlying confidentiality and its limits.

A promise of confidentiality is especially important to adolescents, who, from a developmental perspective, are seeking to achieve autonomy from their parents and are learning to make appropriate decisions about a variety of issues, including healthy behaviors and seeking health care. Failing to afford confidentiality increases the risk of adolescents' delaying seeking or not receiving care until serious consequences arise from undisclosed behaviors (including pregnancy; pelvic inflammatory disease; drug overdose, abuse, or dependence; and alcohol-related motor vehicle injuries).

POLICIES ON CONFIDENTIALITY

Psychologic research suggests that adolescents demonstrate adult reasoning capacity at approximately age 14.

Physicians' professional organizations have long supported the concept of confidential care for adolescents. In 1967, the American Medical Association adopted a position that the epidemic of sexually transmitted diseases among young people required that minors be able to receive treatment for those infections without parental notification. The American Medical Association also opposed regulations that would have required clinicians working in federally funded programs to notify parents when they provided prescription contraceptives to patients under age 18.

In 1988, the American Academy of Pediatrics, the National Medical Association, the American College of Obstetricians and Gynecologists, and the American Academy of Family Physicians jointly endorsed recommendations on confidentiality, concluding that "ultimately, the health risks to adolescents are so impelling that legal barriers and deference to parental involvement should not stand in the way of needed care." The Health Insurance Portability and Accountability Act (1996) and its accompanying Privacy Rule (2001) protect adolescents as much as adults. Adolescents who are legally able to consent to care are generally treated by the Privacy Rule as protected in their own right. The Privacy Rule defers to "state or other applicable law" in terms of parents having access to their children's health information. The specifics of confidentiality protection vary from state to state; hence, clinicians must be knowledgeable about their own state's regulations.

DECIDING WHEN DISCLOSURE IS NECESSARY

Most experts do not recommend a blanket or unconditional assurance of confidentiality, because disclosure is mandated by law in certain circumstances. These include reports of sexual or physical abuse or expression of a clear threat of violence against a readily identifiable individual. Concerns about an adolescent's suicidality also would warrant breaking confidentiality. In such circumstances, the ethical principle of respect for persons, which underlies confidentiality, is overridden by higher ethical principles: "first, do no harm" and obeying the law.

A physician may state "I want to assure you that the information we discuss today is between you and me. It's confidential. In other words, I am not going to tell anyone without your permission, unless there is a situation which I believe might threaten your life or another's life or seriously endanger your health." A belief that a given behavior is wrong in the context of the clinician's own personal, moral, or religious code is not sufficient justification for breaking confidentiality. For example, a personal belief that premarital sex is wrong would not justify disclosing to a parent that an adolescent is sexually active, especially if the adolescent is acting responsibly by taking appropriate steps to protect against sexually transmitted infections or pregnancy.

After a clinician concludes that a breach of confidentiality is warranted, the adolescent should be told in advance and given options about how the disclosure will occur. These might include the adolescent revealing the information to his or her parents in the presence of the clinician, the adolescent telling the parents alone, or the clinician disclosing the information to the parents. In some cases, an adolescent may request that one but not both parents be involved.

In some special circumstances, different rules of confidentiality may apply. For example, the interaction between the adolescent and clinician may be ordered by a court or required as a condition of return to school. Federal and state regulations also may stipulate conditions of confidentiality for adolescents in drug treatment programs. Under these circumstances, the adolescent, the parents, and the clinician should be clear about the nature of the physician–patient relationship, including the boundaries of confidentiality and who will have access to the adolescent's medical record, including any test results.

Drug Testing Adolescents in School

Drug testing was judged to be a rational approach to reducing drug use among students engaged in middle and high school sports programs in the United States as a result of a U.S. Supreme Court's decision, and since that time, more school athletic programs have used drug testing in an attempt to reduce drug use among student athletes. A second U.S. Supreme Court case concerning adolescent drug testing during 2003 extended a school's substance use surveillance to include all extracurricular activities.

The White House Office of National Drug Control Policy actively advocates drug testing in schools and published a booklet: What you need to know about drug testing in schools.

TYPES OF DRUG TESTING

Drug testing can be without cause (e.g., no one suspects the persons of using drugs) or there can be "for cause" testing, based on a person's behavior or after an accident. Most programs, including sports, have used urine testing.

GOAL OF DRUG TESTING

The goal of a drug testing program can vary, depending on the particular population. An adolescent drug testing program within the school more than likely has prevention or deterrence as a primary goal, as well as the potential to uncover substance abuse problems, and provide early onset of appropriate treatment.

Thought of in this way, drug testing young student athletes can be reasoned to be a logical extension of the preparticipation physical examination, a procedure designed to detect and protect adolescents from concurrent injury or disease. This may be considered similar to a physician's report to schools of a medical history, including medication use where some conditions or prescribed medications may limit certain types of activities. These otherwise "confidential" medical records are reported to schools for the child's safety.

LEGAL ISSUES

As previously mentioned, there have been questions of the legality of drug testing, especially with regard to issues of search and seizure. The U.S. Supreme Court and some federal and state courts have determined that the secondary school environment has "a special need," wherein suspicionless student drug testing can be used for safety and discipline and to establish order. The issue for the courts was not whether drug testing was an actual deterrent, shown to effectively reduce substance use or abuse, but whether or not it was a legal policy. In 1995, the U.S. Supreme Court sanctioned drug testing in extracurricular school sport activities, wherein there was a balancing between an individual's rights and the need for drug use regulation in schools. Despite drug testing being legal in federal courts, state courts can agree with or deny use of student drug testing, based on local laws.

DRUG TESTING: THE EVIDENCE

Drug testing is not an established evidence-based policy shown to prevent drug use. Student-athlete and other school-based drug testing have not been adequately evaluated in clinical trials. There have been a few uncontrolled and nonrandomized reports suggesting that drug testing could have a deterrent effect. But the limited evidence from controlled trials that does exist has failed to demonstrate reduction in past-month substance use (drug use or drug and alcohol use), suggesting that more research with randomized controlled studies is needed to establish whether there are clear benefits of testing. Because of the potential risk (increasing risk factors for future drug or alcohol use) of testing and the costs of testing (not only the actual test, but the use of school personnel, lost class time, and more expensive tests [e.g., anabolic-androgenic steroids]), it appears prudent that schools wishing to implement prevention programs should do what they do best and educate their students using evidence-based programs.

CHAPTER 106

Summary Author: Sharon Cirone
Marie E. Armentano • Ramon Solhkhah • Deborah R. Simkin

Co-Occurring Psychiatric Disorders in Adolescents

Adolescents who manifest other psychiatric diagnoses in addition to substance use have elicited increasing concern. Adolescents with substance use disorders (SUDs) exhibit a high prevalence of psychiatric disorders compared to the general population. Studies of treatment-seeking SUD adolescents have documented that 50% to 90% also have non-SUD comorbid psychiatric disorders.

The terms dual diagnosis, comorbidity, and co-occurring disorders refer to patients who meet the criteria for an SUD and for another psychiatric diagnosis on Axis I or II of the *Diagnostic and Statistical Manual of Mental Disorders*, *4th ed.* (*DSM-IV-TR*) of the American Psychiatric Association. Though a high prevalence of comorbidity has been reported among adolescent inpatients with SUDs, it is unclear how many exhibit psychiatric symptoms secondary to the SUDs and how many have a primary or coexisting psychiatric diagnosis.

INCIDENCE AND PREVALENCE

Physicians should know the kinds of comorbidities they are likely to encounter in practice. Until recently, however, large-scale population studies did not focus on adolescents. In one study, 82% of the patients met *DSM-IIIR* criteria for an Axis I psychiatric disorder, 61% had mood disorders, 54% had conduct disorders, 43% had anxiety disorders, and 16% had substance-induced disorder. Three fourths of the patients (74%) had two or more psychiatric disorders.

Another study compared adolescents who had met the criteria for one of six psychiatric diagnoses, including SUDs, before and after they were 14 years of age. Adolescents with early onset of any psychiatric disorder were six times as likely to have one and 12 times as likely to have two additional disorders by the time they were 18 years of age than were those with later onset of psychiatric disorders. This finding suggests that the clinician's index of suspicion for dual diagnosis must be particularly high for younger patients with SUDs.

Yet another study concluded that 15 to 19 years were the peak ages for the onset of depressive disorders in females and for the onset of SUDs and bipolar disorders in both genders.

A large national comorbidity study that included a large noninstitutional sample of persons aged 15 to 24 showed that compared with older adults, 15- to 24-year-olds had the highest prevalence of three or more disorders occurring together and of any disorders, including SUDs.

DIAGNOSIS AND MANAGEMENT

Clinicians should conduct a comprehensive evaluation of each patient including

1. A comprehensive history of alcohol, tobacco, and other drug use
2. An inquiry into psychological and psychiatric symptomatology
3. History and information from multiple sources
4. A mental status examination
5. A high index of suspicion for comorbidity in adolescents whose conditions do not respond to treatment or who present problems in treatment

Management should include

1. Individualized treatment to accommodate both the substance use and psychiatric diagnoses
2. Consultation with an addiction medicine specialist or mental health professional, as necessary
3. Self-help groups such as Al-Ateen, Alcoholics Anonymous, Narcotics Anonymous, or "Double-Trouble" groups for patients with co-occurring psychiatric and addiction disorders

Depressive Disorders

Much has been written about the interplay between depression and substance use. The chief symptom of depression consists of a disturbance of mood, which usually is characterized as sadness or feeling "down in the dumps," and a loss of interest or pleasure. Adolescents may report or exhibit irritability instead of sadness. In addition, their depression may be characterized by guilt, hopelessness, sleep disturbances, appetite disturbances, loss of ability to concentrate, diminution of energy, and thoughts of death or suicide.

To meet *DSM-IV-TR* diagnostic criteria, the patient must exhibit or experience depressed mood most of the day, every day, for 2 weeks. Patients with a substance-induced mood disorder may exhibit the same depressive symptoms.

The emerging concept is that in adolescents and adults, there are two groups that exhibit significant depressive symptoms: those individuals who have a substance-induced mood disorder and those who have a primary depressive disorder. The clinician should consider the importance of distinguishing between primary depressive disorder and substance-induced mood disorder. Studies of adults who abuse substances showed that substance-induced mood disorder dissipates with abstinence, but primary depressive disorders do not and, if left untreated, can interfere with treatment and recovery. Studies of adolescent inpatients on a dual diagnosis unit indicate that between 25% and 35% will have a comorbid major depression, with secondary depressive disorder much more common than primary depressive disorder. Unlike adults, the secondary depression in adolescents may not remit with abstinence. This finding may argue for more vigorous treatment of depressive syndromes in adolescents.

During the mental status examination, depressed adolescents may seem taciturn and show poor eye contact and a sad-looking face. They may be poorly groomed or drably dressed and may become tearful during the interview. Often they deny feelings of sadness, though their demeanor states it eloquently. Depression interferes with treatment through lack of concentration, motivation, and hope, cognitive distortions, as well as the tendency toward isolation.

Some studies show that remission of depression was a stronger predictor of change in drug use than in medication treatment. Although medication may be helpful, depression symptoms may remit in the context of individual outpatient cognitive behavioral therapy (CBT) for SUD without pharmacotherapy. However, if depression does not remit within the 1st month of treatment, it appears that starting fluoxetine, with careful monitoring, even if not yet abstinent, is prudent because ongoing depression may prevent abstinence achievement. Serotonin agents like fluoxetine have a safe profile for side effects and may be appropriate considering reports that young substance abusers may have a preexisting serotonin deficit.

If there are doubts about the diagnosis of depression or about how to treat, consultation with a psychiatrist experienced in treating adolescents with SUDs is indicated. If the primary clinician is concerned about possible suicidal behavior, a consultation should be sought without delay.

Bipolar Disorder

The diagnosis of bipolar disorder may be among the most difficult to make in children and adolescents and is even more difficult in teens who use alcohol or other drugs. Issues such as changes in sleeping patterns or mood swings can be symptoms of bipolar disorder, substance use, or even normal adolescence. The diagnosis of bipolar disorder certainly should be considered in substance-using youth, particularly those with a binge pattern.

In bipolar disorder, which often begins during late adolescence, the initial symptoms of mania include a persistently elevated, expansive, or irritable mood lasting at least 1 week, accompanied by grandiosity or inflated self-esteem, decreased need for sleep, pressured speech, racing thoughts, increased purposeful activity, and excessive involvement in pleasurable activities, such as spending money, sexual indiscretions, or substance use. One study has reported that those with adolescent-onset bipolar disorder had an 8.8 times greater risk of developing an SUD than those with childhood-onset bipolar disorder. Children who were diagnosed and treated appropriately at a younger age had a lower subsequent risk for substance use.

Some patients use substances, particularly alcohol, to calm themselves during a manic phase. With respect to pharmacotherapy, valproic acid, carbamazepine, and other anticonvulsants are used, as are the atypical antipsychotics, such as olanzapine and risperidone. In one treatment study, when lithium was used, not only were the symptoms of mania decreased but the use of alcohol also decreased.

Anxiety Disorders

Anxiety disorders are among the psychiatric conditions most often coexisting in adolescents and adults with SUDs. Typically, these conditions include generalized anxiety disorder, panic disorder, social phobia, obsessive-compulsive disorder, and posttraumatic stress disorder (PTSD). Anxiety disorders often are not detected or treated, especially when present in combination with depression or psychoactive SUDs. In fact, many adolescents (and adults) believe that drugs and alcohol may contribute to reduction of anxiety and stress, and this belief may lead them to initiate or continue use. Studies have demonstrated that the onset of anxiety disorders was more likely to precede SUDs than vice versa. Some well-done studies show that teens who never use drugs or alcohol may be at higher risk for anxiety disorders later in life.

Behavioral treatment, including relaxation training, often is helpful for anxiety disorders. The issue of pharmacotherapy is controversial. Many argue that the use of benzodiazepines is contraindicated in anyone with a history of substance abuse. Buspirone hydrochloride and serotonin reuptake inhibitors have been recommended as nonaddictive antianxiety agents. However, clinical experience and anecdotal reports suggest that for many, buspirone is ineffective. When treating patients who insist that only benzodiazepines are effective, it often is not clear whether the statement represents drug-seeking behavior or a bona fide observation. If abstinence has been established, adequate trials of behavioral or cognitive therapy and alternative medications have failed, and the patient adheres to the treatment and medication regimen; the judicious use of a long-acting benzodiazepine, such as clonazepam, may be justified.

Panic Disorder Panic attacks are periods of intense discomfort that develop abruptly and reach a peak within 10 minutes. Symptoms include palpitations, sweating, trembling, sensations of shortness of breath or choking, chest discomfort, nausea, dizziness, and fears of losing control or dying. As some of these symptoms also might be seen in substance intoxication or withdrawal, it is important to establish abstinence before making a diagnosis.

Social Phobias Sometimes a closer examination of patients who resist attending self-help meetings may reveal a social phobia or agoraphobia. Social phobia and its importance in terms of early diagnosis cannot be overemphasized. Though many children with social phobia are not recognized early because they did not have a behavioral problem in class, children who are referred for evaluation for aggression should be carefully evaluated for social phobia. In one study, the combination of shyness and aggressiveness in boys was a more valid predictor of future cocaine use than a history of aggressiveness alone.

Posttraumatic Stress Disorder In clinical reports on adolescents, the incidence of severe trauma and symptoms of posttraumatic stress disorder is surprisingly high. An adolescent who has been acting out and abusing substances may not have dealt with an earlier trauma, such as physical and sexual abuse or exposure to violence, or with the trauma that may be incurred when abusing substances. Symptoms and memories of trauma may manifest themselves only during abstinence.

Trauma and the symptoms associated with trauma should to be considered and inquired about to ensure adequate treatment of adolescents who abuse substances. Care should be taken to acknowledge the trauma without arousing anxiety that will interfere with abstinence and substance abuse treatment. Groups that support self-care and a first-things-first attitude may be the best approach; the patient needs to learn to stay safe, and treatment for substance abuse is a most important aspect of safety. Treatments that integrate PTSD- and SUD-focused cognitive-behavioral and family treatment for adolescents with comorbid abuse-related PTSD and SUD may optimize outcomes for this population. One treatment example is the Seeking Safety 20 session manualized program that can be used in group or individual therapy.

Substance-Induced Mental Disorders

In some patients, the use of substances—particularly alcohol, methamphetamine, marijuana, cocaine, ecstasy, hallucinogens, and inhalants—is associated with acute and residual cognitive damage. Acute symptoms may include impaired concentration and receptive and expressive language abilities, as well as irritability. Long-term interference with memory and other executive functions may occur.

The possibility of a substance-induced impairment should be considered in adolescents who have difficulty coping with the cognitive and organizational demands of a structured and supportive program. The presence of cognitive deficits, if they persist, should be considered in rehabilitation, educational, and vocational planning. Such patients need neuropsychologic evaluation and follow-up.

Substance-induced psychosis presents, not uncommonly, with cannabis use and occasionally may be observed with PCP-induced delirium.

Learning Disorders

Clinicians should be sure to explore attentional problems and consider other diagnostic possibilities than just ADHD, such as learning disorders. Studies have found that substance abuse at age 14 or 15 could be predicted by academic and social behavior between the ages of 7 and 9. Therefore, early detection of learning disorders is essential in order to reduce the risk of developing an SUD.

Schizophrenia

Patients who simultaneously meet the criteria for schizophrenia and an SUD are less likely to receive treatment in an addiction treatment program than in a psychiatric unit. As the late adolescent years are a time when many schizophrenic disorders begin and the use of substances may precipitate an incipient psychosis, patients with this disorder may seek treatment during the early stages of schizophrenia.

Increasingly, younger schizophrenic patients use substances, some in an attempt to manage or deny their symptoms. Their substance use often interferes with treatment of their psychotic disorder. Such patients are best managed in special dual diagnosis programs for psychotic patients, where the psychosis and the substance use are addressed through integrated mental health and addiction treatment.

Numerous research studies have indicated that there may be a reward deficiency dysfunction in schizophrenia that underlines the use of substances of abuse to compensate and that clozapine and other atypical agents may be effective in the treatment of co-occurring schizophrenia and SUD because they address this reward dysfunction. Marijuana and alcohol are the two most frequently used substances in these patients. Marijuana is known to trigger psychosis in vulnerable individuals (those with a family history or typical premorbid symptoms). Marijuana in these individuals may be associated with earlier and more severe onset of schizophrenia symptoms. There is recent evidence of the emergence of schizophrenia in individuals with no other predisposition but who have a particular genetic allele change and concomitant use of marijuana.

Attention Deficit Hyperactivity Disorder

Many professionals involved in the treatment of adolescents with SUDs have noted that a large number of adolescents also have attention deficit hyperactivity disorder. Treatment of these co-occurring disorders should include behavioral and educational interventions. Pharmacotherapy for adolescents has been controversial. It is prudent to use nonstimulant medications as a first line when treating comorbid ADHD and SUD. It is well documented that treatment of identified ADHD is associated with a decreased risk of subsequent SUDs.

Conduct Disorder and Antisocial Personality Disorder

Conduct disorder and antisocial personality disorder are the diagnoses that most often co-occur with substance abuse, particularly in males. The characteristic symptom of antisocial personality disorder is a pervasive pattern of disregarding and violating the rights of others. The disorder may involve deceitfulness, impulsivity, failure to conform to rules or the law, aggressiveness, and irresponsibility. Conduct disorder has similar criteria but includes manifestations that are likely to be seen in younger persons, such as cruelty to animals, running away, truancy, and vandalism.

Many researchers have noted that adolescent SUD usually occurs as part of a constellation of problem behaviors that may fit into an interesting scheme of hereditary factors on three axes: reward dependence, harm avoidance, and novelty seeking that may account for the interrelationship with externalizing psychiatric diagnoses and the difficulty to treat them.

The interrelationship may perhaps be neurochemically determined and then manifested as difficulty with self-regulation and aggression. Adolescents with conduct disorders and antisocial personality disorder need a strong behavioral program with clear limits.

Borderline and Narcissistic Personality Disorders

Personality disorders are enduring patterns of inner experience and behavior that affect cognition, interpersonal behavior, emotional response, and impulse control. Both borderline and narcissistic personality disorders can present challenges to the clinician and the treatment staff. Powerful negative feelings, conscious and unconscious, are easily aroused by patients who are manipulative and full of rage, who feel entitled, and whose behavior saps the emotional strength of the staff. If the treatment of a patient requires a great deal of emotional energy, personality issues likely are involved. In such situations, it is essential to be aware of the effect that such patients exert and to take care of the clinical staff as well as the patient.

Eating Disorders

The incidence of eating disorders and substance abuse in the adolescent population has increased, so it is not uncommon to find them together. In fact, a fourth of all patients who have an eating disorder either have a history of substance abuse or currently are abusing substances.

Bulimic patients have been found to have a greater risk for substance abuse than restrictive anorexics. Some studies have shown that bulimic women with SUD have higher novelty seeking than bulimic women without SUD. Bulimia involves recurrent episodes of binge eating, sometimes accompanied by compensatory measures (such as vomiting or laxative abuse), and a preoccupation with food and weight. Persons with an eating disorder may abuse amphetamines to lose weight.

Summary Author: John Young
H. Westley Clark • Anton C. Bizzell

Ethical Issues in Addiction Practice

Certain ethical principles are central to medical practice. Foremost among these is the physician's obligation to put the patient's interests first. This is closely followed by respect for the patient's autonomy (which includes the patient's right to make his or her own medical decisions, as well as the right to be left alone) and the patient's privacy or confidentiality. The physician also has a general duty to protect society when the patient's condition poses a threat to others. Physicians who screen, assess, or treat patients for addictive disorders sometimes find themselves in situations where ethical principles are in conflict.

PATIENT AUTONOMY

Medicine places a high value on patient autonomy. Patients consult physicians on their own initiative when they decide they have reached a level of discomfort with a particular problem. The physician can make recommendations but must recognize that the patient has the right to choose among the recommended treatments or to refuse them altogether. Rarely will a physician consider forcing advice on a patient, even if convinced that the patient is making a wrong choice.

When a patient is in denial about his or her abuse of alcohol or drugs, however, the principles of autonomy and privacy can sometimes seem to work against what the physician sees as the patient's best interests.

Dealing with Denial

A physician who screens or assesses patients for addictive disorders is seeking information about lifestyle and personal habits that carry a good deal of stigma. Both the patient and the physician may view such inquiries as intrusions on the patient's autonomy and/or privacy. Nevertheless, when a physician suspects that a patient who presents with another complaint is also abusing drugs or alcohol, he or she must take the initiative if the patient does not raise the issue.

The difficulty is that raising the issue sometimes is not enough, because denial is an integral part of addictive disorders; individuals in denial fail to recognize or are reluctant to acknowledge their problem because they are ambivalent about giving up such use.

Talking with the Patient

To fulfill the ethical responsibility to the patient, the physician must do more than simply raise the issue: he or she should provide relevant information, engage the patient in discussion, and, if the patient shows resistance, follow up in future visits. How far the physician can intrude on the patient's autonomy will depend a great deal on the strength of the physician–patient relationship.

Ordering Laboratory Tests

Screening urine or blood for drugs is not routine practice in primary care settings. A patient confronted with the results of a test he or she did not know about may feel betrayed by the physician, which can damage the doctor–patient relationship and undermine the physician's efforts to induce the patient to acknowledge the problem. The better practice is to obtain the patient's consent for alcohol or drug tests.

A second reason for obtaining the patient's consent before ordering drug screens has to do with the patient's right to privacy. If the physician orders a test, the patient's third-party payer will know about it and perhaps the result as well. The physician's decision to order a drug screen tells the third-party payer a good deal, even if the result is negative.

A third reason is financial. The patient's third-party payer may not cover drug screens, in which case the patient should have the opportunity to decide whether he or she is willing to pay for the test out of pocket.

There is a chance that if the physician asks the patient for permission to perform a drug screen, the patient will refuse. However, this still leaves the door open to further discuss with the patient about possible drug problems.

INFORMED CONSENT

Patients have the right to make decisions about their medical care. Informed consent has three components:

- *Competence*: The patient must be capable of understanding the information and making a decision.
- *Information*: The physician must give the patient the kind and amount of information the patient needs to make an intelligent choice.
- *Voluntariness:* The patient's decision must be a product of his or her free will.

COMPETENCE (DECISION-MAKING CAPACITY)

The concept of informed consent is based on the assumption that the patient has "decisional capacity," meaning that the patient is able to understand the physician's explanation of the diagnosis, prognosis, treatment alternatives, and likely outcome if treatment is refused and is able to go through the process of assessing that information in accordance with his or her personal system of values. The physician may encounter questions about decisional capacity in dealing with two groups: adolescents and older adults.

Issues in Dealing with Adolescents

In states that require parental consent to or notification of treatment for addictive disorders, difficulties arise when an adolescent who seeks assessment or treatment refuses to permit communication with a parent. If the physician believes that the adolescent needs treatment, he or she has three choices:

Choice 1: The Physician Can Treat the Adolescent without Consulting a Parent

Although violation of the parental consent/notification law most likely is not a criminal offense, it could put the physician's professional license at risk or expose him or her to a lawsuit by the adolescent's parents. It is unlikely, however, that a physician treating an adolescent would be faced with either eventuality if the treatment provided is not controversial or intrusive, does not put the adolescent at risk, and is carried out in a responsible, nonnegligent manner. The physician who is considering whether to offer treatment without parental consent or notification in a state that requires it should consider the following factors:

- The adolescent's age. Society accords adolescents more autonomy as they get older.
- The adolescent's maturity. Chronologic age clearly is not the only measure.
- The adolescent's family situation. Adolescents in need of addictive disorder treatment may be estranged from their families and may have good reasons for refusing to permit parental notification.
- The severity of the adolescent's addictive disorder and the danger it poses to his or her life or health
- The kind of treatment to be provided. The more intrusive and intensive the proposed treatment, the more risk the physician assumes.
- The physician's possible liability for refusing to treat the patient. State law may impose a duty to treat patients in need.
- The financial consequences. If the physician treats an adolescent without parental consent, he or she may not be paid.

Choice 2: The Physician Can Refuse to Treat the Adolescent

Refusing to treat the adolescent adheres to the letter of state laws that consider adolescents incompetent to make medical decisions and it shows respect for the patient's privacy, but it may violate the ethical principle that requires the physician to put the patient's health first. In some states, it also violates a law requiring physicians to treat patients in medical need.

Choice 3: The Physician Can Call the Adolescent's Parent to try to Obtain Consent to Treat the Adolescent

Federal confidentiality rules complicate this choice: If the physician is subject to these rules, he or she is prohibited from contacting a parent unless the adolescent consents. The sole exception allows a treatment program director to contact a parent when the life or physical well-being of an adolescent is threatened.

Issues in Dealing with Older Adults

Most older adults are fully capable of understanding medical information, weighing the treatment alternatives, and making and articulating decisions. A small percentage of older patients are incapable of participating in a decision-making process.

Difficulty arises when a physician is screening or assessing an older adult whose mental capacity lies between those two extremes. The patient may have fluctuating capacity or periods of greater or lesser alertness depending on the time of day. Diminished capacity may affect some parts of his or her ability to comprehend information and make complex decisions, but not others. In such situations, there are several possible approaches:

- Present information carefully: Information should be presented in a way that allows the patient to absorb it gradually. The physician can also help the patient identify his or her values and link those values to the alternatives.
- Enlist the help of a health or mental health professional: The physician could suggest a specialist who can help determine why the patient is having difficulty and whether he or she has the capacity to give informed consent.
- Enlist the help of family or close friends: Asking the patient who would be helpful could gain endorsement of this approach.
- Consult a family member or friend: It may be that the patient already has planned for the possibility of incapacity and has signed a durable power of attorney or health care proxy.
- Guardianship: A guardian is a person appointed by a court to manage some or all aspects of another person's life. Anyone seeking appointment of a guardian must show the court that the individual is disabled in some way by disease, illness, or senility and that the disability prevents that individual from performing the tasks necessary to manage one or more areas of his or her life. Guardianship is an expensive process and limits the older adult's autonomy; it should be considered only as a last resort.

INFORMATION

The physician is obligated to give the patient all the information he or she needs to make a decision. This information should include the physician's opinion of the patient's diagnosis, an outline of the available treatment alternatives (including its benefits and risks), an explanation of the consequences should the patient decline treatment altogether, and responses to the patient's questions.

Many managed care contracts create incentives that can impinge on medical judgment. If a physician allows financial incentives or disincentives to influence treatment recommendations, or to discharge a patient who has exhausted benefits under the contract, that physician has placed financial interests before his or her obligation to the patient's health—a clear ethical violation. Ethicists suggest that the physician should inform the patient about any economic issues that could influence either the physician's recommendation or the patient's decision.

VOLUNTARINESS VERSUS COERCION

A number of patients in addiction treatment have been forced into such treatment by their families, employers, or the criminal justice system. Critics of coerced treatment contend that it is unethical because the power imbalance in such circumstances violates the principle of autonomy.

Proponents of coerced treatment counter that although such coercion unquestionably impinges on a patient's autonomy, it does not violate it altogether, even in the criminal context. The patient may not want to enter treatment but always has a choice and retains the right to refuse. He or she may not like the consequences (losing a job or spouse, or being incarcerated on criminal charges) but still retains the autonomy to make the decision. Proponents also point out that patients who stay in treatment for at least 90 days have better outcomes than those who leave earlier. To the extent that coercion raises retention rates, they argue, it works to improve the odds that the patient will have a positive outcome.

CHAPTER 108

Summary Author: John Young
Bonnie B. Wilford

Consent and Confidentiality in Addiction Practice

CONSENT TO TREATMENT

The addiction physician should discuss the risks and benefits of treatment with the patient; if possible, every attempt should be made to involve significant others, family members or guardian, in the treatment process. The treatment plan should be in writing, describing:

- The objectives that will be used to determine treatment success, such as freedom from intoxication, compliance with treatment, and improved physical and psychosocial function
- Whether any further diagnostic evaluations are planned, as well as counseling, psychiatric management, or other ancillary services
- Regular toxicologic testing for therapeutic drug levels and for drugs of abuse
- Number and frequency of all prescription refills
- Alternative treatment options
- Reasons for which drug therapy may be discontinued (i.e., violation of agreement)
- Contingencies for treatment failure

The plan should be reviewed periodically.

Periodic assessment of the patient is necessary to determine effectiveness of the treatment plan and to assess how the patient is handling any prescribed medication. Continuation or modification of opioid therapy should depend on the physician's evaluation of progress toward stated treatment objectives.

CONFIDENTIALITY

Confidentiality is especially important when a patient has an addictive disorder because of the widespread perception that such persons are weak and/or morally impaired, concern that an insurer or HMO might refuse or cancel coverage, and patients' fear that their relationships with others might suffer if they learned about alcohol or drugs problems. This fear can deter patients from admitting to problems with alcohol or drugs and from obtaining treatment for those problems; nevertheless, the right to privacy is not without limits.

Sources of Guidance

Federal Laws In the early 1970s, the Department of Health and Human Services (DHHS) issued regulations protecting the confidentiality of patients in addictive disorder treatment. The federal rules permit disclosures only in very limited circumstances, and apply regardless of whether the person seeking information has a subpoena or search warrant.

Physicians who practice primary care probably are not subject to the federal confidentiality law and regulations; however, when a general care practice includes someone whose primary function is to provide addictive disorder assessment or treatment and the practice benefits from "federal assistance," it must comply with federal rules. The best practice for those not subject to the federal confidentiality rules is voluntary compliance.

In 1996, Congress passed the Health Insurance Portability and Accountability Act (HIPAA), which mandated the establishment of standards for the privacy of "individually identifiable health information." To carry out that mandate, in December 2000, DHHS issued a set of regulations governing patients' privacy that apply to a wide range of "health care providers."

HIPAA regulations are not as restrictive as the federal confidentiality rules. Practitioners who are subject to both sets of rules must follow the more restrictive federal standard.

State Laws Some states have special confidentiality laws that explicitly prohibit practitioners from divulging information about patients without their consent. States often include such prohibitions in professional licensing laws, making unauthorized disclosures grounds for disciplinary action, including license revocation.

Whether a communication (e.g., laboratory test result) is "privileged" or "protected" depends on a number of factors:

- *The type of professional holding the information.* Most state laws do cover licensed physicians.
- *The context in which the information was communicated.* Some states do not protect information disclosed to a physician in the presence of a third party, such as a spouse.
- *The circumstances in which "confidential" information will be or was disclosed.* Some states protect medical information only when that information is sought in a court proceeding.
- *How the right to privacy is enforced.* State legal protection of medical information is useful only when it is backed by enforcement of the law.

States can discipline professionals, allow patients to sue physicians for damages, or criminalize a behavior that violates patients' privacy.

Exceptions Exceptions to any general rule protecting the privacy of information generally include

- *Consent*: All states permit physicians to disclose information if the patient consents; in some states, the consent must be written; in others, it can be oral.
- *Reporting infectious diseases*: All states require physicians to report certain infectious diseases to public health authorities, though states' definitions of reportable diseases vary.
- *Reporting child abuse and neglect*: All states require physicians to report child abuse and neglect to child protective services, though states' definitions of child abuse vary.
- *Duty to warn*: Most states also require physicians to report credible threats a patient makes to harm others.

When Confidentiality Conflicts with Other Principles

The laws may differ depending on whether the physician's obligation is to the patient or another individual or class of individuals.

Employer versus Employee To whom does a physician owe loyalty when treating a patient who has been referred by an employer as a condition of retaining a job? The employer likely will require reports from the physician on the patient's progress in treatment. What should the physician do if the employee is not attending or complying with treatment? This question appears most starkly when the employee is in a safety-sensitive position and the physician is concerned that his or her behavior poses an immediate risk to other employees or to the public.

The best way to avoid having to grapple with this problem is to create agreed-upon ground rules before treatment begins. If an employer requires reports, the physician must have the patient sign a consent form specifying what kinds of information will be reported to the employer. The patient can revoke his or her consent at any time, and the employer must be willing to accept whatever limitations the agreement places on the kinds of information it will receive.

Society versus Patient Most physicians know under what circumstances society has determined that their duty to warn supersedes their duty to protect a patient's privacy. The duty to warn, however, does not completely nullify the patient's right to privacy. The physician can warn others of potential danger in a way that minimizes harm to the patient's privacy, for example, by not disclosing extraneous information about the patient's use of drugs or alcohol.

CHAPTER 109

Summary Author: John Young
Theodore V. Parran, Jr. • Robert L. DuPont • Bruce D. Lamb

Clinical and Legal Considerations in Prescribing Drugs with Abuse Potential

CLINICAL STRATEGIES TO IMPROVE PRESCRIBING

Patient Assessment

An essential first step in appropriate prescribing is obtaining a detailed history of the patient's past use of both prescription and over-the-counter medications. When prescribing a controlled drug to a new patient, many experts recommend additional precautions, including:

- Determining who has been caring for the patient in the past, what drug(s) have been prescribed and for what indications, and what nonpharmaceutical substances the patient has used. Medical records should be obtained.
- In emergency situations, the patient's identity should be verified by obtaining proper identification, and the physician should prescribe no more than 1 day's supply of a drug and arrange for a return visit.
- In nonemergency situations, the physician should prescribe only enough of a controlled drug to meet the patient's needs until the next appointment.

Drug Selection

When the optimum drug has been selected, the dose, schedule, route of administration, and formulation should be determined; these choices are often just as important in optimizing drug therapy as the choice of drug itself.

Most physicians adopt additional safeguards in the use of psychoactive drugs. Physicians typically consider three additional factors before deciding to prescribe:

- The *severity of symptoms*, in terms of the patient's ability to accommodate them
- The patient's *reliability in taking medications*. A physician should assess a patient's susceptibility to drug abuse before prescribing any psychoactive drug and weigh the benefits against the risks. The possible development of dependence in patients on long-term therapy should be monitored through periodic checkups.
- The *dependence-producing potential of the drug*

Patients should be informed that it is illegal to sell, give away, or otherwise share their medication with others, including family members. The patient's obligation extends to keeping the medication in a locked cabinet or otherwise restricting access to it and to safely disposing of any unused supply.

No treatment program should be left open-ended. Where feasible, planned termination of medication therapy is a reasonable goal because it minimizes drug exposure and contains costs.

Monitoring the Patient's Response to Treatment

Simply recognizing the potential for nonadherence, especially during prolonged treatment, is a significant step toward improving medication use. Steps such as simplifying the drug regimen and offering patient education improve adherence, as do phone calls to patients, home visits by nursing personnel, convenient packaging of medication, and monitoring of serum drug levels. Asking the patient to keep a log of signs and symptoms gives him or her a sense of participation in the treatment program and facilitates the physician's review of therapeutic progress and adverse events.

LEGAL STRATEGIES TO IMPROVE PRESCRIBING

Informed Consent

When prescribing controlled drugs, physicians should inform the patient of the risks and benefits of the therapy and of the ethical and legal obligations such therapy imposes on both the physician and the patient. Informed consent should also address the potential for physical dependence and cognitive impairment.

Other factors to be addressed include:

- Agreement to obtain prescriptions from only one physician and, preferably, from one designated pharmacy
- Agreement to take the medication only as prescribed
- Acknowledgment that the patient is responsible for his or her written prescriptions, medications, arranging refills during regular office hours, and planning ahead so as not to run out of medication during weekends or vacations
- Terms for informed consent violations, indicating that continued prescribing may be unsafe
- An understanding that lack of adherence may result in weaning and gradual or abrupt discontinuation of controlled drug therapy

It is helpful to give the patient a copy of the agreement to carry with him or her, to document the source and reason for any controlled drugs in his or her possession. Some physicians provide a laminated card that identifies the individual as a patient of their practice. This is helpful to other physicians who may see the patient and in the event the patient is seen in an emergency department.

Executing the Prescription Order

Under federal law, every prescription order must include at least the following information:

Name and address of the patient
Name, address, and DEA registration number of the physician
Signature of the physician
Name and quantity of the drug prescribed
Directions for use
Refill information

Many states impose additional requirements. In addition, there are special federal requirements for drugs in different schedules of the federal Controlled Substances Act (CSA), particularly those in Schedule II; for example, prescriptions for controlled substances must be signed and dated on the day they are issued.

Drug seekers are constantly on the lookout for blank forms. The physician should immediately report a theft or loss of prescription blanks to the nearest field office of the federal DEA and to the state board of medicine or pharmacy.

When the physician is concerned about a patient's behavior or clinical progress (or the lack thereof), it usually is advisable to seek a consultation with an expert in the disorder for which the patient is being treated, as well as an expert in addiction medicine. Physicians place themselves at risk if they continue prescribing controlled drugs in the absence of such consultations.

The Patient Record

In the event of a legal or regulatory challenge, detailed medical records documenting what was done and why are the foundations of the physician's defense.

At a minimum, patient records should contain the following information:

- *Patient history and physical examination*: The patient record must include a history of all controlled drugs used to treat the patient in the past, any use of illicit substances, and any patient allergies. Regimens tried and failed also should be documented. Documentation should include information about the patient's personal and family histories of alcoholism, drug use, and addiction, as well as any personal history of major depression or other psychiatric disorder. It is wise to obtain the patient's records directly from physicians who have treated him or her in the past.
- *Documentation of the treatment plan*
- *Use of consultants*
- *Prescription orders*, whether written or telephoned; written instructions for the use of all medications should be given to the patient and documented in the record.

- *Informed consent agreement*
- *Monitoring visits*
- *Treatment results*

The importance of accurate and complete documentation cannot be overemphasized, because accurate and up-to-date medical records become the mechanism that protects both the physician and the patient.

CHAPTER 110

Summary Author: John Young
Robert L. DuPont • Bruce A. Goldberger • Mark S. Gold

Clinical and Legal Considerations in Drug Testing

Drug testing identifies recent use of specific drugs; it does not identify addiction. The identification of recent drug use has great value because denial is a cardinal feature of drug abuse and because many drug users do not know which drugs they are taking.

Drug testing has many uses in medicine, even though testing has not been included in the curriculum and practical experience of most physicians. Physician education and expert guidelines are needed.

SCIENCE OF DRUG TESTING

Because the dose of commonly used drugs of abuse needed to produce brain reward is a thousand or more times less than the dose of alcohol, the testing for drugs has been more challenging and more reliant on the evolution of technology. The immunoassay screening test makes use of the remarkable specificity and sensitivity of the antigen-antibody reaction.

For standard drug testing, especially when severe consequences from a single positive test may be imposed and when the testing is controversial, an initial immunoassay screening test is followed by a more specific, sensitive, and expensive confirmation test. This two-step process is required for regulated workplace drug testing. In many clinical settings such as the emergency department, drug treatment, and the criminal justice system, only the initial immunoassay test is required, thus reducing the costs of testing and increasing the speed of obtaining results.

When there are controversies or severe consequences to a drug test result, the ultimate fail-safe is to retain the positive sample in the original collection container in a frozen state for possible retesting. Such repeat testing is easily done with urine testing. The retained positive urine sample is the standard in regulated workplace drug testing today.

With the advent of bench-top mass spectrometry, the confirmation of drugs and drug metabolites by gas chromatography–mass spectrometry (GC-MS) is now compulsory in many settings. The GC-MS identifies the drugs and drug metabolites based primarily on the chemical structure of the compound. It is an accurate method of drug detection and identification. The current highest standard is the gas chromatography–mass spectrometry–mass spectrometry (GC-MS-MS) or liquid chromatography–mass spectrometry–mass spectrometry (LC-MS-MS), which are breathtakingly expensive and sophisticated technologies.

When the two-step process of immunoassay screen and MS confirmation is utilized, the drug identification process is highly accurate. An evaluation by a medical review officer (MRO) can validate whether the drug was in the donor's body as a result of a current medical prescription to the donor. While the highest ("forensic") level of science is desirable in certain cases such as when there are potential legal challenges, even an immunoassay screen alone is highly reliable for many medical purposes.

ON-SITE VERSUS LABORATORY ANALYSIS

Most drug tests are conducted at clinical laboratories following the collection of the sample at some other site; it usually takes a day or two from the time of collection until the result is available. In recent years, more drug testing is done on-site, with the initial immunoassay test done at the point of collection. In forensic settings, the sample that screens positive on-site is sent to a laboratory for a confirming test before being reported as positive. In many clinical settings, such confirmation is unnecessary, especially when the donor admits recent drug use.

Although on-site tests seldom produce false-positive results, false negatives may be more common, a problem that to some extent mitigates the benefits of immediate results. It is possible to define the extent of the problem of false-negative test results with any on-site device by splitting some samples and sending one sample for laboratory-based testing or, in the case of oral fluid testing, by comparing the oral fluid on-site test results with the results of urine samples taken from the same donors at the same time and then analyzed at a laboratory.

CHOICE OF MATRIX

The choice of a testing matrix relates to the duration after use that drugs and their metabolites are typically detectable, the distribution of the drugs and drug metabolites, the ease of specimen collection, and the resistance to cheating.

Urine

Urine is a particularly attractive matrix for drug testing because it is easy to collect, most drugs and metabolites can be readily detected, and drugs and their metabolites are often detectable for longer periods of time in urine when compared to blood and other fluids such as oral fluid.

When urine drug testing first became widespread in drug abuse treatment and criminal justice systems, the standard was to directly observe specimen collection; however, when drug testing came to the workplace, direct observation was considered objectionably intrusive. The change to unobserved urine collection opened the door for cheating. When cheating is suspected, it is useful to use another matrix and/or return to direct observation.

The determinants of the concentration of drug and drug metabolites found in urine after a single use of a drug are complex, including the dose of the drug taken and the duration of time between the last drug use and the urine collection of the sample. Also important is how much drug was used over what periods of time in the days prior to the collection of the test sample. A wild card in urine drug concentrations is the amount of fluid recently consumed; by special order, creatinine determinations can be used to normalize drug concentrations, thus removing the dilution problem.

The federal government's basic five-drug urine test panel, known as the SAMHSA-5, consists of marijuana, cocaine, PCP, amphetamines, and opiates. It is relatively easy and inexpensive to add other drugs to the panel.

Hair

Drugs and drug metabolites are incorporated in hair while it is being formed. Head hair grows approximately one half an inch a month. The typical hair specimen is 1.5 inches long, thus producing a record of drug use for the prior 90 days. However, as it takes about 1 week for the hair to grow from the base of the follicle to the point where it can be snipped at the level of the scalp, there is no record in hair of drug use for the week prior to sample collection. Alcohol is not incorporated in hair, though alcohol's major metabolites, including ethyl glucuronide (EtG), are detectable in hair samples.

Over the course of the 90 days covered by a typical 1.5-inch hair sample, even a few uses of most drugs of abuse are detectable. Marijuana is an exception because concentrations of THC and metabolites from marijuana are in the body, including in the hair, at significantly lower concentrations than most other drugs of abuse. For this reason, it takes marijuana use of about twice a week for the entire 90 days to produce a positive result at the standard cutoff concentrations. Hair tests are absolutely resistant to cheating because hair collection is always under direct observation.

One problem with urine testing is that recent poppy seed consumption can produce a morphine- and/or a codeine-positive test result that is difficult to distinguish from heroin use. Hair samples are not positive for morphine and/or codeine even after repeated consumption of poppy seeds.

Testing of hair is useful in setting where what is being looked for is prior use of drugs and the question of when the drug use occurred is not particularly relevant. An example of this application is preemployment testing, where cheating on the urine test is a major concern because it is a scheduled test.

There are no on-site hair tests at this time; currently, only a handful of commercial laboratories provide hair testing.

Sweat

A patch, similar to a nicotine patch worn in smoking cessation, is applied to the tested person. The patch is removed usually after a week or two for analysis at the laboratory. Sweat testing is prospective from the time the patch is applied, whereas all other drug tests are backward looking from the time of collection. There is no on-site option for the analysis of drugs and drug metabolites in sweat. Sweat testing is resistant to cheating because the patch puckers when removed and reapplied.

Oral Fluid

The liquid content of the oral cavity (e.g., saliva or oral fluid) can be analyzed for drugs of abuse with on-site and laboratory-based techniques. Oral fluid testing is highly resistant to cheating, as the oral fluid sample is collected under direct observation. The major problem with oral fluid testing is that, like hair testing, these tests are relatively insensitive to marijuana use, especially the on-site kits.

Oral fluid testing generally identifies drug use in only 12 to 24 hours prior to sample collection. The panel of drugs identified is usually limited to the SAMHSA-5 in on-site kits.

For many applications, oral fluid testing is widely anticipated to be the standard for future testing; however, the current sensitivity limits of oral fluid testing leaves much to be desired.

Breath

Drugs of abuse are present in the breath at concentrations that are even lower than those in oral fluid. As technology improves, the ultimate in drug testing is likely to be with breath testing, which will be resistant to cheating and far easier to collect than urine, oral fluids, or hair.

Comparing Matrices

Table 110.1 provides comparison of the clinically available test matrices. Clinicians should be familiar with these and with both laboratory-based and on-site testing techniques. In many clinical settings, it is desirable to have access to all of these testing options; it is also desirable to test for a wide variety of drugs from time to time.

Testing for Alcohol

Alcohol is rapidly metabolized, so alcohol concentrations in the blood fall rapidly—typically to zero within a few hours after the last drink. The acute impairing effects of alcohol are related to the blood alcohol concentrations as modified by the moderating effects of tolerance and the subject's familiarity with the task being measured. The urine in the bladder is a reflection of the blood alcohol concentrations over the period of time that the urine was being produced; for this reason, the urine alcohol concentration is lower than the blood alcohol concentration at the time of urine collection during the ascending slope of the blood concentration and higher during the descending slope of blood concentration after drinking stops. The detection window for urine alcohol tests is generally 12 hours or less after drinking has stopped.

The concentration of alcohol in the urine is of limited value in settings such as highway safety. However, in settings in which there is a zero tolerance for alcohol use, such as underage youth, people in drug and alcohol treatment, and people facing legal sanctions for any drinking, urine testing for alcohol can be helpful.

An important recent drug testing option is to test for EtG or ethyl sulfate (EtS), both of which are metabolites of alcohol that are found in urine up to 5 to 7 days following the consumption of alcohol. It is important to warn people who are subject to EtG testing that these tests may be positive when the donor has used an alcohol hand sanitizer or an alcohol-containing mouthwash.

INTERPRETATION OF DRUG TEST RESULTS

In most clinical settings and in the criminal justice system, it is seldom necessary to have an outside medical expert validate the laboratory results of drug tests because the tests are typically part of an ongoing, often long-term, relationship and because the results of a single positive drug test are unlikely to be severe. Though difficult situations do arise, the vast majority of drug test results are easily interpreted and not disputed by the donors. When interpreting a disputed or ambiguous drug test result, it may be wise for the physician to consult the laboratory reporting the result, because the laboratories and drug assay manufacturers have highly qualified forensic toxicologists on staff.

In many nonclinical settings, however, the drug test results may have severe impacts on the tested individual; in these situations, having professional and independent validation of laboratory positive results is often desirable and, under much regulated drug testing, mandatory. In difficult cases, physicians can consult certified

TABLE 110.1 **Comparison of Blood, Urine, Hair, Saliva, and Sweat Patch Testing for Drugs of Abuse**

Characteristic	Blood	Urine	Hair	Saliva	Sweat patch
Immunoassay screen	Yes	Yes	Yes	Yes	Yes
GC/MS confirmation option (laboratory based)	Yes	Yes	Yes	Yes	Yes
Chain-of-custody option	Yes	Yes	Yes	Yes	Yes
Medical review officer option	Yes	Yes	Yes	Yes	Yes
Retest of the same sample	Yes	Yes	Yes	Yes	Yes
Retain positive samples for retest option	Difficult	Possible	Easy	Difficult	Possible
Common surveillance window	3–12 hr	1–3 d	7–90 d+	3–24 hr	1–21 d
Intrusiveness of collection	Severe	Moderate	None	Slight	Slight
Compatibility of new sample if the original test disputed	No	No	Yes	No	No
Number of drugs screened	Unlimited[a]	Unlimited[b]	Large[c]	5 + alcohol	5[d]

Cost/sample (SAMHSA-5)	About $100–$200	About $15–$30	About $40–$65	About $15–$50	About $35
Test can distinguish between light, moderate, and heavy drug use	Yes (short-term)	No	Yes (long-term)	No	Yes (ongoing)
Test resistance to cheating	High	Low	High	High	High
Best application	Postaccident and overdose testing for alcohol and other drugs Blood alcohol concentration	Reasonable-cause testing Frequent testing of high-risk groups such as those in posttreatment follow-up and the criminal justice system Unannounced, random tests with observed collection	Preemployment testing Random and periodic testing Testing to determine severity of drug use for referral to treatment Testing of subjects suspected of seeking to evade urine test detection Opiate addicts claiming poppy seed false positive	Postaccident and overdose testing for alcohol and other drugs Blood alcohol concentration Reasonable-cause testing	Posttreatment testing Maintaining abstinence Opiate addicts claiming poppy seed false positive Compliance testing in DOT and criminal justice system applications

DOT, U.S. Department of Transportation; GC-MS, gas chromatography–mass spectrometry; SAMSHA, Substance Abuse and Mental Health Services Administration.

[a]Blood testing for alcohol is routine, costing about $25/sample, but blood testing for drugs is done by only a few laboratories in the United States. Blood testing for drugs is relatively expensive, costing about $60 for each drug tested for.

[b]Urine tests for nonroutine drugs are available from most reference laboratories, and costs for broad screens are generally <$200.

[c]Hair testing is commonly performed for the SAMSHA-5 (cocaine, opiates, marijuana, amphetamines, and phencyclidine). However, a large number of drugs and metabolites can be detected, and routine broad testing is performed in several toxicology reference laboratories. The cost of nonroutine testing of hair is <$500 in most cases.

[d]Commonly limited to the SAMSHA-5. Tests can also be performed for alcohol.

MROs, who are physicians trained and certified in the interpretation of drug test results. The MRO receives the laboratory positive result (and in regulated workplace testing, negative results as well) before the results go to the individual or the organization requesting the drug test in order to validate that the proper procedures were maintained, including rigorous chain of custody procedures. In addition, the MRO validates that the laboratory positive drug test result was not the result of a legitimate medical prescription for the tested subject.

Today the most common problems with drug testing relate to potentially misleading negative drug tests. Drug tests do not identify recent drug use in general—they only identify recent use of the drugs specified on the particular test. Also, unlike blood and breath alcohol tests, drug tests are commonly reported as either "positive" or "none detected" based on specified cutoff concentrations; therefore, a negative drug test does not guarantee that the tested individual had not recently used that drug.

ETHICAL AND LEGAL ISSUES

Parents now have access to drug testing technology in pharmacies and on the Internet and can choose to pay for testing; drug testing is viewed as prevention by many parents, but those using these tests need education about such issues as how to deal with a positive result.

Some pediatricians consider drug testing a breach of the patient–physician relationship unless the adolescent patient specifically consents to the drug testing. Still, in some situations, such as accidents, depression, learning problems, and suicidal ideation, there appears to be a consensus to test adolescents for drugs of abuse with or without their consent. Even in these settings, there is merit to obtaining consent, especially when testing is done over time, as one of the primary goals of the testing is prevention.

The issue of student drug testing often becomes a question of privacy and a matter subject to litigation, particularly in the public schools where the constitutional protections of the Fourth Amendment apply. In two landmark Supreme Court cases, the Court has upheld mandatory drug testing in public schools when the testing is linked to participation in athletic or extracurricular activities and for all students when it is voluntary on the part of the student and the students' parents. Private schools have no such legal barrier to mandatory drug testing of all students. Similar legal questions have been answered in workplace drug testing, leading to approval by the Supreme Court of drug testing under specified circumstances.

In contrast to drug testing in the workplace and schools, the use of testing in the criminal justice system and as part of routine clinical care has not been held to forensic standards, resulting in drug testing being more flexible and less costly in these settings. Because in these settings funding often is severely limited, the major hurdle for drug testing is not legal but financial—the major question whether or not drug testing is cost-effective. When there are consequences and when the standard is that the patients must be drug free, then drug testing often is vital to the success of the program: drug testing linked to significant consequences for return to any drug use has been identified as a major reason that the nation's physicians' health programs have remarkably high success rates over long periods of time.

CHAPTER 111

Summary Author: John Young
The Hon. Peggy Fulton Hora (Ret.) • The Hon. William G. Schma (Ret.)

Drug Courts and the Treatment of Incarcerated Populations

A NEW APPROACH TO AN OLD PROBLEM

In the past two decades, it has become abundantly clear that incarceration alone is totally ineffective in addressing alcohol and drug abuse and addiction. Society also has come to realize that prison is a scarce resource best employed to isolate violent offenders from the community. These realizations, coupled with an increased knowledge of the neurobiology of addiction and its treatment, have led to an understanding that collaborative projects such as drug treatment courts (DTCs) are the most intelligent way to address this problem.

A DTC is a judicially supervised, treatment-driven program for nonviolent substance-abusing criminal offenders. It is a collaborative effort that involves judges, prosecutors, defense attorneys, probation officers, treatment providers, and other persons or agencies that interact with addicts whose behavior has brought them into the criminal justice system. A criminal defendant in a DTC is given an opportunity to engage in an alternative to the criminal "business as usual" and, in its place, to pursue a program of addiction treatment and recovery. DTCs employ a series of "carrots and sticks" to induce treatment compliance and lifestyle changes in a criminal defendant, the ultimate payoff for the participant being dismissal of the charges, having a sentence set aside, or imposition of a lesser penalty.

The court serves as a convener and coordinator of related services in a continuum of care for substance-abusing individuals, with the courtroom transformed into an arena in which a judge is the central figure of a team that is focused on the participants' recovery. The prosecutor screens each candidate for eligibility and makes sure each candidate is appropriate for participation in the DTC. The defense counsel verifies that clients know of the voluntary nature of DTC participation, are aware of all their legal options, and make a knowing and intelligent waiver of their rights, including their confidentiality rights. A close, interpersonal, and therapeutic relationship develops between the judge and the participant, who is encouraged to develop the tools he or she needs to maintain sobriety and recovery. Participants often enter into written contracts, agreeing to certain behaviors; data show that such contracts are more likely to induce compliance, whether it is taking medication or engaging in addiction treatment. A typical contract includes attending treatment, court dates, self-help meetings, and other appointments on time; complying with all rules; waiving confidentiality; paying fees and fines; taking presumptive urine tests without water loading, adulteration, or counterfeiting; agreeing to refrain from drinking alcohol or taking other drugs or associating with people who do; abstaining from eating poppy seeds, taking over-the-counter or prescription medications without prior approval, or doing other things that could yield a nonnegative result on a urine test; and making a 12- to 18-month commitment to treatment.

Written confidentiality waivers that comply with federal statutes are mandatory, simply because treatment providers, mental health professionals, and physicians must be able to communicate with the court coordinator/case manager and the team. Judges must be able to talk to team members individually throughout the week without inhibition. This team concept of DTCs uniquely facilitates an individual's treatment progress. Police officers, including the bailiff in the courtroom, become supporters and benefactors rather than enemies. Similarly, supporting actors like community-based treatment providers, community policing officers, housing

TABLE 111.1   **Advice on Initiating Treatment with Drug Court Clients**

Set clear goals and expectations. Treatment goals for DTCs are sobriety, program retention, and maintenance of a crime-free lifestyle. Goals are explained in the participants' handbook and the written behavioral contract, as well as by the judge, case coordinator, attorneys, and treatment providers.

Establish treatment attendance. Participants must bring written proof of attendance to each court date. Unverifiable meetings are not allowed except in unusual circumstances. For instance, a participant may be going out of town for a business trip and be allowed to attend Twelve-Step meetings in the area he or she will be visiting. If away for an extended stay, urine testing may be arranged, often with the help of another DTC.

Schedule frequent contacts. Frequent court appearances are a hallmark of DTCs. Daily contact with the case coordinator or treatment provider may be required in volatile relapse situations. At a minimum, weekly contacts are maintained throughout the life of the program in some DTCs.

Use positive incentives to reinforce treatment participation. In the Hayward, CA, DTC, the local Deputy Sheriffs' Association provides the DTC with tickets for Oakland A's games to use as rewards for good performance. There may be a drawing for theater or county fair tickets, a Halloween pumpkin, or a tote bag or tee shirt from the latest conference attended by the judge. To be eligible for the drawing, a participant must have a negative urine test and have attended all meetings. Drawings are held on a random basis and participants who have missed a meeting are quite upset when they are not eligible to participate. One treatment provider awards food vouchers and bus tickets to participants who meet their goals.

Call "no-shows." The court coordinator calls all participants who have failed to appear in court. If there is no response, the bailiff immediately asks the community policing liaison to serve a bench warrant. Through this approach, participants are taught that it is better to appear and test positive than to fail to appear. Program retention and participation lead to negative urine tests; the opposite is not true.

Create a positive environment. Because court appearances are so personalized by the judge, participants develop a positive attitude toward coming to court. Most treatment providers have court meetings so that participants can develop friendships. Participants help each other find jobs and transportation, and even cook Thanksgiving dinner together before marathon holiday meetings. Everyone feels good because of the positive atmosphere in the courtroom.

Enforce "no use" policies for drugs and alcohol. Although there was some initial resistance to uniform "no alcohol" clauses for DTC participants, such requirements now are standard. DTC contracts also include a prohibition on the use of prescription drugs prescribed for others and, of course, prohibit the use of illicit substances.

Establish a daily schedule. Treatment meetings, self-help groups, employment, job training or job seeking, education, volunteer work, and court appointments keep a DTC participant on a tight schedule. Some participants have had to change work shifts and find new employment because working late-night shifts triggered a craving for stimulants to stay awake. Daytime employment and an early bedtime seem to help reduce stimulant craving.

Initiate a schedule for drug testing. Most DTCs require frequent, random, observed urine tests. Night and weekend testing, long-distance testing, and daily testing as a sanction all are employed.

Assess psychiatric comorbidity. Posttraumatic stress disorder and clinical depression are the most commonly observed psychiatric problems among DTC participants. Many DTCs have mutual help groups for co-occurring disorders such a bipolar and schizophrenia. A mental health assessment is ordered for those who are not being program compliant, rather than assuming that the participant is "treatment resistant." The incidence of comorbidity for this population is very high.

Assess associated compulsive sexual behaviors. Treatment providers who work with stimulant abusers in DTCs have special sex addiction groups. DTCs also offer confidential and anonymous HIV testing and education, as well as testing and education for hepatitis B and C and other sexually transmitted diseases (STDs). Many participants have worked as prostitutes, which raises not only STD issues but also posttraumatic stress disorder issues that must be addressed in treatment.

(Continued)

TABLE 111.1	**Advice on Initiating Treatment with Drug Court Clients (*Continued*)**
	Assist with crisis resolution. The court, the case manager, and treatment providers all need to be are aware of the need for suicide and homicide assessment, psychiatric referrals, and necessary medical referrals. Participants may need extra support in times of personal crisis and stepped-up relapse prevention services at these times. The court may order an emergency psychiatric assessment or additional services.

DTC, drug treatment court.

authority personnel, mental health professionals, and physicians have a unique new relationship with the courts and a voice not previously heard.

Using graduated sanctions, the court usually begins with the least restrictive model, as indicated by an assessment tool such as the Addiction Severity Index. The participant is moved to more restrictive placements as needed. Placing a participant in a more restrictive environment is not phrased in terms of punishment; rather, participants are encouraged to see the change as necessary to their recovery. Mental health, housing, physical health, employment, education, and other legal entanglements are addressed. Periods of abstinence, confirmed by weekly, random urine tests, are required for each phase—typically at 30, 90, and 180 days; associated rewards may include an earn-down of program fees, a reduction in the number of court appearances, and awarding of certificates (with much cheering and applause from the audience) to mark the completion of each phase.

Although the judge remains the final arbiter of all issues, he or she receives input from the entire team, including the participant. If a problem arises, such as a use episode, it is not unusual for a participant to arrive in court having already discussed the problem with the treatment provider and a probation officer or court coordinator, who will present a recommendation to the judge. When participants themselves propose the sanctions, they are more likely to comply with them and not to feel coerced by the "system" or the judge. A person who proposes his or her own "punishment" is more likely to think it fair (Table 111.1).

When a participant submits a positive urine test, misses meetings or appointments, fails to participate, or otherwise breaks program rules, sanctions are imposed immediately. Such sanctions may include payment for the urine test, increased meeting attendance, demotion to an earlier phase, requirement to perform volunteer work or short stints of jail time (usually 1 day to no >1 week at a time) or, the ultimate sanction, removal from the program and (in a preplea model) reentry into the criminal system or (after adjudication) sentencing, including incarceration. Consistent noncompliance may trigger a mental health assessment, as many DTC participants have undiagnosed comorbid mental health problems such as clinical depression, posttraumatic stress disorder, bipolar disorder, or schizophrenia. Program dismissal is reserved for the most serious offenses, such as attempts to falsify or adulterate a urine sample, leaving without permission, or being arrested for a violent offense.

Aftercare planning is part of the program, and participants petition the court to "graduate," typically at about 180 days of sobriety. To receive such approval, the participant must have

- A knowledge of addiction
- A clean and sober living environment
- A high school diploma or GED
- Full-time employment or full-time student status
- Paid all fees and fines, or completed substantial amounts of volunteer work
- A drivers' license, insurance, and proof of registration of all vehicles, and be able to show that there are no outstanding tickets or warrants
- A plan for relapse prevention

Graduating participants also must take literacy classes, if they are English speaking, or enroll in a class for students learning English as a second language. The whole person is transformed by the DTC; abstinence alone is not enough.

The participant is invited to become involved in a DTC alumni group.

At any point in this process, the participant may opt out of the DTC and into the traditional criminal justice case processing system, with all the attendant rights and remedies.

WHY DRUG TREATMENT COURTS WORK

There is support for DTCs on many fronts and from all factions of the political spectrum:

- Research indicates that a person coerced to enter treatment by the criminal justice system is likely to do as well as one who volunteers.
- Addiction treatment is as successful as treatment for other chronic diseases and saves $7 for every treatment dollar spent.
- Studies have shown that DTCs save states money, largely from lower recidivism among participants
- Judicial job satisfaction is increased if judges work therapeutically.

DTCs have received endorsement from the U.S. Conference of Chief Justices and the Conference of State Court Administrators. Law enforcement support for DTCs is strong because officers see that recovery presents a long-term solution to a community's and an individual's problems with alcohol or other drugs.

INDEX

Page numbers followed by *f* indicate figures; those followed by *t* indicate tables